Class No. V2 RyD

23/3/01
£24-95
2nd ed.

AN AID TO THE
MRCP SHORT CASES

NLM   WB
Class   18
Mark: R4D
L.G.I.

D1471297

NHS STAFF LIBRARY
CHAPEL ALLERTON

COOKRIDGE MEDICAL LIBRARY

'*MRCP; Member of the Royal College of Physicians . . .*
They only give that to crowned heads of Europe'.

From *The Citadel* by A.J. Cronin

An Aid to the MRCP Short Cases

R.E.J. Ryder, M.A. Mir and E.A. Freeman

Departments of Medicine, City Hospital, Birmingham,
University Hospital of Wales and
University of Wales College of Medicine, Cardiff
and Department of Integrated Medicine,
Royal Gwent and St Woolos Hospitals, Newport

SECOND EDITION

Blackwell
Science

One-third of the royalties from this book will be donated to the
Missionaries of Charity of Mother Teresa of Calcutta

© 1986, 1999 by
Blackwell Science Ltd
Editorial Offices:
Osney Mead, Oxford OX2 0EL
25 John Street, London WC1N 2BL
23 Ainslie Place, Edinburgh EH3 6AJ
350 Main Street, Malden
   MA 02148 5018, USA
54 University Street, Carlton
   Victoria 3053, Australia
10, rue Casimir Delavigne
   75006 Paris, France

Other Editorial Offices:
Blackwell Wissenschafts-Verlag GmbH
Kurfürstendamm 57
10707 Berlin, Germany

Blackwell Science KK
MG Kodenmacho Building
7–10 Kodenmacho Nihombashi
Chuo-ku, Tokyo 104, Japan

The right of the Authors to be
identified as the Authors of this Work
has been asserted in accordance
with the Copyright, Designs and
Patents Act 1988.

All rights reserved. No part of
this publication may be reproduced,
stored in a retrieval system, or
transmitted, in any form or by any
means, electronic, mechanical,
photocopying, recording or otherwise,
except as permitted by the UK
Copyright, Designs and Patents Act
1988, without the prior permission
of the copyright owner.

First published 1986
Reprinted 1988, 1989, 1990, 1991, 1992,
1993, 1994, 1996, 1997
Second edition 1999
Reprinted 2000

Set by Excel Typesetters Company Ltd, Hong Kong
Printed and bound in Great Britain
at the University Press, Cambridge

The Blackwell Science logo is a
trade mark of Blackwell Science Ltd,
registered at the United Kingdom
Trade Marks Registry

DISTRIBUTORS

Marston Book Services Ltd
PO Box 269
Abingdon, Oxon OX14 4YN
(*Orders*: Tel: 01235 465500
       Fax: 01235 465555)

USA
Blackwell Science, Inc.
Commerce Place
350 Main Street
Malden, MA 02148 5018
(*Orders*: Tel: 800 759 6102
       781 388 8250
Fax: 781 388 8255)

Canada
Login Brothers Book Company
324 Saulteaux Crescent
Winnipeg, Manitoba R3J 3T2
(*Orders*: Tel: 204 837-2987)

Australia
Blackwell Science Pty Ltd
54 University Street
Carlton, Victoria 3053
(*Orders*: Tel: 3 9347 0300
       Fax: 3 9347 5001)

A catalogue record for this title
is available from the British Library
and the Library of Congress

ISBN 0-632-03067-4

For further information on
Blackwell Science, visit our website:
www.blackwell-science.com

Contents

Section 4: Experiences, Anecdotes, Tips, Facts and Figures, Quotations, 445

Preface to the second edition

Following publication of the first edition, my co-authors continued making surveys of candidates and accumulated an overwhelming number of questionnaires finding that many candidates, now aware of our book, poured out information to us. These greatly reinforced the information found in our original surveys and presented in the first edition. We found another 50 short cases which we present in this new edition, yet overall the cases seen, mistakes made or avoided, accounts of triumphs, tragedies and downward spirals, remain remarkably constant as each sitting comes and goes. Our much more limited time, now that I have also become a consultant, meant that we were not able to analyse the new surveys to anything like the same extent as in the original edition. Therefore we have not altered the 'frequency of occurrence' figures used in the first edition for the 150 short cases of that edition as we do not believe that a more superficial analysis of the new surveys would be as accurate. It is possible that, for instance, 'old tuberculosis' is occurring in the exam less often than it did as fewer patients who had a thoracoplasty all those years ago are still available (patients with similar signs due to partial or complete pneumonectomy may appear instead, however, and indeed this is one of the new short cases); similarly Fallot's tetralogy with a Blalock shunt. Nevertheless the vast majority of cases seem to maintain a remarkably constant rate of occurrence.

We were able to assign an approximate occurrence rate for each of the additional 50 short cases so that they could be merged in with the original 150. One of the new short cases has come into existence since the first edition because of new College guidelines ('Resuscitation Annie') and one because of the spread of a new condition ('AIDS related'). Some of the new cases are relative rarities which appear in the exam just occasionally. We do not believe that such cases should be excluded from the exam. It would be a shame if clinical awareness of uncommon conditions was extinguished from the physicians of the future just because these conditions are rare. At the same time we do not believe that failure to recognize a rare condition would ever be an important pass/fail factor in the MRCP short cases. A candidate seeing such a case is also likely to see a number of other more usual cases on which the main pass/fail decisions would be made.

Nevertheless there is potential, with rarities, to show a breadth of clinical diagnostic skills which may distinguish a candidate from his/her peers. Before coming to terms with rarities, however, you should ensure you can perform well with the more commonly occurring short cases. In this book we cover them all—the common and rare with rates of frequency of appearance in the clinical exam so that you can ensure that you establish your priorities appropriately. The new surveys have enabled us to considerably expand the experiences and anecdotes in Section 4 and because candidates often 'knew what they were writing for', we have been able to present a number of hardly edited accounts written in the first person.

Acknowledgements

We are grateful to the following for reviewing some or all of the first edition short cases and/or examination routines related to their speciality. We should stress that we did not necessarily always take the advice given but we hope the errors of fact are minimal. G.S. Venables (neurology), S. Sturman (also neurology), K.S. Channer (cardiology), E.E. Kritzinger (medical ophthalmology), P. Stewart (endocrinology), C. Tan (dermatology), D. Honeybourne (respiratory medicine), T. Iqbal (gastroenterology), M. El Nahas (renal medicine), D. Situnayke (rheumatology), D. Bareford (haematology), P. Harper (medical genetics), K.G. Taylor (lipids) and E. McLoskey (Paget's disease). There was also a contribution from A. Jackowski (neurosurgeon). We thank C. Tan for Figs 3.114b and c, and C. Ellis for Fig. 3.156b.

I am particularly grateful to my co-authors for their tolerance with regard to my contribution to the tardiness of the new edition; to colleagues, in particular Ken Taylor and Sharon Jones for their support; to Anne's family, Pete, Lizzie and Jonathan Williams for what they have had to put up with; similarly to Lynda, Farooq, Deborah and Joanne Mir (especially for their wonderful hospitality during some crucial sessions over several days at Afzal's house); similarly and more so to my children Bobby and Anna for what they have had to put up with, but most of all sincere thanks to my wife Anne, without whose support and tolerance, well beyond the call of duty, none of it could ever have happened.

Bob Ryder

Preface to the first edition

The short cases part of the examination for the Membership of the Royal College of Physicians (MRCP) is, by tradition, considered to be the most critical test of bedside behaviour and diagnostic competence. It forms an important milestone in the development of practising physicians. There is, however, no formal syllabus or tutoring and, despite the high failure rate, there is a notable lack of books specifically written to help candidates with this test.

The spectrum of clinical conditions used in the short cases examination is determined by a variety of interchanging factors such as the availability of patients with demonstrable physical signs, the prejudice of the doctors choosing the cases, that of the examiners taking part in the examination and, occasionally, the speciality bias of the examination centre. The cases chosen by the examiners from those assembled on the day in turn determine the problems presented to the candidates and the clinical skills required of them. For this reason we decided to build this book around an extensive survey conducted amongst successful candidates. Our questionnaires yielded information about the cases presented, the questions asked, answers given and the reactions of the examiners. We have thus been able to identify the chief difficulties of candidates in dealing with this practical examination and have attempted to help with these. The advice in Section 1 on how to prepare for the short cases is based on, and illustrated by, the comments received from the candidates. Section 2 is written around the clinical instructions given by the examiners to the candidates, the likely diagnoses under each instruction as revealed in the survey, and details of the examination steps suitable for each command. Section 3 forms the bulk of the book and presents the clinical features of 150 short cases in order of the frequency of their occurrence in the examination as derived from our survey. Thus, priorities are sorted out for the candidates preparing for the examination. In the final section we pass on the experiences and advice of some of the candidates in our survey which we felt would be of interest.

In fulfilling our main task of helping candidates

to improve their performance in clinical examinations we have used three learning techniques which are rather novel to this field. Firstly, the iterative approach which exploits the retentive potential of reinforcement by repeating the main clinical features of a number of conditions whenever any reference to these is made. It is hoped that this method will not only reinforce, but will also alert the candidates to other diagnostic possibilities when looking at a related condition. Secondly, in the examination methods suggested by us we have individualized the inspection to the examination of each subsystem, and have provided a *visual survey* to note the features most likely to be present. This enriches the usual advice to look for everything which often accomplishes nothing unless a specific sign is being looked for. Thirdly, we have reduced our suggested clinical methods to simple steps (*checklists*) which, if practised, may become spontaneous clinical habits, easy to recall and execute.

In the age of superspecialization, the task of summarizing and streamlining a subject as vast and diverse as general medicine to the needs of the short cases examinee has been formidable. We are in no doubt that our attempt will have its inadequacies and would be pleased if you would write to us (c/o Blackwell Scientific Publications) about any errors of fact, or with any suggestions which might be helpful for a future edition, or indeed with any other comments. We would also be interested to hear of any short cases which have occurred in the examination and which are not included on our lists (please give us an idea of your confidence that the case was indeed the condition concerned and why—clinical details, invigilator's confirmation, etc.) or of any Membership experiences which might be of interest.

Medical student note

Although this book has concentrated exclusively on the needs of MRCP candidates, it is noteworthy that the cases included in undergraduate medical short cases examinations are drawn from the same pool as those used in the MRCP examination. Furthermore, physicians are all MRCP trained and tend to use the MRCP style in these examinations. Though clearly the required standard of performance is lower, we feel that medical students preparing for their short cases examinations would also benefit from using this book. It would be a supplement to information gained from more comprehensive textbooks (we assume much basic knowledge) and an aid to practice on the wards.

Acknowledgements

We are indebted to Dr Ralph Marshall and his team (especially Paul Crompton, Keith Bellamy, Steve Young and Adrian Shaw) in the Department of Medical Illustration at the University Hospital of Wales, and Nigel Pearce and Steve Cashmore at the Department of Medical Illustration at the Royal Gwent Hospital. A large proportion of the photographs in the book are from the archives of these departments.

We are grateful to all the patients who gave their consent to the publication of the photographs depicting their medical conditions. Our thanks are due to many colleagues who have allowed us to use photographs from their own collections and photographs of their patients including: T.M. Hayes, C.E.C. Wells, M.S.J. Pathy, R. Marks, R. Hall, J.G. Graham, B.H. Davies, P.J.A. Holt, J. Jessop, M.H. Pritchard, N.W.D. Walshaw, I.S. Petheram, J.M. Swithenbank, M.D. Mishra, B.D. Williams, I.N.F. McQueen, P.E. Hutchinson, J. Rhodes, C.A.R. Pippen, A.J. Birtwell, P.M. Smith, A.G. Knight, S. Richards, A.G. Karseras, J.P. Thomas, C.N.A. Matthews, P.J. Sykes, M.L. Insley, P.I. Williams, B.S.D. Sastry, J.H. Jones, M.Y. Khan, J.D. Spillane, K. Tayton, G.M. Tinker, A. Compston, B.A. Thomas, H.J. Lloyd, G.B. Leitch, B. Calcraft, O.M. Gibby, G.O. Thomas, E. Graham Jones, Byron Evans, D.J. Fisher, G.S. Kilpatrick, L.E. Hughes, P. Harper, G. Griffiths, A.D. Holt-Wilson, D.B. Foster, D.L.T. Webster, J.H. Lazarus, D. Beckingham, J.E. Cawdery, R. Prosser, M.F. Scanlon, I.A. Hughes, O.P. Gray, E. Waddington and L. Beck. Figure 3.42b has already been published in *An Atlas of Clinical Neurology* by Spillane and Spillane (Oxford University Press) and Figs 3.97b and 3.114 from the UHW Medical Illustration archives are also published in *A Picture Quiz in Medicine* by Ebden, Peiras and Dew (Lloyd-Luke Medical Books Ltd). Figures 3.115a (i) and (ii) are published with the permission of the Department of Medical Photography, Leicester Royal Infirmary and Fig. 3.110 with the permission of the University of Newcastle upon Tyne, holders of the copyright.

Our thanks go to colleagues who advised us on points of uncertainty in their fields of interest; especially A.C., B.H.D., M.J.D., L.G.D., R.H., T.M.H., M.H., T.P.K., I.N.F.M., M.D.M., M.F.S., H.S., P.M.S., S.S. and B.D.W.

We are obliged to: Andrea Hill for typing and retyping the manuscript; Janet Roberts for secretarial help with the survey; Jill Manfield for telephoning, chasing and writing again in pursuit of patient consents and for numerous minor secretarial chores; Alan Peiras for some nifty detective work in Edinburgh during the survey; Steve Young for the cover photograph for the book; and to certain pharmaceutical companies for financial assistance (including Astra Pharmaceuticals Ltd, CIBA Laboratories, May and Baker Ltd, Roche Products Ltd, Merck Sharp and Dohme Ltd and Thomas Morson Pharmaceuticals). Our particular thanks to Bayer UK Ltd for sponsoring the colour photographs.

Most of all we thank our long-suffering families without whose forebearance and help the book would never have been finished.

Bob Ryder
Afzal Mir
Anne Freeman

Introduction

'The result comes as a particular shock when you have been sitting exams for many years without failing them'.

The candidate who reaches the MRCP 'clinical' examination has already demonstrated considerable knowledge of medicine by passing the MRCP Part I and MRCP Part II written examinations. The clinical is divided into viva, long case and short cases. Marks are out of 20 for the written exam with 9 being borderline fail, out of 10 for the viva, out of 8 for the long case with 3 being borderline fail and out of 12 for the short cases with 5 being borderline fail. You can compensate for a borderline fail in the written, the long case or short cases by scoring extra marks in other sections of the exam and scoring at least 27 overall (you need only 25 overall if you do not fail any part of the exam). You cannot fail overall simply because of failure in the viva. With regard to the written, the long case and the short cases, a borderline fail in two of these leads to automatic failure overall as does a definite failure in just one of them. Thus, theoretically at least, you could score 0/10 in the viva and still pass if you score highly enough in the other sections of the exam. Similarly you could score 10/10 in the viva and still fail if you score, for instance, only 4/12 (definite fail) in the short cases. The written is a competitive exam, the pass mark being adjusted to ensure 60% of candidates obtain a mark of 10 or more, with 15% obtaining the bare fail mark of 9. Of those candidates who proceed to the clinical and oral examination, the vast majority who fail do so because they fail the short cases. The percentage of candidates who pass varies from time to time, but it is helpful to think in terms of the failure rate for the viva and long case being of the order of 30%. The failure rate for the short cases examination is about 70% (figure from a Membership examiner). Thus all are agreed that the short cases examination is the major hurdle in MRCP Part II. The fact is that many Part II candidates readily pass the written, viva and long case but equally readily fail the short cases (see experience 102, p. 462). For many it is the first examination they have ever failed and it may also be the only examination they have taken that does not have some form of syllabus.

The short cases examination is a practical test which assesses various facets of clinical competence in many subtle ways. Although it is generally accepted that clinical competence cannot be acquired from textbooks, a book such as this can provide indirect help towards that objective. We hope that the examination *routines* (Section 2) together with the *checklists* (Appendix 1) may assist candidates in developing a keen sense of clinical search and detection. The short case *records* (Section 3) should provide the framework, i.e. the main clinical features, the discipline of how to look for them, how to differentiate the diagnostic from the incidental or associated findings, and how and when to be alert to other possibilities. By basing our book on the results of a survey of successful MRCP candidates (see below) we have *created a form of syllabus* which we hope will be of value to future candidates. Not only do the results of the survey advise as to what you are required to know and do, but they also grade these requirements in order of importance.

The short cases examination

'I am sure they assess you very quickly—whether they would like you to be in charge of their patients'.†

Two examiners will take you for approximately 15 minutes each. The College asks them each to record a separate, as well as a combined, mark. Nowadays examiners are encouraged to introduce each case, e.g.: 'This is Mr Smith. His doctor found a heart murmur on routine examination. Please would you examine his heart'. Nonetheless, the old system often prevails: 'Examine this patient's heart'. A striking feature of the examination is the absence of a discussion. The cases are examined, the findings given, and perhaps one or two causes sought whilst moving on to the next case. Only in a minority of the cases is a little time given for the occasional question or brief discussion of causes or complications. The examiners are constantly testing your ability to *elicit and interpret physical signs*. Many examiners say that, in the final analysis, whether a candidate will pass or fail depends very much on the general air of competence or incompetence which prevails during his/her clinical performance. Many candidates who fail feel that the exam is unfair in one way or another (e.g. first person experience 32, p. 487). However, candidates are not in a good position to judge their performance. A candidate who diagnosed the patient with aortic stenosis (which the last three candidates before him all diagnosed correctly) as having mitral stenosis may never know of his error. Furthermore, it is more than just a question of getting the right diagnosis. A candidate recently complained that he had seen a large number of short cases during his exam and knew, because he had a contact at the hospital, that he had got the right diagnosis in all except two of those short cases. He was reporting this during the feedback session of a subsequent mock short cases exam which he had also failed. During that mock exam, after examining the wasted legs of a patient with dystrophia myotonica, his first suggestion as to the cause of the signs in the legs was 'canda equina lesion'. He eventually got to the correct diagnosis but his initial responses left a poor impression on the mock examiners, especially since other candidates in the same mock exam noticed, at once and without prompting, that the patient had gross generalized wasting, indicating that the problem was not one confined to the legs. In similar ways he had performed poorly on other short cases in the mock exam and as a mock examiner one could easily see how he failed in the real exam whilst believing that he usually got the right diagnosis.

As testimony to the precision of the marking system in the MRCP short cases, it is an impressive fact that examiners, though marking independently, rarely differ by more than one mark in the scores they give. As one senior membership examiner put it, the MRCP will usually pick out those who should fail; it will also usually pick out those who should pass — but not necessarily on the current attempt! Given the importance of clinical competence and the fact that this can only be assessed through a clinical exam (and clinical exams by their very nature will always have some in-built inadequacies), it seems unlikely that one could ever improve on this situation. The degree to which the examiners' marks concur suggest that the exam is probably as good as it can be. Our aim in this book, if you are one of those who should pass, is to try to help you to

let the examiners know this on the current attempt or the next, rather than on the next attempt or the one after!

The surveys of MRCP short cases

'Certain "favourite" topics seem to recur. Make sure you know these'.*

First edition

This survey has been introduced in the preface to the first edition. In the first part of this survey, questionnaires were obtained from a number of doctors who had gained the MRCP during the last ten years. In the second part all the successful candidates at a single sitting were circulated. The questionnaires obtained in the two parts of the survey included both the pass and the previous fail attempts of these candidates. Altogether we collected accounts of 248 attempts at the MRCP short cases, covering over 1300 'main focus' short cases as well as over 500 'additional' short cases (see Section 3 for an explanation of these terms). The diagnoses given by these candidates were graded according to the confidence each candidate had in his retrospective assessment. Pass attempt diagnoses were given more weight than fail attempt ones. As a result we hope that the rather complex analysis performed has produced a picture which is as near to the truth as possible. Analysis of the first part of the survey covering candidates' attempts over several years was essentially the same as analysis of the second part. This suggests that the cases used and the skills tested tend to remain constant. This comparison also gives some support to the accuracy of our method of analysis. The main figures from the survey are given in Sections 2 and 3. Some additional figures of interest are collected together under 'Facts and Figures' in Section 4. Apart from figures, the organization of our suggested examination *routines* (Section 2) and the contents of our short case *records* (Section 3) have been closely guided by the survey. For light entertainment, but with ingrained lessons, a number of experiences, anecdotes and quotations from the survey are given in Section 4.

Second edition

As discussed in the preface to the second edition, the original surveys have been embellished for the

*p. 504.

second edition with several surveys conducted since publication of the first edition. We collected accounts of a further 379 attempts covering nearly 2300 additional main focus short cases. Though the second edition surveys were more extensive than those for the first edition, the analysis of them has been more superficial and, therefore, the analysis from the first edition surveys remain the bed rock of this book.

Section 1
Preparation

'Expressionless and without comment they led me away'.

The clinical skills required for the MRCP examination, particularly in relation to the short cases, can only be acquired by thoughtful preparation, experience and purposeful practice. Tutors and examiners alike agree that it is more important to spend time examining patients than reading textbooks. The examiners are not looking for encyclopaedic knowledge, they are just anxious to ascertain that you can be trusted to carry out an adequate clinical examination and make a competent clinical assessment. This book aims to help you organize your overall preparation to meet that objective. We have provided preparatory aids including examination *routines* and short case *records* (see below). We also aim to give you some insight into what most candidates experience in the examination and we hope to help you prepare psychologically. We would like to stress that though the written examination may appear a formidable hurdle, you are very much more likely to pass it than the short cases. You would be wise to err on the side of safety and prepare for the short cases before, during and after your preparations for the written. Thus, we begin with some basic principles of practice and preparations at work.

Clinical experience in everyday work

'Imagine you are seeing the cases in a clinic and carrying out a routine examination'.*
The intention of the College in the examination is to gain a reflection of your usual working day clinical competence for the examiners to judge. In arriving at their final verdict the examiners may take particular note of factors such as your approach to the patient, your examination technique, spontaneity of shifting from system to system in pursuit of relevant clinical signs, fluidity in giving a coherent account of all the findings and conclusions, and your composure throughout. Though you can acquire all this for the day only, as some successful candidates do who are experts at passing examinations, it would be preferable if you could adopt many of these good habits into your everyday clinical approach. In either event, a long, diligent and disciplined practice

is required if your aim is to be able to perform a smooth and polished clinical examination, to display the subtle confidence of a skilled performer, and to suppress signs of anxiety.

One simple approach to the task is that, whatever your job, you should consider all the patients you see as short or long cases (or even viva questions!). Such a practice should not only improve your readiness for the examination but also improve your standard of patient care — the primary objective of every clinician. Look out for all the 'good signs' passing through your hospital and use as many of these as possible as practice short cases. Ask your colleagues to let you know of every heart murmur, every abnormal fundus, every case with abnormal neurology, etc. If you are in, or can get to, a teaching hospital, make regular trips not only to clinical meetings and demonstrations but also, more importantly, to *visit the specialist wards* — neurology, cardiology, chest, rheumatology, dermatology, etc. It is useful to study the signs and conditions even when you know the diagnosis in order to further familiarize yourself with them. It is also a good practice to see cases 'blind' to the diagnosis and to try to simulate the examination situation. Imagine that two examiners are standing over you and there is a need to complete an efficient, once-only examination followed by an immediate response to the anticipated question: 'What are your findings?' or 'What is the diagnosis?'

Simulated examination practice

'I had a lot of practice presenting short cases to a "hawk" of an SR. This experience was invaluable'.†
If a constant effort is made to improve your clinical skills by seeing as many cases as possible, there is no reason why the spontaneity and competence so acquired should not show up on the day. As with all examinations, however, much can be learned about the deficiencies requiring special attention when you put your composite clinical ability to the test in 'mock' examinations. In most district general, and all teaching, hospitals the local postgraduate clinical tutors organize Membership teaching and 'mock'

*p. 509.

†p. 504.

examination sessions, and you should find out about, and join in, as many of these as you can manage. Unfortunately, a lot of these, though useful, tend to teach in groups and discuss management or look at X-rays, rather than provide the intensive 'on the spot' practice on patients that is the ideal preparation for the MRCP short cases. It is, therefore, advisable to supplement these sessions with simulated examination practice arranged by yourself. This requires the cooperation of a 'mock' examiner (consultant, experienced registrar and, on occasion, a fellow examinee) on a *one-to-one basis*. If you can practice with a variety of 'mock' examiners, you will not only broaden the assessment of your imperfections but also learn to respond to the varied approaches of different examiners.

Examination *routines*

'The most important point is to look professional—as if you have done it a hundred times before'. *

The short cases part of the test is very important for the Membership examination because it is designed to test critically two major areas of clinical competence. The first and more important of these is your ability to detect abnormal physical signs, interpret them correctly and put them together into a reasonable diagnosis or differential diagnosis. The second is your competence to conduct a professional and efficient clinical examination (see experience 34, p. 452). As said above, these are generally considered to arise from day-to-day work and your conduct in the examination will reflect your experience in performing clinical tasks, presenting your assessments of patients to your seniors and getting their constant constructive criticism. If you are lucky enough to have worked with a good teacher you may have acquired a firm foundation upon which you could build a structured clinical examination for all systems. As most candidates are engaged in busy clinical jobs and their seniors are often overburdened by administrative chores, etc., useful clinical dialogue between them may be limited. As a result there may be little improvement in the weaknesses acquired during the undergraduate years. The enormous task of preparing for the Membership examination provides an ideal opportunity to remedy any deficiencies in one's clinical methods.

We would suggest that you work out the exact number and sequence of clinical steps for the examination of each subsystem, particularly those you would need to take in response to a particular command from the examiner; then practise going through these steps. Practise them over and over again† on your spouse, or any other willing person, until all the steps become as automatic as driving a car. Practise them on patients until you are confident of being able to pick up or demonstrate any abnormal physical signs. You should be able to maintain the same sequence and run through it rapidly and comprehensively in a way that is second nature to you. The sequence of clinical steps required for the examination of each system or subsystem is collectively referred to as the examination *routine* in this book. In Section 2 we suggest various examination *routines* (which you may wish to adopt or adapt) for you to practise in response to particular commands. In Appendix 1 we provide *checklists* which summarize the major points in each examination *routine*. The *checklists* are designed to help in practising the *routines*.

Short case *records*

'The more practice at presenting short cases the better'. ‡

A knowledge of the possible short cases that may be used in the examination is important so that you can become familiar with the physical signs associated with each, and know what you are looking for as you work through the examination *routine*. Having a good grasp of the clinical features of the case may enable you to score extra marks by looking for additional signs which may be present. Such extra marks identify the above-average candidate from the average ones. Furthermore, by becoming acquainted with descriptions of typical cases you will find it easier to present the case to the examiner using acceptable descriptive terms. In this book, under each short case, we have presented the typical clinical features for you to remember, and to 'regurgitate' what you see (hence the descriptive term *record*), omit what you do not find, and add what you find new. Thus, when confronted with the face of a man with Parkinson's disease which you diagnose at once on seeing his tremor, instead of stuttering and

---

*p. 504.

† MRCP = Methods Require Constant Practice.
‡ p. 504.

stumbling as you try to think of the right words to describe his face, the terms depressed, expressionless, unblinking, drooling and titubation will immediately surface for you to use. In Section 3 we have covered the overwhelming majority of cases which could occur and we have put them in order of priority according to the likelihood of occurrence as assessed from our survey.

Getting 'psyched up'

'Do not be distracted by mistakes made (or imagined) in preceding cases or the examiners' mannerisms or approach (I was and suffered for it). Being very nervous does not necessarily fail you and one bad case should not put you off '.

It is common to hear candidates agonizing over their feeling that they failed to give a performance commensurate with their actual capabilities, simply because they were discouraged by the 'examination ordeal'. Though it is true that knowledge and competence tend to generate confidence and capability, it is also true that extreme anxiety can seriously impair the performance of even the most knowledgeable and competent candidate.

The downward spiral syndrome

'After the first case there was a long pause as if they were waiting for me to say more—I went to pieces after this'.†

The candidate, an otherwise able and experienced doctor, enters the short cases room extremely anxious and lacking in confidence. He is just hovering on the edge of despair and the slightest upset is going to push him over. On one or more of the cases he convinces himself that he is doing badly (whether or not he actually is) and over the edge he goes. The first stage of a rapid 'downward spiral' sets in; the dispirited candidate gets worse and worse and actually gives up before the end in the certainty that he has failed. Months of intensive book work and bedside practice, not to mention the examination fee, go to waste because of *inadequate psychological preparation*. To avoid this there are four basic rules which are well worth noting.

1 You never know you have failed until the list is published

'Don't be put off if you get a few things wrong. I made a lot of mistakes that I know of and still passed'.‡

In the same way as it is said of the greatest saints that they considered themselves to be the greatest sinners, many successful candidates leave the examination centre feeling certain that they have failed. Good candidates may have a heightened awareness of the imperfections of their performance and thereby may exaggerate the impact of their mistakes on the examiner. Furthermore, the 'hawk' examiner may make you feel that you are doing badly, or you may deduce it from his mannerism, regardless of your performance. By the same token the newcomer may slide through the short cases unaware of any errors and with the examiners acting benignly, and then express great surprise as the inevitable 'thin' envelope arrives. It is not really important whether or not you think you have failed during the days between the examination and the arrival of the result. However, if you become convinced that you are failing while you are still sitting the examination, the thought can be disastrous and impair your performance to the extent that your conviction becomes a reality (e.g. see experiences 1 and 2, pp. 447 and 448, anecdote 24, p. 496 and quotation 52, p. 506)

2 Do not be put off by the examiners or their reactions

'The most off-putting aspect of each case is the lack of feedback from the examiners as to whether you are right or wrong. This is much more disconcerting than outright criticism'.§

Many first-timers, despite excellent clinical experience, are stunned by the sombre and restrained atmosphere of the examination which is unlike anything in their past experience (except perhaps the driving test!). It is as well, therefore, to be aware that the examiners tend to wear a 'poker-face' and usually give no feedback or encouragement. The 'hostile hawk' may appear dissatisfied by everything you do and say, but this is not necessarily a guide as to whether you are doing badly or not. A positive

*Quotations 47–54 and 81, pp. 506 and 508.

† p. 506; see also experience 2, p. 448, and p. 491–3.

‡ p. 506.

§ p. 507. This quotation refers to the 'poker-face' examiner (see also quotations 7 and 102, pp. 504 and 509). The candidates in our survey give similar warnings regarding the

'hawk' ('The examiners may appear irritable and unsympathetic—don't worry'—p. 506) and the 'dove' ('Don't be fooled by the apparent relaxed nature of the examiners'—p. 504; see also quotation 112, p. 509) Remember, 'if your examiner challenges, don't assume it means you have said something wrong'—p. 472.

atmosphere is no guide either: the smiling ('smiling death'!) and pleasant ('deadly dove'!) examiner (and the apparently uninterested one), can be as deadly as a black widow spider if you get yourself into a diagnostic maze! Bear in mind that 'hawks' and 'doves' tend to have similar rates of passing and failing candidates. Disregard the atmosphere and concentrate on what the examiner asks you to do rather than on what he looks like, and recall your *routines* and *records*.

3 The cases are easy and you have seen it all before

'My cases were more straightforward than I had been led to believe. Nothing was particularly rare'.*

The psychological scenario of the examination is such that many candidates enter it with the distorted view that behind every case and every question there will be some catch, some clever trap, something never seen before, or a diagnosis never heard of. In fact these suspicions are rarely justified. The *vast majority* of cases and questions are straightforward and a realization of this is likely to produce a confident, straightforward answer from the start instead of the hesitancy born of a mind filled with suspicion and struggling to solve the hidden catch. A study of membership short cases† reveals that there are two broad groups. The first group includes common conditions which you are well used to seeing in everyday clinical practice such as rheumatic heart disease, cirrhosis of the liver, rheumatoid hands and so on. These should surely present little difficulty (especially if you have tailor-made *routines* and *records*). In the second broad group are the rarities with good physical signs such as Osler–Weber–Rendu syndrome, pseudoxanthoma elasticum, Peutz–Jeghers syndrome, etc. You should be well used to these from the study of colour atlases, etc. that you will have done for the MRCP 'pictures' section of the written examination. These too, therefore, should be easy (once you recognize the condition all you have to do is 'play the record'!).

4 You have already passed and you have just got to keep it that way

'It's like skating on thin ice—if you keep going and don't fall through, you make it'.‡

Confidence in one's ability is a very important ingredient in any form of competition. As you go into the examination imagine that you have a clean sheet with 100% mark and that you just have to keep it that way as the examiner shows you a few simple cases such as psoriatic arthropathy, mitral stenosis, cerebellar signs, clubbing, splenomegaly and diabetic retinopathy (a typical combination). Such an attitude should replace the more usual: 'Everybody fails this examination; it's too difficult; how can I possibly pass'. The short cases examination has been well described (Royal Northern course) as 'like walking up a path full of puddles without stepping in the puddles; and you make the puddles yourself'. Remember the way to success is '*Readiness, Routines, Records* and *Right frame of mind*'.

---

* p. 508.
† The 200 covered in this book form a list far more comprehensive than you probably need in order to pass. If you have studied all 200 it would be excessively rare for you to be surprised by a condition not met before.
‡ p. 507.

Section 2
Examination Routines

'Work out the best method for examination and practise it until it is second nature to you'.*

* p. 504.

In this chapter *routines* are suggested for the clinical assessment of various subsystems. These are readily adaptable to your individual methods. The subsystems are arranged according to the examiners' standard instructions (e.g. examine the heart, abdomen, hands, etc.). The choice and order of subsystems have been governed by our first edition surveys.* We have worked out the frequencies of the various instructions and have presented these in their order of priority. Some of the variations of the instruction are also given. Under each subsystem a list of the possible short cases is presented in order of their occurrence in the survey. The percentages given represent our estimate of your chances of each diagnosis being present when you hear the particular instruction.† These lists of diagnoses have guided our suggested *routines*. The latter are broken down into numbered constituents to aid memory and *checklists* are given in Appendix 1 which match up to the numbered points in the examination *routine*. The *checklists* are to help your practice with each subsystem. The idea is to develop a controlled, spontaneous and flawless technique of examination for each subsystem, so that you do not have to keep pausing and thinking what to do next and so that you do not miss out important steps (see experience 36, p. 453). Often you will not need the complete sequence in the examination (for example, it will be rare for you to carry out all the steps in the 'Examine this patient's arms' *routine*; with regard to the 'Examine this patient's chest' *routine*, often the examiner will ask you to only examine 'the back of this patient's chest') but it will certainly increase your confidence if you enter the examination armed with the complete *routines* so that you can adapt them as necessary. The examination methods are supplemented with appropriate hints to avoid common pitfalls and to simplify the diagnostic maze.

Before dealing with the individual subsystems we would make some general points. You should avoid repeating the examiner's command or echoing the last part of it. Refrain from asking questions like: 'Would you like me to give you a running commentary or give the findings at the end?' Such a response wastes invaluable seconds which could be used running through the *checklist* and completing your *visual survey*. It is like a batsman asking a bowler in a cricket match whether he would like his ball hit for a six or played defensively! You must do what you are best at and hope that the examiner does not ask you to do otherwise. As suggested below, a well-rehearsed procedure suited to each subsystem should

<hr/>

* Our second edition surveys were not used to alter the original data as they did not add significantly to the data used for the first edition, except in that we found that the instruction 'examine this patient's cerebellar system' was not uncommon. You should be able to work out a *routine* for this easy instruction from the other *routines* in this section.
† As with all our survey analyses, we graded the confidence of each candidate in his retrospective diagnosis of each short case seen. The percentages are not meant to add up to 100%

because: (i) there are always missing percentages representing those short cases we could not be certain about; (ii) sometimes more than one diagnosis was considered worth counting for one instruction (for example, in order to give you the percentage of 'heart' cases with clubbing, when clubbing was present it was counted as well as the underlying cardiac condition). The figures are best used to give an index of the *relative importance* of the different conditions in terms of frequency of occurrence when you hear a given instruction.

make it possible for you to start purposefully without delay. Your approach to the patient is of great importance; you should introduce yourself to him and ask his permission to examine him. Permission should also be sought for various manoeuvres, such as adjusting the backrest when examining the heart, or before removing any clothing. These polite exchanges will not only please most examiners and patients, but will also provide you with an opportunity to calm your nerves, collect your thoughts and recall the appropriate *checklist*. Although we have continually emphasized the value of looking for signs peripheral to the examiner's instruction (e.g. examine this patient's heart, abdomen, chest), we would like to emphasize too that *dithering* may be counterproductive. In the *visual survey* you should be scanning the patient rapidly and purposefully with a trained eye, not gazing helplessly at him for a long period while you try to decide what to do next. While you are feeling the pulse (heart) or settling the patient lying flat (abdomen), a quick look at the hands should establish whether there are any abnormalities or not. Pondering over normal hands from all angles at great length looks as unprofessional as, indeed, it is. It is of paramount importance to be gentle with the patient. Rough handling (e.g. roughly and abruptly digging deep into the patient's abdomen so that he winces with pain) can bring you instantly to the pass/fail borderline or below it (see also experience 92, p. 459). Make sure that you cover the patient up when you have finished examining him, and thank him.

1 / 'Examine this patient's heart'

Frequency of instruction
97% of candidates in our survey were asked to do this.

Variations of instruction
Listen to this patient's heart
Examine this praecordium
Feel the pulse, then listen to the apex and the base
Examine the heart/cardiovascular system. Don't worry about peripheral pulses— concentrate on the heart
Auscultate the chest
Listen to the apex beat
This patient is short of breath due to cardiovascular disease—examine her
Feel the pulse—listen to the heart sounds
Examine the heart—just listen
This patient has a problem with heart valves—please examine
Listen to the heart. No, don't do that, just listen to the heart
Palpate the apex beat and listen to the heart only
Examine the JVP, apex beat and listen to the apex
Assess the cardiovascular system
Examine the cardiovascular system

This patient has TIAs. Examine the cardiovascular system to elicit a cause

This patient recently had an infarct. Examine the cardiovascular system

This patient has something wrong with his cardiovascular system. Find out in the most expeditious way

Examine the cardiovascular system bit by bit

Examine the cardiovascular system and talk me through it.

Diagnoses from survey in order of frequency

1. Mitral stenosis (lone) 16%
2. Mixed mitral valve disease 13%
3. Combinations of mitral and aortic valve disease 9%
4. Mixed aortic valve disease 8%
5. Aortic incompetence (lone) 7%
6. Mitral incompetence (lone) 5%
7. Aortic stenosis (lone) 5%
8. Ventricular septal defect 3%
9. Prosthetic valves 2%
10. Tricuspid incompetence 2%
11. Mitral valve prolapse 2%
12. Clubbing 2%
13. Patent ductus arteriosus 1%
14. Eisenmenger's syndrome 1%.

Other diagnoses were: atrial septal defect ($<1\%$), coarctation of the aorta ($<1\%$), chronic liver disease due to tricuspid incompetence ($<1\%$), Fallot's tetralogy with a Blalock shunt ($<1\%$), pulmonary stenosis ($<1\%$), cor pulmonale ($<1\%$), complete heart block ($<1\%$), transposition of the great vessels ($<1\%$), repaired thoracic aortic aneurysm ($<1\%$), dextrocardia ($<1\%$) and left ventricular aneurysm ($<1\%$).

Examination *routine*

When asked to 'examine this patient's heart' candidates are often uncertain as to whether they should start with the pulse or go straight to look at the heart. On the one hand it would be absurd to feel all the pulses in the body and leave the object of the examiner's interest to the last minute, whilst on the other hand it would be impetuous to palpate the praecordium straight away. Repeating the examiner's question in the hope that he might clarify it, or asking for a clarification, does nothing but communicate your dilemma to the examiner. You should not waste any time. Bear in mind that our survey has confirmed that the diagnosis is usually mitral and/or aortic valve disease. Approach the right-hand side of the patient and adjust the backrest so that he reclines at 45° to the mattress. If the patient is wearing a shirt you should ask him to remove it so that the chest and neck are exposed. *Meanwhile*, you should complete a *quick*

1 *visual survey*. Observe whether the patient is
   (a) breathless,
   (b) *cyanosed*,
   (c) pale, or
   (d) whether he has a *malar flush* (mitral stenosis).

Look briefly at the earlobes for creases* and then at the *neck* for *pulsations*:

(e) forceful carotid pulsations (Corrigan's sign in aortic incompetence; vigorous pulsation in coarctation of the aorta), or

(f) tall, sinuous venous pulsations (congestive cardiac failure, tricuspid incompetence, pulmonary hypertension, etc.).

Run your eyes down onto the chest looking for

(g) a *left thoracotomy scar* (mitral stenosis†) or a midline sternal scar (valve replacement‡), and then down to the feet looking for

(h) ankle oedema. As you take the arm to feel the pulse complete your *visual survey* by looking at the hands (a quick look; don't be ponderous) for

(i) clubbing of the fingers (cyanotic congenital heart disease, subacute bacterial endocarditis (SBE)) and splinter haemorrhages (infective endocarditis).

If the examiner does not want you to feel the pulse he may intervene at this stage—otherwise you should proceed to

2 note the *rate* and *rhythm* of the **pulse**.

3 Quickly ascertain whether the pulse is **collapsing** (particularly if it is a large volume pulse) or not (make sure you are seen lifting the arm up—see experience 36, p. 453).

Next may be an opportune time to look for

4 **radiofemoral delay** (coarctation of the aorta), though this can be left until after auscultation if you prefer and are sure you will not forget it (see experience 1, p. 447).

5 Feel the brachial pulse followed by the carotid pulses to see if the pulse is a **slow rising** one, especially if the volume (the upstroke) is small.

If the pulsations in the neck present any interesting features you may have already noted these during your initial *visual survey*. You should now proceed to confirm some of these impressions. The Corrigan's sign in the neck (forceful rise and quick fall of the carotid pulsation) may already have been reinforced by the discovery of a collapsing radial pulse. The individual waves of a large venous pulse can now be timed by palpating the opposite carotid. A large *v* wave, which sometimes oscillates the earlobe, suggests tricuspid incompetence and you should later on demonstrate the peripheral oedema and the pulsatile liver using the bimanual technique. If the venous wave comes before the carotid pulsation it is an *a* wave suggestive of pulmonary hypertension (mitral valve disease, cor pulmonale) or pulmonary stenosis (rare). After

6 assessing the height of the **venous pressure** in centimetres vertically above the sternal angle you should move to the praecordium§ and

7 localize the **apex beat** with respect to the mid–clavicular line and ribspaces, firstly by inspection for visible pulsation, and secondly by *palpation*. If the apex

---

* Frank's sign: a diagonal crease in the lobule of the auricle: grade 3 = a deep cleft across the whole earlobe; grade 2A = crease more than halfway across the lobe; grade 2B = crease across the whole lobe, but superficial; grade 1 = lesser degrees of wrinkling. Earlobe creases are associated statistically with coronary artery disease in most population groups.

† NB experiences 4 and 7, pp. 449.

‡ Other scars may also be noted during your *visual survey*—

those of previous cardiac catheterizations may be visible over the brachial arteries.

§ The *visual survey* and the examination steps 2–6 should be completed *quickly* and efficiently particularly if you have been asked to examine the *heart*. The objective should be not only to avoid irritating an impatient examiner but also to accommodate as many short cases as possible in the allotted time.

beat is vigorous you should stand the index finger on it, to localize the point of maximum impulse (PMI) and *assess* the extent of its thrust. The impulse can be graded as just palpable, lifting (diastolic overload, i.e. mitral or aortic incompetence), thrusting (stronger than lifting), or heaving (outflow obstruction).

8 Palpation with your hand placed from the lower left sternal edge to the apex will detect a **tapping** impulse (left atrial 'knock' in mitral stenosis) or *thrills* over the mitral area (mitral valve disease), if present.

9 Continue palpation by feeling the **right ventricular lift** (left parasternal heave). To do this place the flat of your right palm parasternally over the right ventricular area and apply *sustained* and gentle pressure. If right ventricular hypertrophy is present you will feel the heel of your hand lifted by its force (pulmonary hypertension).

10 Next, you should **palpate** the pulmonary area for a *palpable second sound* (pulmonary hypertension), and the aortic area for a palpable *thrill* (aortic stenosis).*

If you feel a strong right ventricular lift quickly recall, and sometimes recheck, whether there is a giant *a* wave (pulmonary hypertension, pulmonary stenosis) or *v* wave (tricuspid incompetence, congestive cardiac failure) in the neck. A palpable thrill over the mitral area (mitral valve disease), or palpable pulmonary second sound over the pulmonary area (pulmonary hypertension) should make you think of, and check for, the other complementary signs. You should by now have a fair idea of what you will hear on auscultation of the heart but you should keep an open mind for any unexpected discovery.

11 The next step will be **auscultation** and you should only stray away from the heart (examiner's command) if you have a strong expectation of being able to demonstrate an interesting and relevant sign (such as a pulsatile liver to underpin the diagnosis of tricuspid incompetence). *Time* the first heart sound with either the apex beat, if this is palpable, or by feeling the carotid pulse (see experience 88, p. 459). It is important to listen to the expected murmurs in the most favourable positions. For example, mitral diastolic murmurs are best heard by turning the patient *onto the left side*, and the early diastolic murmur of aortic incompetence is made more prominent by asking the patient to *lean forwards* with his breath held after expiration.† For low-pitched sounds (mid-diastolic murmur of mitral stenosis, heart sounds) use the bell of your chest-piece but do not press hard, or else you will be listening through a diaphragm formed by the stretched skin! The high-pitched early diastolic murmur of aortic incompetence is very easily missed (see anecdote 37, p. 497). Make sure you specifically listen for it.

If the venous pressure is raised you should check for

12 **sacral oedema** and, if covered, expose the feet to demonstrate any *ankle oedema*.

Auscultation over

13 the **lung bases** for inspiratory crepitations (left ventricular failure), though an essential part of the routine assessment of the cardiovascular system, is seldom required in the examination. You may make a special effort to do this in certain rel-

---

* The thrill of aortic stenosis is best felt if the patient leans forwards with his breath held after expiration.
† With the diaphragm of your chest-piece *ready* in position:

'Take a deep breath in; now out; hold it'. Listen intently for the absence of silence in early diastole. Ask the patient to repeat the exercise if necessary.

evant situations such as a breathless patient, aortic stenosis with displaced PMI or if there are any signs of left heart failure (orthopnoea, pulsus alternans, gallop rhythm, etc.). Similarly, after examination of the heart itself it may (on rare occasions only) be necessary to

14 palpate the **liver** especially if you have seen a large *v* wave and heard a pansystolic murmur over the tricuspid area. In such cases you may be able to demonstrate a *pulsatile* liver by placing you left palm posteriorly and the right palm anteriorly over the enlarged liver.* Finally, you should offer to

15 measure the **blood pressure**. This is particularly relevant in patients with aortic stenosis (low systolic and narrow pulse pressure), and aortic incompetence (wide pulse pressure).

For *checklist* see p. 513.

2 / 'Examine this patient's abdomen'

Frequency of instruction
79% of candidates in our survey were asked to do this.

Variations of instruction
What abnormal structure can you feel in this abdomen?
Palpate this abdomen
Examine this patient's abdomen—look for signs of hepatic failure
Briefly examine the upper abdomen of this man
Examine the abdomen and anything else relevant
Examine this abdomen by palpation only.

Diagnoses from survey in order of frequency
1 Hepatosplenomegaly (not chronic liver disease) 19%
2 Splenomegaly 13%
3 Polycystic kidneys 12%
4 Chronic liver disease 11%
5 Hepatomegaly (without chronic liver disease or splenomegaly) 9%
6 Ascites 6%
7 Single palpable kidney 5%
8 Miscellaneous abdominal masses 4%
9 Hepatosplenomegaly and generalized lymphadenopathy 3%
10 Hepatomegaly and generalized lymphadenopathy 2%
11 Primary biliary cirrhosis 2%.

* An alternative and useful way of demonstrating a pulsatile liver is to place the knuckles of your closed right fist against the inferior border of the liver in the right hypochondrium (warn the patient beforehand!). Your fist will oscillate with each pulsation of the liver.

Other diagnoses were: Crohn's disease (1%), aortic aneurysm (1%), haemo-chromatosis (<1%), polycystic kidneys and a transplanted kidney (<1%), splenomegaly and generalized lymphadenopathy (<1%), abdominal lymphadenopathy (<1%), postsplenectomy (<1%) and normal abdomen (<1%).

Examination *routine*

Analysis of the above list reveals that in nearly 80% of cases the findings in the abdomen relate to a palpable spleen, liver or kidneys. Bearing this in mind you should approach the right-hand side of the patient and position him so that he is lying supine on one pillow (if comfortable), with the whole abdomen and chest in full view. Ideally the genitalia should also be exposed but to avoid embarrassment to patients, who are volunteers and whose genitals are usually normal, we suggest that you ask the patient to lower his garments and ensure that these are pulled down to a level about halfway between the iliac crest and the symphysis pubis. While these preparations are being made you should be performing

  1 a *visual survey* of the patient. Amongst the many relevant physical signs that you may observe in these few seconds are pallor, pigmentation, jaundice, spider naevi, xanthelasma, parotid swelling, gynaecomastia, scratch marks, tattoos, abdominal distension, distended abdominal veins, an abdominal swelling, herniae and decreased body hair. If you use the following *routine* most of these will also be noted during your subsequent examination but at this stage you should particularly note any

  2 **pigmentation**. As the patient is being correctly positioned,

  3 *quickly* **examine the hands*** for

   (a) Dupuytren's contracture,

   (b) clubbing,

   (c) leuconychia,

   (d) palmar erythema, and

   (e) a flapping tremor (if relevant).

After asking you to examine the abdomen many examiners would like, and *expect*, you to concentrate on the abdomen itself without delay, and yet they will not forgive you for missing an abnormal physical sign elsewhere. This emphasizes the importance of a good *visual survey*; a trained eye will miss nothing important on the face or in the hands while the patient is being properly positioned with the hands by his side. Thus, steps 1–3 need not occupy you for more than a few seconds; you may wish to omit steps 5 and 6 if there is no visible abnormality, and steps 7–11 can be completed as part of the *visual survey*.

  4 Pull down the **lower eyelid** to look for *anaemia*. At the same time check the sclerae for *icterus* and look for *xanthelasma*. The guttering between the eyeball and the lower lid is the best place to look for pallor or for any discoloration (e.g. cyanosis, jaundice, etc.).

  5 Look at the lips for cyanosis (cirrhosis of the liver) and shine your pen torch into the **mouth†** looking for swollen lips (Crohn's), telangiectasis (Osler–Weber–Rendu), patches of pigmentation (Peutz–Jeghers) and mouth ulcers (Crohn's).

---

* For a full list of the signs that may be visible in the hands in chronic liver disease, see p. 84.
† Though a brief examination of the mouth is usefully included as part of the full 'examine the abdomen' *routine*, it is worth noting that in our survey when there were the findings mentioned, the candidates were given a more specific instruction such as 'Look at this patient's mouth'.

6 Palpate the neck and supraclavicular fossae for *cervical lymph nodes.** If you do find lymph nodes you should then proceed to examine the axillae and groins for evidence of generalized lymphadenopathy (lymphoma, chronic lymphatic leukaemia). As you move from the neck to the chest, check for

7 gynaecomastia (palpate for glandular breast tissue in obese subjects),

8 spider naevi (may have been noted already on hands, arms and face and may also be present on the back), and

9 scratch marks (may have been noted on the arms, and may also be found on the back and elsewhere). Next,

10 look at the chest (in the male) and in the axillae for **paucity of hair** (if diminished note facial hair in the male; pubic hair if not visible, may be noted later).

11 Observe the abdomen in *three segments* (epigastric, umbilical and suprapubic) for any visible signs such as *pulsations*, generalized *distension* (ascites) or a *swelling* in one particular area. Note any scars or fistulae (previous surgery; Crohn's). Look for distended *abdominal* veins (the flow is away from the umbilicus in portal hypertension but upwards from the groin in inferior vena cava obstruction).

With practice the examination to this point can be completed very rapidly and will provide valuable information which may be overlooked if proceeding carelessly straight to palpation of the abdomen (see experience 2, p. 448). If the examiner insists that you start with abdominal palpation† it suggests that there is little to be found elsewhere, but you should nevertheless be prepared to use your 'wide-angled lenses' in order not to miss any of the above features.

12 Palpation of the abdomen should be performed in an orthodox manner; any temptation to go straight for a visible swelling should be resisted. Put your palm gently over the abdomen and ask the patient if he has any tenderness and to let you know if you hurt him. First systematically examine the whole of the abdomen with *light palpation*. Palpation should be done with the *pulps* of the fingers rather than the tips, the best movement being a gentle flexion at the metacarpophalangeal joints with the hand flat on the abdominal wall. Next, examine specifically for the *internal organs*. For both liver and spleen start in the right iliac fossa (you cannot be frowned upon for following this orthodox procedure‡), working upwards to the right hypochondrium in the case of the *liver* and diagonally across the abdomen to the left hypochondrium in the case of the *spleen*. The organs are felt against the radial border of the index finger and the pulps of the index and middle fingers as they descend on inspiration, at which time you can gently press and move your hand upwards to meet them. The *kidneys* are then sought by bimanual palpation of each lateral region. Palpation of the internal organs may be difficult if there is

---

* The supraclavicular lymph nodes, particularly on the left side, may be enlarged with carcinoma of the stomach (*Troisier's sign*; NB *Virchow's node* behind the left sternoclavicular joint) or carcinoma of any other abdominal organ or with carcinoma of the bronchus.

† Some examiners admit to being irritated at seeing candidates examine normal hands for a long time after being asked to examine the abdomen. They argue that the information obtainable from the face, mouth and hands can be gathered without delay during the inspection part of the examination (see anecdote 25, p. 496).

‡ Even though it is the time-honoured, orthodox procedure, many clinicians, these days, are opposed to this practice. They argue that a grossly enlarged spleen will be picked up on the initial light palpation which makes the approach from the right iliac fossa unnecessary. If they do not feel a mass in the left hypochondrium on initial palpation, they start deep palpation a few centimetres below the left costal edge.

ascites. In this case the technique is to press quickly, flexing at the wrist joint, to displace the fluid and palpate the enlarged organ ('dipping' or 'ballotting'). In a patient well chosen for the examination, a mass in the left hypochondrium may present a problem of identification (see experiences 23 and 30, pp. 451 and 452; anecdotes 25 and 29, p. 496); the examiner (testing your confidence) may ask you if you are sure that it is a spleen and not a kidney or vice versa. Do not forget to establish whether you can *get above* the mass and *separate* it from the costal edge, whether you can *bimanually* palpate it and whether the percussion note over it is *resonant* (all features of an enlarged kidney, see also p. 80). Palpate *deeply* with the pulps to look for the *ascending* and *descending colons* in the flanks, and use *gentle* palpation to feel for an *aortic aneurysm* in the midline. Complete palpation by feeling for *inguinal lymph nodes*, noting obvious herniae and, at the same time, adding information about the distribution and thickness of pubic hair to that already gained about the rest of the body hair.

13 Percussion must be used from the nipple downwards on both sides to locate the upper edge of the liver on the right and the spleen on the left (NB the left lower lateral chest wall may become dull to percussion before an enlarged spleen is palpable). The lower palpable edges of the spleen and liver should be defined by percussion in an orthodox manner, proceeding from the resonant to dull areas. If you suspect free fluid in the peritoneum you must establish its presence by demonstrating

14 shifting dullness. Initially check for *stony dullness* in the flanks. There is no need to continue with the procedure of demonstrating shifting dullness if this is not present. By asking the patient with ascites to turn on his side you can shift the dullness from the upper to the lower flank. Before you conclude the palpation and percussion of the abdomen, ask yourself whether you have found anything abnormal. If there are no abnormal physical signs make sure that you have not missed a polycystic kidney or a palpable splenic edge (or occasionally a mass in the epigastrium or iliac fossae); during your auscultation listen carefully for a bruit over the aorta and renal vessels. Generally speaking

15 auscultation has very little to contribute in the examination setting, but as part of the full *routine* you should listen to the bowel sounds, check for renal artery bruits and for any other sounds such as a rub over the spleen or kidney or a venous hum (both excessively rare).

Examination of the

16 external genitalia is not usually required in the examination for the reasons given above, and we have never heard of a case where

17 a rectal examination was required. You should, however, comment that you would like to complete your examination of the abdomen by examining the external genitalia (especially in the male with chronic liver disease—small testes; or cervical lymphadenopathy — drainage of testes to para-aortic and cervical lymph nodes) and rectum. You may of course never get this far since the examiner may interrupt you at an appropriate stage to ask for your findings. If you are allowed to conclude the examination and you have found nothing abnormal despite your careful search, on rare occasions the diagnosis of a normal abdomen will be accepted (see p. 444).

For *checklist* see p. 513.

3 / 'Examine this patient's fundi'

Frequency of instruction
67% of candidates in our survey were asked to do this.

Variations of instruction
Examine the left eye with the ophthalmoscope provided

Look at the normal fundus on the left, then look at the abnormal fundus on the right

Examine the ocular movements and fundi.

Diagnoses from survey in order of frequency
1 Diabetic retinopathy 36%
2 Optic atrophy 14%
3 Hypertensive retinopathy 9%
4 Retinitis pigmentosa 5%
5 Papilloedema 5%
6 Cataracts 4%
7 Choroidoretinitis 4%
8 Retinal vein thrombosis 3%
9 Myelinated nerve fibres 2%
10 Retinal artery occlusion 1%

Other diagnoses were: normal fundi in a patient with multiple sclerosis (<1%), large optic cup due to glaucoma (<1%), retinal detachment (<1%), iridodonesis (fluttering of the iris) due to a removed lens (<1%), lupus retinopathy (<1%) and calcified embolus (<1%).

Special note
Two-thirds of the candidates in our survey received this instruction. Though there are only a limited number of possibilities, it is clear from the survey that a lot of candidates experience more difficulty with a fundus than with any other short case. On our questionnaire a considerable number of candidates reported 'I said optic atrophy . . .', or 'I said diabetic retinopathy . . . but I hadn't got a clue what it was' (see experiences 51 and 52, p. 454). Clearly there is not a lot that a book like this can do to help other than to warn you in advance of the problem, to provide you with a list of the likely conditions and to describe them (see individual short cases). Other than this the art of fundoscopy and fundal diagnosis can only be acquired with practice. With a moderate degree of clinical expertise and common sense most candidates ought to be able to overcome this hurdle.

Examination *routine*
Almost invariably if you are asked to look at the fundus the diagnosis must be in the fundus. However, it is a good practice to precede fundoscopy with
1 a **quick general look** at the patient (this will rarely help but the occasional diabetic in the examination may also have *foot ulcers* or *necrobiosis lipoidica* or may be

wearing a *medic-alert* bracelet or neck chain), at his eyes (*arcus lipidus* at an inappropriately young age may suggest diabetes), and at his pupils (usually, but not always, dilated for the examination).

Turning to ophthalmoscopy, it may be your practice to focus immediately on the fundus and, in the vast majority of cases, this will provide the diagnosis. However, it would be preferable to cultivate the habit (if you can gain sufficient expertise to do it quickly and efficiently) of looking first at

2 the structures in front of the fundus, particularly the **lens** (diabetics will often reward you with early *cataract* formation; your examiner will sometimes not have noticed it, but as long as you are right when he checks you may score points). Adjust the lenses of the ophthalmoscope so that you move down through

3 the **vitreous** noting any *opacities* (e.g. asteroid hyalinosis, p. 374), *haemorrhages*, *fibrous tissue* or *new vessel formation* (diabetes) until you get to

4 the **fundus**. Localize the disc and examine it and its margins for *optic atrophy*,* *papillitis* (p. 82) or *papilloedema* (p. 166) and for *myelinated nerve fibres* (p. 248). Trace the

5 **arterioles** and **venules** out from the disc noting particularly their calibre, light reflex (*silver wiring*) and arteriovenous (AV) crossing points (*AV nipping*, see p. 136).

6 Examine **each quadrant** of the fundus and especially the **macular area** and its temporal aspect.† You are looking particularly for *haemorrhages* (dot, blot, flame-shaped), *microaneurysms*, *exudates* both hard (well-defined edges; increased light reflex) and soft (fluffy with ill-defined edges; *cotton-wool spots*). If hard exudates are present see if these form a ring (*circinates* in diabetes).

If you see haemorrhages you must look specifically for

(a) dot haemorrhages/microaneurysms,

(b) new vessel formation, and

(c) photocoagulation scars.

If you diagnose diabetic retinopathy your examiner will expect you to be able to comment on the presence or absence of all of these (see experiences 53 and 90, pp. 455 and 459). If you cannot find these diagnostic clues you may have noted the features that suggest hypertensive rather than diabetic retinopathy (silver wiring, AV nipping, more soft exudates than hard, haemorrhages which are mainly flame-shaped, early disc swelling with loss of venous pulsation‡ or frank papilloedema).

In the patient with diabetic retinopathy, it is of particular clinical significance to assess whether lesions (especially haemorrhages and hard exudates) involve or threaten (i.e. are near to) the macula.§

---

* There are normal variations in disc colour; in both infancy and old age it is naturally pale, as is the enlarged disc of a myopic eye. The advice of a well-known neurologist and experienced MRCP teacher to his MRCP candidates was: 'Don't diagnose optic atrophy unless it is a "barn door" optic atrophy'. It is well worth bearing this advice in mind (see experience 52, p. 454). Temporal pallor of the disc due to a lesion in the papillomacular bundle is often seen in multiple sclerosis. However, temporal pallor is not always pathological.

† The macula will come in to view if you ask the patient with a dilated pupil to look at the ophthalmoscopic light. Ideally, you should use the dot light for this, if it is available in your ophthalmoscope.

‡ Observation of venous pulsation is an expertise which comes with much practice of looking at normal as well as abnormal fundi. Though it could be useful if you have acquired this expertise before the examination, do not get bogged down studying the venous pulsation for too long if you are not used to it. See also p. 166.

§ European diabetic retinopathy screening guidelines suggest that patients with haemorrhages or hard exudate within one disc diameter of the macula should be considered for referral to an ophthalmologist (p. 68).

It would be useful if you knew that the patient was a diabetic (see experience 106, p. 466; quotation 46, p. 506) but if you remain in doubt remember that diabetes and hypertension often coexist in a patient, and that it is more important that you have checked comprehensively for the above features, and report your findings honestly (mentioning the features in favour of one diagnosis or the other), than to guess or make up findings.*

We leave you to master the findings of the other fundal short cases and to ensure that you would recognize each (see individual short cases). The final point in this important *routine* is to

7 stay examining until you have finished and are **ready** to present your findings. Do not be put off by the impatient words or mumblings of your examiner; these will be forgotten when you present accurate findings and get the diagnosis right. Conversely, it is too late to go back and check if the examiner asks whether you saw a . . . and you are not sure (experiences 53 and 90, pp. 455 and 459). You need to be able to give a clear and unequivocal 'Yes' or 'No'. Thus, the best tip we can offer as you look around the fundus is to stop at the disc, the macula, and in each quadrant of each eye and ask yourself the question: 'Are there any abnormalities? What are they?' before moving on to the next area.

For *checklist* see p. 513.

4 / 'Examine this patient's hands'

Frequency of instruction
58% of candidates in our survey were asked to do this.

Variations of instruction
Look at this man's hands
Look at this patient's hands and then, after you have made a diagnosis, look at the face
Examine this man's hands, commenting on positive or negative features as you go
Examine the wrists and hands
What do you think of these hands? Describe them to me.

Diagnoses from survey in order of frequency
1 Rheumatoid hands 22%
2 Systemic sclerosis (calcinosis, Raynaud's phenomenon, sclerodactyly and telangiectasis (CRST)) 13%
3 Wasting of the small muscles of the hand 12%
4 Psoriatic arthropathy/psoriasis 11%

---

* Making up findings is strictly inadvisable and can result in failure whereas missing one short case need not fail you.

5 Ulnar nerve palsy 9%
6 Clubbing 7%
7 Raynaud's 3%
8 Vasculitis 3%
9 Steroid changes (especially purpura) 3%
10 Acromegaly 2%
11 Motor neurone disease 2%
12 Xanthomata 2%
13 Cyanosis 2%
14 Chronic liver disease 2%
15 Thyroid acropachy 2%
16 Carpal tunnel syndrome 2%
17 Osteoarthrosis 2%
18 Osler–Weber–Rendu syndrome 1%
19 Tophaceous gout 1%.

Other diagnoses were: neurofibromatosis (<1%), systemic lupus erythematosus (<1%), cervical myelopathy (<1%), dermatomyositis ('examine hands and face'; <1%), nail–patella syndrome ('examine hands and knees', <1%), Charcot–Marie–Tooth disease (<1%), superior vena cava obstruction (<1%), facioscapulohumeral muscular dystrophy (<1%), Addison's disease (<1%) and Marfan's syndrome (<1%).

Examination *routine*

Analysis of the list given above suggests that when you hear this instruction, rheumatoid arthritis is likely to be present in about a quarter of the cases, and either scleroderma, wasting of the small muscles of the hand, psoriasis, ulnar nerve palsy or clubbing in about a further half. As you approach the patient you should bear this in mind and look specifically at

1 the **face** for the typical expressionless facies, with adherent shiny skin, sometimes with telangiectasis (*systemic sclerosis*). It is clear from the survey list that a variety of other conditions may show signs in either the face or in the general appearance, particularly *cushingoid* facies (steroid changes in a patient with rheumatoid arthritis), *acromegalic* facies, *arcus senilis* or *xanthelasma* (xanthomata), *icterus* and *spider naevi* (chronic liver disease), or *exophthalmos* (thyroid acropachy). We leave you to consider the changes you may note as you approach the patient with the other conditions on the list (see individual short cases). Even if the diagnosis is not immediately clear on looking at the face it is likely that in many cases it will become rapidly apparent as you

2 **inspect the hands**. Run quickly through the six main conditions that make up 75% of cases:

(a) *rheumatoid arthritis* (proximal joint swelling, spindling of the fingers, ulnar deviation, nodules),

(b) *systemic sclerosis* (sclerodactyly with tapering of the fingers, sometimes with gangrene of the fingertips, tight, shiny, adherent skin, calcified nodules, etc.),

(c) generalized *wasting* of the small muscles of the hand, perhaps with dorsal guttering,

(d) *psoriasis* (pitting of the nails, terminal interphalangeal arthropathy, scaly rash),

(e) *ulnar nerve palsy* (may be a typical claw hand or may be muscle wasting which spares the thenar eminence; often this diagnosis will only become apparent when you have made a sensory examination), and

(f) *clubbing.*

The changes that you may see in the other conditions in the list are dealt with under the individual short cases, but if in these first few seconds you have not made a rapid spot diagnosis, study first the dorsal and then the palmar aspects of the hands, looking specifically at

3 the **joints** for swelling, deformity or Heberden's nodes;

4 the **nails** for pitting, onycholysis, clubbing, nail-fold infarcts (vasculitis — usually rheumatoid) or splinter haemorrhages (unlikely);

5 the **skin** for *colour* (pigmentation, icterus, palmar erythema), for *consistency* (tight and shiny in scleroderma; papery thin, perhaps with purpuric patches in steroid therapy; thick in acromegaly), and for *lesions* (psoriasis, vasculitis, purpura, xanthomata, spider naevi, telangiectasis in Osler–Weber–Rendu and systemic sclerosis, tophi, neurofibromata, other rashes);

6 the **muscles** for isolated *wasting* of the thenar eminence (median nerve lesion), for generalized wasting especially of the first dorsal interosseous but sparing the thenar eminence (ulnar nerve lesion), for generalized wasting from a T1 lesion or other cause (p. 162) or for *fasciculation* which usually indicates motor neurone disease, though occasionally it can occur in other conditions such as syringomyelia, old polio or Charcot–Marie–Tooth disease.

Before leaving the inspection it is worth looking specifically for *skin crease pigmentation* (see experience 84, p. 458) before moving to

7 **palpation** of the hands for Dupuytren's contracture, nodules (may be palpable in the palms in rheumatoid arthritis), calcinosis (scleroderma/CRST), xanthomata, Heberden's nodes or tophi. In the vast majority of cases you will have, by now, some findings demanding either specific further action (see below) or a report with a diagnosis. Nonetheless, you should be prepared to continue with a full neurological examination of the hands to confirm a suspected neurological lesion, or if you have still made no diagnosis. If the hands appear normal it may be that there is a sensory defect. In these cases, it is more efficient, therefore, to commence the examination by testing

8 **sensation**. If you feel the examiners will not object, ask the patient if there has been any numbness or tingling in his hands and if so, when (?worse at night — carpal tunnel syndrome) and where. Bearing in mind the classical patterns of sensory defect in ulnar and median nerve lesions (Fig. 2.1) and the dermatomes (see Fig. 2.3, p. 41) seek and define an area of deficit to *pinprick* and *light touch* (dab cotton wool lightly), and check the *vibration* and *joint position* sense. With incomplete sensory loss due to either an ulnar or a median nerve defect, if you stroke the medial border of the little finger and the lateral border of the index finger with your fingers simultaneously, the patient may sense that the one side feels different from the other.

9 Check the **tone** of the muscles in the hand by flexing and extending all the joints including the wrist in a 'rolling wave' fashion.

10 The **motor** system of the hands can be tested with the instructions:

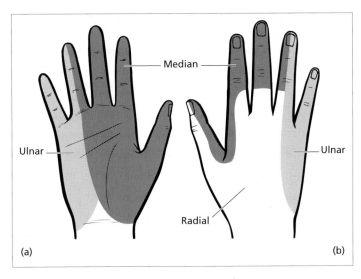

Fig. 2.1 Dermatomes in the hand.

(a) 'Open your hands; now close them; now open and close them quickly' (dystrophia myotonica)*

(b) 'Squeeze my fingers'—offer two fingers (C8, T1),†

(c) 'Hold your fingers out straight' (demonstrate); 'stop me bending them' (C7)

(d) 'Spread your fingers apart' (demonstrate); 'stop me pushing them together' (dorsal‡ interossei—ulnar nerve)

(e) 'Hold this piece of paper between your fingers; stop me pulling it out' (palmar‡ interossei—ulnar nerve)

(f) 'Point your thumb at the ceiling; stop me pushing it down' (abductor pollicis brevis—median nerve)

(g) 'Put your thumb and little finger together; stop me pulling them apart' (opponens pollicis—median nerve)

Finally, for the sake of completeness, check the

11 radial pulses.

The action you take after finding an abnormality at any stage during the above *routine* will depend on what you find. Most commonly an abnormality found during the inspection will lead to most of the above being skipped in favour of a search for other evidence of the condition you suspect. It is worth emphasizing that there may be clues at

12 the **elbows** in several of the common conditions: rheumatoid arthritis (nodules), psoriatic arthropathy (psoriatic plaques), ulnar nerve palsy (scar, filling of the ulnar groove, restriction of range of movement at the elbow or evidence of fracture) and xanthomata. On the evidence of our survey you will need to examine

---

* Alternatively, you could miss this step out and go straight to step (b), but then issue the instruction 'Let go' and if there is any suspicion of dystrophia myotonica move to step (a).

† Some neurologists prefer to test the deep finger flexors by trying to extend flexed fingers, whilst steadying the wrist (flexor digitorum profundus C8).

‡ Remember DAB and PAD: DAB = dorsal abduct, PAD = palmar adduct.

the elbows in over 40% of cases (do not be put off by rolled-down sleeves). It is worth considering where else you would look, what for and what other tests you would do with the other conditions on the list (see individual short cases), but in particular remember to look for *tophi* on the ears if you suspect gout, and if you have diagnosed acromegaly seek an associated *carpal tunnel syndrome* (see experience 9, p. 449). If on inspection you suspect a neurological deficit in the hand, you may wish to confirm it by performing only that part of the above *routine* relevant to that lesion, e.g. testing abduction and opposition of the thumb and seeking the classical sensory pattern if you see lone wasting of the thenar eminence and suspect carpal tunnel syndrome.

For *checklist* see p. 513.

5 / 'Examine this patient's legs'

Frequency of instruction
54% of candidates in our survey were asked to do this.

Variations of instruction
Examine this patient's lower limbs
Examine this patient's legs neurologically
Look at these legs
Look at these legs and make a few general observations
Examine this patient's legs. What else would you like to examine?
Show me how you would examine the reflexes in the legs
Examine the motor system of this man's legs
Examine this man's legs from the end of the bed.

Diagnoses from survey in order of frequency

Group 1 (spot)	Group 2 (neurological)
Paget's disease 13%	Spastic paraparesis 13%
Erythema nodosum 4%	Peripheral neuropathy 12%
Pretibial myxoedema 4%	Hemiplegia 5%
Diabetic foot 3%	Cerebellar syndrome 4%
Necrobiosis lipoidica diabeticorum 3%	Cervical myelopathy 4%
Erythema ab igne 2%	Diabetic foot 3%
Vasculitis 2%	Motor neurone disease 3%
Swollen knee 1%	Old polio 3%
Pemphigoid/pemphigus <1%	Absent leg reflexes and extensor plantars 3%
Deep venous thrombosis (DVT)/ruptured Baker's cyst <1%	Friedreich's ataxia 2%
Ankle swelling (nephrotic syndrome) <1%	Subacute combined degeneration of the cord 2%
Multiple thigh abscesses <1%	Charcot–Marie–Tooth disease 1%

Vasculitic leg ulcers <1%

Pyoderma gangrenosum <1%

Stigmata of sickle-cell disease <1%

Mycosis fungoides <1%

Diabetic ischaemia <1%

Ehlers–Danlos syndrome <1%

Bilateral below-knee amputation <1%

Polymositis <1%

Lateral popliteal (common peroneal) nerve palsy <1%

Tabes <1%

Diabetic amyotrophy <1%

Examination *routine*

An analysis of the conditions in our survey shows that they roughly fall into the two broad groups shown above:

Group 1: a spot diagnosis

Group 2: a neurological diagnosis.

Either way initial clues may be gained by first performing a brief

1 *visual survey* of the patient as a whole. Look at the head and face for signs such as *enlargement* (Paget's disease), *asymmetry* (hemiparesis), *exophthalmos* with or without *myxoedematous facies* (pretibial myxoedema), or obvious *nystagmus* (cerebellar syndrome). Run your eyes over the patient for other significant signs such as thyroid *acropachy* (pretibial myxoedema), *rheumatoid hands* (swollen knee), nicotine-stained fingers (leg amputations), *wasted hands* (motor neurone disease, Charcot–Marie–Tooth disease, syringomyelia), and for muscle *fasciculation* (usually motor neurone disease).

Turning to the legs, look at the skin, joints and general shape and for any

2 **obvious lesion**, especially from the list of disorders in group 1. If such a lesion is visible a further full examination of the legs will not be required in most cases. You will be able to begin your description and/or diagnosis immediately (see individual short cases). If there is no obvious lesion look again specifically for

3 **bowing** of the tibia (see experience 80, p. 458), with or without enlargement of the skull. Though the changes of vascular insufficiency (absence of hair, shiny skin, cold pulseless feet, peripheral cyanosis, digital gangrene, painful ulcers) barely occurred in our survey, these should be *briefly* looked for (because they will direct you to examine the pulses, etc. rather than the neurological system).

Observing the legs from the neurological point of view note whether there is

4 **pes cavus** (Friedreich's ataxia, Charcot–Marie–Tooth disease) or

5 **one leg smaller** than the other (old polio, infantile hemiplegia). Next note

6 **muscle bulk**. Bear in mind that some generalized disuse atrophy may occur even in a limb with upper motor neurone weakness (e.g. severe spastic paraparesis — see experience 2, p. 448). There may be unilateral loss of muscle bulk (old polio), muscle wasting that stops part of the way up the leg (Charcot–Marie–Tooth disease), isolated anterior thigh wasting (e.g. diabetic amyotrophy) or generalized proximal muscle wasting (polymyositis) or muscle wasting confined to one peroneal region (lateral popliteal nerve palsy). Look specifically for

7 **fasciculation** (nearly always motor neurone disease).

8 Examine the **muscle tone** in each leg by passively moving it at the hip and knee joints (with the patient relaxed roll the leg sideways, backwards and forwards

on the bed; lift the knee and let it drop, or bend the knee and partially straighten in an irregular and unexpected rhythm).

    9 Test **power:***
        (a) 'Lift your leg up; stop me pushing it down' (L1,2)
        (b) 'Bend your knee; don't let me straighten it' (L5,S1,2)
        (c) (Knee still bent) 'Push out straight against my hand' (L3,4)
        (d) 'Bend your foot down; push my hand away' (S1)
        (e) 'Cock up your foot; point your toes at the ceiling. Stop me pushing your foot down' (L4,5).

Moving smoothly into testing

10 coordination, take your hand off the foot and run your finger down the patient's shin below the knee saying

        (f) 'Put your heel just below your knee then run it smoothly down your shin; now up your shin, now down . . .' etc.†

11 Check the knee (L3,4) and ankle (S1,2) **jerks**‡ and if there is any possibility of pyramidal disease try to demonstrate *ankle clonus* (and patellar clonus).

12 Test the **plantar response** remembering that in slight pyramidal lesions an extensor plantar is more easily elicited on the outer part of the sole than the inner.§

13 Turning to **sensation,** dermatomes L2 to S1 on the leg (Fig. 2.2) are tested if you examine *light touch* (dab cotton wool lightly), and *pinprick* once each on the outer thigh (L2), inner thigh (L3), inner calf (L4), outer calf (L5), medial foot (L5) and lateral foot (S1). The most common sensory defect is a peripheral neuropathy with stocking distribution loss. Demonstrate this with light touch (usually the most sensitive indicator) and pinprick:

Test above the sensory level:
    'Does the pin feel sharp and prickly'—'Yes'.
Test on the feet:
    'Does the pin feel sharp and prickly'—'No'.
    'Tell me when it changes'.

Work up the leg to the sensory level and confirm afterwards by demonstrating the same level medially and laterally.‖ The level of the peripheral neuropathy may be different on the two legs. *Vibration* should be tested on the medial malleoli (and knee, iliac crest, etc., if it is impaired), and *joint position* sense in the great toes (remember to explain to the patient what you mean by 'up' and 'down' in his toes

---

* The screen of instructions from a to e will identify most legs in which there are abnormalities of motor function. You may wish to embellish these, where necessary, with instructions to test hip extension, hip adduction, hip abduction and hip rotation.

† If there is possible or definite cerebellar disease, you may wish to demonstrate dysdiadochokinesis in the foot by asking the patient to tap his foot quickly on your hand.

‡ One study has suggested that the plantar strike technique for examining ankle jerks may be more reliable than the better known tendon strike technique, especially in the elderly (*Lancet* 1994, **344**: 1619–20).

§ In slight pyramidal disease the extensor plantar is first elicited on the dorsilateral part of the foot (*Chaddock's manoeuvre*). As the degree of pyramidal involvement increases the area in which a *Babinski's sign* may be elicited increases first to cover the whole sole and then spreads beyond the foot until *Oppenheim's sign* (extensor response when the inner border of the tibia is pressed heavily; Fig. 3.69b, p. 212) or *Gordon's reflex* (extensor response on pinching the Achilles tendon) can be elicited. In such cases the big toe may be seen to go up as the patient takes his socks off.

‖ The same method can be used for rapid demonstration of a higher sensory level: normal sensation is demonstrated above the lesion, e.g. on the shoulder or chest. The pin is then rapidly moved up the whole body from the foot until the patient announces that the sensation is changing to normal. That area is then worked over rapidly to detect the actual sensory level.

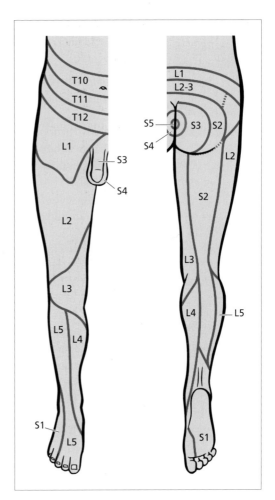

Fig. 2.2 Dermatomes in the lower limb (after Foerster, 1933, Oxford University Press, *Brain* **56**: 1). There is considerable variation and overlap between the cutaneous areas supplied by each spinal root so that an isolated root lesion results in a much smaller area of sensory impairment than the diagram indicates.

before you get him to close his eyes'; whilst testing the position sense hold the toe by the lateral aspects).

Sometimes the examiner will stop you before you get this far. If the lesion is predominantly motor he may break in before you have tested sensation, and if predominantly sensory he may lead you to test sensation earlier or stop you at this point. You should, however, be sufficiently deft to perform the full examination described above quickly and efficiently, and be prepared to complete it by examining the patient's

14 gait (check the patient can walk by asking for either his or the examiner's permission to examine the gait). First, watch his *ordinary walk* to a defined point and back (see p. 186) and then watch him walk *heel-to-toe* (ataxia), on his *toes* and on his *heels* (foot-drop). Finally perform

15 Romberg's test with the feet together and the arms outstretched. You must be ready to catch the patient if there is any possibility of ataxia. Romberg's test is only positive (sensory ataxia, e.g. subacute combined degeneration, tabes dorsalis) if the patient is more unsteady (tends to fall) with the eyes closed than open.

For *checklist* see p. 514.

6 / 'Examine this patient's chest'

Frequency of instruction
49% of candidates in our survey were asked to do this.

Variations of instruction
Listen to this man's chest

Examine the respiratory system of this man's chest. Is there anything else you would look for?

Examine the right side of this man's chest

Listen to the back of this patient's chest

Examine this lady's chest but could you confine yourself to her back

Listen to and percuss the posterior aspect of this gentleman's chest

Examine this man's chest from the front

This lady is short of breath. Examine the respiratory system from behind

Listen to the back of the chest. What two other signs would you seek?

Diagnoses from survey in order of frequency
1 Dullness at the lung base 27%
2 Fibrosing alveolitis 15%
3 Old tuberculosis 12%
4 Carcinoma of the bronchus 10%
5 Bronchiectasis 8%
6 Chronic bronchitis and emphysema 8%
7 Radiation burn on the chest 4%
8 Pneumonia or chest infection 4%
9 Heart murmurs* 2%
10 Ankylosing spondylitis 2%
11 Cor pulmonale 1%
12 Superior vena cava obstruction <1%
13 Pancoast's syndrome <1%
14 Pneumothorax <1%
15 Systemic sclerosis <1%
16 (Kypho)scoliosis <1%.

Examination *routine*
While approaching the patient, asking for his permission to examine him and settling him reclining at 45° to the bed with his chest bare, you should observe

 1 his **general appearance**. Note any evidence of *weight loss*. The features of conditions such as superior vena cava obstruction (p. 239), systemic sclerosis (p. 96) and lupus pernio (p. 224) may be readily apparent as should be severe kyphoscoliosis. However, *ankylosing spondylitis* is easily missed with the patient lying down (see experiences 3 and 31, pp. 448 and 452). Observe specifically whether the patient

---

* Though a small number of candidates in our survey reported that they were asked to 'examine the chest' in patients with heart murmurs, we suspect that the examiners gave some further suggestive clue that they meant the heart to be examined.

2 is **breathless** at rest or from the effort of removing his clothes,

3 **purses** his lips (chronic small airways obstruction), or

4 has central **cyanosis*** (cor pulmonale, fibrosing alveolitis, bronchiectasis). Central cyanosis may be difficult to recognize; it is always preferable to look at the oral mucous membranes (see below). Observe

5 if the **accessory muscles** are being used during breathing (chronic small airways obstruction, pleural effusion, pneumothorax, etc.),

6 if there is generalized **indrawing** of the intercostal muscles or supraclavicular fossae (hyperinflation) or if there is indrawing of the lower ribs on inspiration (due to low, flat diaphragms in emphysema). Localized indrawing of the intercostal muscles suggests bronchial obstruction.

Listen to the breathing with unaided ears whilst you observe the chest wall and hands (but do not dither). This will allow a dual input whereby a collaboration of what you hear and what you see may help you form a diagnostic impression. You should listen to whether *expiration* is more *prolonged* than inspiration (normally the reverse), and difficult (chronic airways obstruction), whether it is *noisy* (breathlessness) and if there are any additional noises such as *wheezes* or *clicks*. Difficult and noisy inspiration is usually caused by obstruction in the major bronchi (mediastinal masses, retrosternal thyroid, bronchial carcinoma, etc.) while the more prolonged, noisy and often wheezy expiration is caused by chronic small airways obstruction (asthma, chronic bronchitis). While you are listening observe.

7 the *movement* of the **chest wall**. It may be mainly *upwards* (emphysema), or *asymmetrical* (fibrosis, collapse, pneumonectomy, pleural effusion, pneumothorax). In the context of the examination it is particularly important to look for localized *apical flattening* suggestive of underlying fibrosis due to old tuberculosis (p. 108) or pneumonectomy (p. 288). You may also note a thoracotomy or thoracoplasty *scar* (pp. 108 and 289) or the presence of *radiotherapy field markings* (Indian ink marks) or radiation *burns* on the chest (intrathoracic malignancy, p. 313).

Check the hands for

8 **clubbing** (p. 201), *tobacco staining*, coal dust tattoos, or other conditions which affect the hands and may be associated with lung disease such as rheumatoid arthritis (nodules, p. 73) or systemic sclerosis (p. 96).

9 Feel the **pulse** and if it is bounding, or if the patient is cyanosed, check for a *flapping tremor* of the hands (CO_2 retention). If there is doubt about the presence of cyanosis you could at this point check the tongue and the buccal mucous membranes over the premolar teeth before moving to the neck to look for

10 **raised venous pressure** (cor pulmonale) or fixed distension of the neck veins (superior vena cava obstruction). Next examine

11 the **trachea**. Place the index and ring fingers on the manubrium sternae over the prominent points on either side. Use the middle finger as the exploring finger to gently feel the tracheal rings to detect either *deviation* or a *tracheal tug* (i.e. the

---

* Occurs with mean capillary concentration of $\geq 4\,g\,dl^{-1}$ of deoxygenated haemoglobin (or $0.5\,g\,dl^{-1}$ methaemoglobin). Alternatively, the presence of cyanosis may be supported by demonstrating a low arterial oxygen saturation ($<85\%$) non-invasively with an ear oximeter applied to the antihelix of the ear. Central cyanosis is more readily detected in patients with polycythaemia than in those with anaemia—because of the low haemoglobin, patients with anaemia require a much lower oxygen saturation to have $4\,g\,dl^{-1}$ of unsaturated haemoglobin in capillary blood.

middle finger being pushed upwards against the trachea by the upward movement of the chest wall). Check the *notch–cricoid* distance.*

12 Feel for **lymphadenopathy** (carcinoma, tuberculosis, lymphoma, sarcoidosis) in the cervical region and axillae. As the right hand returns from the left axilla look for

13 the **apex beat** (difficult to localize if the chest is hyperinflated) which in conjunction with tracheal deviation may give you evidence of mediastinal displacement (collapse, fibrosis, pneumonectomy, effusion, scoliosis).

14 To look for **asymmetry** rest one hand lightly on either side of the front of the chest to see if there is any diminution of movement (effusion, fibrosis, pneumonectomy, collapse, pneumothorax). Next grip the chest symmetrically with the fingertips in the ribspaces on either side and approximate the thumbs to meet in the middle in a straight horizontal line in order

15 to assess **expansion** first in the inframammary and then in the supramammary regions. Note the distance between each thumb and the midline (may give further information about asymmetry of movement) and between both thumbs and try to express the expansion in centimetres (it is better to produce a tape measure for a more accurate assessment of the expansion in centimetres). Comparing both sides at each level

16 **percuss** the chest from above downwards starting with the supraclavicular fossae and over the clavicles† and do not forget to percuss over the axillae. Few clinicians now regularly map out the area of cardiac dullness. In healthy people there is dullness behind the lower left quarter of the sternum which is lost together with normal liver dullness in hyperinflation. Complete palpation by checking for

17 **tactile vocal fremitus** with the ulnar aspect of the hand applied to the chest.

18 Auscultation of the **breath sounds** should start *high* at the apices and you should remember to listen in the *axillae*. You are advised to cover both lung fields first with the bell‡ before using the diaphragm (if for no other reason than that this allows you a chance to check the findings without appearing to backtrack!). In the nervousness of the examination harsh breathing heard with the diaphragm near a major bronchus (over the second intercostal space anteriorly or below the scapula near the midline posteriorly) may give an impression of bronchial breathing, particularly in thin people. Compare corresponding points on opposite sides of the chest. Ensure that the patient breathes with the mouth open, regularly and deeply, but not noisily (see experience 55, p. 455). Auscultation is completed by checking

19 **vocal resonance** in all areas; **if** you have found an area of bronchial breathing (the sounds may resound close to your ears—aegophony) check also for whispering pectoriloquy. The classical timings of crackles/crepitations of various origins are

(a) *Early inspiratory*: chronic bronchitis, asthma

(b) *Early and mid-inspiratory and recurring in expiration*: bronchiectasis (altered by coughing)

---

* The length of trachea from the suprasternal notch to the cricoid cartilage is normally three or more finger breadths. Shortening of this distance is a sign of hyperinflation.
† Percussion on the bare clavicle may cause discomfort to the patient.

‡ Many physicians prefer to use the diaphragm in their routine examination of the chest though some believe that as the respiratory auscultatary sounds are usually of low pitch, the bell is preferable.

(c) *Mid/late inspiratory*: restrictive lung disease (e.g. fibrosing alveolitis*) and pulmonary oedema.

20 To **examine the back** of the chest sit the patient forward (it may help to cross the arms in front of the patient to pull the scapulae further apart) and repeat steps 14–19. You may wish to start the examination of the back by palpating for cervical nodes from behind (particularly the scalene nodes between the two heads of sternomastoid).

Though with sufficient practice this whole procedure can be performed rapidly without loss of efficiency, often in the examination you will only be asked to perform some of it—usually 'examine the back of the chest'. As always when forced to perform only part of the complete *routine*, be sure that the partial examination is no less thorough and professional. Be prepared to put on your 'wide-angled lenses' so as not to miss other related signs (see experience 1, p. 447; anecdotes 11 and 12, p. 495).

Though by now you will usually have sufficient information to present your findings, occasionally you will wish to check other features on the basis of the findings so far. Further purposeful examination gives an impression of confidence but it should not be overdone. For example, looking for evidence of Horner's syndrome, or wasting of the muscles of one hand† in a patient with apical dullness and a deviated trachea, will suggest professional keenness; whereas routinely looking at the eyes and hands after completion of the examination may only suggest to the examiner that you do not have the diagnosis and are hoping for inspiration! If you suspect airways obstruction the examiner may be impressed if you perform a bedside respiratory function test—the *forced expiratory time* (FET).‡

For *checklist* see p. 514.

7 / 'What is the diagnosis?'

Frequency of instruction
41% of candidates in our survey were asked to do this.

---

* In fibrosing alveolitis late inspiratory crackles may become reduced if the patient is made to lean forward; thereby the compressed dependent alveoli (which crackle-open in late inspiration) are relieved of the pressure of the lungs.
† A good *visual survey* may reveal such signs at the beginning.
‡ Ask the patient to take a deep breath in and then, on your command (timed with the second hand of your watch), to breathe out as hard and as fast as he can until his lungs are completely empty. A normal person will empty his lungs in less than 6 seconds (1 second for every decade of age, e.g. a

normal 30-year-old will do it in 3 seconds). An FET of >6 seconds is evidence of airways obstruction. You need to practise this test with patients if it is to be slick. As with peak flow rate (PFR) and forced expiratory volume in 1 second (FEV$_1$) etc., it is important to make sure that certain patients, particularly females, *are* blowing as hard and as fast as they can ('don't worry about what you look like—give it everything you've got—like this'—give a demonstration) and empty their lungs completely ('keep going, keep going . . . keep going, well done!')

Variations of instruction

First, look generally at this man. What do you notice?

What is wrong with this patient?

Ask the patient to look at the ceiling—what is the diagnosis?

Look at this patient

Look at this man and at his hands

I would like you to look at him and tell me what's the matter

What do you notice from here? (end of the bed)

Look at this patient. What other specific things would you like to examine?

Observe this patient

What is that?

Comment on this patient's appearance

Diagnosis please

Give me as many diagnoses as you can and listen to the heart

What do you think this man is suffering from and why?

What do you think?

Do you notice anything about this patient's appearance?

Come and have a look at this man

What do you notice? Now examine the abdomen

On general appearance what's wrong with this man?

This man is breathless. Observe him

What observations do you make?

What do you notice looking at this patient that is in the MRCP curriculum?

Look at this man from the end of the bed. What would you like to do now?

Look at this patient and then examine the relevant parts.

Diagnoses from survey in order of frequency

1 Acromegaly 11%
2 Parkinson's disease 5%
3 Hemiplegia 5%
4 Goitre 5%
5 Jaundice 5%
6 Dystrophia myotonica 4%
7 Pigmentation 4%
8 Graves' disease 4%
9 Exophthalmos 4%
10 Paget's disease 3%
11 Ptosis 3%
12 Choreoathetosis 3%
13 Drug-induced parkinsonism 3%
14 Breathlessness 2%
15 Purpura 2%
16 Hypopituitarism 2%
17 Addison's/Nelson's 2%
18 Cushing's syndrome 2%
19 Psoriasis 2%
20 Hypothyroidism 2%
21 Systemic sclerosis/CRST 2%

22 Sturge–Weber syndrome 2%
23 Spider naevi and ascites 1%
24 Marfan's syndrome 1%
25 Neurofibromatosis 1%
26 Cyanotic congenital heart disease 1%
27 Pretibial myxoedema 1%
28 Uraemia and dialysis scars 1%
29 Horner's syndrome 1%
30 Cachexia 1%
31 Osler–Weber–Rendu syndrome 1%
32 Ankylosing spondylitis 1%
33 Ulnar nerve palsy 1%
34 Turner's syndrome 1%
35 Down's syndrome 1%
36 Bilateral parotid enlargement/Mikulicz's syndrome 1%
37 Old rickets 1%
38 Torticollis 1%
39 Congenital syphilis 1%
40 Syringomyelia <1%
41 Herpes zoster <1%
42 Pemphigoid/pemphigus <1%
43 Bell's palsy <1%
44 Necrobiosis lipoidica diabeticorum <1%
45 Primary biliary cirrhosis <1%.

Examination *routine*

Advice commonly given by the candidates in our survey as a result of their Membership experiences was to 'keep calm'. When you stand before a patient with a condition from the above list and hear the instruction under consideration you are being asked to do what you do every day of your medical life. There are two differences, however, between everyday medical life and the examination: (i) the patients in the examination usually have classical, often florid, signs and should be easier to diagnose than most patients seen in the clinic; and (ii) in the examination, you may be overwhelmed by nerves and as a result make the most fundamental errors. You must indeed try to keep calm and remind yourself that this is likely to be an easy case, and that you will not only make a diagnosis (as you would with ease in the clinic), but will also find a way of scoring some extra marks. Unlike some of the instructions requiring long examination *routines*, the 'spot diagnosis' may be solved in seconds leaving time for something extra which you may be able to dictate, rather than leaving it to the examiner to lead. You should start with

1 a *visual survey* of the patient, running your eyes from the head via the neck, trunk, arms and legs to the feet, seeking the areas of abnormality, and thereby the diagnosis. We would suggest that you rehearse presenting the *records* for the various possibilities on the list (see individual short cases). If you are well prepared with the features of these short cases, then in the majority of instances you should be able to make a diagnosis, or likely diagnosis, which you can confirm or highlight by demonstrating additional features (see below). If you have scanned the patient briefly and not found any obvious abnormality, then

2 retrace the same ground scrutinizing each part more thoroughly and asking yourself at each stage, 'Is the head normal?', 'Is the face normal?', etc. If it is not normal describe the abnormality to yourself in the mind trying to match it up with one of the short case *records*. In this way cover the

(a) head (think especially of *Paget's* and *dystrophia myotonica* with frontal balding),

(b) face (think especially of *acromegaly*, *Parkinson's*, the facial asymmetry of *hemiplegia*, the long lean look of dystrophia myotonica, tardive dyskinesia, hypopituitarism, Cushing's, hypothyroidism, systemic sclerosis),

(c) eyes (*jaundice*, *exophthalmos*, ptosis, Horner's, xanthelasma),

(d) neck (*goitre*, Turner's, ankylosing spondylitis, torticollis),

(e) trunk (pigmentation, ascites, purpuric spots, spider naevi, wasting, pemphigus, etc.),

(f) arms (choreoathetosis, psoriasis, Addison's, spider naevi, syringomyelia),

(g) hands (acromegaly, *tremor*, clubbing, sclerodactyly, arachnodactyly, claw hand, etc.),

(h) legs (bowing, purpura, pretibial myxoedema, necrobiosis), and

(i) feet (pes cavus).

If you still do not have the diagnosis

3 specifically consider **abnormal colouring** such as *pigmentation*, *icterus* or pallor, and then cover the same ground again but in even more detail

4 breaking down each part into its constituents, scrutinizing them, and continually asking yourself the question: 'Is it normal?' This procedure is most profitable on the face (see p. 38).

Once you have the diagnosis, the natural impulse for most people is to give it in one word, and then stand back and wait for the applause. However, it is worth remembering that the majority of the candidates, who have all worked hard and prepared for the examination, are likely to 'spot' the diagnosis and yet only a few end up with the diploma. Do not let this opportunity pass you by; try to make more of the case yourself by proceeding to

5 look for **additional** and **associated features**, and then by making your presentation more elaborate. Describe the findings in detail (see individual short cases) and highlight the key features to support your diagnosis (lenticular abnormalities in dystrophia myotonica and Marfan's; thyroid bruit in Graves' disease; webbed neck in Turner's syndrome, and so on). It is worth going through the diagnoses on the list yourself, and considering what additional features you would look for, and how you could really go to town on an easy case. For example, if you diagnose acromegaly you could demonstrate the massive sweaty palms, commenting on the increased skin thickening and on the presence or absence of thenar wasting (carpal tunnel syndrome — see experience 19, p. 449), and then proceed to test the visual fields. If you suspect Parkinson's disease, take the hands and test for cog-wheel rigidity at the wrist, demonstrate the glabellar tap sign (despite its unreliability) and then ask the patient to walk. If you diagnose hemiplegia, confirm that facial weakness is upper motor neurone (see p. 106), and then check for atrial fibrillation. If you see a goitre, examine it and then assess the thyroid status.

For *checklist* see p. 514.

8 / 'Examine this patient's eyes'

Frequency of instruction
32% of candidates in our survey were asked to do this.

Variations of instruction
Tell me about this patient's eyes
Look at these eyes
Examine the eye movements.

Diagnoses from survey in order of frequency
1 Exophthalmos 27%
2 Ocular palsy 23%
3 Nystagmus 11%
4 Diabetic retinopathy 8%
5 Optic atrophy 7%
6 Myasthenia gravis 4%
7 Visual field defects 3%
8 Ptosis 3%
9 Retinitis pigmentosa 2%
10 Horner's syndrome 2%
11 Holmes–Adie pupil 1%
12 Argyll Robertson pupils 1%
13 Cataracts 1%
14 Papilloedema 1%.

Other diagnoses were: buphthalmos in a patient with Sturge–Weber syndrome (1%), normal eyes in a patient who was supposed to have internuclear ophthalmoplegia (1%) and retinal detachment (<1%).

Examination routine
A study of the above list maps out your examination steps when you hear this instruction. It is basically going to be a part of your cranial nerves *routine* (p. 55) but carried out in slightly more detail. It should be your habit to commence all examination *routines* by *scanning* the whole patient. The patient with nystagmus due to cerebellar disease (p. 142) may have an *intention tremor* which will occasionally be noticeable even with minor movements. The patient with exophthalmos may have *pretibial myxoedema* or *thyroid acropachy*. A number of other conditions with stigmata elsewhere on the body may cause eye signs. Though these conditions were not prominent in our survey, they should be borne in mind as you complete this *visual survey*: face and hands of acromegaly, foot ulcers in diabetes, pes cavus in Friedreich's ataxia, the long, lean look of dystrophia myotonica, etc. As you finish your *visual survey* briefly look again at
1 the **face** (e.g. myasthenic facies, tabetic facies, facial asymmetry in hemiparesis), and then concentrate on
2 the **eyes**. Ask yourself if there is

(a) exophthalmos,

(b) strabismus,

(c) ptosis, or

(d) other abnormalities such as xanthelasma or arcus senilis.

Look at

3 the **pupils** for inequality of size and shape; whether one or both are small (Argyll Robertson, Horner's) or large (Holmes–Adie, IIIrd nerve palsy). Next, it is traditional to check

4 the **visual acuity** by asking the patient to read a newspaper or other print which you hold up, and by asking him to look at the clock on the wall (see p. 56); alternatively it would be preferable to pull out a pocket-sized Snellen's chart.* In the traditional *routine* you should next test

5 visual fields (see p. 48). However, in the majority of cases the important findings are on testing

6 eye movements (see p. 56). We leave you to decide if you wish to follow the traditional *routine* or check eye movements before acuity and visual fields (see experience 37, p. 453; quotation 57, p. 506). You are looking for

(a) ocular palsy (p. 117),

(b) diplopia,

(c) nystagmus, or

(d) lid lag.

In order to test

7 the **pupillary light reflex**, take out your pen torch and shine the light twice (*direct* and *consensual*) in each eye. Then test

8 the **accommodation–convergence reflex** — hold your finger close to the patient's nose:

'Look into the distance';

then suddenly

'Now look at my finger'.†

Finally, examine

9 the **fundi**.

As usual, when you have the diagnosis, think what else you could look for (e.g. cerebellar signs in a patient with nystagmus; sympathectomy scar over the clavicle in a patient with Horner's syndrome; absent limb reflexes in Holmes–Adie pupil) before shouting out the diagnosis even if it is obvious (e.g. exophthalmos).

For *checklist* see p. 514.

---

* We advise you to take a pocket-sized Snellen's chart (like the one provided in Appendix 4). It will enable you to put an approximate value on the patient's visual acuity while taking no extra time.

† Some neurologists believe that as this traditional method of examining the accommodation-convergence reflex may involve a change in optical axis and luminance, it is better to get the patient to follow a target down the optical axis over 2 m.

9 / 'Examine this patient's face'

Frequency of instruction
20% of candidates in our survey were asked to do this.

Variations of instruction
Look at this patient's face
What is wrong with this patient's face?
Comment on the facial appearance
You are good at looking at the face and making a diagnosis; can you do that in this patient?

Diagnoses from survey in order of frequency
1 Lower motor neurone VIIth nerve lesion 12%
2 Lupus pernio 8%
3 Ptosis 7%
4 Sturge–Weber syndrome 7%
5 Hypothyroidism 7%
6 Osler–Weber–Rendu syndrome 7%
7 Dystrophia myotonica 4%
8 Jaundice 4%
9 Horner's syndrome 4%
10 Systemic sclerosis/CRST 3%
11 Peutz–Jeghers syndrome 3%
12 Upper motor neurone facial weakness 3%
13 Systemic lupus erythematosus 3%
14 Parkinson's disease 3%
15 Cushing's syndrome 2%
16 Neurofibromatosis 2%
17 Superior vena cava obstruction 2%
18 Plethora (polycythaemia rubra vera) 2%
19 Hypopituitarism 2%
20 Vitiligo and a goitre 2%
21 Cyanosis 2%
22 Paget's disease 1%
23 Bilateral parotid enlargement 1%
24 Exophthalmos 1%
25 Acromegaly 1%
26 Dermatomyositis (hands and face) 1%
27 Xanthelasma and arcus senilis 1%
28 Acne rosacea 1%
29 Dermatitis herpetiformis 1%
30 Malar flush 1%.

Examination *routine*

This instruction is really just a variation on the 'spot diagnosis' theme, only easier because you are told where the abnormalities lie. In a way similar to that described in the 'What is the diagnosis?' *routine*,

1 *survey* the patient from head to foot and then

2 **scan the face** and skull. The abnormality will usually be obvious (see above list) but if you find none then proceed to

3 **break down the parts** of the face into their constituents and scrutinize each, asking the question to yourself: 'Is it normal?' Thus if you have scanned the eyes and have not been struck by any obvious abnormality (e.g. ptosis or an abnormal pupil), you should look at all the structures such as the *eyelids* (mild degree of ptosis, heliotrope rash on the upper lid in dermatomyositis), *eyelashes* (sparse in alopecia*), *cornea* (arcus senilis, ground-glass appearance in congenital syphilis), *sclerae* (icteric, congested in superior vena cava obstruction and polycythaemia), *pupils* (small, large, irregular, dislocated lens in Marfan's, cataract in dystrophia myotonica) and *iris* ('muddy iris' in iritis)† on both sides. Look at the *face* for any erythema or infiltrates (lupus pernio, systemic lupus erythematosus (SLE), dermatomyositis, malar flush), around the *mouth* for tight, shiny, adherent skin (systemic sclerosis) or pigmented macules (Peutz–Jeghers) and, if indicated, in the mouth for telangiectases (Osler–Weber–Rendu), cyanosis or pigmentation (Addison's). The whole face can be rapidly covered in this manner. Having spotted the abnormality and, you hope, made the diagnosis you should, if appropriate, try to score extra points by demonstrating

4 **additional features** in the same way as described under 'What is the diagnosis?' Go through each diagnosis on the list and work out what additional features you would see elsewhere. Thus, if you find a lower motor neurone VIIth nerve lesion, demonstrate the weakness in the upper as well as the lower part of the face (see p. 198), then be seen to examine the ears for evidence of herpes zoster (Ramsay Hunt syndrome).

If despite carrying out the above routine there is still no apparent abnormality then examine the facial musculature (see 'Examine this patient's cranial nerves') for evidence of a VIIth nerve lesion which is not obvious.

For *checklist* see p. 515.

10 / 'Examine this patient's arms'

Frequency of instruction

15% of candidates in our survey were asked to do this.

---

* May be associated with the organ-specific autoimmune diseases—see p. 279.

† Another uncommon but important sign which may occur in the iris is neovascularization in diabetes (rubeosis iridis). However, it is unlikely that this would occur in the context of 'examine this patient's face' at the examination.

Variations of instruction

This lady has noticed weak arms. Examine her
Look at this patient's forearms
Examine this patient's forearms.

Diagnoses from survey in order of frequency

1 Wasting of the small muscles of the hand 26%
2 Motor neurone disease 19%
3 Hemiplegia 7%
4 Cerebellar syndrome 6%
5 Cervical myelopathy 6%
6 Neurofibromatosis 4%
7 Muscular dystrophy 4%
8 Psoriasis 4%
9 Purpura due to steroids 4%
10 Parkinson's disease 3%
11 Syringomyelia 3%
12 Hemiballismus 3%
13 Lichen planus 3%
14 Pseudoxanthoma elasticum 3%
15 Old polio 3%
16 Rheumatoid arthritis 3%
17 Axillary vein thrombosis 3%
18 Contracture of the elbow in a case of haemophilia 3%
19 Ulnar nerve palsy 1%
20 Pancoast's syndrome 1%
21 Herpes zoster 1%
22 Mycosis fungoides 1%
23 Polymyositis 1%.

Examination *routine*

Consideration of the above list from the survey reveals that the vast majority (over 80%) of conditions behind this instruction are neurological with a handful of spot diagnoses which will usually be obvious. If the diagnosis is not an obvious 'spot' (and you should make sure that you would recognize each on the list—see individual short cases) your *routine* should commence in the usual way by scanning the whole patient but in particular looking at

1 the **face** for obvious abnormalities such as *asymmetry* (hemiplegia), *nystagmus* (cerebellar syndrome), *wasting* (muscular dystrophy), sad, immobile, unblinking facies (*Parkinson's* disease), or *Horner's* syndrome (syringomyelia, Pancoast's syndrome). You may return to seek a less obvious Horner's or nystagmus later, if necessary. In search of obvious abnormalities run your eyes down to

2 the **neck** (pseudoxanthoma elasticum, lymph nodes), and then scan down the arms looking in particular at

3 the **elbows** which should be particularly inspected for *psoriasis, rheumatoid nodules* and *scars* or *deformity* underlying an ulnar nerve palsy. Before picking up the hands look for

4 a **tremor** (Parkinson's disease), then briefly inspect

5 the **hands** in the same way as you have practised under 'Examine this patient's hands', looking at

(a) the joints (swelling, deformity),

(b) nail changes (pitting, onycholysis, clubbing, nail-fold infarcts), and

(c) skin changes (colour, consistency, lesions).

If you have not already been led towards a diagnosis requiring specific action, start a full neurological examination by studying first

6 the **muscle bulk** in the upper arms, lower arms and hands, bearing in mind that in about one-quarter of cases there will be wasting of the small muscles of the hands (see p. 162), and in one-fifth of cases there will be motor neurone disease which means wasting and

7 fasciculation.

8 Test the **tone** in the arms by passively bending the arm (with the patient relaxed) to and fro in an irregular and unexpected fashion, and in the hands by flexing and extending all the joints, including the wrist in the classic 'rolling wave' fashion used to detect cog-wheel rigidity (Parkinson's disease).

9 Ask the patient: 'Hold your **arms out in front** of you' (look for *winging* of the scapulae, involuntary movements or the *myelopathy hand sign**); 'Now close your eyes' (look for *sensory wandering* — parietal drift or pseudoathetosis (Fig. 3.69c, p.212)).

Next test

10 power:

(a) 'Put your arms out to the side' (demonstrate this to the patient yourself — arms at 90° to your body with elbows flexed); 'Stop me pushing them down' (deltoid—C5)

(b) 'Bend your elbow; stop me straightening it' (biceps—C5,6)

(c) 'Push your arm out straight'—resist elbow extension (triceps—C7)

(d) 'Squeeze my fingers'—offer two fingers (C8,T1)†

(e) 'Hold your fingers out straight' (demonstrate); 'Stop me bending them' (if the patient can do this there is nothing wrong with motor C7 or the radial nerve)

(f) 'Spread your fingers apart' (demonstrate); 'Stop me pushing them together' (dorsal interossei—ulnar nerve)

(g) 'Hold this piece of paper between your fingers; stop me pulling it out' (palmar interossei—ulnar nerve)

(h) 'Point your thumb at the ceiling; stop me pushing it down' (abductor pollicus brevis—median nerve)

(i) 'Put your thumb and little finger together; stop me pulling them apart' (opponens pollicis—median nerve).

11 Test **coordination**

(a) 'Can you do this?'—demonstrate by flexing your elbows at right angles and then pronating and supinating your forearms as rapidly as possible

(b) 'Tap quickly on the back of your hand' (demonstrate)

---

* With the hands outstretched and supinated, passive abduction of the little finger indicates a pyramidal lesion or ulnar nerve palsy (sensory testing should distinguish). The sign is common in, but not specific for, cervical pyramidal lesions—as the lesion becomes more severe, adjacent fingers also passively abduct.

† See footnote, p. 23.

(c) 'Touch my finger; touch your nose; backwards and forwards quickly and neatly' (demonstrate if necessary—vary the target).

12 Check the biceps (C5,6), triceps (C7), supinator (C5,6) and finger (C8) **reflexes**.

13 Finally perform a **sensory screen** with *light touch* and *pinprick* bearing in mind the dermatomes shown in Fig. 2.3 and the areas of sensation covered by the ulnar, median and radial nerves in the hand (see Fig. 2.1, p. 23). Finally, check *vibration* and *joint position* sense.

We leave you to consider where else you could look with each of the conditions given on the list in order to find additional information (see individual short cases). For example, you could look for nystagmus should you find cerebellar signs, or for a Horner's syndrome should you suspect syringomyelia or Pancoast's syndrome.

For *checklist* see p. 515.

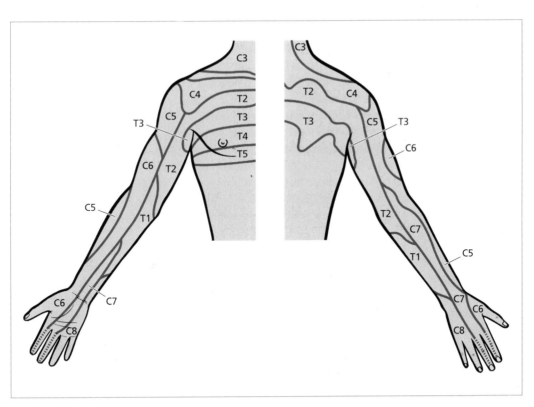

Fig. 2.3 Dermatomes in the upper limb (after Foerster, 1933, Oxford University Press, *Brain* **56**: 1). There is considerable variation and overlap between the cutaneous areas supplied by each spinal root so that an isolated root lesion results in a much smaller area of sensory impairment than the diagram indicates.

11 / 'Examine this patient's neck'

Frequency of instruction
12% of candidates in our survey were asked to do this.

Variations of instruction
Examine this patient's neck. Do you think she is euthyroid?
Feel the mass in this patient's neck.

Diagnoses from survey in order of frequency
1 Goitre 46%
2 Generalized lymphadenopathy 17%
3 Graves' disease 12%
4 Jugular vein pulse (JVP) abnormality 6%
5 Bilateral parotid enlargement/Mikulicz's syndrome 4%
6 Supraclavicular mass with a Horner's syndrome 4%
7 Facioscapulohumeral muscular dystrophy 4%
8 Ankylosing spondylitis 2%
9 Hypothyroidism 2%.
10 Acanthosis nigricans <1%.

Examination *routine*
As usual the first step is to
1 *survey* the patient quickly from head to foot (exophthalmos, myxoedematous facies, ankle oedema, etc.) and then to
2 **look at the neck.** According to the survey the reason for the instruction in half of the cases will be a *goitre*. If another abnormality is visible your further action will be dictated by what you see and we suggest you go through the list and establish a sequence of actions for each abnormality (e.g. if you see giant *v* waves you would wish to examine the heart and liver—see p. 214). If you do see a goitre, offer a drink to the patient:
   'Take a sip of water and hold it in your mouth';
look at the neck:
   'Now swallow'.
Watch the movement of the goitre, or the *appearance* of a *nodule* not visible before swallowing (behind sternomastoid—see Fig. 13.29c, p. 127). Next ask the patient's permission to feel the neck, and then approach him from behind. If there has been no evidence of a goitre so far you may wish to palpate the neck for lymph nodes *before* feeling for a goitre. Otherwise
3 **palpate** the thyroid. With the right index and middle fingers feel below the thyroid cartilage where the isthmus of the thyroid gland lies over the trachea. Then palpate the two lobes of the thyroid gland which extend laterally behind the sternomastoid muscle. Ask the patient to swallow again while you continue to palpate the thyroid, ensuring that the neck is slightly flexed to ease palpation. Remember that if there is a goitre, when you give your presentation you are going to want to comment on its *size*, whether it is *soft*, or *firm*, whether it is *nodular* or

diffusely enlarged, whether it *moves* readily on swallowing, whether there are *lymph nodes* (see below) and whether there is a vascular *murmur* (see below). Extend palpation upwards along the medial edge of the sternomastoid muscle on either side to look for a *pyramidal lobe* which may be present. Apologize for any discomfort you may cause because the deep palpation necessary to feel the thyroid gland causes pain,* particularly in patients with Graves' disease. Next palpate laterally to examine

4 for **lymph nodes**. If you find lymph node enlargement check not only in the *supraclavicular fossae* and right up the neck but also in the *submandibular, postauricular* and *suboccipital* areas, ensuring that the head is slightly flexed on the side under palpation to allow access and scrutiny of slightly enlarged lymph nodes. Ascertain whether the lymph nodes are *separate* (reactive hyperplasia, infectious mononucleosis, lymphoma, etc.) or *matted* together (neoplastic, tuberculous), *mobile* or *fixed* to the skin or deep tissues (neoplastic), or whether they are *soft, fleshy, rubbery* (Hodgkin's disease) or *hard* (neoplastic). Particularly if you find lymph nodes without a goitre, examine for lymph nodes in the axillae and groins (lymphoma, chronic lymphatic leukaemia, etc.) and, if allowed, feel for the spleen.

5 **Auscultate** over the thyroid for evidence of increased vascularity. You may need to occlude venous return to rule out a venous hum, and listen over the aortic area to ensure that the thyroid bruit you hear is not, in fact, an outflow obstruction murmur conducted to the root of the neck.

6 If there is any evidence of thyroid disease begin an assessment of **thyroid status** (see 'Examine this patient's thyroid status') by feeling and counting the pulse (NB do not miss *atrial fibrillation* whether slow or fast). The examiner will soon stop you if he wishes to hear your description of a multinodular goitre in a euthyroid patient.

For *checklist* see p. 515.

12 / 'Ask this patient some questions'

Frequency of instruction
8% of candidates in our survey were asked to do this.

Variations of instruction
Talk to this patient
Examine this patient's speech
Converse with this patient.

---

* In viral thyroiditis (rare) the patient may complain of a painful thyroid and the thyroid may be overtly tender on light palpation.

Diagnoses from survey in order of frequency

1 Dysphasia 24%
2 Cerebellar dysarthria 16%
3 Raynaud's 11%
4 Systemic sclerosis/CRST 8%
5 Pseudobulbar palsy 8%
6 Myxoedema 5%
7 Graves' disease 5%
8 Crohn's disease 5%
9 Ankle oedema due to nephrotic syndrome 5%
10 Senile dementia 5%
11 Parkinson's disease 3%.

Examination *routine*

Inspection of the list of cases in our survey which provoked this instruction reveals that they fall into four groups, each with a very different reason for the instruction:

Group 1: to spot the diagnosis and confirm it by eliciting *revealing answers* 39%
Group 2: to demonstrate and diagnose the type of a dysarthria 32%
Group 3: to diagnose a dysphasia 24%
Group 4: to assess higher mental function 5%.

With the group 1 patients you may have been given a lead such as 'Look at the hands' (Raynaud's) or 'Look at the face' (systemic sclerosis, myxoedema, etc.) before the instruction 'Ask this patient some questions'. At any rate you should start your examination as usual with

  1 a *visual survey* of the patient from head to foot, particularly looking for evidence of: (i) the spot diagnosis in group 1 patients (Raynaud's, systemic sclerosis/CRST, hypo- or hyperthyroidism, Crohn's, nephrotic syndrome); (ii) a *hemiplegia* which may be associated with dysphasia; or (iii) any of the conditions associated with dysarthria (see p. 260) especially *nystagmus* or *intention tremor* (which may be revealed by even minor movements) in cerebellar disease, *pes cavus* in Friedreich's ataxia and the *facies/tremor* of Parkinson's disease.

  In the group 1 patients once you are on to the diagnosis the sort of
  2 **specific questions** the examiners are looking for (see also the individual short cases) are: *Raynaud's* (see also anecdote 20, p. 495):
    'Do your fingers change colour in the cold?'
    'What colour do they go?' ('Is there a particular sequence of colours?')
    'How long have you had the trouble?'
    'What is your job?' (vibrating tools, etc.)
and if there is any possibility of connective tissue disease
    'Do you have any difficulty with swallowing?' etc.
Systemic sclerosis:
    'Do you have any difficulty with swallowing?'
    'Do your fingers change colour in the cold?'
    'Do you get short of breath?' (on hills? on flat? etc.)
We leave you to work out the straightforward questions you would ask the slow croaking patient with *myxoedematous facies*, the patient with *exophthalmos*, or the

one who has *lid retraction* and is *fidgety*, or the patient who has *multiple scars* and *sinuses* on his abdomen. In the young patient who may have nephrotic syndrome you would be looking for the history of a sore throat.

If there are no features suggesting a group 1 patient, it is likely that the problem is either a dysarthria or dysphasia, and, as already mentioned, there may be clues pointing to one of these. You need to ask the patient

3 some **general questions** to get him *talking*:

'My names is . . . Please could you tell me your name?'

'What is your address?'

If you still need to hear a patient speak further ask

4 **more questions** which require *long answers* such as

'Please could you tell me all the things you ate for breakfast/lunch.'

To test

5 **articulation** ask the patient to repeat the traditional words and phrases such as 'British Constitution', 'West Register Street', 'biblical criticism' and 'artillery'. As well as testing articulation such

6 **repetition** is useful for assessing speech when the patient only gives one-word answers to questions. If necessary ask the patient to repeat long sentences after you. Information gained from repetition may also be useful in your assessment of dysphasia (see below).

If the problem is *dysarthria*, it is really a spot diagnosis to test your ability to recognize and demonstrate the features of the different types (see p. 260). It is recommended that you find as many patients as possible with the conditions causing the various types of dysarthria and listen to them speak so that, as with murmurs, the diagnosis is a question of instant recognition. This is particularly true of the ataxic dysarthria of cerebellar disease. When you have heard enough to make the diagnosis, you should either describe the speech (p. 260) and, with supporting signs seen on inspection, give the diagnosis, or proceed to look for

7 **additional signs** (in the same way as you might do after the 'What is the diagnosis' instruction).

If the patient has a *dysphasia* (see p. 261) you may wish to demonstrate that

8 **comprehension** is good (expressive dysphasia) or impaired (receptive dysphasia). Perform a few simple commands *without gesturing*, e.g.

'Please put your tongue out'.

'Shut your eyes'.

'Touch your nose', etc.

Assuming these are performed adequately proceed to look for expressive dysphasia by asking the patient to name some everyday items, e.g. a comb, pen, coins. If the patient is unable to name the objects test for

9 **nominal dysphasia**. Hold up your keys:

'What is this?'—patient does not answer

'Is this a spoon'—'No'.

'Is it a pen'—'No'.

'Is it keys'—'Yes'.

If the patient is able to name objects, test the ability to form sentences by asking the patient to describe something in more detail, e.g.

'Could you tell me where you live and how you would get home from here?'

'Could you tell me the name of as many objects in this room as possible?'

If there are expressive problems you should check to see if the problem is true expressive dysphasia or whether there is

10 orofacial dyspraxia. * Ask the patient to perform various orofacial movements (assuming there is no receptive dysphasia). These should be tested first by command *without gesture*, e.g.

'Please show me your teeth'.

'Move your tongue from side to side'.

Subsequently ask the patient to obey the same commands but *with gesture*, i.e. so the patient can mimic. This should give some idea as to whether the patient has either ideational or ideomotor dyspraxia.†

Our survey showed that it is extremely rare for candidates to be asked to assess **11 higher mental functions.**‡ This is, however, an assessment which every Membership candidate should be equipped to make. The following is the 'abbreviated mental test' (AMT)—more than four of the questions wrong suggests a well-established dementia:

1 Age
2 Time (to nearest hour)
3 Address for recall at end of test — this should be repeated by the patient to ensure it has been heard correctly: 42 West Street
4 Year
5 Name of this place
6 Recognition of two persons (doctor, nurse, etc.)
7 Date of birth (day and month sufficient)
8 Year of First World War
9 Name of present Monarch
10 Count backwards from 20 to 1.

Agnosia, apraxia, dyslexia, dysgraphia and dyscalculia are considered on p. 106.

For *checklist* see p. 515.

13 / 'Examine this patient's pulse'

Frequency of instruction
7% of candidates in our survey were asked to do this.

Variations of instruction
Feel this pulse
Examine this patient's pulse—look for the cause
Examine this patient's pulses.

---

* It is important to make this distinction so that the type of speech therapy is appropriate—in orofacial dyspraxia the therapist needs to work on mouth movements rather than concentrating only on linguistic problems. It has recently been established that the lesion which leads to orofacial dyspraxia is in the operculum.

† Again it is relevant to therapy to establish if the patients can make movements when aided by gesture.
‡ Rare at the time of writing (see anecdote 38, p. 497): it is conceivable that any examiners who see this book will be given ideas as to the areas they are neglecting!

Diagnoses from survey in order of frequency

1 Irregular pulse 44%
2 Slow pulse 12%
3 Graves' disease 12%
4 Aortic stenosis 9%
5 Complete heart block 9%
6 Brachial artery aneurysm 9%
7 Impalpable radial pulses due to low output cardiac failure 9%
8 Tachycardia 6%
9 Takayasu's disease 3%
10 Hypothyroidism 3%
11 Fallot's tetralogy with a Blalock shunt 3%.

Examination *routine*

As you approach the patient from the right and ask for his permission to examine him you should

1 look at his **face** for a *malar flush* (mitral stenosis, myxoedema) or for any signs of *hyper-* or *hypothyroidism*. As you take the arm to examine the right radial pulse, continue the *survey* of the patient by looking at

2 the **neck** (Corrigan's pulse, raised JVP, thyroidectomy scar, goitre) and then the *chest* (thoracotomy scar). Quickly run your eyes down the body to complete the *survey* (ascites, clubbing, pretibial myxoedema, ankle oedema, etc.) and then concentrate on

3 the **pulse** and note

4 its **rate** (count for at least 15 seconds), volume and

5 its **rhythm**. A common diagnostic problem is presented by *slow atrial fibrillation* which may be mistaken for a regular pulse. To avoid this concentrate on the *length of the pause* from one beat to another and see if each pause is equal to the succeeding one (see also p. 189). This method will reveal that the pauses are variable from beat to beat in controlled slow atrial fibrillation.

6 Assess whether the **character** (waveform) of the pulse (information to be gained from radial, brachial and carotid) is normal, *collapsing, slow rising*, or jerky. To determine whether there is a collapsing quality put the palmar aspect of the four fingers of your left hand on the patient's wrist just below where you can easily feel the radial pulse. Press gently with your palm, lift the patient's hand above his head and then place your right palm over the patient's axillary artery. If the pulse has a *water-hammer* character you will experience a flick (a sharp and tall up-stroke and an abrupt down-stroke) which will *run* across all four fingers and at the same time you may also feel a flick of the axillary artery against your right palm. The pulse does not merely become palpable when the hand is lifted but its character changes and it imparts a sharp knock. This is classical of the pulse that is present in haemodynamically significant aortic incompetence and in patent ductus arteriosus. If the pulse has a collapsing character but is not of a frank water-hammer type then the flick runs across only two or three fingers (moderate degree of aortic incompetence or patent ductus arteriosus, thyrotoxicosis, fever, pregnancy, moderately severe mitral incompetence, anaemia, atherosclerosis). A *slow rising* pulse can best be assessed by palpating the brachial pulse with your left thumb and, as you press *gently*, you may feel the anacrotic notch (you will need practice to appreciate this) on the up-stroke against the pulp of your thumb. In mixed aortic valve disease the combination of plateau and collapsing effects can produce a bisferiens pulse. Whilst feeling the brachial pulse look for any catheterization *scars* (indicating valvular or ischaemic heart disease).

7 Proceed to feel the **carotid** where either a slow rising or a collapsing pulse can be confirmed.

8 Feel the **opposite radial pulse** and determine if both radials are the same (e.g. Fallot's with a Blalock shunt—p. 284), and then feel

9 the **right femoral pulse** checking for any *radiofemoral delay* (coarctation of the aorta). If you are asked to examine the pulses (as opposed to the pulse) you should continue to examine

10 all the other **peripheral pulses**. It is unlikely that the examiner will allow you to continue beyond what he thinks is a reasonable time to spot the diagnosis that he has in mind. However, should he not interrupt continue to look for

11 **additional diagnostic clues**. Thus, in a patient with atrial fibrillation and features suggestive of thyrotoxicosis you should examine the thyroid and/or eyes. In a patient with atrial fibrillation and hemiplegia or atrial fibrillation and a mitral valvotomy scar, proceed to examine the heart.

For *checklist* see p. 515.

14 / 'Examine this patient's visual fields'

Frequency of instruction
6% of candidates in our survey were asked to do this.

Variation of instruction
See p. 523.

Diagnoses from survey in order of frequency
1 Homonymous hemianopia 25%
2 Optic atrophy 21%
3 Bitemporal hemianopia 21%
4 Unilateral hemianopia 7%
5 Partial field defect in one eye due to retinal artery branch occlusion 7%
6 Bilateral homonymous quadrantic field defect 4%
7 Acromegaly 4%.

Examination *routine*
Ask the patient to sit upright on the side of the bed while you position yourself in visual confrontation about a metre away. This apposition will help you to test the visual fields of his left and right eyes against those of your right and left respectively. As he is doing this perform

1 a *visual survey* (acromegaly, hemiparesis, cerebellar signs in multiple sclerosis)

of the patient. Test both temporal fields together so that you do not miss any *visual inattention*. Ask the patient to look at your eyes while you place your index fingers just inside the outer limits of your temporal fields. Then move your fingers in turn and then both at the same time, and ask him:

'Point to the finger which moves'.

If there is visual inattention, the patient will only point to one finger when you move both at the same time. Next test each eye individually and ask him to cover his right eye with his right index finger, and close your left eye:

'Keep looking at my eye'.

2 Examine his **peripheral visual fields**. Test his left temporal vision against your right temporal by moving your wagging finger from the periphery towards the centre:

'Tell me when you see my finger move'.*

The temporal field should be tested in the horizontal plane and by moving your finger through the upper and lower temporal quadrants. Change hands and repeat on the nasal side. By comparing his visual field with your own, any areas of field defect are thus mapped out. The visual fields of his right eye are similarly tested.

3 A **central scotoma** is tested for with a red-headed hat pin. If you have already found a field defect which does not require further examination, or if the examiner does not wish you to continue, he will soon stop you. Otherwise comparing your right eye with his left, as before, move the red-headed pin from the temporal periphery through the central field to the nasal periphery, asking the patient:

'Can you see the head of the pin? What colour is it? Tell me if it disappears or changes colour'.

If there is no scotoma find his blind spot and compare it with your own.

Having found the field defect, look for

4 **additional features** (e.g. acromegaly, hemiparesis, nystagmus and cerebellar signs) if appropriate. Recall the possible causes for each type of field defect as this question, at the end of the case, is almost inevitable (see p. 131).

For *checklist* see p. 516.

15 / 'Examine this patient's skin'

Frequency of instruction
5% of candidates in our survey were asked to do this.

---

* This will pick up most gross visual field defects rapidly. Moving objects are more easily detected and therefore your moving finger will be immediately noticed by the patient as it moves out of the blind area into his field of vision. Remember that his area of blindness to a stationary object may be greater than that to a moving object. In the dysphasic patient you should ask him to point at the moving finger when he sees it rather than telling you he sees it.

Variations of instruction

Look at this skin

Examine the skin

Look at this skin lesion.

Diagnoses from survey in order of frequency

1 Psoriasis 15%
2 Vitiligo 10%
3 Systemic sclerosis/CRST 10%
4 Radiation burn on the chest 10%
5 Epidermolysis bullosa dystrophica 10%
6 Purpura 5%
7 Pseudoxanthoma elasticum 5%
8 Localized scleroderma 5%.

Examination *routine*

This instruction is a rather more specific variation of the 'spot diagnosis' *routine*. You should

1 perform a *visual survey* of the patient, from scalp to sole, with regard to the fact that most dermatological lesions have a predilection for certain areas. It is as well to remember some of the regional associations as you *survey* the patient:

Scalp	Psoriasis (look especially at the hairline for redness, scaling, etc.), alopecia,* ringworm (very uncommon)
Face	Systemic sclerosis (tight shiny skin, pseudorhagades, beaked nose, telangiectasis), discoid lupus erythematosus (raised, red, scaly lesions with telangiectasis, scarring and altered pigmentation), xanthelasma, dermatomyositis (heliotrope colour to eyelids), Sturge–Weber, rodent ulcer (usually below the eye or on the side of the nose, raised lesion with central ulcer, the edges being rolled and having telangiectatic blood vessels)
Mouth	Osler–Weber–Rendu, Peutz–Jeghers, lichen planus (white lace-like network on mucosal surface), pemphigus, candidiasis (white exudate inside the mouth usually associated with a disease requiring multiple antimicrobial therapy, or an immunosuppressive disorder, e.g. leukaemia, AIDS, etc.), herpes simplex, Behçet's
Neck	Pseudoxanthoma elasticum, tuberculous adenitis with sinus formation (?ethnic origin)
Trunk	Radiotherapy stigmata, morphoea, neurofibromatosis, dermatitis herpetiformis (itching blisters over scapulae, buttocks, elbows, knees), herpes zoster along the intercostal nerves, pityriasis rosea, Addison's (areolar and scar pigmentation), pemphigus (trunk and limbs)
Axillae	Vitiligo, acanthosis nigricans (pigmentation and velvety thickening of axillary skin, perianal, areolar and lateral abdominal skin, 'tripe palms', mucous membranes involved, maybe underlying insulin resistance or malignancy)

* Some causes of alopecia:
1 Diffuse—male pattern baldness, cytotoxic drugs, hypothyroidism, hyperthyroidism, iron deficiency.
2 Patchy—alopecia areata, ringworm; with scarring—discoid lupus erythematosus, lichen planus.

Elbows	Psoriasis (extensor), pseudoxanthoma elasticum (flexor), xanthomata (extensor), rheumatoid nodules (extensor), atopic dermatitis (flexor), olecranon bursitis, gouty tophi
Hands	Systemic sclerosis (sclerodactyly, infarcts of finger pulps, prominent capillaries at nail folds), lichen planus (wrists), dermatomyositis (heliotrope lesions—Gottron's papules—on the joints of the dorsum of the fingers/hands, nail-fold capillary dilatation and infarction), Addison's (skin crease pigmentation), granuloma annulare, erythema multiforme (polymorphic eruption, 'target' lesions, mucous membrane involvement, macules, vesicles, bullae, etc.), SLE (erythematous patches over the dorsal surface of the phalanges), scabies (not in MRCP clinical!)
Nails	Psoriasis (pitting, onycholysis), iron deficiency (koilonychia), fungal dystrophy, tuberous sclerosis (periungal fibromata)
Genitalia	Behçet's (iridocyclitis, uveitis, pyodermas, ulcers, etc.), lichen sclerosus (white plaques), candidiasis
Legs	Leg ulcer (diabetic, venous, ischaemic, pyoderma gangrenosum), necrobiosis lipoidica diabeticorum, pretibial myxoedema, erythema nodosum, Henoch–Schönlein purpura, tendon xanthomata in Achilles, erythema ab igne, pemphigoid (legs and arms), lipoatrophy
Feet	Pustular psoriasis, eczema, verrucae, keratoderma blenorrhagica (?eyes, joints, etc.).

During this *survey* you should consider

2 the **distribution** of the lesions (psoriasis on extensor areas, lichen planus in flexor areas, candidiasis in mucous membranes, tuberous sclerosis on nails and face, necrobiosis lipoidica diabeticorum usually bilateral, gouty tophi in the joints of hands, elbows and on the ears, etc.). Then after the *survey* (which should take a few seconds)

3 examine the **lesions** (see 'Examine this patient's rash') looking in particular for the *characteristic* features, e.g. scaling in psoriasis, shiny purple polygonal papules with Wickham's striae in lichen planus, etc. If you have made a diagnosis consider whether you need to look for any

4 associated lesions (arthropathy and nail changes with psoriasis, evidence of associated autoimmune disease with vitiligo, etc.). Go through the skin conditions which our survey has suggested occur in the exam (see also Appendix 6) and make sure that you would recognize each, would know what else to look for, and what to say in your presentation.

For *checklist* see p. 516.

16 / 'Examine this patient's gait'

Frequency of instruction
4% of candidates in our survey were asked to do this.

Variations of instruction

Look at this patient's gait

Watch this patient walk

Watch this patient walk. What do you think the diagnosis is?

Diagnoses from survey in order of frequency

1 Ataxia 45%

2 Spastic paraparesis 20%

3 Parkinson's disease 10%

4 Charcot–Marie–Tooth disease 5%

5 Ankylosing spondylitis 5%.

Examination *routine*

As you approach the patient perform

1 a *quick visual survey* noting any *cerebellar signs* (nystagmus, intention tremor) or obvious signs of conditions such as *Parkinson's* disease (facies, tremor), *Charcot–Marie–Tooth* disease (peroneal wasting, pes cavus, etc.) or *ankylosing spondylitis*. Introduce yourself to the patient and ask him

2 **whether he can walk** without help (*cerebellar dysarthria* heard during his reply may be a useful clue). If he reports difficulty reassure him that you will stay with him in case of any problems.

3 **Ask him to walk** to a defined point and back whilst you look for any of the classical abnormal gaits (see p. 186), particularly ataxic (cerebellar or sensory), spastic, steppage (Charcot–Marie–Tooth) or parkinsonian (?pill-rolling tremor). As the patient walks make sure you note specifically

4 the **arm swing** (Parkinson's) and

5 any *clumsiness* on **the turns** (ataxia, Parkinson's). Next test

6 **heel-to-toe** gait (demonstrate as you ask the patient to do this) which will *exacerbate* ataxia (note the side to which the patient tends to fall). Ask the patient to walk

7 **on his toes** (S1) and then

8 **on his heels** (L5; foot-drop — lateral popliteal nerve palsy, Charcot–Marie–Tooth disease). If he has a spastic gait or a hemiparesis he may find both these tests difficult to perform.

9 Now ask him to stand with his *feet together, arms out* in front; when you are satisfied with the degree of steadiness with the eyes open, ask him to *close his eyes* (you should be standing nearby to catch him if he shows a tendency to fall). **Romberg's test** is only positive (*sensory ataxia*) if the patient is more unsteady (tends to fall) with the eyes closed than with them open (dorsal column disease, e.g. subacute combined degeneration, tabes dorsalis, etc.).

10 If you suspect sensory ataxia a further test is to ask the patient to **close his eyes while walking** (he will become *more* ataxic). Again you should be ready to catch the patient should he fall. As always be ready to look for

11 **additional features** of the conditions on the list if appropriate (see individual short cases, and consider what you would do with each).

For *checklist* see p. 516.

17 / 'Examine this patient's rash'

Frequency of instruction
4% of candidates in our survey were asked to do this.

Variations of instruction
Examine the skin rash.

Diagnoses from survey in order of frequency
1 Psoriasis 20%
2 Purpura 10%
3 Vasculitis 10%
4 Neurofibromatosis 10%
5 Juvenile chronic arthritis (Still's disease) 10%
6 Xanthomata 5%
7 Necrobiosis lipoidica diabeticorum 5%
8 Radiation burn on the chest 5%.

Examination *routine*
This *routine* is generally the same as that discussed under 'Examine this patient's skin'.

1 You should quickly conduct a *visual survey* as described under 'skin' and note if there are any similar or related lesions elsewhere. Look at the
2 **distribution** of the lesions, whether confined to a single area (morphoea, erythema nodosum, rodent ulcer, melanoma, alopecia areata, etc.) or present in other areas such as psoriasis, neurofibromatosis, acanthosis nigricans, dermatomyositis, etc. While concentrating on the lesion in question, it is important to look at the
3 **surrounding skin** for any helpful clues such as *scratch marks* as evidence of itching,* *radiotherapy field markings* on the skin in the vicinity of a radiation burn, or *paper-thin skin* with purpura (corticosteroid therapy), etc. You should now
4 **examine the lesion** in detail. To determine the *extent* of the lesion you may have to ask the patient to undress, a procedure which will provide you with a little more time to survey other areas. Decide if the rash is *pleomorphic* or *monomorphic* (all the lesions are similar). If so examine one typical lesion carefully in terms of:

    (a) *Colour*, e.g. erythematous or pigmented
    (b) *Size*
    (c) *Shape*, e.g. oval, circular, annular, etc.
    (d) *Surface*, e.g. scaling or eroded
    (e) *Character*, e.g. macule, papule, vesicle, pustule, ulcer, etc.
    (f) *Secondary features*, e.g. crusting, lichenification, etc.

It is advisable to be familiar with the correct use of the terms to describe rashes (especially if you do not recognize the lesion!). To say 'skin lesion' or 'skin rash'

---

* Some causes of itching:
1 Dermatological—scabies, dermatitis herpetiformis, lichen planus, eczema.

2 Medical—cholestasis, chronic renal failure, lymphoma, polycythaemia rubra vera.

conveys no diagnostic meaning. In your presentation you should be able to describe the lesion with respect to the above six features, especially if you do not know the diagnosis. The following are some of the useful terms employed in describing skin lesions:

Macules: flat, circumscribed lesions, not raised above the skin — size and shape varies

Papules: raised, circumscribed, firm lesions up to 1 cm in size

Nodules: like papules but larger; usually lie deeper in skin

Tumours: larger than nodules, elevated or very deeply placed in the skin

Weals: circumscribed elevations associated with itching and tingling

Vesicles: small well-defined collections of fluid

Bullae: large vesicles

Pustules: circumscribed elevations containing purulent fluid which may, in some cases, be sterile (e.g. Behçet's)

Scales: dead tissue from the horny layer which may be dry (e.g. psoriasis) or greasy (e.g. seborrhoeic dermatitis)

Crusts: these consist of dried exudate

Ulcers: excavations in the skin of irregular shape; remember that every ulcer has a shape, an edge, a floor, a base and a secretion, and it forms a scar on healing

Scars: the result of healing of a damaged dermis.

5 Finally, if indicated, look for **additional features** (arthropathy in psoriasis or Still's disease, cushingoid facies if purpura is due to steroids, clubbing with radiation burns on the chest, etc.).

For *checklist* see p. 516.

18 / 'Examine this patient's legs and arms'

Frequency of instruction
3% of candidates in our survey were asked to do this.

Variations of instruction
Examine the limbs neurologically—motor function only.

Diagnoses from survey in order of frequency
1 Motor neurone disease 29%
2 Cervical myelopathy 14%
3 Syringomyelia 14%
4 Friedreich's ataxia 14%
5 Parkinson's disease 7%.

As appropriate from 'Examine this patient's arms' (p. 39) and 'Examine this patient's legs' (p. 24).

19 / 'Examine this patient's cranial nerves'

Frequency of instruction
3% of candidates in our survey were asked to do this.

Variations of instruction
Look at this patient's cranial nerves.

Diagnoses from survey
Bulbar palsy
Cerebellopontine angle syndrome
Myasthenia gravis
Ocular palsy and dysarthria
Unilateral VIth, VIIth nerve palsies and nystagmus and possibly a XIIth nerve palsy*
Unilateral IXth, Xth, XIth and XIIth nerve lesions (suggesting jugular foramen syndrome†).

Examination *routine*
Perhaps surprisingly this instruction was comparatively rare in our survey. It is one of the most feared instructions but at the same time it can provide an opportunity to score highly. More than in any other system, the well-rehearsed candidate can appear competent and professional compared to the unrehearsed. Detailed examination of the individual nerves is not usually required but rather a quick and efficient screen like that used by neurologists at the bedside or in out-patients (it is well worth attending neurology out-patients to watch quick and efficient examination techniques, if for nothing else). Not only can you look good but also the abnormalities are usually easy to detect. Although it is to be hoped that your practised *routine* will not miss out any nerves, it is preferable to perform a smooth, professional examination, which accidentally misses out a nerve, than to test your examiner's patience through a hesitant and meditative examination which takes a long time to start and may never finish! Since the examination is most easily carried out face to face with the patient it is best, if possible, to get him to sit on the edge of the bed facing you. First

   1 take a good general and *quick* **look** at the patient; in particular his face, for any obvious abnormality. Next ask him about

* The candidate diagnosed a XIIth nerve palsy and passed
(experience 1, p. 447) but see footnote, p. 57.
† This diagnosis was not made by the candidate.

2 his sense of smell and taste:

'Do you have any difficulty with your sense of smell?' (I). Although you should have the ability to examine taste and smell formally if equipment is provided, usually questioning (or possibly the judicious use of a bedside orange) is all that is required. All the examination referable to the eyes is best performed next. Unless there is a Snellen's chart available ask the patient to look at the clock on the wall or some newspaper print to give you a good idea of his

3 visual acuity:

'Do you have any difficulty with your vision?'

'Can you see the clock on the wall?' (if he has glasses for long sight he should put them on).

'Can you tell me what time it says?' (II)

A portable Snellen's chart will enable you to perform a more formal test (see Appendix 4).

Now test

4 visual fields (see p. 48), including for *central scotoma*, with a red-headed hat pin. Follow this by examining

5 eye movements (move your finger in the shape of a cross, from side to side then up and down):

'Look at my finger; follow it with your eyes (III, IV, VI),

asking the patient at the extremes of gaze whether he sees one or two fingers. If he has diplopia establish the extent and ask him to describe the 'false' image. As you test eye movements note at the same time any

6 nystagmus (VIII, cerebellum or cerebellar connections—see Fig. 3.49, p. 173) or

7 ptosis (III, sympathetic).

Remember that either extreme abduction of the eyes or gazing at a finger that is too near can cause nystagmus in normal eyes (optikokinetic). Now examine

8 the pupils for the direct and consensual *light reflex* (II → optic tract → lateral geniculate ganglion → Edinger–Westphal nucleus of III → fibres to ciliary muscle) and for the *accommodation–convergence* reflex (cortex → III) with your finger just in front of his nose:

'Look into the distance'.

Now look at my finger' (see also footnote, p. 36).

Finally examine the optic discs (II) by

9 fundoscopy (this can be left until last if you prefer). Having finished examining the eyes examine

10 facial movements:

'Raise your eyebrows'
'Screw your eyes up tight'
'Puff your cheeks out'   } VII
'Whistle'
'Show me your teeth'

'Clench your teeth'—feel masseters and
    temporalis   } motor V
'Open your mouth; stop me closing it'

11 then palatal movement:

'Keep your mouth open; say aah' (IX, X)

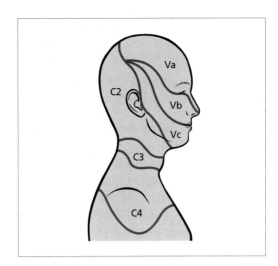

Fig. 2.4 Dermatomes in the head and neck.

12 and **gag reflex***—touch the back of the pharynx on both sides with an orange stick (IX, X). Look at

13 the **tongue** as it lies in the floor of the mouth for *wasting* or *fasciculation* (XII):
  'Open your mouth again'
then get the patient to:
  'Put your tongue out'—note any deviation†—'waggle it from side to side' (XII).

14 Test the **accessory nerve**:‡
  'Shrug your shoulders; keep them shrugged'—push down on the shoulders (XI).
  'Turn your head to the left side—now to the right'—feel for the sternomastoid muscle on the side opposite to the turned head.

Finally test

15 **hearing**:
  'Any problem with the hearing in either ear?'
  'Can you hear that?'—rub finger and thumb together in front of each ear in turn (VIII—proceed to the Rinné and Weber tests§ if there is any abnormality, and look in the ear if you suspect disease of the external ear, perforated drum, wax, etc.), and

16 test **facial sensation** including *corneal reflex* (sensory V—Fig. 2.4).

For *checklist* see p. 516.

---

* This can be unpleasant, so ask the examiner's permission, explain to the patient and ask for his permission as well.
† In unilateral facial paralysis the protruded tongue, though otherwise normal, may deviate so that unilateral hypoglossal paralysis is suspected (see p. 198). In unilateral lower motor neurone XIIth nerve palsy there is wasting (?fasciculation) on the side of the lesion and the tongue curves to that side.
‡ Painless neck weakness has only four causes: myasthenia gravis (p. 269), dystrophia myotonica (p. 159), polymyositis (p. 329) and motor neurone disease (p. 123).

§ *Weber test*: sound from a vibrating tuning fork held on the centre of the forehead is conducted towards the ear if it has a conductive defect (e.g. wax or otitis media) and away from the ear if it has a nerve deafness. *Rinné test*: a positive test (normal) is when the sound of the tuning fork is louder by air conduction (prongs by external auditory meatus) than by bone conduction (base of fork on mastoid process). Negative is abnormal.

20 / 'Examine this patient's thyroid status'

Frequency of instruction
2% of candidates in our survey were asked to do this.

Variations of instruction
Assess thyroid status clinically
Examine this patient's neck; do you think she is euthyroid?
Do you think this lady is thyrotoxic now just looking at her?

Diagnoses from survey in order of frequency
1 Euthyroid Graves' disease 42%
2 Hyperthyroidism 17%
3 Euthyroid simple goitre 8%.

Examination *routine*
Although the patient usually has signs of thyroid disease (exophthalmos, goitre), you are not being asked to examine these, but rather to assess whether the patient is clinically hypo-, eu- or hyperthyroid. Perform a speedy

1 *visual survey* looking specifically for *signs of thyroid disease* (exophthalmos, goitre, thyroid acropachy, pretibial myxoedema—all can occur in association with *any* thyroid status), and ask yourself if the facies are in any way myxoedematous. Observe the patient's

2 **composure**, whether *hyperactive*, *fidgety* and *restless* (hyperthyroid); normal, composed demeanour (euthyroid); or if she is somewhat *immobile* and *uninterested* in the people around her (hypothyroid).

3 Take the **pulse** and *count* it for 15 seconds, noting the presence or absence of *atrial fibrillation* (slow, normal rate, or fast). If the pulse is slow (less than 60), or if you suspect hypothyroidism, proceed immediately to test

4 for **slow relaxation** of the ankle,* supinator or other jerks. To test the reflexes you will require the patient's cooperation and the ensuing conversation may provide you with helpful clues (slow hesitant speech, slow movements, etc.). Otherwise

5 feel the **palms**, whether *warm* and *sweaty* or cold and sweaty (anxiety) and then

6 ask the patient to stretch out his hands to full extension of the wrist and elbow. If the **tremor** is not obvious, place your palm against his outstretched fingers to feel for it. Alternatively, you can place a piece of paper on the dorsum of his out-stretched hands—it will oscillate if a fine tremor is present.

7 Look at the **eyes**, noting exophthalmos (sclera visible above the lower lid—a sign not related to thyroid status) but looking specifically for *lid retraction* (sclera visible above the cornea). Test for lid lag (lid lag and retraction may diminish as the hyperthyroid patient becomes euthyroid).

---

* The slow relaxing ankle jerk in hypothyroidism is best demonstrated with the patient kneeling on a chair or bed with the feet hanging over the edge, and the examiner standing behind the patient. However, this manoeuvre (which is useful for the dressed patient in the out-patient department) is not necessary in the MRCP examination unless the jerk cannot be elicited by the usual procedure.

8 Examine the **thyroid** as described under 'Examine this patient's neck', remembering the steps are (i) look, (ii) palpate, and (iii) auscultate.*

Putting the above findings together it should be possible to provide a definite conclusion about thyroid status; this is considered a very basic skill and it will not be taken lightly if, in your state of nerves, you make fundamental errors. Though the examiner may put you under pressure to test your confidence, keep calm and be particularly wary of being led to diagnose hypo- or hyperthyroidism in the presence of a normal pulse rate (see experience 91, p. 459).

9 Be prepared with the **standard questions** for assessment of thyroid status (temperature preference, weight change, appetite, bowel habits, palpitations, change of temper, etc. — see pp. 114 and 152) should the examiner wish you to question the patient. Indeed, if there is any doubt about the thyroid status after the above examination, offer to ask the patient these questions.

For *checklist* see p. 516.

---

* A thyroid bruit is good evidence of thyroid overactivity; if present it can be heard over the isthmus and lateral lobe of the thyroid; it will not be obliterated by occluding the internal jugular vein (venous hum) or by rotation of the head and it will not be influenced by pressure of the stethoscope (use light pressure to avoid causing non-thyroid bruits).

Section 3
200 Short Case Records

*'Be professional in presentation. I agree it's an easy exam—it's easy to fail'.**

*p. 505.

In this section we present aides-mémoire (clinical descriptions for presentation to the examiner) for 200 short cases. We have called these aides-mémoire *records*. The order has been determined by the frequency with which, according to our surveys, these short cases have appeared in the examination. Thus short case no. 1 occurred most commonly, followed by short case no. 2 and so on. The percentages given represent your chance of meeting a particular short case in any one attempt at the MRCP short cases examination. They range from diabetic retinopathy (34%) to pyoderma gangrenosum (0.1%) which means that on average you will see a diabetic fundus in one out of every three attempts at the examination, but you may have to go through a thousand attempts before you meet pyoderma gangrenosum! Sometimes in the survey a particular short case was an additional feature of another short case. For example, a case of Graves' disease could also have a goitre, exophthalmos or pretibial myxoedema. With each short case we have pinpointed what the main focus was of that case. In the previous example, if the examiner asked for examination of the eyes, and all the attention was on the eyes, the main focus would be exophthalmos. If additional features (e.g. in this case goitre and pretibial myxoedema) were present, these were counted separately and the percentages for them are also given.* It cannot be overstressed that the first short cases we have dealt with occurred very commonly and the last very rarely, with all grades in between. The implications for your priorities are obvious.

The style of each *record* imagines you to be in the examination situation with the patient displaying the typical features of a particular condition; you are 'churning out' these to the examiner along with the answers to various anticipated questions. Thus, you play the *record* of the condition to the examiner. Of course the cases in the actual examination will only have some of the features (the *record* tends to describe the 'full house' case) and it is hoped that by becoming familiar with the whole *record* you will be well equipped:

1 To pick up all the features present in the cases you meet on the day by scanning through the *records* in your mind; and

2 To adapt the *record* for the purpose of presenting those features which are present.

To facilitate quick revision, the main points of each short case are highlighted in italics. The small print is a mixed bag of additional features and facts, lists of differential diagnoses and answers to some of the questions that might be asked.†

---

* We believe that candidates did not always mention all the additional features in their reports to us. As an extreme example, not every candidate who reported meeting a case of mitral stenosis mentioned whether or not the pulse was irregular. Thus our appraisal of when 'irregular pulse' was an additional feature is likely to be an underestimate of its real frequency. Similarly ptosis was not always mentioned as being present in cases of Horner's syndrome or in association with a IIIrd nerve palsy. Consequently we believe

that these 'additional features' figures tend to be underestimates.

† As already mentioned, questions and discussion of cases are only a very minor feature of the short cases examination. Obviously the questions that could be asked are legion and a comprehensive coverage is beyond the scope of this book. However, where our survey did point to the possibility of certain questions we have included the answers in the small print.

With the lists of differential diagnoses we have tended to put the most important ones (which you should consider first) in large print with longer lists in the small print. The lists are not necessarily meant to be comprehensive. Next to the diagnoses on these lists we have used brackets to give some of the features of the conditions concerned, or perhaps one or two features you could look for (indicated by ?). The ? is put there as a cue for you to look for important diagnostic features. We make no apology for repeating some of the features often, in the hope that by constant reinforcement they will become more firmly embedded in your memory. When unilateral signs could affect either side we have not usually specified the side in the *record* but have indicated this by R/L. In these cases, however, each R/L in the *record* refers to the same side. Also . . . is occasionally used for a sign in the lung fields or retina which could occur in any zone or to indicate the size of an organ or sign where the size is unspecified.

Presentation to the examiner

Becoming familiar with the short case *records* will arm you for the examination, though obviously it will not always be necessary, or desirable, for you to use them. Sometimes it may be appropriate just to give the diagnosis—even so it may still be possible to enrich it with some of the well-known features from the *record*. If the examiner's question is: '*What is the diagnosis?*' you could answer 'mitral stenosis' and await his reaction. On the other hand, if you are certain of your diagnosis, it would be better to say: 'The diagnosis is mitral stenosis because there is a rough, rumbling mid-diastolic murmur localized to the apex of the heart, there is a sharp opening snap and a loud first heart sound, a tapping impulse, an impalpable left ventricular apex, a left parasternal heave and a small volume pulse. Furthermore, the chaotic rhythm suggests atrial fibrillation and the patient has a malar flush'.

If you enlarge your response to 'What is the diagnosis?' by giving the features in this way, it is best to give the evidence in order of its importance to the diagnosis (as shown in the example). However, if the question is: '*What are your findings?*' it is best to give them in the order they are elicited: 'The patient has a malar flush and is slightly breathless at rest. The pulse is irregular in rate and volume. The jugular venous pressure is not elevated and the cardiac apex is not palpable but there is a tapping impulse parasternally on the left side and there is a left parasternal heave. The first heart sound is loud and there is an opening snap followed closely by a mid-diastolic rumble which is localized to the apex. These signs suggest that the patient has mitral stenosis'.

Remember, if you are talking in front of the patient, to avoid using words like 'cancer', 'motor neurone disease' and 'multiple sclerosis'. Use euphemisms such as 'neoplastic disease', 'anterior horn cell disease' and 'demyelinating disease'.

Remember that you can influence any discussion that follows by what you say. For example, the words: 'The diagnosis is aortic incompetence' may produce an interrogation by the examiner, or you may just be moved on to the next case. However, if you say: 'He has aortic incompetence for which there are several causes', this invites the examiner to ask you the causes. It is, therefore, a good answer—as long as you know them!

1 / Diabetic retinopathy

Frequency in survey: 34% of attempts at MRCP short cases.

Survey note: this is the commonest short case; it is also one of the easiest to fail. Some candidates who saw haemorrhages failed to note whether there were also microaneurysms. The uninitiated failed to recognize photocoagulation scars. The commonest forms reported in the survey were background diabetic retinopathy (40%) and proliferative retinopathy treated with photocoagulation (40%). Most of the rest were fundi with untreated proliferative retinopathy. Advanced diabetic eye disease was only rarely reported.

Record 1

There are *microaneurysms*, *blot haemorrhages* and *hard exudates* (due to lipid deposition in the retina).*
  The patient has background diabetic retinopathy.

Record 2

The above plus: in the R/L eye there is a *circinate formation* of *hard exudates* (indicating oedema) *near*† the R/L *macula* suggesting that macular oedema is present or imminent. It would be important to assess the patient's visual acuity.

Record 3

Any of the above plus: there are *cotton-wool spots*, *flame-shaped haemorrhages* (both indicating ischaemia), and leashes of *new vessels* (say where). *Photocoagulation scars* are seen (say where).
  The patient has proliferative diabetic retinopathy treated by photocoagulation.

Record 4

Any of the above plus: *vitreous haemorrhage/vitreous scar/retinal detachment* (widespread and impairing vision) indicate advanced diabetic eye disease.
  NB With diabetic retinopathy there may also be:
1 Cataracts (p. 251).
2 AV nipping (indicating either coexistent hypertension or arteriosclerosis).

Indications for photocoagulation are the sight-threatening forms of retinopathy:
1 *Maculopathy* (especially type II = non-insulin-dependent diabetes): warning signs are hard exudates often in rings (indicating oedema) encroaching on the macula, sometimes with multiple haemorrhages (indicating ischaemia). Macular oedema itself is difficult to recognize with the direct oph-

* Say where the lesions are; particularly in relation to the macula—see criteria for referral to an ophthalmologist.
† If you use the tiny spotlight of the ophthalmoscope and ask the patient to *look at* the light while you look in, you will be looking at the macula and this may help you assess whether there are hard exudates or haemorrhages involving the macula.

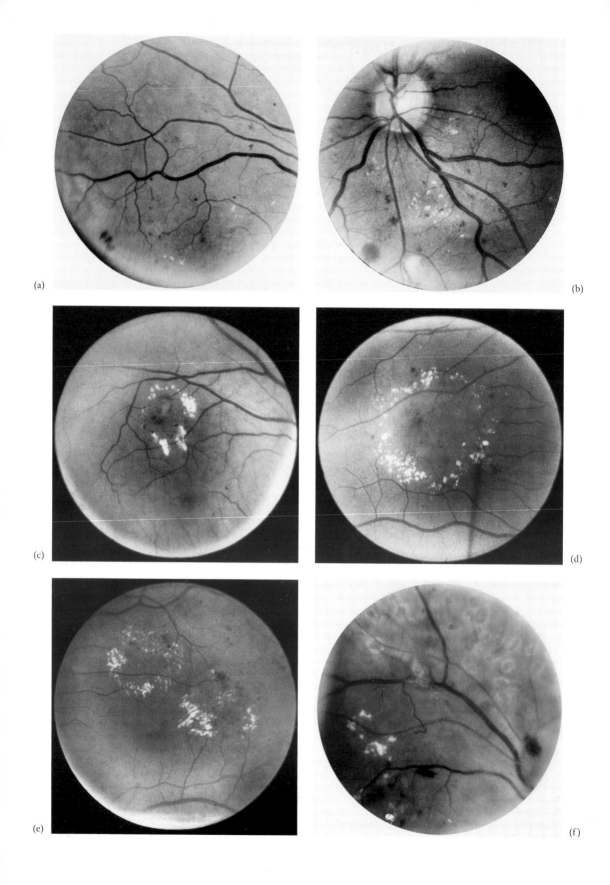

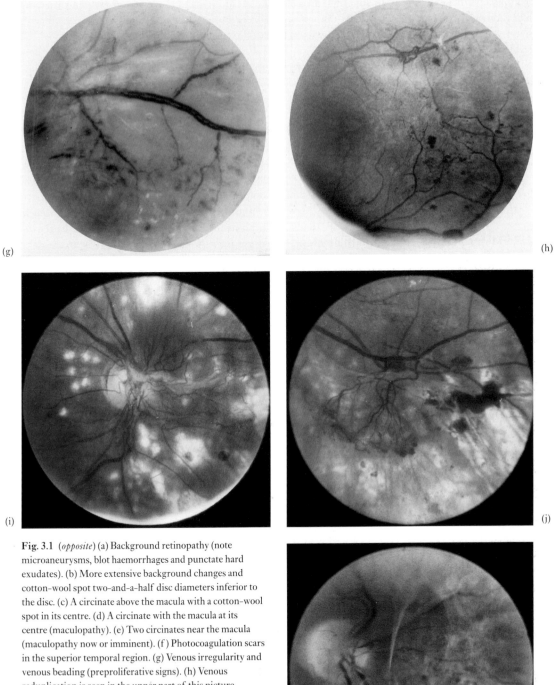

(g)

(h)

(i)

(j)

(k)

Fig. 3.1 (*opposite*) (a) Background retinopathy (note microaneurysms, blot haemorrhages and punctate hard exudates). (b) More extensive background changes and cotton-wool spot two-and-a-half disc diameters inferior to the disc. (c) A circinate above the macula with a cotton-wool spot in its centre. (d) A circinate with the macula at its centre (maculopathy). (e) Two circinates near the macula (maculopathy now or imminent). (f) Photocoagulation scars in the superior temporal region. (g) Venous irregularity and venous beading (preproliferative signs). (h) Venous reduplication is seen in the upper part of this picture (a preproliferative sign). (i) Leashes of new vessels with a leash of fibrous tissue (healing following haemorrhage of some of the new vessels into the vitreous) projecting into the vitreous and photocoagulation scars in the background. (j) Leashes of peripheral new vessels which are haemorrhaging. Photocoagulation scars in the background (same patient as (i)). (k) Advanced diabetic eye disease (note vitreous scar).

thalmoscope though signs of an abnormal greyish reflection or discoloration at the macula are suggestive. Even slight visual deterioration is highly significant if there is any suspicion of maculopathy

2 *Preproliferative and proliferative retinopathy* (commonly type I = insulin-dependent diabetes): preproliferative lesions suggesting that neovascularization is imminent are:

Multiple cotton-wool spots
Multiple large blot haemorrhages
Venous beading
Venous loops
Arterial sheathing
Atrophic looking retina.

Criteria for referral to an ophthalmologist

(according to European diabetic retinopathy screening guidelines):

1 Proliferative retinopathy (new vessels on disc or elsewhere; preretinal haemorrhage; fibrous tissue)

2 Advanced diabetic eye disease (vitreous haemorrhage; fibrous tissue; recent retinal detachment; rubeosis iridis)

3 Preproliferative retinopathy (venous irregularities—beading, reduplication, loops; multiple haemorrhages; multiple cotton-wool spots; intraretinal microvascular abnormalities (IRMA))

4 Non-proliferative retinopathy with macular involvement (reduced visual acuity not corrected by pinhole, i.e. suggesting macular oedema; haemorrhages and/or hard exudates within one disc diameter of the macula, with or without visual loss

5 Non-proliferative retinopathy without macular involvement (large circinate or plaque of hard exudates within the major temporal vasular arcades).

For colour photographs see pp. 527–9.

2 / Hepatosplenomegaly

Frequency in survey: main focus of a short case in 24% of attempts at MRCP short cases. Additional feature in a further 8%.

Record

There is hepatosplenomegaly, the *spleen* is enlarged . . . cm below the left costal margin. The *liver* is palpable at . . . cm below the right costal margin; it is non-tender, firm and smooth (now look for clinical *anaemia*, *lymphadenopathy* and signs of *chronic liver disease*).

Likely causes to be considered are:

No other signs or clinical anaemia only

1 Myeloproliferative disorders (p. 80)
2 Lymphoproliferative disorders (p. 81)
3 Cirrhosis of the liver with portal hypertension (less likely if there are no other signs of chronic liver disease).

Hepatosplenomegaly plus palpable lymph nodes*

1 Chronic lymphatic leukaemia
2 Lymphoma.

Other conditions to be considered would include infectious mononucleosis (?throat), infective hepatitis (?icterus) and sarcoidosis.

Signs of chronic liver disease

Cirrhosis of the liver with portal hypertension (p. 84).

Other causes of hepatosplenomegaly

Hepatitis B or C† (?icterus, tattoo marks, needle marks)
Brucellosis ('examine this farmer's abdomen')
Weil's disease (?icterus, sewerage worker or fell into canal)
Toxoplasmosis (glandular fever-like illness)
Cytomegalovirus infection (glandular fever-like illness)

Pernicious anaemia and other megaloblastic anaemias (NB SACD – p. 314. NB Associated organ-specific autoimmune disease–p. 279)
Storage disorders (e.g. Gaucher's – spleen is often huge; glycogen storage disease)
Amyloidosis (?underlying chronic disease)‡
Other causes of portal hypertension (e.g. Budd–Chiari syndrome = hepatic vein thrombosis—see pp. 84 and 191)

---

*These conditions can also occur without palpable lymph nodes.
†NB Hepatitis serology heads the list of investigations of icterus of uncertain cause.
‡Though hepatosplenomegaly can occur in primary and myeloma associated amyloidosis, it is commoner in the secondary form. Other organs particularly involved in secondary amyloidosis are kidneys (nephrotic syndrome),

adrenals (clinical adrenocortical failure may occur) and alimentary tract (rectal biopsy). Conditions associated with secondary amyloidosis include rheumatoid arthritis (including juvenile type), tuberculosis, leprosy, chronic sepsis, Crohn's disease, ulcerative colitis, ankylosing spondylitis, paraplegia (bedsores and urinary infection), malignant lymphoma and carcinoma. See also footnote on p. 134.

Infantile polycystic disease (in some variants of this, children have relatively mild renal involvement but hepatosplenomegaly and portal hypertension).

Common causes on a worldwide basis
Malaria
Kala–azar
Schistosomiasis
Tuberculosis.

3 / Mitral stenosis (lone)

Frequency in survey: 20% of attempts at MRCP short cases.

Record

There is a *malar flush* and a *left thoracotomy scar*. The pulse is *irregularly irregular* (give rate) in rate and volume (if sinus rhythm the volume is usually small). The venous pressure is not raised, and there is no ankle or sacral oedema (unless in cardiac failure). The cardiac impulse is *tapping* (palpable first heart sound) and the apex is not displaced. There is a *left parasternal heave*. The *first heart sound* is *loud*, there is a loud pulmonary second sound and an *opening snap* followed by a *mid-diastolic rumbling murmur* (with *presystolic accentuation* if the patient is in sinus rhythm) *localized* to the apex and heard most loudly with the patient in the *left lateral* position.*

The diagnosis is mitral stenosis. The patient has had a valvotomy in the past. There are signs of pulmonary hypertension.

Other signs which may be present

Giant v waves (tricuspid incompetence — usually secondary; may be primary—see p. 214)

Graham Steell† murmur — rare (secondary pulmonary incompetence; a high-pitched, brief, early diastolic whiff in the presence of marked signs of pulmonary hypertension and a pulse which is not collapsing).

The opening snap

soon after the second sound‡ in tight mitral stenosis (<0.09 seconds — mean left atrial pressure above 20 mmHg); longer after the second sound in mild mitral stenosis (>0.1 seconds — mean left atrial pressure below 15 mmHg); absent if the mitral valve is calcified (first heart sound soft).

Indications for considering surgery

Significant symptoms which limit normal activity

An episode of pulmonary oedema without a precipitating cause

Recurrent emboli

Pulmonary oedema in pregnancy (emergency valvotomy)

Deterioration due to atrial fibrillation which does not respond to medical treatment

Haemoptysis.

Criteria for valvotomy§

Mobile valve (loud first heart sound, opening snap, absence of calcium on X-ray screening and thin mobile cusps on echocardiography)

Absence of mitral incompetence.

For colour photograph see p. 531.

---

*If unsure about the presence of the murmur, it can be accentuated by exercise—get the patient to touch her toes and then recline 10 times.

† Though associated eponymously with Graham Steell, the original source of the observation was probably George Balfour of Edinburgh, for whom Steell worked as house physician (*Journal of the Royal College of Physicians* 1991, 25: 66–70).

‡ The interval from the second sound to the opening snap varies with heart rate. If the interval is ≤0.07 seconds with the heart rate < 100, the mitral stenosis is usually of haemodynamic significance.

§ Should be considered, particularly in the young female who has a desire for pregnancy. Sometimes it can be performed before the development of significant symptoms.

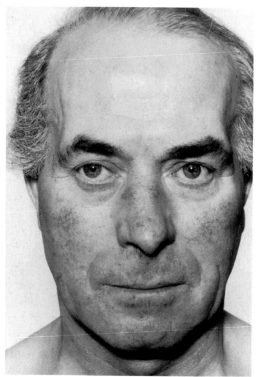

(a)

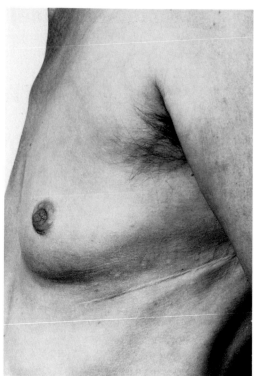

(b)

Fig. 3.3 (a) Mitral facies. (b) Thoracotomy scar for mitral valvotomy.

4 / Rheumatoid hands

Frequency in survey: main focus of a short case in 17% of attempts at MRCP short cases. Additional feature in a further 7%.

Record

There is a *symmetrical deforming arthropathy*. There is *spindling* of the fingers due to soft tissue swelling at the *proximal interphalangeal* joints and *metacarpophalangeal joints*. There is generalized *wasting* of the *small muscles* of the hand and use is restricted by weakness, deformity and pain. There are *nodules* at the elbow, over the extensor tendons, and in the palm. There is *ulnar deviation* of the fingers (consequent upon subluxation and dislocation at the metacarpophalangeal joints). The *terminal interphalangeal joints* are *spared*. There are arteritic lesions* in the nail folds.

The patient has rheumatoid arthritis.

The ratio of males to females is 1:3.

Other features which may occur

'Swan neck' deformity (*hyperextension of proximal interphalangeal* joint with fixed flexion of metacarpophalangeal and terminal interphalangeal joints)

Boutonnière deformity (flexion deformity of proximal interphalangeal joint with *extension contracture of terminal interphalangeal* and metacarpophalangeal joints)

Z deformity of the thumb

Triggering of the finger (flexor tendon nodule)

Palmar erythema

Iatrogenic Cushing's (?facies, thin atrophic skin, purpura)

Swollen or deformed knees (p. 297)

Cervical spine disease (upper cervical spine, especially atlantoaxial joint — subluxation can occur with *spinal cord compression*; a lateral X-ray centred on the odontoid peg with the neck in full flexion, shows the distance from the odontoid to the anterior arch of the atlas as abnormal at more than 3 mm—general anaesthesia is dangerous and requires extreme care in neck handling)

Anaemia (five causes†)

Chest signs (?pleural effusions; fibrosing alveolitis‡)

Neurological signs (?peripheral neuropathy, mononeuritis multiplex, carpal tunnel syndrome)

Eye signs (episcleritis, painful scleritis, scleromalacia perforans, cataracts due to chloroquine or steroids)

Sjögren's syndrome (?dry eyes, dry mouth)

Felty's syndrome (?spleen—p. 435)

---

* As well as causing nail-fold infarcts and chronic leg ulceration, the vasculitis (p. 241) which is immune complex-induced and may affect small, medium or large vessels, may also lead to digital gangrene. A purpuric rash may occur due to capillaritis. Raynaud's phenomenon (p. 350) may occur. Pyoderma gangrenosum (p. 431) is a rare cause of ulceration.

† Five causes of anaemia in rheumatoid arthritis are:

1 Anaemia of chronic disease (normochromic normocytic)

2 Gastrointestinal bleeding related to nonsteroidal anti-inflammatory agents

3 Bone marrow suppression (gold, phenylbutazone, indomethacin, penicillamine)

4 Megaloblastic anaemia (folic acid deficiency or associated pernicious anaemia, see organ-specific autoimmune disease, p. 279 and footnote)

5 Felty's syndrome (p. 435).

‡ The lungs may also be affected in other ways. Rheumatoid nodules may occur in the lung fields on chest X-ray and in patients exposed to certain dusts—especially coal miners—nodules may be accompanied by massive fibrotic reactions (Caplan's syndrome). Obliterative bronchiolitis is a severe but rare complication which may be associated with penicillamine therapy.

Leg ulceration (vasculitic)*

Cardiac signs (pericarditis is present in up to 40% of patients at autopsy but is rarely apparent clinically; myocarditis, conduction defects and valvular incompetence are rare consequences of granulomatous infiltration)

Secondary amyloidosis (?proteinuria, hepatosplenomegaly, etc.—see footnote, p. 69)

Other autoimmune disorders (see pp. 142, 269 and 279).

For colour photographs see pp. 537–8.

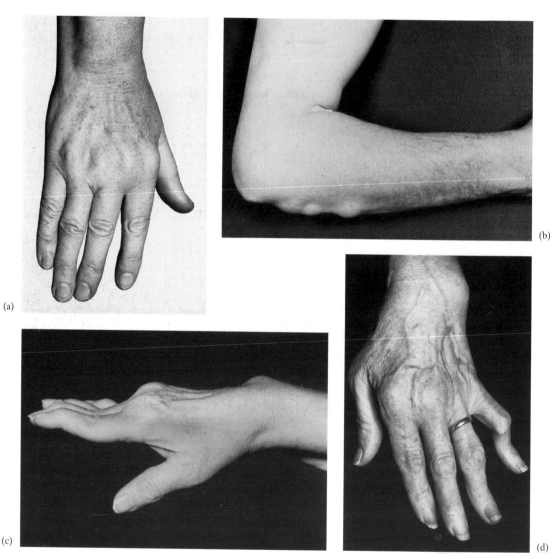

(a)

(b)

(c)

(d)

Fig. 3.4 (a) Early changes—swelling of the metacarpophalangeal joints, slight ulnar deviation.

(b) Rheumatoid nodules. (c) 'Swan neck' deformity.
(d) Boutonnière deformity.

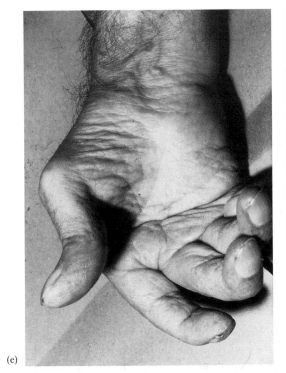

(e)

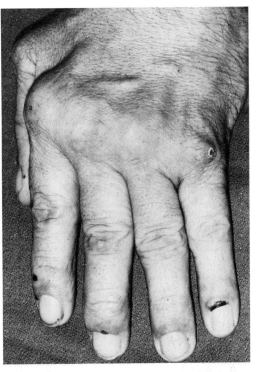

(f)

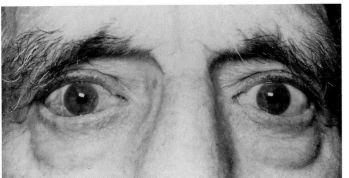

Fig. 3.4 (*continued*) (e) Z-shaped thumb. (f) Vasculitis. (g) Episcleritis.

(g)

5 / Mixed mitral valve disease

Frequency in survey: 16% of attempts at MRCP short cases.

Record 1

There is a *malar flush* and a *left thoracotomy scar*. The pulse is irregularly irregular (give rate) in rate and volume and the venous pressure is not raised. The cardiac impulse is *tapping* and the apex beat is *not displaced*. There is a *left parasternal heave*. On auscultation there is a *loud* first heart sound, a *pansystolic murmur** radiating to the axilla, a loud pulmonary second sound, and an *opening snap* followed by a *mid-diastolic rumbling murmur* localized to the apex.

The patient has mixed mitral valve disease. In view of the tapping cardiac impulse, the loud first heart sound and the undisplaced apex, I think this is predominant mitral stenosis. There are signs of pulmonary hypertension.

Record 2

There is a left thoracotomy scar. The pulse is irregularly irregular (give rate) in rate and volume and the venous pressure is not raised. The apex beat is *thrusting* and *displaced* to the sixth intercostal space in the anterior axillary line and there is a *left parasternal heave*. On auscultation the first heart sound is *soft* and there is a loud *pansystolic murmur* at the left sternal edge and/or apex radiating to the axilla. There is a loud pulmonary second sound and with the patient in the left lateral position I could hear a *mid-diastolic rumbling murmur* following an opening snap.†

The patient has mixed mitral valve disease with pulmonary hypertension. In view of the soft first heart sound and displaced and vigorous apex beat, I think this is predominant mitral incompetence.

If it is not clear clinically which lesion is predominant (e.g. loud first heart sound but enlarged left ventricle) and the examiners wish your opinion, point out the factors in favour of each (Table 3.5) then come down in favour of the one you think most likely, but point out that in this case cardiac catheter studies would be required to be certain, e.g. 'It is difficult in this case. The loud first heart sound would suggest predominant mitral stenosis; however, the enlarged left ventricle suggests mitral incompetence as the more important lesion. I think cardiac catheter studies would be required to resolve the issue'.

---

*In the patient with severe pulmonary hypertension when a very large right ventricle displaces the left ventricle posteriorly, the murmur of tricuspid incompetence (p. 214) can mimic that of mitral incompetence. The murmur of tricuspid incompetence is ordinarily heard best at the lower left sternal border, increases with inspiration and is not heard in the axilla or over the spine posteriorly. In tricuspid incompetence giant *v* waves will be present.

† In severe mitral incompetence without mitral stenosis a mid-diastolic flow murmur may be heard without an opening snap. The presence of a third heart sound is incompatible with any significant degree of mitral stenosis.

Table 3.5 Factors pointing to a predominant lesion in mixed mitral valve disease

	Mitral stenosis	Mitral incompetence
Pulse	Small volume	Sharp and abbreviated
Apex	Not displaced; tapping impulse present	Displaced, thrusting
First heart sound	Loud	Soft
Third heart sound	Absent	Present

6 / Dullness at the lung base

Frequency in survey: main focus of a short case in 14% of attempts at MRCP short cases. Additional feature in a further 4%.

Record

The pulse is regular and the venous pressure is not elevated. The trachea is central,* the expansion is normal, but the percussion note is *stony dull* at the R/L base(s), with *diminished* tactile *fremitus* and vocal *resonance*, and *diminished breath sounds*. There is (may be) an area of bronchial breathing above the area of dullness.

The diagnosis is R/L pleural effusion.

Causes of pleural effusion

Exudate (protein content $> 30\,\text{g}\,\text{l}^{-1}$)

Bronchial carcinoma (?nicotine staining, clubbing, radiation burns on chest, lymph nodes)

Secondary malignancy (?evidence of primary especially breast, lymph nodes, radiation burns)

Pulmonary embolus and infarction (?deep venous thrombosis; blood-stained fluid will be found at aspiration)

Pneumonia (bronchial breathing/crepitations, fever, etc.)

Tuberculosis

Rheumatoid arthritis (?hands and nodules)

Systemic lupus erythematosus (?typical rash)

Lymphoma (?nodes and spleen)

Mesothelioma (asbestos worker, ?clubbing).

Transudate (protein content $< 30\,\text{g}\,\text{l}^{-1}$)

Cardiac failure (?JVP ↑, ankle and sacral oedema, large heart, tachycardia, S_3 or signs of a valvular lesion)

Nephrotic syndrome (?generalized oedema, patient may be young—p. 322)

Cirrhosis (?ascites, generalized oedema, signs of chronic liver disease—p. 84).

Other causes of pleural effusion

Meigs' syndrome (ovarian fibroma)

Subphrenic abscess (?recent abdominal disease or surgery)

Peritoneal dialysis

Hypothyroidism (?facies, pulse, ankle jerks)

Pancreatitis (more common on the left; fluid has high amylase)

Dressler's syndrome (recent myocardial infarction, ?pericardial friction rub)

Trauma

Asbestos exposure

Yellow nail syndrome (yellowish-brown beaked nails usually associated with lymphatic hypoplasia, see p. 423)

Chylothorax (trauma or blockage of a major

---

*The trachea may be deviated if the effusion is very large. A large effusion without any mediastinal shift (clinically and on chest X-ray) raises the possibility of collapse as well as effusion.

intrathoracic lymphatic—usually by a neoplastic process).

Other causes of dullness at a lung base
Raised hemidiaphragm (e.g. hepatomegaly, phrenic nerve palsy)
Basal collapse

Collapse/consolidation (if the airway is blocked by, for example, a carcinoma there may be no bronchial breathing)
Pleural thickening (e.g. old tuberculosis or old empyema or a mesothelioma).

7 / Splenomegaly (without hepatomegaly)

Frequency in survey: main focus of a short case in 14% of attempts at MRCP short cases. Additional feature in a further 2%.

Record

The spleen is palpable at . . . cm.
or
There is a *mass* in the *left hypochondrium*. On palpation I *cannot get above* the mass, it has a *notch*, and on inspiration moves diagonally across the abdomen. The *percussion note* is *dull* over the left lower lateral chest wall and over the mass.

I think this is the spleen enlarged at . . . cm. Likely causes* to be considered are:

Very large spleen†

1 Chronic myeloid leukaemia (Philadelphia chromosome positive in 90%)
2 Myelofibrosis
and in other parts of the world
3 Chronic malaria
4 Kala–azar.

Spleen enlarged 4–8 cm (2–4 finger breadths)

1 Myeloproliferative disorders‡ (e.g. chronic myeloid leukaemia and myelofibrosis)
2 Lymphoproliferative disorders§ (e.g. lymphoma and chronic lymphatic leukaemia)
3 Cirrhosis of the liver with portal hypertension (spider naevi, icterus, etc.—p. 84).

Spleen just tipped or enlarged 2–4 cm (1–2 finger breadths)

1 Myeloproliferative disorders‡

---

* To help you remember some common causes to mention in the examination we have given the three or four most common causes of a spleen of a particular size. An alternative way of dividing up splenomegaly which can be found in many textbooks is:
1 Infectious and inflammatory splenomegaly (e.g. SBE, infectious mononucleosis, sarcoidosis)
2 Infiltrative splenomegaly
  (a) benign (e.g. Gaucher's, amyloidosis)
  (b) neoplastic (e.g. leukaemias, lymphoma).
3 Congestive splenomegaly (e.g. cirrhosis, hepatic vein thrombosis)
4 Splenomegaly due to reticuloendothelial hyperplasia (e.g. haemolytic anaemias, immune thrombocytopenias).
† *Gaucher's* disease and *rapidly progressive lymphoma*

(especially high-grade lymphoma) may also cause a huge spleen. *Chronic congestive splenomegaly* (Banti's syndrome = splenomegaly, pancytopenia, portal hypertension and gastrointestinal bleeding) may also cause massive splenomegaly. A huge spleen developing in a patient with *polycythaemia rubra vera* is usually due to the development of myelofibrosis.
‡ When listing the causes of splenomegaly or hepatosplenomegaly in the limited time of the examination, to use the term 'myeloproliferative disorders' in its broadest interpretation is a useful way of covering several conditions in one phrase. If asked to explain it (unlikely), one strict definition covers a group of related disorders of haemopoietic stem cell proliferation: chronic myeloid leukaemia (CML), myelofibrosis, polycythaemia rubra vera and essential

2 Lymphoproliferative disorders§ (?palpable lymph nodes)
3 Cirrhosis of the liver with portal hypertension
4 Infections such as:

    (a) glandular fever (?throat, lymph nodes)

    (b) infectious hepatitis (?icterus)

    (c) subacute bacterial endocarditis (?heart murmur, splinter haemorrhages, etc.).

Other causes of splenomegaly

Polycythaemia rubra vera (?plethoric, middle-aged man)

Brucellosis ('examine this farmer's abdomen')

Sarcoidosis (?erythema nodosum or history of; lupus pernio; chest signs)

Haemolytic anaemia (?icterus)

Pernicious anaemia and other megaloblastic anaemias (?pallor; NB SACD—p. 314; NB Associated organ-specific autoimmune diseases, especially autoimmune thyroid disease, diabetes, Addison's, vitiligo, hypoparathyroidism — see p. 279)

Idiopathic thrombocytopenic purpura (?young female, purpura)

Felty's syndrome (?hands, nodules)

Amyloidosis (?underlying chronic disease, other organ involvement—see p. 69)

SLE (?typical rash)

Lipid storage disease (spleen may be enormous — e.g. Gaucher's)

Myelomatosis

Chronic iron deficiency anaemia

Thyrotoxicosis

Other infections (subacute septicaemia, typhoid, disseminated tuberculosis, trypanosomiasis, echinococcosis)

Other causes of congestive splenomegaly* (hepatic vein thrombosis, portal vein obstruction, schistosomiasis, congestive heart failure).

thrombocythaemia. The term can be used more broadly to cover acute myeloid leukaemia as well. A small spleen is more likely to be due to acute leukaemia than CML or myelofibrosis because splenic enlargement in the latter conditions is often already marked at the time of presentation.

§ The lymphoproliferative disorders are chronic lymphatic leukaemia, lymphoma, myelomatosis, Waldenström's macroglobulinaemia, acute lymphatic leukaemia and hairy cell leukaemia. Of these, the first two and Waldenström's macroglobulinaemia are usually associated with lymphadenopathy and hepatomegaly. Multiple myeloma seldom causes palpable spenomegaly.

8 / Optic atrophy

Frequency in survey: main focus of a short case in 14% of attempts at MRCP short cases. Additional feature in a further 4%.

Record

The disc is *pale* and *clearly delineated* and (in the severe case) the *pupil reacts consensually* to light but *not directly*.* Field testing with the head of a hat pin (maybe) reveals a *central scotoma*.

The diagnosis is optic atrophy. The well-defined disc edge suggests that it is not secondary to papilloedema† (yellow/grey disc with blurred margins). Common causes of primary optic atrophy are:

1 Multiple sclerosis (may be temporal pallor only; ?nystagmus, scanning speech, cerebellar ataxia, etc.—p. 433)
2 Compression of the optic nerve by:
  (a) tumour (e.g. pituitary—?bitemporal hemianopia)
  (b) aneurysm
3 Glaucoma (?pathological cupping).

Other causes

Ischaemic optic neuropathy (abrupt onset of visual loss in an elderly patient; may be painful; thrombosis or embolus of posterior ciliary artery; temporal arteritis is sometimes the cause)

Leber's optic atrophy (males:females = 6:1)

Retinal artery occlusion (p. 277)

Toxic amblyopia (lead, methyl alcohol, arsenic, insecticides, quinine)

Nutritional amblyopia (famine, etc., tobacco–alcohol amblyopia, vitamin B_{12} deficiency, diabetes mellitus‡)

Freidreich's ataxia (?cerebellar signs, pes cavus, scoliosis, etc.—p. 234)

Tabes dorsalis (?Argyll Robertson pupils, etc. —p. 330)

Paget's disease (?large skull, bowed tibia, etc.—p. 87)

Consecutive optic atrophy.†

For colour photograph see p. 528.

---

* In early unilateral optic neuritis before the direct reflex is lost, it may simply become more sluggish than the consensual reflex. In this situation it may be possible to demonstrate the *Marcus Gunn* phenomenon. In this the direct reflex may at first appear to be brisk. However, when the light is alternated from one side to the other, the pupil on the affected side may be seen to dilate slowly when exposed to the light. The mechanism is as follows: when the light shines in the healthy eye a rapid constriction occurs in both eyes. As the light then moves to the affected eye, this fails to transmit the message to continue constriction as quickly as normal. As a result the pupils have time to recover and dilate, despite the light shining on the abnormal eye.

† Optic atrophy can be divided into primary, secondary and consecutive. Consecutive optic atrophy follows damage to the parent ganglion cells of the retina as in widespread choroidoretinitis, retinitis pigmentosa, and retinal artery occlusion.

‡ Optic atrophy in diabetes mellitus may also occur in the DIDMOAD syndrome—with diabetes insipidus, diabetes mellitus, and deafness. It is a rare, recessively inherited disorder.

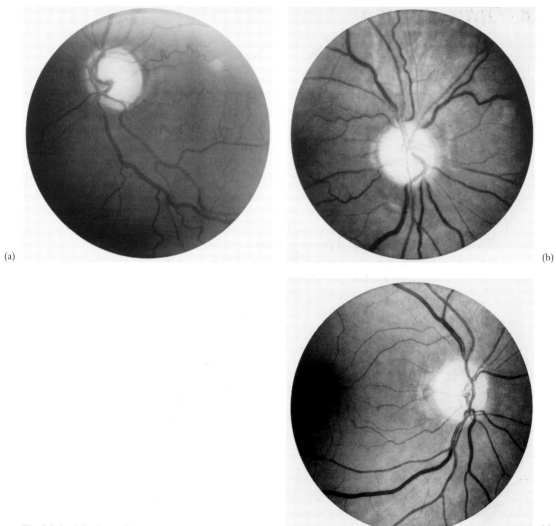

(a)

(b)

(c)

Fig. 3.8 (a–c) Optic atrophy.

9 / Chronic liver disease

Frequency in survey: main focus of a short case in 13% of attempts at MRCP short cases. Additional feature in a further 3%.

Record

The patient is *icteric*, *pigmented* and *cyanosed* (due to pulmonary venous shunts). He has *clubbing, leuconychia, palmar erythema, Dupuytren's contracture** and there are several *spider naevi*. He has a flapping tremor of the hands (suggesting some portosystemic encephalopathy). There are scratch marks on the forearms and back, and there is purpura. There is *gynaecomastia, scanty body hair* and his *testes* are *small*. There is 5 cm *hepatomegaly* and 3 cm *splenomegaly*. He has *ascites* and *ankle oedema*, and there are *distended abdominal veins* in which the flow is away from the umbilicus.

The diagnosis is likely to be cirrhosis of the liver with portal hypertension.

Possible causes

1 Alcohol
2 Viral hepatitis
    (a) hepatitis B (?health or clinical laboratory worker)
    (b) hepatitis C (the major cause of post-transfusion hepatitis)
    (c) hepatitis D (unusual; requires antecedent or simultaneous hepatitis B virus infection)
3 Lupoid hepatitis (pubertal or menopausal female, steroid responsive; associated with diabetes, inflammatory bowel disease, thyroiditis and pulmonary infiltrates; ?smooth muscle antibodies)
4 Primary biliary cirrhosis (middle-aged female, scratch marks, xanthelasma; ?antimitochondrial antibody—p. 222)
5 Haemochromatosis (male, slate-grey pigmentation—p. 253)
6 Cryptogenic.

Other causes

Cardiac failure (?JVP ↑, *v* waves, *S3* or a valvular lesion, tender pulsatile liver if tricuspid incompetence)
Constrictive pericarditis† (JVP raised, abrupt *x* and *y* descent, loud early *S3* ('pericardial knock' — a valuable sign but only present in < 40% of cases) though heart sounds often normal, slight 'paradoxical pulse', *no signs in lung fields*, chest X-ray may show calcified pericardium; rare but important cause of ascites as response to treatment may be dramatic)

* Twenty signs which may be present in the hands of the patient with chronic liver disease are clubbing, Dupuytren's contracture, palmar erythema, spider naevi, flapping tremor, leuconychia, scratch marks, icterus, pallor, pigmentation, cyanosis, xanthomata, purpura, koilonychia, paronychia, abscesses, oedema, muscle wasting, tattoos (?HBsAg-positive), needle marks (intravenous drug abuse—more likely in antecubital fossa).

† The spleen may be palpable. In the absence of evidence of *bacterial endocarditis* or *tricuspid valve disease*, the presence of splenomegaly in a patient with congestive heart failure should arouse suspicion of *constrictive pericarditis* or *pericardial effusion with tamponade*.

Budd–Chiari syndrome (in the acute phase ascites develops rapidly with pain, there are no cutaneous signs of chronic liver disease and the liver is smoothly enlarged and tender; if the inferior vena cava is involved there is no hepatojugular reflux)

Biliary cholestasis (bile obstruction with or without infection)

Toxins and drugs (methotrexate, methyldopa, isoni-azid, carbon tetrachloride, amiodarone, aspirin, phenytoin, propylthiouracil, sulphonamides)

Wilson's disease (?Kayser–Fleischer rings, tremor, rigidity, dysarthria)

Alpha$_1$ antitrypsin deficiency (?lower zone emphysema)

Other metabolic causes (galactosaemia, tyrosinaemia, type IV glycogenosis).

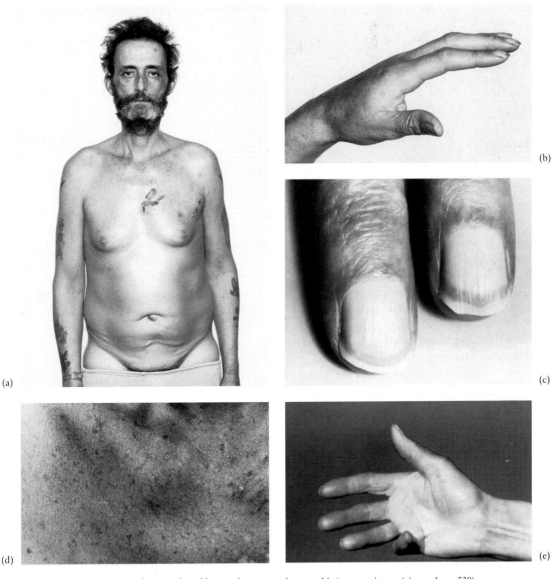

(a)

(b)

(c)

(d)

(e)

Fig. 3.9 (a) Note from above downwards: spider naevi, herpes zoster (debilitated patient), gynaecomastia, tattoo marks, everted umbilicus, swelling of the flanks, abdominal wall veins and paucity of hair. (b) Clubbing of the fingers and leuconychia (same patient as (a); see also p. 530).
(c) Leuconychia. (d) Spider naevi (close up). (e) Dupuytren's contracture.

10 / Polycystic kidneys

Frequency in survey: main focus of a short case in 12% of attempts at MRCP short cases. Additional feature in a further 2%.

Record

There are *bilateral masses* in the *flanks* which are *bimanually ballotable*. I can *get above* them and the percussion note is *resonant* over them.* I suspect, therefore, that they are renal masses and a likely diagnosis is polycystic kidneys (?*uraemic facies*; the *blood pressure* may be raised). The *arteriovenous fistula/shunt* on his arm indicates that the patient is being treated with haemodialysis (about 5% develop renal failure).

Other causes of bilateral renal enlargement include:
1 Bilateral hydronephrosis
2 Amyloidosis (?underlying chronic disease, hepatosplenomegaly, etc.—see p. 69)
3 Tuberous sclerosis (?adenoma sebaceum, p. 308)
4 Von Hippel–Lindau disease.†

Polycystic disease of the liver in adults may cause a nodular liver enlargement (liver function may be normal despite massive hepatomegaly). About 50% have renal involvement. Cystic liver is a major feature of infantile polycystic disease (autosomal recessive) but a minor feature of adult polycystic kidney disease (autosomal dominant).

Other features of adult polycystic kidney disease

Cysts may also occur in other organs—most important are sacular aneurysms (berry aneurysms) of the cerebral arteries (10%) which, in combina-

tion with the hypertension, leads to serious risk of intracranial haemorrhage (cause of death in 10% of cases according to some authorities). There may be focal neurological defects

Mitral valve prolapse (p. 207) may occur in 25% as a further manifestation of the systemic collagen defect. Patients often have palpitations and atypical chest pain

It may present with flank pains, bleeding, urinary tract infection, nephrolithiasis or obstructive uropathy

Renal cell carcinoma may be more common than in the general population but this is uncertain.

*Look for abdominal scars from previous peritoneal dialysis or cyst aspiration. The latter is performed to relieve obstruction of the outflow tract by the cyst, intractable pain or haematuria.

† An autosomal dominant condition in which patients develop retinal haemangiomata, cerebellar haemangioblastomata and phaeochromocytomata. Hepatic, renal, pancreatic and epididymal cysts may occur.

11 / Paget's disease

Frequency in survey: main focus of a short case in 12% of attempts at MRCP short cases. Additional feature in a further 1%.

Survey note: candidates were often asked follow-up questions on investigation, complications, treatment, etc.—NB experience 80, p. 458.

Record

There is (in this elderly patient) *enlargement* of the *skull*. There is also *bowing* of the R/L *tibia* (or femur) which is *warmer* (due to increased vascularity) than the other and the patient is (may be) *kyphotic* (vertebral involvement leads to *loss of height* and kyphosis from disc degeneration and vertebral collapse).

The diagnosis is Paget's disease. (There may be evidence of complications, e.g. a *hearing aid*—see below.)

Paget's disease occurs in 3% (autopsy series) of the population over the age of 40, rising to 10% over the age of 70, though it is not clinically important in the vast majority of these. Though it is often asymptomatic, patients may have symptoms such as bone pain, headaches, tinnitus and vertigo. Serum *alkaline phosphatase* and *urinary hydroxyproline* are elevated except sometimes in very early disease. Serum calcium and phosphate concentrations are usually normal in mobilized patients but may be increased or decreased. Urinary calcium and hydroxyproline rise in immobilized patients. High serum uric acid and erythrocyte sedimentation rate may also occur. There is growing ultrastructural and immuno-histochemical evidence that Paget's disease may represent a 'slow' virus infection in susceptible individuals—paramyxoviruses (which include respiratory syncytial virus, measles and distemper) have been implicated. Specific therapies which can be considered if indicated* include bisphosphonates, calcitonin and mithramycin.

Complications

Progressive closure of skull foramina may lead to:
1 Deafness (also results from Pagetic involvement of the ossicles†)
2 Optic atrophy‡
3 Basilar invagination (platybasia causing brainstem signs).
Other complications include:
1 High output cardiac failure (?bounding pulse—occurs when more than 30–40% of the skeleton is involved)
2 Pathological fractures
3 Urolithiasis
4 Sarcoma (incidence is probably <1%; increase in pain and swelling may occur; 'explosive rise' in alkaline phosphatase occurs only occasionally).

---

* Bisphosphonates are now the first-line treatment with short courses leading to long-term suppression of disease activity and improvement in bone pain, etc. Indications for specific therapy in Paget's disease are: bone pain; osteolytic lesions in weight-bearing bones; neurological complications (except deafness); delayed or non-union of fractures; immobilization hypercalcaemia; before and after orthopaedic surgery.

† Although hearing loss is frequently attributed to compression of the VIIIth cranial nerve in the canal in the temporal bone, this is unlikely to be the major cause because the facial nerve, which follows the same course, is rarely affected.
‡ The other ophthalmological finding which may occur in Paget's disease is angioid streaks in the retina (see p. 542).

Causes of 'bowed tibia'

True bowing due to soft bone:
Paget's disease (asymmetrical)
Rickets (bilateral, symmetrical—p. 394).

Apparent bowing due to thickening of the anterior surface of the tibia secondary to periostitis:
Congenital syphilis (?saddle nose, bulldog jaw, rhagades, Hutchinson's teeth, Moon's molars, etc.—p. 331)
Yaws.

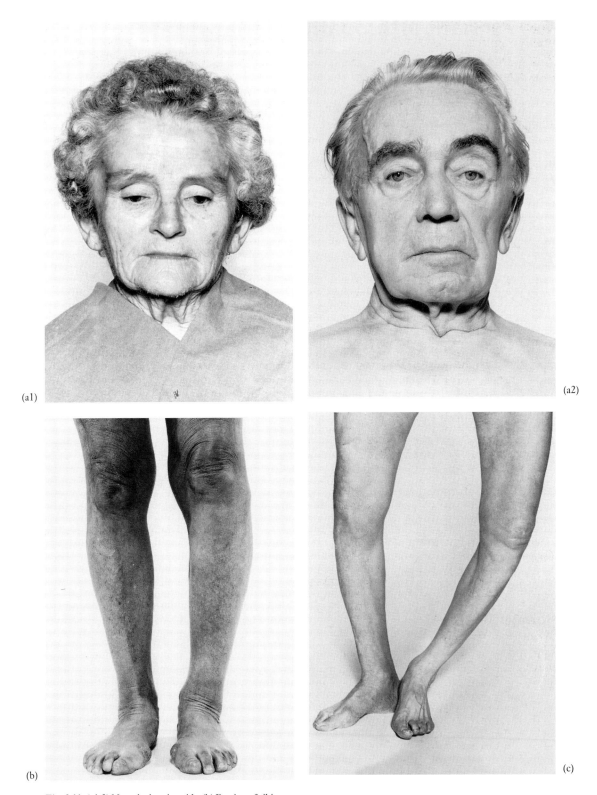

Fig. 3.11 (a1,2) Note the hearing aids. (b) Bowing of tibiae.
(c) Gross deformity.

12 / Psoriatic arthropathy/psoriasis

Frequency in survey: main focus of a short case in 11% of attempts at MRCP short cases. Additional feature in a further 1%.

Survey note: patients had arthropathy and/or skin lesions. Questions such as treatment only occasionally asked.

Record

There is an *asymmetrical arthropathy* involving mainly the *terminal interphalangeal joints*. There is *pitting* of the fingernails and *onycholysis*. Some of the nail plates (say which) are thickened and there is a thick scale (*hyperkeratosis*) under them. There are patches of psoriasis at the *elbows*. The plaques are circular with well-defined edges and they are *red* with a *silvery scaly* surface.

The patient has psoriatic arthropathy.

Psoriatic arthropathy (even if severe) can occur with minimal skin involvement.* If there is no obvious psoriasis at the elbows the following areas should particularly be checked for skin lesions:

1 Extensor aspects
2 Scalp
3 Behind the ears
4 In the navel.

Other forms of psoriatic arthropathy

Arthritis mutilans (see Fig. 3.12f and p. 530)
Arthritis clinically indistinguishable from rheuma-
   toid arthritis but consistently seronegative
Asymmetrical oligo- or monoarthropathy
Ankylosing spondylitis occurring alone or in con-
   junction with any of the other forms.

Treatment

Treatments of the skin lesions include sunlight, UV light, coal tar, dithranol, local steroids, calipotriol, PUVA (psoralen and UVA light). Systemic treat-ment with acitretin (a retinoid) or antimetabolites (methotrexate, azathioprine, hydroxyurea), because of their side-effects, should be reserved for severe widespread disease unresponsive to topical mea-sures. Analgesic anti-inflammatory agents are used for the pain of the arthropathy. Sulphasalazine and methotrexate are becoming established as effective agents for the treatment of psoriatic arthropathy. Gold and penicillamine may be useful, but few con-trolled studies have been done. Cyclosporin may also have a place in refractory disease. Choroquine is contraindicated as it may exacerbate the skin lesions (exfoliative dermatitis). Intra-articular steroids are useful for a single inflamed troublesome joint.

Incidence

1–5% of Caucasians in north-western Europe and USA. Uncommon among Japanese, North Ameri-can Indians and Afro-Americans.

For colour photograph see p. 530.

---

* There is no evidence of a link between the activity of the skin lesions and the arthropathy.

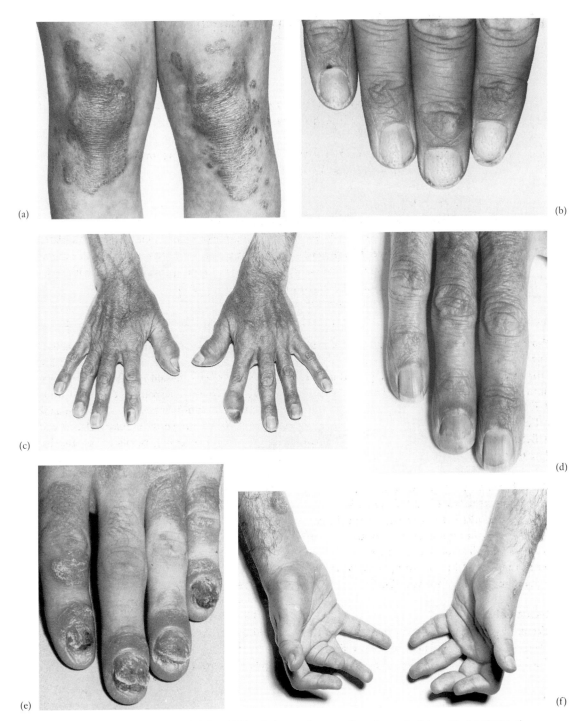

Fig. 3.12 (a) Typical plaques. (b) Nail pitting. (c) Terminal interphalangeal arthropathy and nail changes. (d) Onycholysis. (e) Advanced nail changes (note the psoriatic plaques and hyperkeratosis of the nail beds). (f) Note the typical plaque on the forearm and telescopic middle finger.

(g1)

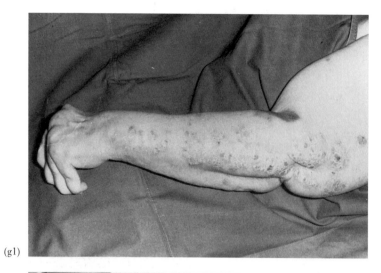

(g2)

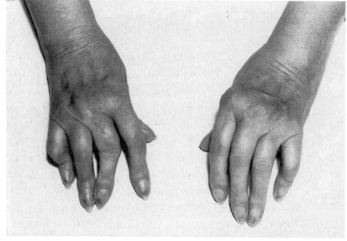

Fig. 3.12 (*continued*) (g1,2) indistinguishable from rheumatoid arthritis. Note plaques in (1) and nails in (2).

13 / Other combinations of mitral and aortic valve disease

Frequency in survey: 11% of attempts at MRCP short cases.

Survey note: patients with any combination of aortic and mitral valve disease may be found in the examination (including, very rarely, lesions of one valve in combination with a prosthetic valve—see p. 228). Whenever you are examining the heart it is essential that, having found some obvious murmurs, you go in search of the others which may be present and less obvious, before presenting your findings (see experience 83, p. 458; anecdote 37, p. 497).

If the examiner seeks an opinion as to which are the main lesions, or if you feel confident to offer, the criteria used are the same as those described under mixed mitral valve disease (p. 76) and mixed aortic valve disease (p. 94). The example here is of a *record* of mixed mitral and aortic valve disease.

Record

There is a left thoracotomy scar, and the patient has a malar flush. The pulse is irregularly irregular (give rate) and *slow rising* (can be difficult to assess if the patient is in atrial fibrillation) in character. The venous pressure is not elevated. The apex is . . . (give appropriate word on the basis of what you find; e.g. thrusting, heaving, lifting, etc.) in the anterior axillary line and there is a *left parasternal heave*. There is a *systolic thrill* at the apex, in the aortic area and in the neck. The first heart sound is *loud*, there is a harsh *ejection systolic murmur* in the aortic area radiating into the neck, a *pansystolic murmur* at the lower left sternal edge radiating to the *apex* and to the *axilla*, an *early diastolic murmur* just audible in the aortic area and down the *left sternal edge* with the patient *sitting forward* in *expiration*, and an *opening snap* followed by a *mid-diastolic rumbling murmur* localized to the apex.

The findings suggest mixed aortic and mitral valve disease. The slow rising pulse suggests aortic stenosis is the dominant aortic valve lesion. It is not possible to ascertain clinically which is the major mitral valve lesion.* Further investigation involving echocardiography, probably leading on to cardiac catheterization with left ventricular angiography would be required to assess the haemodynamic significance of each lesion.

---

* In the case of severe mitral stenosis the signs of significant aortic stenosis may be underestimated. A displaced apex in the above setting would tend to suggest that mitral incompetence is haemodynamically dominant.

14 / Mixed aortic valve disease

Frequency in survey: 11% of attempts at MRCP short cases.

Record 1

The pulse is regular (give rate) and *slow rising* (may have a *bisferiens* character). The venous pressure is not raised. The apex beat is palpable 1 cm to the left of the mid-clavicular line as a *forceful, sustained heave*. There is a *systolic thrill* palpable at the apex, in the aortic area and also in the carotid. There is a *harsh ejection systolic murmur* in the aortic area radiating into the neck, the *aortic component* of the second sound is *soft*, and there is an *early diastolic murmur* down the *left sternal edge* audible when the patient is sitting forward in expiration.

The diagnosis is mixed aortic valve disease. Since the pulse is slow rising rather than collapsing, there is a systolic thrill, the second sound is soft and the apex has a forceful heaving quality, I think this is predominant aortic stenosis. (Systolic blood pressure will be low with a low pulse pressure.)

Record 2

The pulse is regular (give rate), of *large volume* and *collapsing* (may have a *bisferiens* character). The venous pressure is not raised. The apex beat is *thrusting* in the *anterior axillary line* in the sixth intercostal space. There is a harsh *ejection systolic murmur* in the aortic area radiating into the neck and an *early diastolic murmur* down the *left sternal edge* (loudest with the patient sitting forward in expiration).

The diagnosis is mixed aortic valve disease. Since the pulse is collapsing rather than plateau in character and the apex is displaced and thrusting, I think the predominant lesion is aortic incompetence. (Blood pressure will show a wide pulse pressure.)

Often mixed aortic murmurs will be due to either aortic stenosis with incidental aortic incompetence or severe aortic incompetence with a systolic flow murmur.* In such cases commenting on dominance is easy. If it is not clear clinically which lesion is predominant and the examiners wish your opinion, point out the factors in favour of each (Table 3.14), stress that you would like to measure the blood pressure and how this would help and lean towards or, if possible, come down in favour of the one you think most likely, giving the reasons; but point out that in this case cardiac catheter studies with left ventricular angiography and an aortogram to show the aortic regurgitation would be required to be certain (see p. 76 for an example of how this might be done in the case of mixed mitral valve disease). Echocardiography may help but Doppler valve gradient is inaccurate in the presence of significant aortic incompetence.

---

*NB The causes of aortic incompetence in this latter case—
see p. 104.

Table 3.14 Factors pointing to a predominant lesion in mixed aortic valve disease

	Aortic incompetence	Aortic stenosis
Pulse	Mainly collapsing	Mainly slow rising
Apex	Thrusting, displaced	Heaving, not displaced much
Systolic thrill	Absent	Present
Systolic murmur	Not loud, not harsh	Loud, harsh
Blood pressure		
systolic	High	Low
pulse pressure	Wide	Narrow

15 / Systemic sclerosis/CRST syndrome

Frequency in survey: main focus of a short case in 11% of attempts at MRCP short cases. Additional feature in a further 1%.

Record

The *skin* over the *fingers* and *face* (of this middle-aged female) is *smooth*, *shiny* and *tight*. There is *sclerodactyly*, the *nails* are *atrophic* and there is evidence of *Raynaud's phenomenon* (p. 350). There is atrophy of the soft tissues at the ends of the fingers. There is *telangiectasia* of the face and pigmentation. There are nodules of *calcinosis** palpable in some of the fingers.

The diagnosis is systemic sclerosis or CRST† syndrome.

Other signs which may be present

Skin ulcers

Vitiligo (p. 279)

Dry eyes and dry mouth (Sjögren's syndrome—see p. 221)

Dyspnoea or inspiratory crackles (diffuse interstitial fibrosis‡—decreased pulmonary diffusion capacity is the first sign; overspill pneumonitis may also occur).

Other systems which may be involved

Oesophagus (dysphagia or other oesophageal symptoms are present in 45–60%; oesophageal manometry is abnormal and shows diminished peristalsis in 90%)

Kidney (renal failure occurs in 20%—it is late but often fatal; it may be associated with malignant hypertension which tends to be responsive to ACE inhibitors but is otherwise resistant to therapy)

Heart (pericardial effusion is not an uncommon finding if careful echocardiography is performed; cardiomyopathy may occur but is rare)

Musculoskeletal (inflammatory arthritis or myositis —their presence raises the possibility of mixed connective tissue disease§ and therefore increased likelihood of improvement with steroid therapy)

Intestine (rarely hypomotility with a dilated second part of the duodenum leads to bacterial overgrowth, which in turn leads to steatorrhoea and malabsorption; wide-mouthed colonic diverticuli, and the rare pneumatosis cystoides are other abnormalities which may occur)

Liver (may be associated with primary biliary cirrhosis—p. 222).

For colour photograph see p. 532.

---

* If there is diffuse deposition of calcium in subcutaneous tissue in the presence of acrosclerosis this is termed the Thibierge–Weissenbach syndrome.

† CRST or CREST is the association of calcinosis, Raynaud's, oesophageal involvement, sclerodactyly and telangiectasia. It may be a variant of systemic sclerosis associated with a more benign prognosis.

‡ Pulmonary hypertension may develop independent of parenchymal changes, suggesting primary pulmonary vessel disease which may respond to steroids. Renal failure has now been replaced by pulmonary complications as the major cause of death in systemic sclerosis. Pleural effusions, pulmonary hypertension, interstitial lung disease, progressive pulmonary fibrosis and obstructive airways disease, all contribute to respiratory failure. Pulmonary hypertension can develop suddenly; all patients should be followed closely for the changes in P_2. The appearance of tricuspid regurgitation is evidence of established pulmonary hypertension. Aggressive vasodilation therapy should be used to treat pulmonary hypertension.

§ Mixed connective tissue disease is a clinical overlap between systemic sclerosis, SLE and polymyositis. The serum has a high titre of antiribonuclear protein antibody. The fluorescent antinuclear antibodies are typically distributed in a speckled pattern.

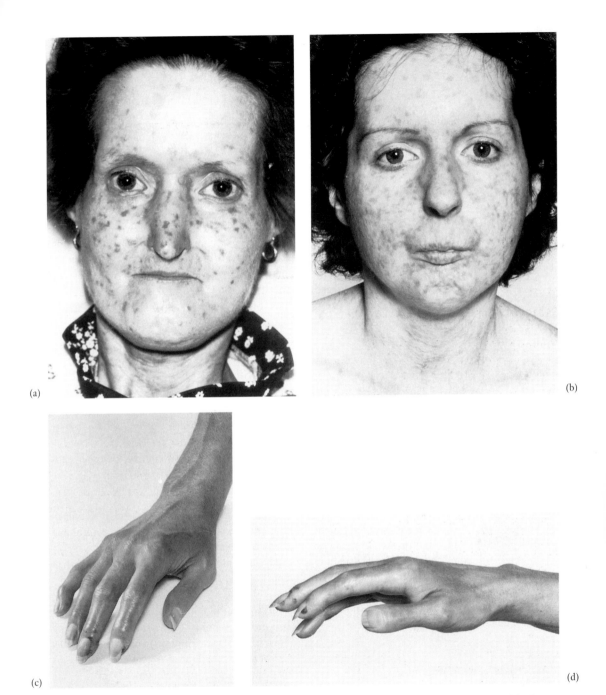

(a)

(b)

(c)

(d)

Fig. 3.15 (a) Note telangiectasia, pinched nose and adherent skin. (b) Perioral tethering with pseudorhagades. (c) Tight, shiny, adherent skin and vasculitis. (d) Atrophy of the finger pulps.

16 / Exophthalmos

Frequency in survey: main focus of a short case in 11% of attempts at MRCP short cases. Additional feature in a further 8%.

Record 1

There is (may be) bilateral *swelling* of the *medial caruncle* and *vascular congestion of the lateral canthus* with exophthalmos (protrusion of the eye revealing the *sclera above the lower lid* in the position of forward gaze) which is greater on the R/L side. Likely causes include:

1 Hyperthyroid Graves' disease* (?lid retraction or lag, tachycardia, bruit over the goitre; exophthalmos usually symmetrical)

2 Euthyroid Graves' disease (?no lid lag, *normal* pulse rate, no sweating or tremor, etc.)

3 Hypothyroid Graves' disease (?facies, scar of thyroidectomy, hoarse voice, slow pulse, ankle jerks, etc.).

Record 2

There is severe exophthalmos, *chemosis, corneal ulceration* and *ophthalmoplegia†* which is reducing the upward and lateral gaze most and which is responsible for the *diplopia*. Convergence (check for this) is also impaired. Testing the eye movements caused the patient discomfort (or pain).

The diagnosis is Graves' malignant exophthalmos (patient may be hyper-, eu- or hypothyroid).

Graves' malignant exophthalmos (congestive ophthalmopathy) can cause severe pain and the patient is at risk of blindness due to pressure on the optic nerve, if not treated. The condition may require large doses of systemic steroids and sometimes *tarsorrhaphy* (which may be in evidence in the examination patient) or even orbital decompression may be necessary. Radiotherapy has also been successfully used.

Other causes of exophthalmos

Bilateral (though asymmetrical) with conjunctival oedema:

Cavernous sinus thrombosis (follows infection of the orbit, nose and face; eyeball is painful and there is extreme venous congestion)

Caroticocavernous fistula (pulsating exophthalmos).

Unilateral:

Retro-orbital tumour (the protrusion measured with the Hertel exophthalmometer is usually >5mm more than the unaffected eye by the time of presentation, whereas Graves' eyes rarely achieve a difference of 5mm‡)

Orbital cellulitis.

---

* There are some studies that suggest that radioactive iodine therapy for Graves' disease may worsen exophthalmus though this is a controversial area.

† The ophthalmoplegia is due to infiltration, oedema and subsequent fibrosis of the external ocular muscles. It may occur with oedema of the lids and conjunctivae and precede the exophthalmos. For this reason the term 'congestive

ophthalmopathy' may be preferable to 'malignant exophthalmos'.

‡ Unless the diagnosis is unquestionably Graves' disease, the possibility of a retro-orbital tumour should always be investigated with computed tomographic (CT) scan, etc., regardless of the Hertel exophthalmometer measurement.

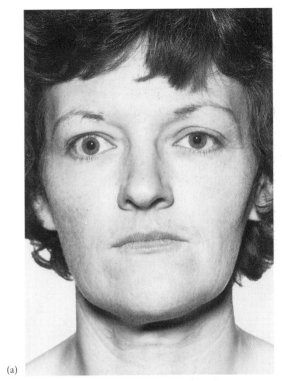

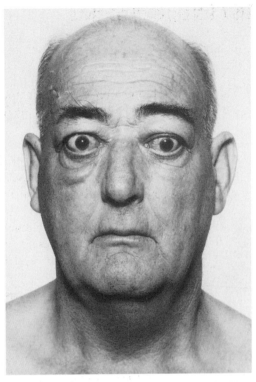

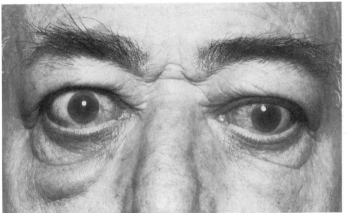

Fig. 3.16 (a) Unilateral
exophthalmos. (b1,2) Bilateral
exophthalmos (note proptosis,
ophthalmoplegia, conjunctival
congestion, swelling of the medial
caruncle and periorbital swelling).

(c)

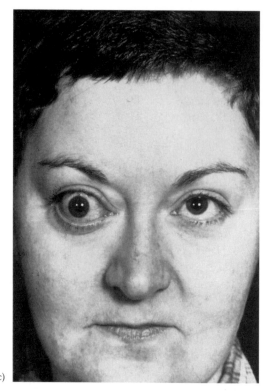

(d)

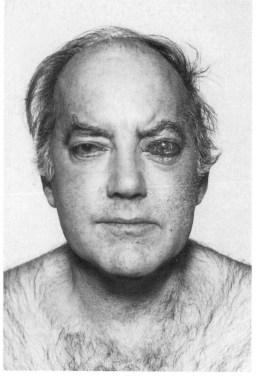

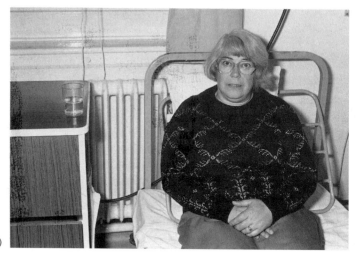

(e)

Fig. 3.16 (*continued*) (c)
Ophthalmoplegia of the right eye.
(d) Severe congestive
ophthalmopathy, chemosis and
corneal ulceration. (e) Tell-tale glass
of water (for examination of the
goitre) in a patient with
exophthalmos.

17 / Hepatomegaly (without splenomegaly)

Frequency in survey: main focus of a short case in 10% of attempts at MRCP short cases. Additional feature in at least a further 9%.

Record

The liver is palpable at . . . cm below the right costal margin (*?icterus, ascites*, signs of *cirrhosis* (do not miss gynaecomastia), *pigmentation, lymph nodes*).

Common causes

Cirrhosis—usually alcoholic (?spider naevi, gynaecomastia, etc.—p. 84)

Secondary carcinoma (?hard and knobbly, cachexia, evidence of primary)

Congestive cardiac failure (?jugular venous pulse (JVP) ↑, ankle oedema, *S3* or cardiac murmur; tender pulsatile liver with giant *v* waves in the JVP in tricuspid incompetence).

Other causes of hepatomegaly

Infections such as hepatitis A, glandular fever, Weil's disease and hepatitis B (remember hepatitis serology heads list of investigations in icterus of uncertain cause)

Primary tumours both malignant (hepatoma may complicate cirrhosis) and benign (liver cell adenoma is associated with oral contraceptive use)

Lymphoproliferative disorders (?lymph nodes)

Primary biliary cirrhosis (?middle-aged female, scratch marks, xanthelasma, etc.—p. 222)

Haemochromatosis (?male, slate-grey pigmentation, etc.—p. 253)

Sarcoidosis (?erythema nodosum or history of, lupus pernio, chest signs)

Amyloidosis (?rheumatoid arthritis or other underlying chronic disease—see footnote, p. 69)

Hydatid cyst (?Welsh connection — NB patient's name)

Amoebic abscess (?tropical connection — name, appearance)

Budd–Chiari syndrome (?icterus, ascites, tender hepatomegaly)

Riedel's lobe

Emphysema (apparent hepatomegaly).

Hard and knobbly hepatomegaly— possible causes

Malignancy—primary or secondary

Polycystic liver disease (?kidneys—p. 86)

Macronodular cirrhosis (following hepatitis B with widespread necrosis)

Hydatid cysts (may be eosinophilia; rupture may be associated with anaphylaxis)

Syphilitic gummas (late benign syphilis; there is usually hepatosplenomegaly and anaemia; rapid response to penicillin).

18 / Spastic paraparesis

Frequency in survey: main focus of a short case in 10% of attempts at MRCP short cases. Additional feature in a further 2%.

Record

The *tone* in the legs is *increased* and they are *weak* (in chronic immobilized cases there may be some disuse atrophy, and in severe cases there may be contractures). There is bilateral *ankle clonus*, patellar clonus and the *plantar* responses are *extensor*. (?Abdominal reflexes.)

The patient has a spastic paraparesis.* The most likely causes are:

1 Multiple sclerosis (?obvious nystagmus, incoordination or staccato speech from the end of the bed; ?impaired rapid alternate motion of arms when you check at the end of your leg examination—p. 433)

2 Cord compression (?sensory level; root, back or neck pain; no signs above level of lesion. NB Cervical spondylosis—see p. 211)

3 Trauma (?scar or deformity in back)

4 Birth injury (cerebral palsy—Little's disease)

5 Motor neurone disease (?no sensory signs, muscle fasciculation, etc.—p. 123).

Other causes

Syringomyelia (?kyphoscoliosis, wasted hands, dissociated sensory loss, Horner's syndrome, etc.—p. 305)

Anterior spinal artery thrombosis (sudden onset, ?dissociated sensory loss up to the level of the lesion)

Friedreich's ataxia (?pes cavus, cerebellar signs, kyphoscoliosis, etc.—p. 234)

Hereditary spastic paraplegia

Subacute combined degeneration of the cord† (?posterior column loss, absent ankle jerks,‡ peripheral neuropathy, anaemia—p. 314)

Parasagittal cranial meningioma

Human T-cell lymphotrophic virus type 1 (HTLV-1) infection§ (Afro-Caribbean populations—tropical spastic paraparesis)

Acquired immune deficiency syndrome (AIDS) myelopathy (late phase—direct human immunodeficiency virus (HIV) central nervous system involvement, p. 365)

General paralysis of the insane (?dementia, vacant expression, trombone tremor of the tongue, etc. —see p. 381)

Taboparesis (?Argyll Robertson pupils, posterior column loss, etc.—p. 381).

---

* A clue to the underlying cause of spastic paraparesis may be:
Cerebellar signs: Multiple sclerosis
               Friedreich's ataxia (?pes cavus)
Wasted hands: Cervical spondylosis (?inverted reflexes)
               Syringomyelia (?Horner's)
               Motor neurone disease (?prominent fasciculation)
† Stocking sensory loss (with or without absent ankle jerks) in association with a spastic paraplegia, i.e. extensor plantars, is strongly suggestive of subacute combined degeneration of the cord.
‡ Absent ankle jerks and upgoing plantars—p. 340.
§ The other main HTLV-1 associated disease is *adult T-cell*

leukaemia / lymphoma which is especially found in southern Japan and the Caribbean Islands. The clinical course is often associated with a high white count, *hypercalcaemia* and cutaneous involvement. Measurement of HTLV-1 antibodies should always be considered in the patient with unexplained hypercalcaemia. Other HTLV-1 associated diseases include polymyositis, infective dermatitis—a chronic generalized eczema of the skin—and B-cell chronic lymphocytic leukaemia.

HTLV-2 has been found in some patients with T-cell hairy cell leukaemia and in parenteral drug abusers but remains a true orphan virus, without, at the time of writing, clear disease association.

19 / Fibrosing alveolitis

Frequency in survey: main focus of a short case in 10% of attempts at MRCP short cases. Additional feature in a further 1%.

Record

There is *clubbing* of the fingers, (may be) *cyanosis*, and there are *fine inspiratory crackles* (or crepitations—whichever term you prefer) at both bases.

The likely diagnosis is (cryptogenic*) fibrosing alveolitis (CFA).

Conditions which may be associated with cryptogenic fibrosing alveolitis

Rheumatoid arthritis (?hands, nodules)

Systemic lupus erythematosus (?typical rash)

Systemic sclerosis (?typical mask-like facies, telangiectasia, sclerodactyly—p. 98)

Sjögren's syndrome (?dry eyes and dry mouth)

Polymyositis (?proximal muscle weakness and tenderness—p. 329)

Dermatomyositis (?heliotrope rash on eyes/hands and polymyositis—p. 293)

Ulcerative colitis (?colostomy)

Chronic active hepatitis (?icterus, hepatosplenomegaly)

Raynaud's phenomenon

Digital vasculitis.

Conditions in which alveolitis and pulmonary fibrosis occur

Sarcoidosis (?erythema nodosum or history of, lupus pernio)

Extrinsic allergic alveolitis (?farmer, pigeon racer, etc.)

Asbestosis (?lagger, etc.)

Silicosis (?slate worker or granite quarrier, etc.)

Drug reactions (e.g. bleomycin, busulphan, nitrofurantoin, amiodarone)

Chemical inhalation (e.g. beryllium, mercury)

Poison ingestion (e.g. paraquat)

Radiation fibrosis

Mitral valve disease

Uraemia

Adult respiratory distress syndrome (complicating acute severe illness often with septicaemia).

---

* In the absence of an identifiable causal agent the fibrosing alveolitis is termed 'cryptogenic'. Occupational exposure to metal or wood dust is commoner in CFA patients than controls.

Frequency in survey: main focus of a short case in 9% of attempts at MRCP short cases. Additional feature in a further 1% (not counting where additional to other valve lesions).

Record

The pulse is regular* (give rate), of large volume and *collapsing* in character. The venous pressure is not raised but *vigorous arterial pulsations* can be seen in the neck (Corrigan's sign†). The apex beat is *thrusting* in the anterior axillary line, in the sixth intercostal space. There is an *early diastolic murmur* audible down the left sternal edge and in the aortic area; it is *louder* in *expiration* with the patient *sitting forward*. (The blood pressure may be wide with a high systolic and low diastolic. In severe cases it may be 250–300/30–50.)

The diagnosis is aortic incompetence (now consider looking for *Argyll Robertson pupils, high-arched palate* or *marfanoid* appearance, or obvious features of an arthropathy especially *ankylosing spondylitis*. If these are not present the aortic incompetence is likely to be rheumatic in origin — rheumatic fever and infective endocarditis are the commonest identifiable causes).

The early diastolic murmur can be difficult to hear and is easily overlooked (see anecdote 37, p. 497). It should be specifically sought with the patient sitting forward in expiration. Listen for the 'absence of silence' in the early part of diastole. The murmur is usually best heard over the mid-sternal region or at the lower left sternal edge. In some cases, particularly syphilitic aortitis, it is loudest in the aortic area. There is often an accompanying systolic murmur due to increased flow which does not necessarily indicate coexistent aortic stenosis (see p. 94).

If there is a mid-diastolic murmur at the apex it may be an Austin Flint murmur‡ or it may represent some associated mitral valve disease. These two may be clinically indistinguishable, though the presence of a loud first heart sound and an opening snap suggest the latter. Though the first heart sound in the Austin Flint may be loud, it is never palpable (i.e. no tapping impulse).

Causes of aortic incompetence

Rheumatic fever

Infective endocarditis (usually occurs on a deformed valve)

Syphilitic aortitis (?Argyll Robertson pupils; there may be an aneurysm of the ascending aorta)

Ankylosing spondylitis (?male with fixed kyphosis and stooped 'question mark' posture — p. 184; aortic incompetence may also occur in the other seronegative arthropathies — psoriatic, ulcerative colitic and Reiter's syndrome)

Rheumatoid arthritis (?hands, nodules)

---

* The pulse is usually regular unless there is associated mitral valve disease.

† Other physical signs which result from a large pulse volume and peripheral vasodilatation include de Musset's sign (the head nods with each pulsation) and Quincke's sign (capillary pulsation visible in the nail beds). Of greater clinical value is Duroziez's sign—the femoral artery is compressed and auscultated proximally with a stethoscope; a diastolic murmur implies retrograde flow and aortic incompetence of at least moderate severity.

‡ The Austin Flint murmur occurs in severe aortic incompetence. It is probably attributable to (i) the regurgitant jet interfering with the opening of the anterior mitral valve leaflet, and (ii) the left ventricular diastolic pressure rising more rapidly than the left atrial diastolic pressure.

Marfan's syndrome (?tall with long extremities, arachnodactyly and high-arched palate, etc. — p. 267)

Hurler's syndrome

Severe hypertension (by causing aortic dilatation; complications of hypertension such as ascending aortic aneurysm or dissecting aneurysm may also cause aortic incompetence)

Coarctation of the aorta (late complication)

Associated ventricular septal defect (loss of support for valve).

Indications for surgery

Although patients tolerate aortic incompetence longer than aortic stenosis (p. 112), the clinician's aim is to replace the valve *before* serious left ventricular dysfunction occurs. Every effort should be made to recognize any reduction in left ventricular function or reserve as early as possible. Serial chest X-rays, echocardiograms and radionuclear angiography will show a gradual increase in cardiac size. Radionuclear angiography can be particularly useful in showing evidence of early left ventricular dysfunction in asymptomatic patients. The left ventricular ejection fraction, though normal at rest, may show a subnormal rise during exercise. Aortic valve replacement may have to be undertaken as a matter of urgency in patients with infective endocarditis in whom the leaking valve causes rapidly progressive left ventricular dilatation.

21 / Hemiplegia

Frequency in survey: main focus of a short case in 9% of attempts at MRCP short cases. Additional feature in a further 3%.

Record

There is a R/L *upper motor neurone* weakness of the facial muscles.* The R/L *arm* and *leg* are *weak* (without wasting) with *increased tone* and *hyperreflexia*. The R/L plantar is *extensor* and the *abdominal reflexes* are *diminished* on the R/L side.

This is a R/L hemiplegia.

There is also (may be) *hemisensory loss* on the R/L side. Visual field testing reveals (may be) a R/L homonymous hemianopia. The most likely causes are:

1 Cerebrovascular accident due to cerebral
   (a) thrombosis (?hypertension)
   (b) haemorrhage (?hypertension)
   (c) embolism (?atrial fibrillation, murmurs, bruits)
2 Brain tumour (?insidious onset, papilloedema, headaches; ?evidence of primary e.g. clubbing).

A right-sided hemiplegia associated with dysphasia would suggest (in a right-handed patient) that the causative lesion is affecting the speech centres in the dominant hemisphere (see p. 261) as well as the motor cortex (precentral gyrus) and if there are sensory signs, the sensory cortex (postcentral gyrus). If cerebrovascular in origin the causative lesion is likely to be in the *carotid* distribution.

The presence of signs such as nystagmus, ocular palsy, dysphagia (?nasogastric or PEG (percutaneous endoscopic gastrostomy) feeding tube) and cerebellar signs suggest that the hemiparesis is due to a brainstem lesion. If cerebrovascular in origin the lesion is likely to be in *vertebrobasilar* distribution (see p. 438 for the eponymous syndromes†).

Parietal lobe and related signs‡

Agnosia. Though peripheral sensation is intact (tactile, visual, auditory) the patient fails to appreciate the significance of the sensory stimulus without the aid of other senses.

Tactile agnosia or astereognosis (contralateral posterior parietal lobe)—inability to recognize a familiar object placed in the hand (e.g. pen, keys) with the eyes closed. Opening the eyes or hearing the keys rattle may allow recognition.

Visual agnosia (parieto-occipital lesions—especially in the left hemisphere of right-handed patients) — the patient is not able to identify the familiar object by sight (e.g. a pen, surroundings) but may do at once when he is allowed to handle it.

Auditory agnosia (temporal lobe of dominant hemisphere)—the patient may only be able to recognize the sound of a voice, telephone or music when he is allowed to use the senses of vision or touch.

Autotopagnosia (usually a left hemiplegia in a right-handed person)—difficulty in perceiving or identifying the various parts of the body; the patient may be unaware of the left side of his body. It may be associated with anosognosia in which case

---

* In an upper motor neurone lesion, the lower face is much weaker than the upper because the muscles frontalis, orbicularis oculi and corrugator superficialis ('raise your eyebrows', 'screw your eyes up tight', 'frown') are bilaterally innervated and are all only minimally impaired.

† These are in fact rarely used in everyday practice.
‡ These did not occur in our survey of MRCP short cases.

there is no appreciation of a disability (e.g. hemiplegia, blindness) on the same side.

Apraxia. Whereas in agnosia the difficulty is in recognition, in apraxia it is in execution. Though power, sensation and coordination are all normal, the patient is unable to perform certain familiar activities. It may affect:

The upper limbs — e.g. difficulty using a pen, comb or toothbrush, winding a watch, dressing or undressing ('dressing apraxia'§).

The lower limbs — may mimic ataxia or weakness‖ — the patient may appear unable to lift one foot in front of the other (gait apraxia).

The trunk — the patient may have difficulty seating himself on a chair or lavatory seat, getting on to his bed, or in turning over in bed.

The face — the patient may be unable to whistle, put out his tongue or close his eyes.

The lesions (tumours or atrophy) tend to be in the corpus callosum, parietal lobes and premotor areas. Dominant lobe lesions may produce bilateral apraxia. Unilateral left-sided apraxia may be caused by a lesion in the right posterior parietal region or in the corpus collosum of a right-handed patient. The lesion in 'dressing apraxia' is usually in the right parieto-occipital region. In 'constructional apraxia' (most often seen in patients with hepatic encephalopathy) the patient is unable to construct simple figures such as triangles, squares or crosses from matchsticks.

Dyslexia (impairment of reading ability), **dysgraphia** (impairment of writing ability) and **dyscalculia** (difficulty with calculating) usually represent lesions in the posterior parietal lobe.

---

§ Some authorities consider this to be a visuospatial right hemisphere disorder and not a true apraxia.
‖ A parietal lobe lesion may cause ataxia, hemiparesis or marked astereognosis. In hemiparesis of parietal origin, the limbs are often hypotonic with an absent plantar response, rather than spastic. The limb muscles may even waste (like a lower motor neurone lesion). Often the patient is disinclined to move the limb rather than actually paralysed.

22 / Old tuberculosis

Frequency in survey: 8% of attempts at MRCP short cases.

Record 1

The trachea is *deviated* to the R/L. The R/L upper chest shows *deformity* with *decreased expansion, dull percussion* note, *bronchial breathing* and *crepitations*. The apex beat is (may be) *displaced* to the R/L. There is a *thoracotomy scar* posteriorly with evidence of rib resections.

     The patient has had a R/L thoracoplasty for treatment of tuberculosis before the days of chemotherapy.

Record 2

The tracheal deviation to the R/L and the diminished expansion and crackles at the R/L apex suggest R/L apical fibrosis.

    Old tuberculosis is the likely cause.

Record 3

Expansion is diminished on the R/L with dullness and reduced/absent breath sounds at the R/L lung base. There is a R/L supraclavicular scar (there may also be crepitations).

    The patient has had a phrenic nerve crush for tuberculosis before the days of chemotherapy.

23 / Acromegaly

Frequency in survey: main focus of a short case in 8% of attempts at MRCP short cases. Additional feature in a further 1%.

Survey note: candidates were sometimes asked questions on subjects such as presentation, investigation and complications.

Record

The patient has prominent *supraorbital ridges* and a *large lower jaw*. The facial wrinkles are exaggerated and the lips are full. There is *poor occlusion* of the teeth, the *lower teeth overbiting* in front of the upper (prognathism). The *nose, tongue* and *ears* are enlarged and the patient is *kyphotic*. The *hands* are *large*, doughy and spade-shaped,* and the *skin* over the back of them is *thickened* (shake hands and examine the dorsum). There is (may be) loss of the thenar eminence bilaterally with impaired sensation in the median nerve distribution (*carpal tunnel syndrome*). The patient is *sweating* excessively and is mildly *hirsute* (one-third of cases). The *voice* is husky and cavernous. There is a *bitemporal peripheral visual field defect*.

The diagnosis is acromegaly.

Other physical signs which may be present

Bowed legs
Rolling gait
Goitre
Gynaecomastia
Galactorrhoea
Small gonads
Greasy skin
Acne
Acanthosis nigricans
Osteoarthrosis
Prominent superficial veins of extremities
Proximal muscle weakness
Cardiomegaly (hypertension and cardiomyopathy)
IIIrd nerve palsy.

Other features

Diabetes mellitus (glycosuria, glucose intolerance or frank diabetes may occur; it is usually mild and ketoacidosis is rare; it is somewhat resistant to insulin)
Hypertension (20–50%)
Hypercalciuria (common)
Hypercalcaemia† (occasionally)
Diabetes insipidus (normally due to hypothalamic pressure effect; if there is impaired cortisol secretion symptoms may be masked)
Hypopituitarism (p. 297)
Osteoporosis.

---

* Shaking hands with the patient may give the impression of losing one's hands in a mass of dough.

† In some this disappears when the acromegaly is successfully treated. In others it is due to associated hyperparathyroidism as part of *multiple endocrine adenopathy (MEA) type 1* (Werner's syndrome) which is two or more of:
1 Pituitary tumour (eosinophil or chromophobe)
2 Islet-cell tumour (gastrin or insulin)
3 Primary hyperparathyroidism (adenoma or hyperplasia)
4 Adrenocortical adenoma (see also p. 231 and footnote).
MEA type 1 should probably be regarded as a complex of separate genetic abnormalities rather than as a consequence of a single primary disease. It should not be confused with MEA type 2 which is usually an autosomal dominant trait with a high degree of penetrance (see footnot, p. 128).

Symptoms before presentation‡

Excessive sweating

Increasing size of shoes, gloves, hats, dentures and rings

Paraesthesiae of hands and feet

Digital pain and stiffness (of slowly expanding fingers and toes)

Arthralgia

Hypogonadism (amenorrhoea, loss of libido)

Headache (may be severe; may occur without clinically detectable enlargement of the pituitary tumour; the mechanism is not clear)

Visual field or acuity disturbance.

Investigations

Comparative study of old photographs of the patient

Skull X-ray

CT scan or magnetic resonance imaging (MRI) scan of pituitary fossa

X-ray for heel pad thickness (increased) is rarely carried out nowadays

Visual fields

Glucose tolerance test with growth hormone response (lack of suppression; sometimes a paradoxical rise)

Tests of anterior pituitary function (*adrenocorticotroph*: short Synacthen test,§ insulin tolerance test; *thyrotroph*: thyroid-stimulating hormone (TSH) plus total or free T_4; *gonadotroph*: menstrual history plus oestrodiol, luteinizing hormone (LH) and follicle-stimulating hormone (FSH) (female), potency plus testosterone (male); *lactotroph*: prolactin‖).

Treatments

Trans-sphenoidal hypophysectomy

Transfrontal hypophysectomy in some cases with large extensive adenomata

External irradiation (especially if surgery fails; takes 1–10 years to take effect)

Radioactive gold or yttrium implants (very restricted in terms of availability)

Bromocriptine (50% respond but the size of the tumour is not reduced; useful for growth hormone hypersecretion after surgery)

Long-acting somatostatin analogues (require parenteral administration); effective in lowering growth hormone until surgery/radiotherapy; tumour may shrink in some cases.

---

‡ The mean age of onset has been estimated at about 27 years whereas the mean age of presentation is over 40 years, i.e. there is an average pre-presentation lapse of 13–14 years.
§ In hypopituitarism, the adrenal cortex does not respond sufficiently in the short Synacthen test. It needs to be primed continually by adrenocorticotrophic hormone (ACTH) from a functioning pituitary in order to be responsive.

‖ The prolactin may be low in hypopituitarism. However, production may also be elevated because (i) some growth hormone secreting pituitary tumours co-secrete prolactin, and (ii) any pituitary macroadenoma which presses on the pituitary stalk will interfere with dopamine suppression of prolactin production and lead to hyperprolactinaemia.

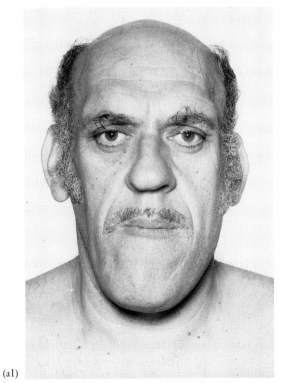
(a1)

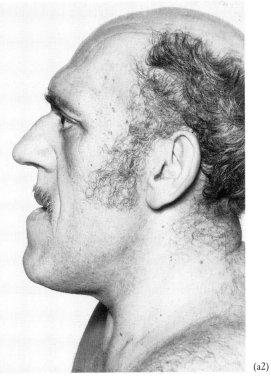
(a2)

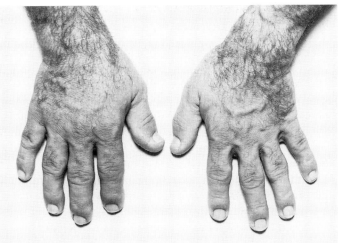
(b)

Fig. 3.23 (a1,2) Acromegalic facies.
(b) Large hands with thickened skin.

Frequency in survey: 8% of attempts at MRCP short cases.

Record 1

The *pulse* is regular (give rate), of *small volume* and *slow rising*. The venous pressure is not raised (unless there is cardiac failure). The apex beat is palpable 1 cm to the left of the mid-clavicular line in the fifth intercostal space (the apex position is normal or only slightly displaced in pure aortic stenosis unless the left ventricle is starting to fail) as a forceful *sustained heave*.* There is a *systolic thrill* palpable over the aortic area and the carotids (may be felt over the apex). Auscultation reveals a *harsh ejection systolic murmur* in the aortic area *radiating* into the *neck*, and the *aortic second sound* is *soft* (or absent). (The blood pressure is usually low normal with a decreased difference between systole and diastole—pulse pressure.)

The diagnosis is aortic stenosis.

Possible causes

1 Rheumatic heart disease (mitral valve is usually involved as well and aortic incompetence is often present)

2 Bicuspid aortic valve (commoner in males; typically presents in the sixth decade)

3 Degenerative calcification (in the elderly; the stenosis is usually relatively mild)

4 Congenital (may worsen during childhood and adolescence due to calcification).

In the late stages of aortic stenosis when cardiac failure with low cardiac output supervenes, the murmur may become markedly diminished in intensity. The murmur of associated mitral stenosis should be carefully sought, particularly in the female patient, because the association of these two obstructive lesions tends to diminish the physical findings of each. Mitral stenosis is easily missed and the severity of aortic stenosis underestimated. As with all valvular heart diseases, echocardiography is of great value in a situation like this.

Indications for surgery

In the adult patient valve replacement is indicated for symptoms or a systolic pressure gradient greater than 50–60 mmHg (lower when the left ventricle has

failed), as without operation the outlook for these patients is poor. Critical coronary lesions can be bypassed at the same time. Asymptomatic children and young adults can be treated with valvotomy if the obstruction is severe, as the operative risk appears to be less than the risk of sudden death. This is only temporary but may postpone the need for valve replacement for many years.

Record 2

The *carotid pulses* are *normal*, the apical impulse is just palpable and not displaced. There are *no thrills*. There is an *ejection systolic murmur* which is not (usually) harsh or loud and is audible in the aortic area but only faintly in the neck. The aortic component of the second sound is well

---

* There may also be a presystolic impulse due to left atrial overactivity (this is also felt in moderately severe cases of hypertrophic obstructive cardiomyopathy). The result is a double apical impulse best felt in the left lateral recumbent

position. Other signs which may be present include: a fourth heart sound; a single second sound or even paradoxical splitting of the second sound which are both due to prolonged left ventricular ejection.

heard. The blood pressure is normal (or may be hypertensive).

These findings suggest aortic sclerosis (or minimal aortic stenosis) rather than significant aortic stenosis. (NB The differentiation of this from the other causes of a short systolic murmur: prolapsing mitral valve, p. 209; trivial mitral incompetence and hypertrophic obstructive cardiomyopathy, p. 436.)

25 / Graves' disease

Frequency in survey: main focus of a short case in 8% of attempts at MRCP short cases. Additional feature in a further 8%.

Record 1

The patient (usually female) is *thin*, has *sweaty palms*, a *fine tremor* of the outstretched hands, a *tachycardia*,* and she is *fidgety* and nervous. There is a small diffuse *goitre* with a *bruit*, and she has *exophthalmos* (p. 98) with *lid lag*.†

This patient is *thyrotoxic* and has Graves' disease.

Record 2

There is *exophthalmos* (?chemosis, ophthalmoplegia, diplopia, lateral tarsorrhaphy), *thyroid acropachy*,‡ and the lesions on the front of the shins are *pretibial myxoedema* (p. 275). The pulse is regular* and the *pulse rate* is *normal* (give rate), the palms are *not sweaty*, and there is *no hand tremor* or *lid lag*. There is a *thyroidectomy scar*.

The diagnosis is *euthyroid* Graves' disease,§ the patient having been treated by thyroidectomy in the past.

Male to female ratio is 1 : 5.

Record 3

This patient with *exophthalmos* (?chemosis, ophthalmoplegia, diplopia, lateral tarsorrhaphy, goitre, thyroidectomy scar, pretibial myxoedema, thyroid acropachy) has *hypothyroid facies*, a *hoarse voice*, *slow pulse** and *slowly relaxing reflexes*.

The patient has Graves' disease and is clinically *hypothyroid*. It is likely that she had hyperthyroidism treated in the past (?thyroidectomy or radioactive iodine) and is probably now on inadequate thyroxine replacement. (Because of the close links between the autoimmune thyroid diseases—see below — patients with Graves' disease occasionally go on to develop hypothyroidism spontaneously.)

---

*The pulse may be regular or irregular—the patient may have sinus rhythm or atrial fibrillation whatever the thyroid status (hyperthyroid; eu- or hypothyroid due to treatment).

† Graves' disease may be present in the absence of the eye signs and in an elderly male patient. There may be evidence of the humoral autoimmunity, more specifically a circulating antibody to the thyrotrophin (TSH) receptor. The thyroid gland may even have a nodular enlargement but its radio iodine uptake is uniformly increased throughout the gland between the nodules in autoimmune disease (Graves' disease). The patient with nodular goitre and thyrotoxicosis due to autonomous hypersecretion of nodule(s) that does not have an autoimmune (thyrotoxicosis) basis, will have some nodules with increased uptake (hot nodules) on the isotope scan. Such patients are more likely to relapse after antithyroid drug therapy than patients with Graves' disease.

‡ Thyroid acropachy may resemble finger clubbing in hypertrophic pulmonary osteoarthropathy (HPOA). However, in thyroid acropachy new bone formation seen on X-ray has the appearance of soap bubbles on the bone surface with coarse spicules. In HPOA new bone is formed in a linear distribution. Sometimes the new bone formation in acropachy is both visible and palpable along the phalanges.

§ Graves' exophthalmos is due to increased retro-orbital fat and enlarged intraorbital muscles infiltrated with lymphocytes and containing increased water and mucopolysaccharide. It may develop in the absence of hyperthyroidism and remit, persist or develop further despite successful treatment of hyperthyroidism. Pretibial myxoedema tends to develop after the hyperthyroidism has been treated—especially with radioactive iodine.

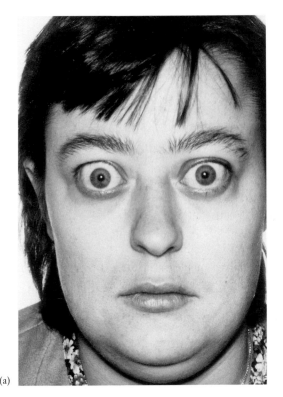

(a)

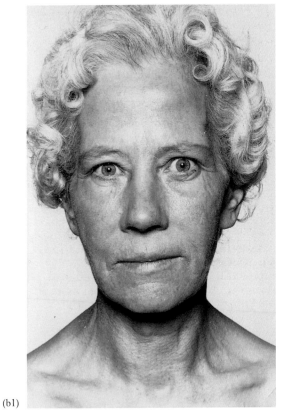

(b1)

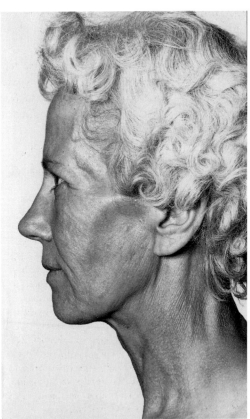

(b2)

Fig. 3.25 (a) Graves'disease. (b1,2) Hyperthyroidism in a patient who presented with the complaint that she had noticed a staring appearance of her left eye (note thinning of the hair in the temporal region).

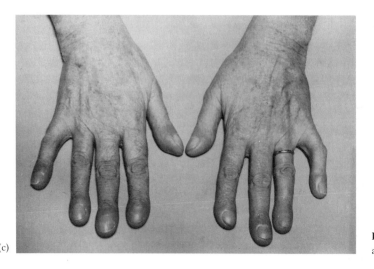

(c)

Fig. 3.25 (*continued*) (c) Thyroid acropachy.

Other signs which may occur

Fever (rarely hyperpyrexia)

Systolic hypertension with wide pulse pressure

Cutaneous vasodilatation

Systolic murmur due to increased blood flow

Proximal muscle weakness (thyrotoxic myopathy)

Hyperactive reflexes

Choreoathetoid movements (in children)

Fine thin hair (females may show temporal recession of the hairline)

Onycholysis (Plummer's nails, typically found bilaterally on the fourth finger)

Palmar erythema

Spider naevi

Splenomegaly (minimal)

Hepatomegaly (minimal)

Palpable lymph nodes (especially axillae)

Thyrotoxic osteoporosis (only rarely causes kyphosis or loss of height).

Important symptoms of hyperthyroidism (if asked to ask the patient some questions) are heat intolerance, weight loss, increased appetite, diarrhoea, exertional dyspnoea, undue fatiguability, 'can't keep still', irritability and nervousness.

The other organ-specific autoimmune diseases (see also p. 279) of which autoimmune thyroid disease‖ is an example include:

1 Pernicious anaemia

2 Atrophic gastritis with iron deficiency anaemia

3 Diabetes mellitus

4 Addison's disease

5 Idiopathic hypoparathyroidism

6 Premature ovarian failure

7 Renal tubular acidosis

8 Fibrosing alveolitis

9 Chronic active hepatitis

10 Primary biliary cirrhosis.

All of these diseases show a *marked female preponderance*. Premature greying of the hair, alopecia areata and vitiligo (see also p. 279) are all associated with this group of diseases. Autoimmune thyroiditis is also associated with:

1 Sjögren's syndrome

2 Myasthenia gravis

3 Systemic sclerosis

4 Mixed connective tissue disease

5 Cranial arteritis

6 Polymyalgia rheumatica.

‖ Graves' disease is one of the three closely related autoimmune thyroid diseases—the others being Hashimoto's thyroiditis and its atrophic variant, myxoedema. Among patients with one of these three it is typical to find relatives with one of the other two. Some patients appear to have a combination which has been termed 'hashitoxicosis'.

26 / Ocular palsy

Frequency in survey: main focus of a short case in 8% of attempts at MRCP short cases. Additional feature in a further 3%.

Record 1

The patient has a *convergent strabismus* at rest. There is *impairment* of the *lateral movement* of the R/L eye and *diplopia* is worse on looking to the R/L (the outermost image comes from the affected eye).

The patient has a *VIth nerve palsy*.

Possible causes

1 The causes of mononeuritis multiplex*
2 Multiple sclerosis (?ipsilateral facial palsy because the VIth and VIIth nuclei are very close in the pons; ?nystagmus, cerebellar signs, pyramidal signs, pale discs, etc.—p. 433)
3 Raised intracranial pressure (?papilloedema) causing stretching of the nerve (a false localizing sign) during its long intracranial course
4 Neoplasm (?papilloedema; associated ipsilateral facial palsy if pontine tumour)
5 Myasthenia gravis (see below)
6 Vascular lesions (probably common as a cause of 'idiopathic' VIth nerve palsy)
7 Compression by aneurysm (ectatic basilar artery; uncommon)
8 Subacute meningitis (carcinomatous; lymphomatous; fungal (NB AIDS); tuberculous; meningovascular syphilis—see p. 381).

Record 2

There is *ptosis*. Lifting the eyelids reveals *divergent strabismus* and a *dilated pupil*. The eye is fixed in a *down and out position* (and there is *angulated diplopia*).

The diagnosis is complete (NB the condition is often partial) *IIIrd nerve palsy*.

Possible causes

1 Unruptured aneurysm† of posterior communicating (or internal carotid) artery (painful)
2 The causes of mononeuritis multiplex*
3 Vascular lesion† (if there is a contralateral hemiplegia the diagnosis is Weber's syndrome—p. 438).

---

* The causes of mononeuritis multiplex include diabetes mellitus, polyarteritis nodosa and Churg–Strauss syndrome, rheumatoid disease, SLE, Wegener's granulomatosis, sarcoidosis, carcinoma, amyloidosis, leprosy, Sjögren's syndrome and Lyme disease.
† If the ophthalmoplegia is predominant compared to the ptosis/pupil dilatation, the cause is likely to be vascular (intrinsic). If the ophthalmoplegia is minimal compared to the ptosis/pupil dilatation, the cause is more likely to be extrinsic compression by aneurysm, pituitary tumour, meningioma, etc.

4 Midbrain demyelinating lesion‡ (?cerebellar signs, staccato speech, pale discs, etc.—p. 433)

5 Myasthenia gravis (see below).

Other causes of a IIIrd nerve palsy

Subacute meningitis (carcinomatous; lymphomatous; fungal (NB AIDS); tuberculous; meningovascular syphilis — at one time the commonest cause, now very rare—p. 381)

Ophthalmoplegic migraine (similar to posterior communicating artery aneurysm except that it begins in childhood or adolescence, recovery is more rapid and is always complete; recovery is never complete with an aneurysm)

Parasellar neoplasmta†

Sphenoidal wing meningiomata†

Carcinomatous lesions of the skull base.†

Other causes of ocular palsy

Internuclear ophthalmoplegia (adduction impaired bilaterally but abduction normal or vice versa; ataxic nystagmus is present and distinguishes it from bilateral VIth nerve palsy—see p. 171; ?cerebellar signs)

Exophthalmic ophthalmoplegia (exophthalmos and diplopia — upward and outward gaze most often reduced)

Myasthenia gravis (?ptosis, variable strabismus, facial weakness with a snarling smile, proximal muscle weakness, weak nasal voice, all of which worsen with repetition—p. 269. NB It may superficially resemble IIIrd or VIth nerve palsy)

Cavernous sinus and superior orbital fissure syndromes (total or subtotal ophthalmoplegia which is often painful, together with sensory loss over the first division of the Vth nerve—absent corneal reflex; it is due to a tumour or carotid aneurysm affecting the IIIrd, IVth, Vth and VIth nerves as they travel together through the cavernous sinus into the superior orbital fissure — see Fig. 3.29d, p. 128)

Fourth nerve palsy (adducted eye cannot look downwards—the patient experiences 'one above the other' diplopia when attempting to do this; angulated diplopia occurs when looking down and out; the diplopia is worse when reading and going down stairs)

Ocular myopathy (see p. 226 and footnote, p. 345).

‡ IIIrd nerve palsy is rare in demyelinating disease; internuclear ophthalmoplegia (pp. 171 and 433) is a much commoner result of this condition.

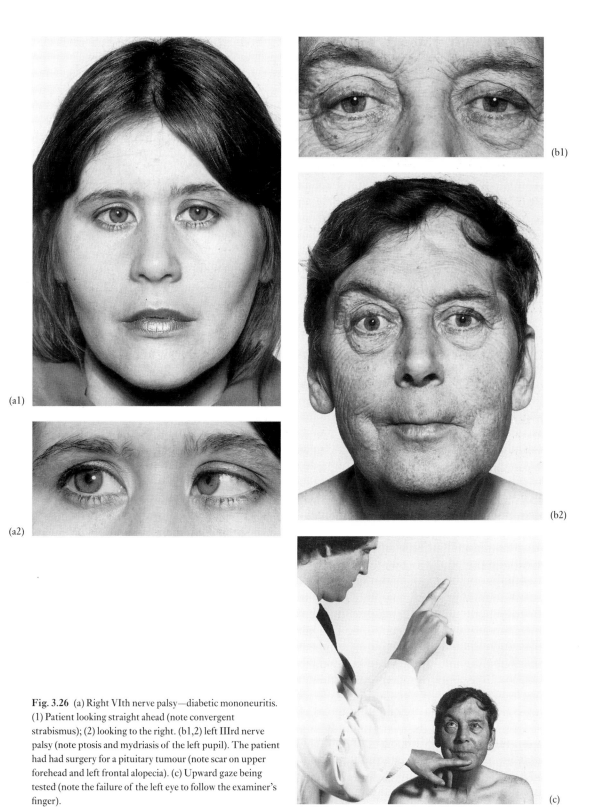

Fig. 3.26 (a) Right VIth nerve palsy—diabetic mononeuritis. (1) Patient looking straight ahead (note convergent strabismus); (2) looking to the right. (b1,2) left IIIrd nerve palsy (note ptosis and mydriasis of the left pupil). The patient had had surgery for a pituitary tumour (note scar on upper forehead and left frontal alopecia). (c) Upward gaze being tested (note the failure of the left eye to follow the examiner's finger).

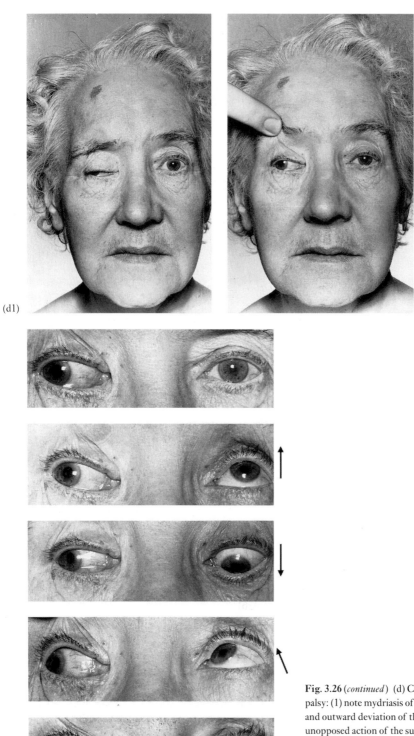

(d1)

(d2)

Fig. 3.26 (*continued*) (d) Complete right IIIrd nerve palsy: (1) note mydriasis of the right pupil and the down and outward deviation of the right eye (due to the unopposed action of the superior oblique and lateral rectus muscles innervated by the IVth and VIth nerves, respectively); (2) testing eye movements (note the failure of the right eye to look straight, upwards, downwards, upwards and laterally, and medially).

27 / Mitral incompetence (lone)

Frequency in survey: 7% of attempts at MRCP short cases.

Record

The pulse is regular (give rate). The venous pressure is not raised and there is no ankle or sacral oedema (unless in cardiac failure). The apex beat is *thrusting* in the sixth intercostal space in the anterior axillary line, and there is (may be) a systolic thrill. There is a left *parasternal heave*. The *first heart sound* is *soft*, and there is a *third heart sound* (both suggest severe mitral incompetence). There is a loud *pansystolic murmur* at the apex, *radiating* to the *axilla*.

The diagnosis is mitral incompetence with signs of pulmonary hypertension.

Causes of mitral incompetence*

1 Rheumatic heart disease (males more commonly than females; contrast with mitral stenosis which affects females more commonly than males)

2 Previous mitral valvotomy for mitral stenosis (left thoracotomy scar)

3 Papillary muscle dysfunction (ischaemia, infarction or other disease of papillary muscles or adjacent myocardium)

4 Severe left ventricular dilatation (due to any cause — lateral displacement of the papillary muscles and sometimes possibly dilatation of the mitral annulus† interfere with coaptation of the valve leaflets)

5 Mitral valve prolapse (p. 209).

Other physical signs (*which may occur in severe mitral incompetence*)

Mid-diastolic rumbling murmur‡ (brief)

Sharp and abbreviated peripheral pulse (lack of sustained forward stroke volume because of the regurgitant leak)

Wide splitting of the second sound (early closure of the aortic valve because the regurgitant loss shortens the left ventricular ejection time)

Fourth heart sound (acute severe regurgitation with sinus rhythm).

Other causes of mitral incompetence*

Infective endocarditis (fever, splenomegaly, petechiae, splinter haemorrhages, clubbing, Osler's nodes, Janeway's lesions, Roth spots, etc.)

Annular calcification (especially in the elderly female)

Hypertrophic obstructive cardiomyopathy (see p. 436)

---

* Regardless of the aetiology, mitral incompetence is a condition which gradually worsens spontaneously ('mitral incompetence begets mitral incompetence')—enlargement of the left atrium and left ventricle both worsen the incompetence and a vicious circle is set up.

† Left ventricular dilatation is common but the frequency of dilatation of the mitral valve annulus is an uncertain and controversial point. The mitral valve ring is a thick fibrous structure, so that if significant dilatation does occur, it probably indicates severe left ventricular disease.

‡ A short mid-diastolic murmur in the context of mitral incompetence could indicate associated mitral stenosis, or it could represent a flow (left atrium to left ventricle) murmur. The presence of an opening snap in such cases indicates mitral stenosis. In the absence of an opening snap the mid-diastolic murmur has two possible causes: (i) severe mitral incompetence with an increased flow murmur, or (ii) associated mitral stenosis and a calcified mitral valve. In the former there is often a third heart sound. In the latter the murmur is usually longer.

Rupture of the chordae tendinae§ (usually causes acute severe mitral incompetence; causes include infective endocarditis, rheumatic mitral valve disease, mitral valve prolapse, trauma)

Connective tissue disorders

    (a) SLE (Libman–Sachs endocarditis—p. 237)

    (b) rheumatoid arthritis (?hands, ?nodules)

    (c) ankylosing spondylitis (?male with fixed kyphosis and stooped posture; aortic valve more commonly affected—p. 237)

Congenital with or without other abnormalities

    (a) ostium primum atrial septal defect (p. 430)

    (b) Marfan's syndrome (?tall with long extremities, arachnodactyly, high-arched palate, etc.—p. 267)

    (c) Ehlers–Danlos syndrome (?hyperextensible skin and joints, thin scars, etc.—p. 263)

    (d) pseudoxanthoma elasticum (?loose skin or 'chicken skin' appearance in anticubital fossae, inguinal regions, neck, etc.—p. 311)

    (e) osteogenesis imperfecta (?blue sclerae, deformity from old fractures, etc.—p. 348)

Endomyocardial fibrosis (10% of cardiac admissions in East Africa; also occurs in West Africa, Southern India and Sri Lanka; the aetiology is unknown).

Indications for surgery

Improvements in surgical techniques and artificial valves, and the reduction in operative mortality, have reduced the threshold of physicians for considering surgery in moderately disabled patients (i.e. breathlessness caused by normal activity)—particularly if cardiomegaly and an elevated end-systolic left ventricular volume ($\geqslant 30$ ml m^{-2} body surface area) persists despite medical therapy (digoxin, diuretics, vasodilators). Repair and reconstruction of the valve (annuloplasty), if feasible (mostly in children and young adults), is preferable because of its low perioperative mortality. Asymptomatic patients should not be considered for surgery since the condition progresses slowly;* they may live for many years with little noticeable deterioration in their condition. Acute severe mitral incompetence (e.g. infective endocarditis, ruptured chordae tendinae) may require emergency valve replacement.

§ If the posterior leaflet is predominantly involved the systolic murmur is best heard at the left sternal edge whereas if the anterior leaflet is involved the murmur is best heard over the spine.

28 / Motor neurone disease

Frequency in survey: main focus of a short case in 7% of attempts at MRCP short cases. Additional feature in a further 1%.

Record

This patient has *weakness*, *wasting* and *fasciculation* of the muscles of the hand (p. 162), arms and shoulder girdle (*progressive muscular atrophy* in its pure form is characterized by minimal pyramidal signs), but the upper limb reflexes are exaggerated (reflexes in motor neurone disease may be increased, decreased or absent depending on which lesion is predominant). There is upper motor neurone *spastic weakness* with *exaggerated reflexes* in the legs (*amyotrophic lateral sclerosis**). There is ankle clonus and the patient has bilateral *extensor plantar* responses. The patient also has (may have) indistinct *nasal speech*, a *wasted fasciculating tongue* and *palatal paralysis* (*progressive bulbar palsy*— p. 257). There are *no sensory signs*.

The diagnosis is motor neurone disease.

Other conditions in which fasciculation may occur

Cervical spondylosis (see below)

Syringomyelia (fasciculation less apparent, dissociated sensory loss, etc.—p. 305)

Charcot–Marie–Tooth disease (fasciculation less apparent, atrophy which stops abruptly part of the way up the legs, pes cavus, sometimes palpable lateral popliteal and ulnar nerves, etc.—p. 249)

Acute stages of poliomyelitis (and rarely also in old polio; see below)

Neuralgic amyotrophy (pain, wasting and weakness of a group of muscles in a limb, sometimes following a viral infection; usually C5, C6 innervated muscles—shoulder)

Thyrotoxic myopathy (tachycardia, tremor, sweating, goitre with bruit, lid lag, etc.—p. 117)

Syphilitic amyotrophy (see below)

Chronic asymmetrical spinal muscular atrophy (see below)

After exercise in fit adults

After Tensilon test (p. 269)

Benign giant fasciculation.

Differential diagnosis of motor neurone disease

Cervical cord compression (p. 211) is the most important condition to be excluded in the diagnosis of motor neurone disease. Bulbar palsy and sensory signs should be carefully sought but a myelogram is often required to exclude it. *Syphilitic amyotrophy* (slowly progressing wasting of the muscles of the shoulder girdle and upper arm with loss of reflexes and no sensory loss; fasciculation of the tongue may occur) should always be excluded in the investigation of motor neurone disease as it is amenable to treatment. Occasionally patients with *old polio*, after many years, develop a progressive wasting disease (with prominent fasciculation) which is indistinguishable from progressive muscular atrophy motor neurone disease. Also, in immunologically incompetent patients (carcinoma, lymphoma, steroid therapy) a pure amyotrophy may develop that progresses over several months and is found at autopsy to be chronic poliomyelitis. The diagnosis of *chronic asymmetrical spinal muscular atrophy* (CASMA), a condition which appears to be distinct from classical

---

* Glutamate toxicity has been implicated as a factor leading to neuronal damage in amyotrophic lateral sclerosis. Trials suggest riluzole may retard progression and lengthen survival.

motor neurone disease, is favoured by age of onset under 40 years, absence of pyramidal or bulbar involvement after 3 or more years of symptoms, and depressed or absent reflexes. CASMA is only slowly progressive and carries a considerably better prognosis than classical motor neurone disease. CASMA may be inherited and there are reports of patients with this condition having relatives with Werdnig–Hoffmann disease—a fatal early infantile form of spinal and bulbar muscular atrophy that appears to be a single genetic entity.

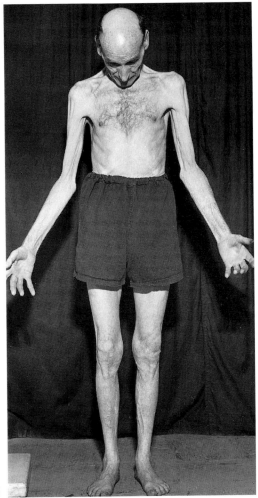

(a1)

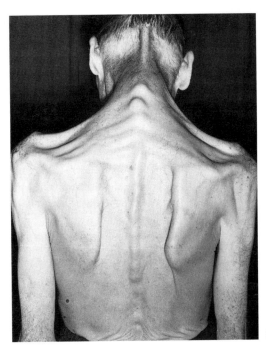

(a2)

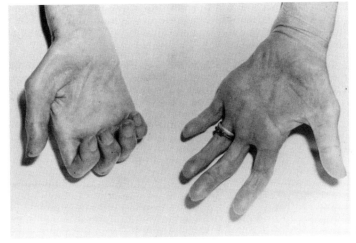

(b)

Fig. 3.28 (a1,2) Generalized muscle wasting (note weakness of the extensors of the neck). (b) Wasting of the small muscles of the hand.

29 / Goitre

Frequency in survey: main focus of a short case in 7% of attempts at MRCP short cases. Additional feature in a further 6%.

Record 1

There is a *multinodular* goitre, the R/L lobe being enlarged more than the R/L. There are *no lymph nodes* palpable, there is *no retrosternal* extension, there is *no bruit* and the patient is clinically *euthyroid* (having checked pulse, palms, tremor, lid lag, tendon reflexes).

The diagnosis (in this middle-aged or elderly patient) is likely to be simple multinodular goitre.

Simple multinodular goitre is due to relative iodine deficiency in a susceptible person. The multinodular nature suggests that it is long standing. If there has been no recent rapid increase in size and if the gland is not causing symptoms or worrying the patient then no further investigation or treatment is required. The patient should be observed in 6 months or a year to confirm that there is still no change. Fine-needle aspiration should be undertaken if there is any doubt.

Record 2

There is a *firm, diffusely enlarged* goitre without retrosternal extension (check for bruit and if allowed feel the pulse and assess thyroid status).

Possible causes

Simple goitre (euthyroid, no bruit, relative iodine deficiency, especially females, ?puberty, ?pregnancy)

Treated Graves' disease* (?exophthalmos ± bruit, patient is euthyroid—normal pulse, no tremor or sweatiness — or even hypothyroid — slow pulse, facies, ankle jerks)

Hyperthyroid Graves' disease* (?bruit, tachycardia,

exophthalmos, tremor, sweatiness, etc.)

Hashimoto's disease* (goitre usually, but not always, finely micronodular, firm and symmetrical; ?hypothyroid facies, pulse, ankle jerks, etc.)

De Quervain's (viral) thyroiditis (thyroid tender ± constitutional upset; absent radioactive iodine uptake on scan though the serum thyroxine may be elevated with TSH supressed†)

Goitrogens (e.g. lithium, iodide in large doses, phenylbutazone, para-aminosalicylic acid and others are all rare causes)

Dyshormonogenesis (six different types of congenital enzyme defect, all rare).

Record 3

There is a *solitary nodule* in the thyroid (check for lymphadenopathy).

Possible causes

Only one palpable nodule in a multinodular goitre

Thyroid adenoma (scan may show decreased, normal or increased (subclinical toxic nodule) uptake)

Toxic adenoma (hot nodule on scan, tachycardia, sweaty palms, lid lag, etc.)

*NB The possibility of associated autoimmune disease adding extra interest to the case of goitre in the Membership (see experience 19, p. 451); e.g. diabetes mellitus, rheumatoid arthritis, Addison's disease, pernicious anaemia. About 7% of patients with Graves' disease have vitiligo. About 5% of

patients with myasthenia gravis have thyrotoxicosis at some time. (See also pp. 114, 152 and 279.)

† By contrast, when the goitre and raised serum thyroxine is due to Graves' disease there is high radioactive iodine uptake on scan.

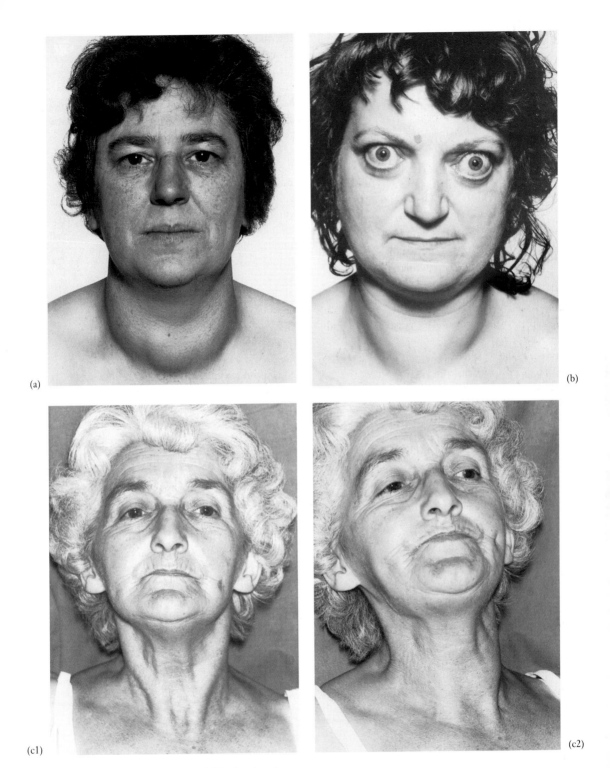

(a)

(b)

(c1)

(c2)

Fig. 3.29 (a) Multinodular goitre. (b) Diffusely enlarged thyroid (Graves' disease). (c1,2) solitary nodule only made obvious by swallowing (right).

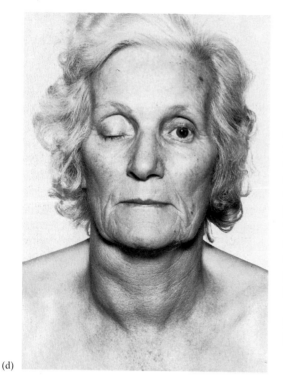

(d)

Fig. 3.29 (*continued*) (d) Follicular carcinoma of the thyroid with secondaries in the cavernous sinus (total ophthalmoplegia and absent corneal reflex on the right).

Thyroid cyst
Thyroid carcinoma (?hard, lymph nodes, recent change, cold on scan).

As well as assessment of thyroid function, fine-needle aspiration to attempt to establish histological diagnosis should be undertaken in most cases of solitary thyroid nodule. As an adjunct the nodule may be scanned radioisotopically though this is not usually necessary. If the nodule is hot it is not malignant but if it is cold it may be. In an older patient in whom the nodule has been present without changing for a long time, observation only (perhaps with full dose thyroxine therapy which will reduce many nodules) may sometimes be justified initially. In any case of doubt, exploration of the neck and biopsy of the nodule are indicated, proceeding to subtotal lobectomy if the nodule is benign.

Types of thyroid carcinoma

Papillary carcinoma is the commonest form. It occurs in children and the middle-aged. It spreads to regional lymph nodes but is often resectable and has a good prognosis. It is often TSH-dependent and may respond to thyroxine

Follicular carcinoma is the next commonest and tends to arise later in life. Blood-borne metastases may occur, but following surgery and suppressive thyroxine treatment, the prognosis is fair. It and its secondaries often take up and respond to radioactive iodine

Anaplastic carcinoma tends to arise in the elderly and is highly malignant

Medullary carcinoma‡ is rare, tends to arise in young adults, secretes calcitonin and sometimes ACTH, but usually carries a good prognosis

Lymphoma generally arises in a gland affected by Hashimoto's thyroiditis. A rapidly enlarging mass in the thyroid of a patient with Hashimoto's should arouse suspicion.

‡ MEA (multiple endocrine adenopathy) type IIa (Sipple's syndrome, also known as MEN (multiple endocrine neoplasia) syndrome) describes the association of
1 Medullary cell carcinoma of the thyroid
2 Phaeochromocytoma
3 Parathyroid hyperplasia (50%).
In MEA type IIb, medullary cell carcinoma of the thyroid and sometimes phaeochromocytoma are associated with a variety of neurological abnormalities including mucosal neuromas (lumpy, bumpy lips and eyelids), marfanoid habitus,

hyperplastic corneal nerves, skin pigmentation, proximal myopathy and intestinal disorders such as megacolon and ganglioneuromatosis. Parathyroid hyperplasia is less common. In MEA type IIa medullary carcinoma may occasionally secrete other substances such as ACTH, histaminase, vasoactive intestinal peptide (VIP), prostaglandins and serotonin whereas in MEA type IIb production of hormones other than calcitonin is rare. Both are autosomal dominant. Type IIb is sometimes called type III.

30 / Ulnar nerve palsy

Frequency in survey: 7% of attempts at MRCP short cases.

Record

The hand shows *generalized muscle wasting** and *weakness* which *spares* the *thenar eminence*. There is sensory loss over the *fifth finger*, the *adjacent half* of the *fourth finger* and the dorsal and palmar aspects of the *medial side* of the *hand*.† (Look for hyperextension at the metacarpophalangeal joints with flexion of the interphalangeal joints in the fourth and fifth fingers—the *ulnar claw hand*.)‡

The patient has an ulnar nerve lesion. (Now examine the elbow for a cause.)

Likely causes

1 Fracture or dislocation at the elbow (?scar or deformity; history of injury)
2 Osteoarthrosis at the elbow with osteophytic encroachment on the ulnar nerve in the cubital tunnel ('filling in' of the ulnar groove due to palpable enlargement of nerve; limitation of elbow movement is often seen; certain occupations predispose to osteoarthrosis at the elbow—see below).

Other causes

Occupations with constant leaning on elbows (clerks, secretaries on telephone, etc.)

Occupations with constant flexion and extension at the elbow (bricklayer, painter/decorator, carpenter, roofer—shallow ulnar groove will predispose; these occupations may also lead to osteoarthrosis—see above)

Excessive carrying angle at elbow (malunited fracture of the humerus or disturbance of growth leading to cubitus valgus and, over the years, 'tardy ulnar nerve palsy')

Injuries at the wrist or in the palm (different degrees of the syndrome depending on which branches of

the nerve are damaged; e.g. occupations using screwdrivers, drills, etc.)

The causes of mononeuritis multiplex (diabetes, polyarteritis nodosa and Churg–Strauss syndrome, rheumatoid, SLE, Wegener's, sarcoid, carcinoma, amyloid, leprosy, Sjögren's syndrome, Lyme disease).

NB Other causes of wasting of the small muscles of the hand (p. 162) may sometimes resemble ulnar nerve palsy. The major features pointing to ulnar nerve palsy as the cause are *sparing of the thenar eminence* and the characteristic sensory loss pattern. The main distinguishing features of the differential

---

*(i) The *hypothenar eminence wastes*, though in the manual worker with thickened skin the hand contour may be preserved and the wasting may only be detected on palpation. Loss of the other small muscles is seen from (ii) *loss of the first dorsal interosseous* in the dorsal space between the first and second metacarpals and (iii) *guttering of the dorsum* of the hand—which becomes more prominent as the lesion advances.

† *Record* (continuation): there is *weakness* of *abduction* and *adduction* of the *fingers*, and *adduction* of the *extended thumb* against the palm (inability to grip a piece of paper between thumb and index finger without flexing the affected thumb—

Froment's 'thumb sign'). Flexion of the fourth and fifth fingers is weak. When the proximal portions of these fingers are held immobilized, flexion of the terminal phalanges is not possible. There is also *wasting* of the *medial aspect* of the *forearm* (flexor carpi ulnaris and half of the flexor digitorum profundus). When the hand is flexed to the ulnar side against resistance the tendon of flexor carpi ulnaris is not palpable.

‡ The ulnar claw hand or partial *main-en-griffe* is due to the unopposed action of the long extensors and is only seen in the fourth and fifth fingers because the radial lumbricals are supplied by the median nerve.

diagnoses which may mimic the muscle wasting of ulnar paralysis are:

Syringomyelia—dissociated sensory loss extending beyond the ulnar zone; loss of arm reflexes; ?Horner's

C8 lesion (e.g. Pancoast syndrome)—sensory loss involves radial side of fourth finger, ?Horner's

Cervical rib — objective sensory disturbances are usually slight or absent and without characteristic ulnar distribution.

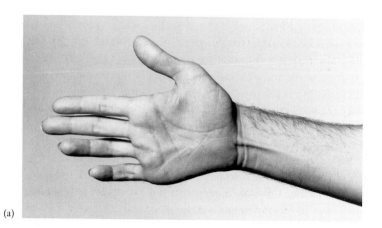

(a)

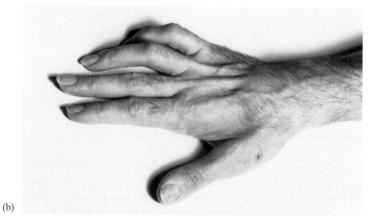

(b)

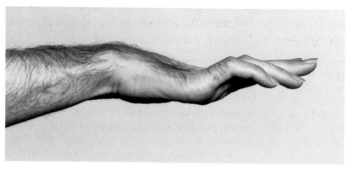

(c)

Fig. 3.30 (a) Loss of hypothenar eminence. (b) Dorsal guttering. (c) Typical ulnar claw hand.

31 / Visual field defect

Frequency in survey: main focus of a short case in 6% of attempts at MRCP short cases. Additional feature in a further 3%.

Record 1

There is an *homonymous hemianopia*. This suggests a lesion of the *optic tract* behind the optic chiasma (with sparing of the macula and hence normal visual acuity).

Likely causes

1 Cerebrovascular accident (?ipsilateral hemiplegia, atrial fibrillation, heart murmurs or bruits, hypertension)
2 Tumour (?ipsilateral pyramidal signs, papilloedema).

Record 2

There is a *bitemporal* visual field defect worse on R/L side. This suggests a lesion at the *optic chiasma*. (NB There may be optic atrophy, sometimes with a central scotoma, on the R/L side due to simultaneous compression of the optic nerve by the lesion.)

Possible causes

1 Pituitary tumour (?acromegaly, hypopituitarism, gynaecomastia, galactorrhoea, menstrual disturbance, etc.)
2 Craniopharyngioma (?calcification on skull X-ray)
3 Suprasellar meningioma
4 Aneurysm.
Rarer causes are glioma, granuloma and metastasis.

Record 3

The visual fields are considerably constricted, the central field of vision being spared. This is *tunnel vision*.* I would like to examine the fundi, looking for evidence of retinitis pigmentosa, glaucoma (pathological cupping) or widespread choroidoretinitis. (Hysteria may occasionally be a cause; papilloedema causes enlargement of the blind spot and peripheral constriction.)

Record 4

There is a *central scotoma*. (NB The discs may be pale (atrophy), swollen and pink (papillitis), or normal (retrobulbar neuritis).)

Causes to be considered

Demyelinating diseases (?nystagmus, cerebellar signs, etc.; however, multiple sclerosis frequently causes retrobulbar neuritis without other signs)

---

* The Committee on the Safety of Medicine has received reports of visual field defects associated with the anti-epileptic drug *vigabatrin* including three cases of severe, symptomatic, persistent visual field constriction (tunnel vision).

Compression†
Ischaemia
Leber's optic atrophy (males : females = 6 : 1)
Toxins (e.g. methyl alcohol)
Macular disease
Nutritional (famine, etc., tobacco–alcohol ambly-
opia, vitamin B_{12} deficiency, diabetes mellitus).

Record 5

There is *homonymous upper quadrantic visual field
loss*. This suggests a lesion in the temporal cortex.

NB Field defects may sometimes originate from
retinal damage, e.g. occlusion of a branch of the
retinal artery or a large area of choroidoretinitis.

---

† There may be clues as to the site of the compression. (i) A
lesion in the frontal lobe which compresses the optic nerve
may cause dementia. (ii) It may also cause contralateral
papilloedema (the *Foster–Kennedy syndrome* due to a frontal
tumour or aneurysm, e.g. olfactory groove meningioma). (iii)
A lesion in front of the chiasma involving crossing fibres that
loop forward into the opposite optic nerve may cause a
contralateral upper temporal quadrantic field defect. (iv) A
lesion at the chiasma may cause a bitemporal field defect. (v)
A lesion at the lateral chiasma (pituitary tumour, aneurysm,
meningioma) involving the terminal optic tract as well as the
optic nerve may cause an homonymous hemianopia.

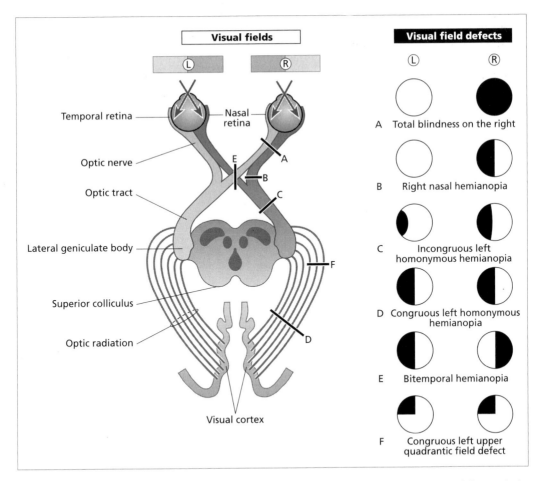

Fig. 3.31 The visual pathways and visual field defects resulting from different lesions. If there is exact overlap of the field defects from both eyes the defect is said to be congruous. If not, it is incongruous. The defects in B and E above are incongruous. Though the complete homonymous hemianopia in D is congruous, lesions of the optic tract (C), which are comparatively rare, produce characteristic incongruous visual changes. The fibres serving identical points in the homonymous half fields do not fully commingle in the anterior optic tract so lesions encroaching on this structure produce incongruous and usually incomplete homonymous hemianopias. Lesions of the geniculate ganglia, visual radiations or visual cortex produce congruous visual field defects. F represents a lesion of the temporal loop of the optic radiation.

32 / Peripheral neuropathy

Frequency in survey: main focus of a short case in 6% of attempts at MRCP short cases. Additional feature in a further 5%.

Record

There is *impairment* of *sensation* to light touch, vibration sense, joint position sense and pinprick over a *stocking* and, to a lesser extent, a *glove distribution* (much less common).

The patient has a peripheral neuropathy.

Most likely causes

1 Diabetes mellitus (?fundi, amyotrophy)
2 Carcinomatous neuropathy (?evidence of primary, cachexia, clubbing)
3 Vitamin B_{12} deficiency (subacute combined degeneration not always present; ?plantars)
4 Vitamin B deficiency (alcoholics*)
5 Drugs (e.g. isoniazid, vincristine, nitrofurantoin, gold, ethambutol, phenytoin, hydrallazine, metronidazole, amiodarone, chloramphenicol, cyclosporin)
6 Idiopathic (in 10–20% of patients with chronic peripheral neuropathy for >1 year, no cause can be found).

There are many rare causes (see below).

Leprosy is a cause of major importance worldwide.

Important rare causes

Guillain–Barré syndrome (also motor involvement, absent reflexes, ?bilateral lower motor neurone VIIth nerve palsy; ?peak flow rate—p. 286)
Polyarteritis nodosa (?arteritic lesions)
Rheumatoid arthritis and other collagen disease (hands, facies)
Amyloidosis (?thick nerves, autonomic involvement)†
AIDS.‡

Causes of predominantly motor neuropathy

Carcinomatous neuropathy (?evidence of primary, cachexia)
Lead (wrists mainly)
Porphyria
Diphtheria
Charcot–Marie–Tooth disease (?atrophy of peronei, pes cavus, etc.—p. 249).

* Can also occur with nutritional deficiencies from other causes, e.g. dialysis for chronic renal failure, prison camp victims.
† Neuropathy is a feature of primary and myeloma-associated amyloidosis (it is exceptional in secondary amyloidosis). Carpal tunnel syndrome is not uncommon. Sensory or mixed sensory and motor neuropathy are commonest. Signs of autonomic involvement would be orthostatic hypotension, impotence, impairment of sweating and diarrhoea. The other organs mainly involved in primary and myeloma-associated amyloidosis include heart (cardiomyopathy), tongue (dysarthria), skeletal and visceral muscle and alimentary tract (rectal biopsy). See also footnote on p. 69.
‡ Acute (Guillain–Barré type) or chronic inflammatory neuropathy may be the presenting feature of HIV infection but with a cerebrospinal fluid pleocytosis which is not usually seen in these conditions. A distal sensory neuropathy may also occur in AIDS, sometimes but not always caused by cytomegalovirus infection.

Other rare causes of peripheral neuropathy

Myxoedema (?facies, pulse, reflexes, etc.—p. 152)

Acromegaly (?facies, hands, etc.—p. 109)

Sarcoidosis (?lupus pernio, chest signs)

Uraemia (?pale brownish yellow complexion)

Lyme disease

Tetanus

Botulism (can be mistaken for Guillain–Barré, encephalitis, stroke or myasthenia gravis; electromyograph (EMG) resembles Eaton–Lambert)

Paraproteinaemia

Hereditary ataxias

Refsum's disease (cerebellar ataxia, pupillary abnormalities, optic atrophy, deafness, retinitis pigmentosa, cardiomyopathy, ichthyosis)

Arsenic poisoning (e.g. pesticides; Mee's transverse white lines may occur on the fingernails and raindrop pigmentation may occur on the skin)

Other chemical poisoning (e.g. tri-ortho-cresyl phosphate).

33 / Hypertensive retinopathy

Frequency in survey: main focus of a short case in 6% of attempts at MRCP short cases. Additional feature in a further 1%.

Record

The retinal arterioles are *narrow* (normal ratio of vein to artery is 1.1 : 1), they are (may be) *tortuous* and (may) vary in calibre (localized constriction followed by segments of arteriolar dilatation) with increased light reflex (copper or *silver wiring*) and *AV nipping* (these changes all occurring with ageing and arteriosclerosis as well as with hypertension). There are *flame-shaped* and (less frequently) *blot haemorrhages*, and *cotton-wool exudates* (all indicating grade 3 retinopathy and a diagnosis of malignant (accelerated) hypertension *even without* papilloedema), and there is *papilloedema* (indicating cerebral oedema; papilloedema may occur in malignant hypertension even without haemorrhages and exudates).

This is grade 4 hypertensive retinopathy.

Causes of hypertension

Essential—94% (cause unknown)

Renal — 4% (renal artery stenosis — *?bruit*, acute nephritis, pyelonephritis, glomerulonephritis, polycystic disease, systemic sclerosis, SLE, hydronephrosis, renin secreting tumour, and renoprival—after bilateral nephrectomy)

Endocrine — 1%* (Cushing's, Conn's, phaeochromocytoma,† acromegaly, hyperparathyroidism, hypothyroidism and oral contraceptive use)

Miscellaneous — <1% (coarctation of the aorta — *?radiofemoral delay*, polycythaemia, acute porphyria, pre-eclampsia).

NB Cerebral tumour or raised intracranial pressure from any cause may lead to secondary hypertension (Cushing's reflex).

For colour photographs see p. 528.

---

*The figure 1% does not include hypertension due to oral contraceptive use.

† All patients with phaeochromocytomata should be screened for multiple endocrine neoplasia (MEN) type II (p. 128) and von Hippel–Lindau disease (p. 86) to avert further morbidity and mortality in the patients and their families. All patients in families with MEN-II or von Hippel–Lindau disease should be screened for phaeochromocytoma even if they are asymptomatic.

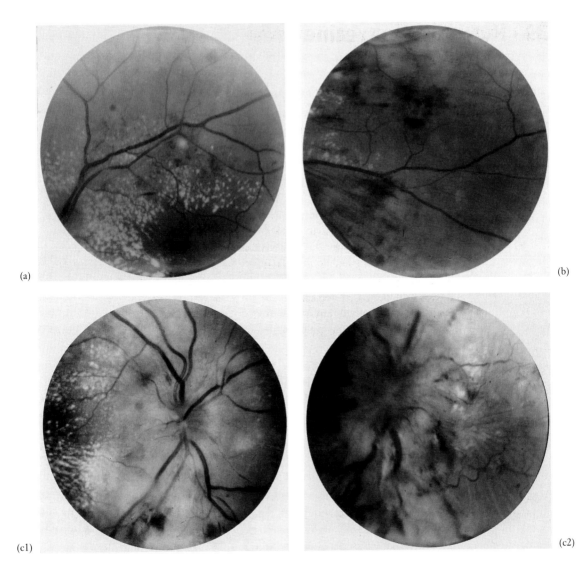

Fig. 3.33 (a) Thin, irregular arterioles, AV nipping, haemorrhages and exudates forming a macular star in hypertension. (b) Flame-shaped haemorrhages in hypertension. (c1,2) Papilloedema—hypertension.

34 / Resuscitation Annie

Frequency in survey: 7% of attempts at MRCP short cases.

A change from a live patient to an inanimate model can be unsettling not only for the candidates but also for the examiners. Many candidates feel awkward and self-conscious while shouting at the dummy such things as, 'Are you all right?', or 'Annie, Annie' or 'Help—call an ambulance'; and when they attempt to demonstrate various components of cardiopulmonary resuscitation on the manikin. From the candidates' experiences reported to us, the main concern of the examiners seemed to be whether the candidates could perform various steps competently and show that they had done it all before. We have selected seven anecdotes (from our surveys) here which highlight the examiners' concern, but we would suggest that it would be advisable to practise on a manikin before going for the clinical examination. Nevertheless candidates who regularly take part in the cardiac arrest team as part of their everyday job, should have no difficulty with this short case.

Anecdote 1

'Now we will move onto the fourth case', said the examiner sternly after a candidate had struggled through a difficult cardiac short case. 'This next subject isn't a patient', he continued. They walked into the adjacent room and he was confronted by a resuscitation manikin. 'Now, I would like you to imagine that you are in a town centre and somebody has just collapsed in the street. Using this manikin, I would like you to demonstrate what you would do and explain your actions as you proceed'.

He reports: 'Assessment of responsiveness was the first thought that came to my mind. Talk in detail about each component of ABC (airway, breathing, circulation), I thought, and allow yourself to collect your ideas about the European Resuscitation Council Guidelines* for basic life support'. He explained that he would first take care that there was no direct danger to himself or other helpers at the scene of the collapse and would shout to the casualty to assess her level of consciousness. 'Do it', the examiner said and the candidate found himself shouting, 'Are you all right?', while shaking the manikin's shoulders in a rather self-conscious way.

'Your patient is unconscious', he was told. He turned to the other examiner and asked her to go and phone for an ambulance (much to the delight of her colleague!). 'I now need to open the airway and check for breathing and for the presence of a pulse'. The examiner asked him to be specific and the candidate mentioned 'the carotid artery', upon which he was asked to demonstrate how to locate and palpate this artery. 'Assuming both pulse and respiration are absent, what would you do?' The candidate explained how he would first ensure that there was a clear airway and demonstrated the opening of the airway by tilting the head and lifting the chin. He was very familiar with in-hospital resuscitation using

* *British Medical Journal* 1993, **306**: 1587–9.

Ambu bags and endotracheal tubes, but had not performed mouth-to-mouth resuscitation since his life-saving awards for swimming. He opened the manikin's mouth (with the head still extended), took a deep breath, and placed his mouth over that of the manikin to make a good seal. He was about to exhale, but something didn't feel right! At the last moment he remembered to pinch the manikin's nose with the fingers of his left hand. It was a great relief to see that the chest wall rose and the yellow light illuminated to indicate adequate ventilation.

Having given two breaths of expired air ventilation, he started chest compressions. He demonstrated the correct position over the middle of the lower half of the sternum. 'Why are you placing your hands on the sternum rather than over the apex of the heart?', asked the other examiner somewhat abruptly. 'To reduce trauma to the chest wall, and to provide the most effective thoracic compression and thus cerebral blood flow', the candidate replied. He was allowed to continue regular compressions, a little over one each second (approximately $80 \, min^{-1}$) aiming to depress the sternum about 4–5 cm (2 inches) on each occasion. 'What ratio of compressions to ventilation would you give?', asked the examiner. The candidate said '15 to 2' upon which the examiner lead him on to the next case.

Anecdote 2

'This 55-year old woman had a heart attack yesterday and is on the CCU. She has lost consciousness with this ECG trace (asystole) and there is no one else around. Show me what you would do next'. The candidate approached the resuscitation doll and proceeded to confirm that there was no pulse and no respiration. She commenced external cardiac massage and demonstrated mouth-to-mouth inflation of the lungs (the test console lights went on). The examiners altered the ECG tracing to ventricular fibrillation and asked her what she would do. She said she would give a DC shock and a lignocaine bolus followed by an infusion. She was then asked to show where she would place the defibrillation paddles which she did.

Anecdote 3

A candidate was taken up to Resuscitation Annie and told: 'Your friend collapses whilst eating lunch in a restaurant'. The candidate told us that she approached Annie calling 'Annie, Annie'. She checked for respiration and pulses and then shouted: 'Help, call an ambulance'. She went through the motions of moving food and tilting the head; she gave two puffs of mouth-to-mouth resuscitation then started 15 : 2 cardiopulmonary resuscitation which she told us was being marked by a computer!

Anecdote 4

A candidate was taken to a resuscitation doll and told: 'Show me how you would resuscitate this patient'. The examiner was producing a carotid pulsation by a little hand-held bulb which the candidate said he hadn't seen and was not expecting. At first he missed the pulsation which was present but he soon got the hang of it. He was asked about what drugs he would give for a bradycardia and at what dose.

Anecdote 5

A candidate reported that half-way through his short cases a second examiner—a sterner looking woman—took over. She took the candidate to a side ward and said that the next patient would be a shock because the patient had just arrested. The candidate felt cheered up as he had been practising resuscitation for the exam. He found Resuscitation Annie laid out on the bed and started basic life support and then asked the observing examiner to call the cardiac arrest team—the examiner nodded assent. The candidate reported that there was a meter with lights which showed green if the massage and ventilation were effective though he was not able to see the lights. He was told that enough had been done after two cycles of inflation and chest massage. He was asked when he would stop resuscitation in real life. The candidate replied that this would be when the cardiac arrest team took over with advanced life support with other helpers to perform massage and ventilate the patient. The examiner pointed out that the candidate had not delivered the precordial thump. The candidate replied that there were two opinions with regard to whether this should form part of basic life support—one opinion was against, on the grounds that the precordial thump could provoke the R on T phenomena leading to ventricular tachycardia, therefore worsening the situation if no defibrillator was available; the other opinion suggesting that it was safe in the hospital setting as the precordial thump could convert a ventricular tachycardia to sinus rhythm. The candidate told the examiners that he did not usually include the precordial thump as part of his own basic life support.

Anecdote 6

The candidate was shown Resuscitation Annie and asked: 'Have you seen one of these before?' He was then shown the following rhythms and asked what they were: atrial fibrillation, supraventricular tachycardia, ventricular tachycardia, ventricular fibrillation. When ventricular fibrillation was shown, the candidate was asked what he would do. The candidate commenced resuscitation after which the examiner commented: 'Goodness you managed to get the right lights to go!—I can't!' A discussion took place on how to put in an internal jugular line as this was the candidate's preferred method at a cardiac arrest; the candidate reports that 'Neither examiner was familiar with it!' Apparently this short case was very relaxed and informal.

Anecdote 7

The candidate was taken to a resuscitation dummy and told: 'You walk onto a ward and a nurse calls you to a patient who has collapsed and who has "arrested"—what would you do? Show us.' The candidate said he would check to see if the patient had truly arrested, that he would call the 'crash team', he would give a sternal blow, start resuscitation with an Ambu bag and mask combined with cardiac massage, whilst taking a history, obtaining an ECG trace and undertaking defibrillation, etc. The examiners challenged him with various 'What if' scenarios such as 'Suppose the nurse faints'; 'Suppose it happened in the street would you be concerned with regard to AIDS and mouth-to-mouth resuscitation?' The candidate discussed each of these and said he would not be worried about AIDS and mouth-to-mouth resuscitation! The candidate reported that the examiners were checking that he was getting 'the right light' on the control panel during resuscitation and he reported that the lights were green for correct ventilation, and orange for correct cardiac massage with red being for incorrect resuscitation. The candidate was asked about the damage that could be caused by incorrect resuscitation technique. The candidate was asked if he had had much experience with cardiac arrests to which the candidate replied that he had over a year's experience on 'acute crash teams'. He was asked what his immediate success rate was and replied that this varied with circumstances and depending on whether the resuscitation was taking place on the coronary care unit or, for instance, a surgical ward; and also depending on the patient's pathology, etc. Apparently the examiners spent quite a long time discussing these aspects. The candidate reckoned that his initial resuscitation success rate was probably around 30% to spontaneous rhythm.

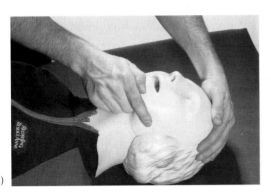

(a)

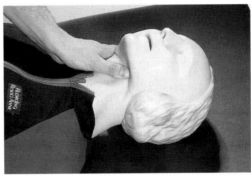

(b)

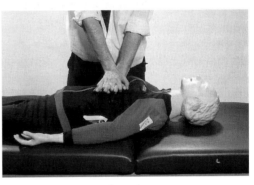

(c)

Fig. 3.34 Resuscitation Annie. (a) Head tilt. (b) Locating the carotid artery. (c) Cardiac massage.

35 / Cerebellar syndrome

Frequency in survey: main focus of a short case in 6% of attempts at MRCP short cases. Additional feature in a further 6%.

Record 1

There is nystagmus to the R/L and there is ataxia with the eyes open as shown by impairment of rapid alternate motion on the same side (*dysdiadochokinesis*). The *finger–nose test* is impaired on the R/L with *past pointing* to that side and an *intention tremor* (increases on approaching the target). The *heel–shin test* is *impaired* on the R/L and the *gait* is *ataxic* with a tendency to fall to the R/L. There is *ataxic dysarthria* with explosive speech (staccato).

The patient has a R/L cerebellar lesion.

Causes include

1 Multiple sclerosis (?internuclear ophthalmoplegia, optic neuritis or atrophy, etc. —p. 433)
2 Brainstem vascular lesion
3 Posterior fossa space-occupying lesion (?papilloedema; e.g. tumour or abscess*)
4 Cerebellar syndrome of malignancy (?clubbing, cachexia, etc.)
5 Alcoholic cerebellar degeneration (nutritional†)
6 Friedreich's ataxia (?scoliosis, pes cavus, pyramidal and dorsal column signs, absent ankle jerks, etc.—p. 234)

Other causes of cerebellar ataxia include

Hypothyroidism (?facies, pulse, reflexes, etc. — p. 152)
Anticonvulsant toxicity (especially phenytoin which can cause gross multidirectional nystagmus)
Ataxia–telangiectasia (recessive; from childhood onwards progressive ataxia, choreoathetosis and oculomotor apraxia; later telangiectases on conjunctivae, ears, face and skin creases; low IgA leads to repeated respiratory tract infections; lymphoreticular malignancies common; death usually in second or third decade of life)
Other cerebellar degeneration syndromes.‡

Other cerebellar signs

Ipsilateral hypotonia and reduced power
Ipsilateral pendular knee jerk
Skew deviation of the eyes (ipsilateral down and in, contralateral up and out)
Failure of the displaced ipsilateral arm to find its original posture (ask the patient to hold his arms out in front of him and keep them there. If you push the ipsilateral arm down it will fly past the starting point on release without reflex arrest).

* NB Otitis media may underlie a cerebellar abscess. Intracranial abscesses may result from direct spread from the upper respiratory passages (nasal sinuses, middle ear, mastoid). Less often the cause is haematogenous spread (e.g. intrathoracic suppuration), congenital heart disease or fracture of the base of the skull. Abscesses secondary to otitis occur in the temporal lobe about twice as often as they do in the cerebellum.

† Other causes of nutritional deficiency such as pellagra, amoebiasis and protracted vomiting may cause a similar syndrome.
‡ The names associated with these other rare hereditary ataxias apart from Friedreich are Charcot, Marie, Déjèrine, Alajouanine, André Thomas, Gowers and Holmes.

Record 2 (vermis lesion)

There is a wide-based *cerebellar ataxia* (ataxic gait and Rombergism more or less the same with eyes open and closed; cf. sensory ataxia—worse with eyes closed), but there is little or no abnormality of the limbs when tested separately on the bed. This suggests a lesion of the cerebellar vermis.

36 / Retinitis pigmentosa

Frequency in survey: 6% of attempts at MRCP short cases.

Record

There is *widespread* scattering of *black pigment* in a pattern resembling *bone corpuscles*. The macula is spared. There is *tunnel vision*.

The diagnosis is retinitis pigmentosa.

The patient may well have presented with night blindness. The condition progresses remorselessly with increasing retinal pigmentation, deepening disc pallor of consecutive optic atrophy as the ganglion cells die, and increasing constriction of visual field. It may occur on its own although it is often associated with other abnormalities such as cataracts,* deaf–mutism and mental deficiency. Pigmentary degeneration of the retina may also occur in many conditions such as:

Laurence–Moon–Biedl syndrome (autosomal recessive; ?obesity, hypogonadism, dwarfism, mental retardation and polydactyly—p. 358)

Refsum's disease (autosomal recessive; ?pupillary abnormalities, cerebellar ataxia, deafness, peripheral neuropathy, cardiomyopathy and icthyosis)

as well as some of the

Hereditary ataxias

Familial neuropathies

Neuronal lipidoses (ceroid lipofuscinosis).

For colour photograph see p. 528.

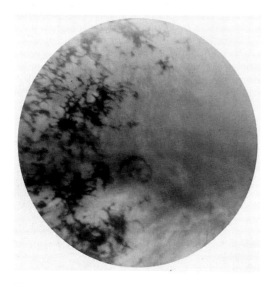

Fig. 3.36 Peripheral pigmentation resembling bone corpuscles.

* Visual acuity may sometimes be considerably improved by cataract removal.

37 / Carcinoma of the bronchus

Frequency in survey: main focus of a short case in 5% of attempts at MRCP short cases. Additional feature in a further 4%.

Survey note: candidates reported a variety of signs. The three *records* given are typical.

Record 1

There is *clubbing* of the fingers which are *nicotine-stained*. There is a hard *lymph node* in the R/L supraclavicular fossa. The pulse is 80/min and regular, and the venous pressure is not raised. The trachea is central, chest expansion normal, but the percussion note is *stony dull* at the R/L base and *tactile fremitus*, *vocal resonance* and *breath sounds* are all *diminished* over the area of dullness.

The likely diagnosis is carcinoma of the bronchus causing a *pleural effusion*.

Record 2

The patient is *cachectic*. There is a *radiation burn* on the R/L upper chest wall. There is *clubbing* of the fingers which are *nicotine-stained*. The pulse is 80/min, venous pressure not elevated and there are no lymph nodes. The *trachea* is *deviated* to the R/L and *expansion* of the R/L upper chest is *diminished*. *Tactile vocal fremitus* and *resonance* are *increased* over the upper chest where the *percussion note* is *dull* and there is an area of *bronchial breathing*.

It is likely that this patient has had radiotherapy for carcinoma of the bronchus which is causing *collapse* and *consolidation of the R/L upper lung*.

Record 3

There is a *radiation burn* on the chest. There are *lymph nodes* palpable in the R/L axilla. The trachea is central. I did not detect any abnormality in expansion, vocal fremitus, vocal resonance or breath sounds, but there is *wasting* of the *small muscles* of the R/L *hand*, and *sensory loss* (plus pain) over the *T1** dermatome. There is a R/L *Horner's syndrome* (p. 180).

The diagnosis is *Pancoast's syndrome* (due to an apical carcinoma of the lung involving the lower brachial plexus and the cervical sympathetic nerves).

Other complications of carcinoma of the bronchus

1 Other local effects such as:

Superior vena cava obstruction (?oedema of the face and upper extremities, suffusion of eyes, fixed engorgement of neck veins and dilatation of superficial veins, etc.—p. 239)

Stridor (often associated with superior vena cava obstruction; dysphagia may occur)

2 Metastases and their effects (pain, ?hepatomegaly, neurological signs, etc.)

3 Non-metastatic effects such as:

Hypertrophic pulmonary osteoarthropathy (?clubbing plus pain and swelling of wrists and/or

---

* The weakness, sensory loss and especially pain may be more widespread (C8,T1,T2).

ankles — subperiosteal new bone formation on X-ray)

Neuropathy (peripheral neuropathy — sensory, motor or mixed; cerebellar degeneration and encephalopathy; proximal myopathy, polymyositis, dermatomyositis, reversed myasthenia — Eaton–Lambert syndrome)

Endocrine (inappropriate antidiuretic hormone, ectopic ACTH, ectopic parathormone or parathormone-related peptide,† carcinoid)

Gynaecomastia (if rapidly progressive and painful may be a human chorionic gonadotrophin (HCG) secreting tumour)

Thrombophlebitis migrans (?deep venous thrombosis)

Non-bacterial thrombotic endocarditis

Anaemia (usually normoblastic; occasionally leuco-erythroblastic from bone marrow involvement)

Pruritus

Herpes zoster (p. 325)

Acanthosis nigricans (grey–brown/dark brown areas in the axillae and limb flexures, in which skin becomes thickened, rugose and velvety with warts — p. 419)

Erythema gyratum repens (irregular wavy bands with a serpiginous outline and marginal desquamation on the trunk, neck and extremities).

Record 4 (lobectomy)

There is a R/L *thoracotomy scar*. The *trachea* is *deviated* to the R/L. On the R/L side *chest expansion* is *diminished*, percussion note more resonant and breath sounds are harsher. The patient has had a R/L lobectomy to remove a tumour, resistant lung abscess or localized area of bronchiectasis.

---

† Hypercalcaemia may also be due to bone secondaries.

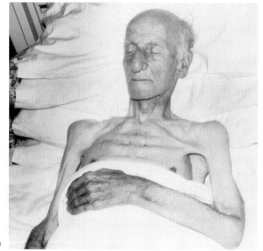

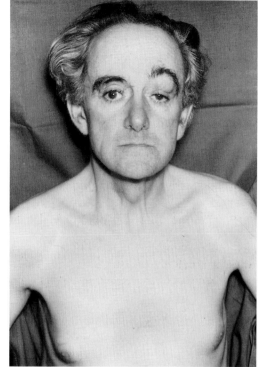

Fig. 3.37 (a) Cachexia due to carcinoma of the bronchus (note radiotherapy ink marks). (b) Pancoast's tumour (note gynaecomastia and left Horner's syndrome).

(a)

(b)

38 / Parkinson's disease

Frequency in survey: 5% of attempts at MRCP short cases.

Record

This man has an *expressionless, unblinking face* and slurred *low volume monotonous speech*. He is drooling (due to excessive salivation and some dysphagia) and there is *titubation*. He has difficulty starting to walk ('freezing') but once started, progresses with quick shuffling steps as if trying to keep up with his own centre of gravity. As he walks he is *stooped* and he *does not swing his arms* which show a continuous *pill-rolling tremor*. (He has poor balance and tends to fall, being unable to react quickly enough to stop himself.) His arms show a *lead-pipe rigidity* at the elbow but *cog-wheel rigidity* (combination of lead pipe rigidity and tremor—i.e. worse with anxiety) at the wrist. He has a positive glabellar tap sign (an unreliable sign) and his signs generally are *asymmetrical*—note the greater tremor in the R/L arm. (The tremor is decreased by intention but hand-writing may be small, tremulous and untidy). There is *blepharoclonus* (tremor of the eyelids when the eyes are gently closed).

The diagnosis is Parkinson's disease.

Male to female ratio is 3:1.

The features of Parkinson's disease are

1 Tremor
2 Rigidity
3 Bradykinesia.

Bradykinesia (the most disabling) can be demonstrated by asking the patient to touch his thumb successively with each finger. He will be slow in the initiation of the response and there will be a progressive reduction in the amplitude of each movement and a peculiar type of fatiguability. He will also have difficulty in performing two different motor acts simultaneously.

Other causes of the parkinsonian syndrome

Drug-induced (p. 220)
Postencephalitic (increasingly rare; definite history of encephalitis — encephalitis lethargica pandemic 1916–1928; there may be ophthalmoplegia, pupil abnormalities and dyskinesias; poor response to L-dopa)
Brain damage from anoxia (e.g. cardiac arrest), carbon monoxide or manganese poisoning (dementia and pyramidal signs likely with all)

Neurosyphilis
Cerebral tumours affecting the basal ganglia.

Other conditions which may have some extrapyramidal features

Arteriosclerotic Parkinson's (stepwise progression, broad-based gait, pyramidal signs; may be no more than simply two common conditions occurring in the same patient—cerebral arteriosclerosis and idiopathic parkinsonism)
Normal pressure hydrocephalus (may have a number of causes including head injury, meningitis or subarachnoid haemorrhage though in many instances the cause cannot be determined; the classic triad is *urinary incontinence, gait apraxia* and *dementia*; diagnosed by CT or MRI scan; important to diagnose because it may respond to ventriculosystemic shunting)
Steele–Richardson–Olszewski syndrome (supranuclear gaze palsy, axial rigidity, a tendency to fall backwards, pyramidal signs, subtle dementia or frontal lobe syndrome)
Shy–Drager syndrome (idiopathic orthostatic hypotension, impotence, urinary incontinence,

anhidrosis, cerebellar and pyramidal signs and peripheral neuropathy; L-dopa contraindicated)

Alzheimer's disease (severe dementia, mild extrapyramidal signs)

Olivopontocerebellar degeneration (sometimes familial; cerebellar and extrapyramidal signs)

Wilson's disease (Kayser–Fleischer rings, cirrhosis, chorea, psychotic behaviour, dysarthria, dystonic spasms and posturing; leading, if untreated, to dementia, severe dysarthria and dysphagia, contractures and immobility)

Jakob–Creutzfeldt disease (prion protein encephalopathy leading to rapidly progressive dementia with myoclonus and multifocal neurological signs including aphasia, cerebellar ataxia, cortical blindness and spasticity)

Hypoparathyroidism (basal ganglia calcification).

NB A condition which is often misdiagnosed as Parkinson's disease in the elderly is *benign essential tremor* (often autosomal dominant, intention tremor worse with stress, no other neurological abnormality; usually improves when alcohol is taken and sometimes with diazepam or propranolol).

(a)

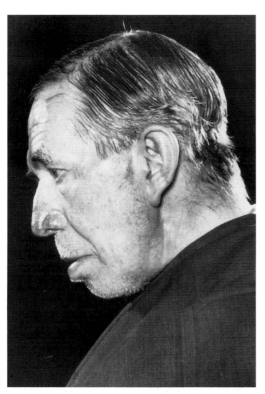

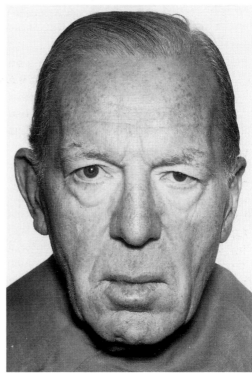

(b)

Fig. 3.38 (a,b) Parkinson's disease.

39 / Chronic bronchitis and emphysema

Frequency in survey: main focus of a short case in 5% of attempts at MRCP short cases. Additional feature in a further 1%.

Survey note: usually the patients in the examination fall between the extremes of the classical *records* below.

Record 1

This thin man (with an anxious, drawn expression) presents the classic 'pink puffer' appearance. He has *nicotine staining* of the fingers. He is tachypnoeic at rest with *lip pursing* during expiration, which is *prolonged*. The suprasternal notch to cricoid distance is reduced (a sign of hyperinflation; normally >3 finger breadths). His chest is *hyperinflated*, *expansion* is mainly *vertical* and there is a *tracheal tug*. He uses his *accessory muscles* of respiration at rest and there is *indrawing* of the *lower ribs* on inspiration (due to a flattened diaphragm). The percussion note is hyper-resonant, obliterating cardiac and hepatic dullness, and the breath sounds are quiet (this is so in classical pure emphysema—frequently, though, wheezes are heard due to associated bronchial disease).

These are the physical findings of a patient with emphysema (inspiratory drive often intact).*

Record 2

This (male) patient (who smokes, lives in a foggy city, works amid dust and fumes, and has probably had frequent respiratory infections) presents the classic 'blue bloater' appearance. He has *nicotine staining* on the fingers. He is stocky and *centrally cyanosed* with suffused conjunctivae. His chest is *hyperinflated*, he uses his *accessory muscles* of respiration; there is *indrawing* of the *intercostal muscles* on inspiration and there is a *tracheal tug* (both signs of hyperinflation). His pulse is 80/min, the venous pressure is not elevated (may be raised with ankle oedema and hepatomegaly if cor pulmonale is present), the trachea is central, but the suprasternal notch to cricoid distance is reduced. *Expansion* is equal but *reduced* to 2 cm and the percussion note is resonant; on auscultation the expiratory phase is prolonged and he has widespread *expiratory rhonchi* and (may be) coarse inspiratory crepitations. (His forced expiratory time—p. 31—is 8 seconds.) There is no flapping tremor of the hands (unless he is in severe hypercapnoeic respiratory failure in which case ask to examine the fundi—? papilloedema).

These are the physical findings of advanced chronic bronchitis† (inspiratory drive often reduced) producing chronic small airways obstruction (and, if ankle oedema, etc., right heart failure due to cor pulmonale).

---

* Emphysema is, however, a pathological diagnosis.
† Chronic bronchitis, though, is defined as sputum production (not due to specific disease such as bronchiectasis or tuberculosis) on most days for 3 months of the year on 2 consecutive years.

Causes of emphysema

Smoking (usually associated with chronic bronchitis; mixed centrilobular and panacinar)

Alpha$_1$ antitrypsin deficiency (?young patient; lower zone emphysema, panacinar in type; ?icterus, hepatomegaly, etc. of hepatitis or cirrhosis)

Coal dust (centrilobular emphysema — simple coal worker's pneumoconiosis — only minor abnormalities of gas exchange)

Macleod's (Swyer–James) syndrome—rare (unilateral emphysema following childhood bronchitis and bronchiolitis with subsequent impairment of alveolar growth; breath sounds diminished on affected side — more likely to meet this in the 'pictures' section of MRCP Part 2 written examination).

Record 1 (continuation)

The decreased breath sounds over the . . . zone of the R/L lung of this patient with emphysema raises the possibility of an emphysematous bulla.

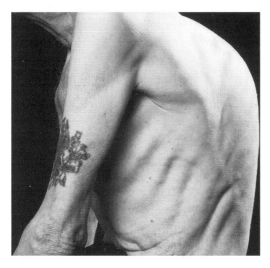

Fig. 3.39 Hyperinflated rib cage. Note indrawing of intercostal muscles.

Frequency in survey: main focus of a short case in 5% of attempts at MRCP short cases. Additional feature in a further 1%.

Record 1

The patient is *overweight* with myxoedematous facies (*thickened* and *coarse facial features*, *periorbital puffiness* and pallor). The *skin* is rough, *dry, cold* and inelastic with a distinct yellowish tint (due to carotenaemia), and there is generalized *non-pitting swelling* of the subcutaneous tissues. The patient's voice is *hoarse* and *croaking*, she is somewhat hard of hearing and her movements are *slow*. There is *thinning* of the *hair* which is *dry* and *brittle* and there is (may be) loss of the outer third of the eyebrows (not a reliable sign). The pulse is *slow* (give rate). There is no palpable goitre. The relaxation phase of the *ankle jerks* (and other reflexes) is delayed and *slow*.

This patient has *myxoedema** (?evidence of associated autoimmune disease—see below).

Record 2

As appropriate from the above plus: in view of the symmetrical, firm, finely micronodular (the typical features of a Hashimoto's goitre though there are many exceptions) *goitre* the likely diagnosis is hypothyroidism due to *Hashimoto's thyroiditis** (?associated autoimmune disease—see below).

Record 3

As appropriate from the above plus: in view of the *exophthalmos* it is likely that this patient was treated in the past for *Graves' disease* by radioactive iodine (or thyroidectomy, if scar) and is now hypothyroid (occasionally Graves' disease progresses spontaneously to hypothyroidism—see p. 98).

Associated autoimmune diseases†
Pernicious anaemia (?spleen, SACD)
Addison's disease (?buccal + scar pigmentation)
Vitiligo
Rheumatoid arthritis (?hands, nodules)
Sjögren's syndrome (?dry eyes and mouth)
Ulcerative colitis
Idiopathic (presumed to be autoimmune) chronic active hepatitis (?icterus, etc.)
Systemic lupus erythematosus (?rash)

Haemolytic anaemia
Diabetes mellitus (?fundi)
Graves' disease
Hypoparathyroidism
Premature ovarian failure.

Important symptoms (if asked to ask the patient some questions—NB deafness and hoarse voice):
Cold intolerance
Tiredness and depression

* In hypothyroidism, accumulation of hyaluronic acid in the dermis as well as other tissues alters the composition of the ground substance. This material binds water, producing the mucinous oedema that is responsible for the thickened features and puffy appearance of full blown hypothyroidism which is termed myxoedema. Hypothyroidism due to autoimmune thyroiditis may present as primary thyroid atrophy (*record* 1) or Hashimoto's disease (*record* 2).
† See also p. 279.

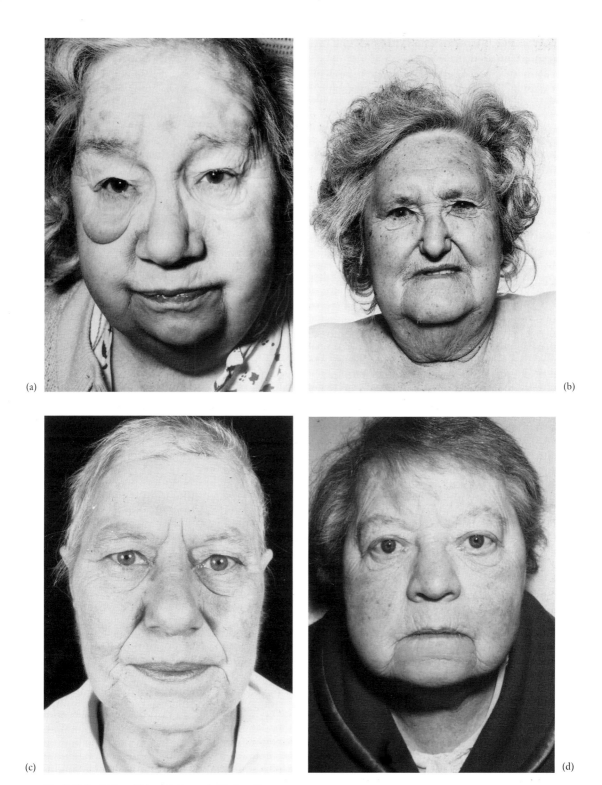

Fig. 3.40 (a–d) Note thickened skin, periorbital swelling, sparse eyebrows and alopecia. The patient in (d) had a malar flush (see also p. 531).

Constipation (may occasionally present to the sur-
geons with faecal impaction)
Angina (treatment may unmask, therefore start with
low doses if age >50, or if patient has angina)
Menorrhagia (middle-aged females)
Primary or secondary amenorrhoea (younger
patients).

Other features

Anaemia (normochromic, iron deficient — atrophic
gastritis, or megaloblastic — frank pernicious
anaemia; slight macrocytosis may occur in
hypothyroidism without a megaloblastic change
in the marrow)
Carpal tunnel syndrome (p. 333)
Peripheral cyanosis (there may be a malar flush)
Raynaud's phenomenon

Hypertension
Accident proneness (may present to the casualty
department)
Hypothermia (especially the elderly living alone)
Hoffman's syndrome (pain, aching and swelling in
muscles after exertion together with signs of
myotonia)
Psychosis (myxoedematous madness)
Hypothyroid coma.

A variety of other central nervous system disorders
may occur,* such as peripheral neuropathy, cerebellar ataxia, pseudodementia, drop attacks and
epilepsy.

For colour photograph see p. 531.

---

* Always exclude concomitant vitamin B_{12} deficiency as the
association with pernicious anaemia is strong. If you find
peripheral neuropathy think also of concomitant diabetes
mellitus before putting it down to the hypothyroidism.

41 / Osler–Weber–Rendu syndrome

Frequency in survey: 5% of attempts at MRCP short cases.

Record

There is *telangiectasia* on the face, around the *mouth*, on the lips, on the *tongue* (look under the tongue), the buccal and nasal mucosa and on the fingers, of this (?clinically anaemic) patient (who has none of the features of systemic sclerosis—p. 96).

The diagnosis is Osler–Weber–Rendu syndrome (hereditary haemorrhagic telangiectasia). The lesions may occur elsewhere, especially in the gastrointestinal tract, and may bleed. Patients may present with *epistaxis* (the most common and sometimes the only site of bleeding), *gastrointestinal haemorrhage*, chronic iron deficiency *anaemia* and occasionally with haemorrhage elsewhere (e.g. haemoptysis).

Usually considered to be autosomal dominant. In fact it is a family of disorders caused by mutations in various genes.

The telangiectasis consists of a localized collection of non-contractile capillaries and shows a prolonged bleeding time if punctured. In some variants (the pattern in individual families tends to be constant) pulmonary arteriovenous aneurysms are common and increase in frequency (as do the telangiectases) with advancing age. These cases may have *cyanosis* and *clubbing*, and *bruits* over the lung fields. The neurological complications include haemorrhage and the formation of bland or mycotic aneurysms. In the eye there may be bloody tears (conjunctival telangiectasia); retinal haemorrhage or detachment may occur. Cirrhosis (due to telangiectasia or multiple transfusions) and massive intrahepatic shunting may occur.

Treatment

Chronic oral iron therapy may be required. Oestrogens (inducing squamous metaplasia of the nasal mucosa) may be helpful if epistaxis is the main symptom. Also for epistaxis, a low dose of the antifibrinolytic agent, aminocaproic acid, may be successful but should not yet be considered the standard approach. Individual lesions should not be cauterized.

For colour photographs see p. 534.

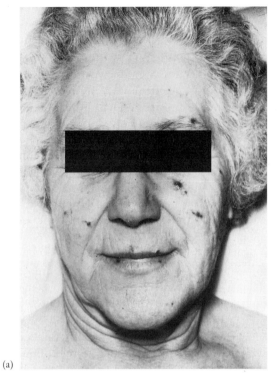

(a)

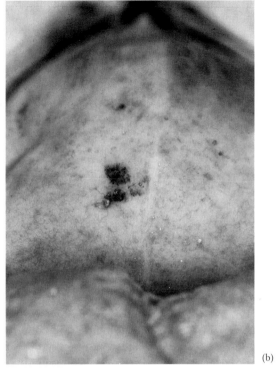

(b)

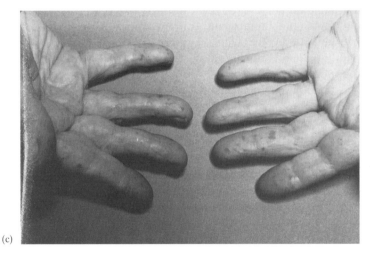

(c)

Fig. 3.41 (a,b) Note palatal telangiectasia in (b). (c) Telangiectasiae of the fingers.

42 / Abdominal mass

Frequency in survey: main focus of a short case in 4% of attempts at MRCP short cases. Additional feature in a further 3%.

Survey note: discussion usually concerned differentiation from/of enlarged organs (spleen, kidney, liver) or differential diagnosis.

Record 1

In this young (?somewhat pale-looking) adult patient there is a freely mobile 5 × 4 cm (measure) firm non-tender mass in the *right iliac fossa*. None of the abdominal organs is enlarged, and there are no fistulae.

The diagnosis could be Crohn's disease (p. 207).

Other causes of a mass in the right iliac fossa

1 Ileocaecal tuberculosis (?ethnic origin, chest signs)
2 Carcinoma of the caecum (?older person, non-tender and hard mass, lymph nodes)
3 Amoebic abscess (?travelled abroad)
4 Lymphoma (?hepatosplenomegaly, lymph nodes elsewhere)
5 Appendicular abscess
6 Neoplasm of the ovary
7 Ileal carcinoid (rare).

Record 2

A freely mobile tender 6 × 5 cm mass is palpable in the *left iliac fossa* in this elderly patient. None of the other organs is palpable.

It is probably a diverticular abscess (usually tender).

Other causes of a mass in the left iliac fossa

1 Carcinoma of the colon (?non-tender, hepatomegaly)
2 Neoplasm of the left ovary
3 A faecal mass (no other signs)
4 Amoebic abscess.

Record 3

In this thin and pale patient there is a round, hard 8 × 6 cm non-tender mass with ill-defined edges in the *epigastrium*. It does not move with respiration. Neither the liver nor the spleen is enlarged (check neck for lymph nodes).

The probable diagnosis is a neoplasm such as:
1 Carcinoma of the stomach (?Troisier's sign)
2 Carcinoma of the pancreas (?icterus. NB Courvoisier's sign)
3 Lymphoma (?generalized lymphadenopathy, spleen).

Record 4

In this elderly patient there is a *pulsatile* (pulsating anteriorly as well as transversely), 6×4 cm firm mass* palpable 2 cm above the umbilicus and reaching the epigastrium. Both femoral pulses are palpable just before the radials (no evidence of dissection) and there are no bruits heard either over the mass or over the femorals. (Look for evidence of peripheral vascular insufficiency in the feet.)

This patient has an aneurysm of his abdominal aorta (the commonest cause is arteriosclerosis†).

If you find a mass in either upper quadrant you should define its:

- Size
- Shape
- Consistency
- Whether you can get above it
- Whether it is bimanually ballotable
- Whether it moves with respiration
- Whether it is tender.

In either upper quadrant it has to be differentiated from a renal mass (pp. 86 and 109); if in the left hypochondrium it has to be differentiated from a spleen (p. 80) and in the right hypochondrium from a liver (p. 101). Other causes of an upper quadrant mass include:

- Carcinoma of the colon
- Retroperitoneal sarcoma
- Lymphoma (?generalized lymphadenopathy, spleen)
- Diverticular abscess (?tender).

---

* Pulsations without a mass may be transmitted from a normal aorta. A mass from a neighbouring structure may overlie the aorta and transmit (only anterior) pulsations.

† Mycotic aneurysms (see anecdote 39, p. 497) are a major complication (2.5% of patients with valvular infections) of infective endocarditis and are most commonly associated with relatively non-invasive organisms such as *Streptococcus viridans*. They may occur at any age, either during the active phase or months (sometimes years) after the endocarditis has been successfully treated. More common sites of mycotic aneurysms are brain (2–6% of all aneurysms in the brain), sinuses of Valsalva, and ligated ductus arteriosus. Clinical manifestations of abdominal aortic aneurysms (e.g. backache) appear after the lesions have started to leak slowly. Surgical treatment is almost always indicated.

43 / Dystrophia myotonica

Frequency in survey: 4% of attempts at MRCP short cases.

Record

The patient has *myopathic facies* (drooping mouth and long, lean, sad, lifeless, somewhat sleepy expression) frontal *balding* (in the male), *ptosis* (may be unilateral) and *wasting* of the *facial muscles*, temporalis, masseter, *sternomastoids*, shoulder girdle and quadriceps. The forearms and legs are involved and the *reflexes* are *lost*. The patient has *cataracts*. After he made a fist he was unable to quickly open it, especially when asked to do this repetitively (this gets worse in the cold and with excitement). He has difficulty opening his eyes after firm closure. When he shook hands there was a delay before he released his grip* (these are all features of *myotonia*). When dimples and depressions are induced in his muscles by percussion, they fill only slowly (*percussion myotonia*—e.g. tongue and thenar eminence).

The diagnosis is dystrophia myotonica.

Males > females.
Autosomal dominant.

Other features

Cardiomyopathy (?small volume pulse, low blood pressure, splitting of first heart sound in mitral area; low voltage P wave, prolonged PR interval, notched QRS and prolonged QT_c on the ECG; dysrythmias; sudden death may occur)

Intellect and personality deterioration

Slurred speech due to combined tongue and pharyngeal myotonia

Testicular atrophy (small soft testicles but secondary sexual characteristics preserved; usually develops after the patient has had children and thus the disease is perpetuated; evidence regarding ovarian atrophy is indefinite)

Diabetes mellitus (end-organ unresponsiveness to insulin)

Nodular thyroid enlargement, small pituitary fossa but normal pituitary function, dysphagia, abdominal pain, hypoventilation, and postanaesthetic respiratory failure may also occur.

The condition may show 'anticipation'—progressively worsening signs and symptoms in succeeding generations; e.g. presenile cataracts may be the sole indication of the disorder in preceding generations.

Myotonia congenita (Thomsen's disease)

There is difficulty in relaxation of a muscle after forceful contraction (myotonia) but none of the other features of dystrophia myotonica (e.g. weakness, cataracts, baldness, gonadal atrophy, etc.) The *reflexes are normal*. Some patients have a 'Herculean' appearance from very developed musculature (?related to repeated involuntary isometric exercise). Myotonia congenita is usually autosomal dominant.

---

*There may be absence of grip myotonia in advanced disease because of progressive muscle wasting. Though myotonia can be relieved by phenytoin, quinine or procainamide, it is weakness (for which there is no treatment) rather than the myotonia which is the main cause of disability in dystrophia myotonica.

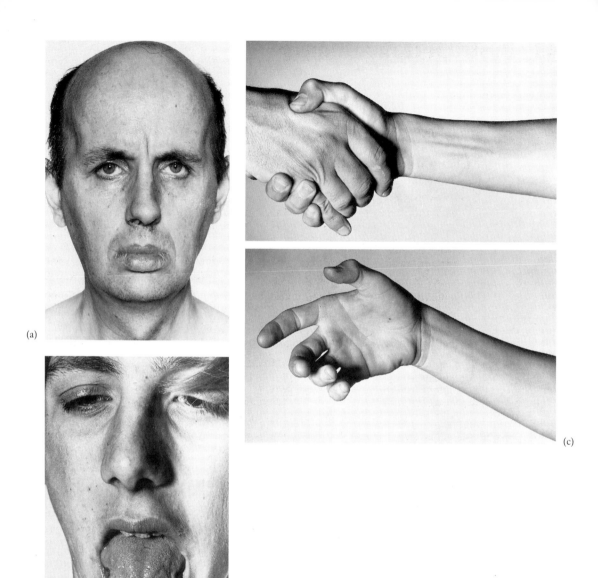

(a)

(b)

(c)

Fig. 3.43 (a–c) Note balding, ptosis, myotonia of the tongue and hands.

44 / Bronchiectasis

Frequency in survey: main focus of a short case in 4% of attempts at MRCP short cases. Additional feature in a further 1%.

Record

This patient (who may be rather *underweight*, *breathless* and *cyanosed*) has *clubbing* of the fingers (not always present) and a frequent *productive cough* (the patient may cough in your presence;* there may be a *sputum pot* by the bed). There are (may be) *inspiratory clicks* heard with the unaided ear. There are *crepitations* over the . . . zone(s) (the area(s) where the bronchiectasis is) and (may be) widespread *rhonchi*.

The diagnosis could well be bronchiectasis. The frequent productive cough and inspiratory clicks are in favour of this. Other possibilities (clubbing and crepitations) are:

1 Carcinoma of the lung (?heavy nicotine staining, lymph nodes, etc.)
2 Fibrosing alveolitis* (marked sputum production and clicks are against this)
3 Lung abscess.

Possible causes of bronchiectasis

Respiratory infection in childhood (especially whooping cough, measles, tuberculosis)

Cystic fibrosis (young, thin patient, may have malabsorption and steatorrhoea, p. 411)

Bronchial obstruction due to foreign body, carcinoma, granuloma (tuberculosis, sarcoidosis) or lymph nodes (e.g. tuberculosis)

Fibrosis (complicating tuberculosis, unresolved or suppurative pneumonia with lung abscess, mycotic infections or sarcoidosis)

Hypogammaglobulinaemia (congenital and acquired)

Allergic bronchopulmonary aspergillosis (proximal airway bronchiectasis)

Marfan's syndrome (?tall, long extremities, high arched palate, p. 267)

Yellow nail syndrome (?excessively curled yellow nails with bulbous fingertips; lymphoedema of extremities, p. 423)

Congenital disorders such as sequestrated lung segments, bronchial atresia, and Kartagener's syndrome.†

---

* It is worth asking the patient to 'give a cough' as it may help you differentiate brochiectasis from fibrosing alveolitis.
† The features of Kartagener's syndrome are dextrocardia, situs inversus, infertility, dysplasia of frontal sinuses, sinusitis and otitis media. Patients have ciliary immotility.

45 / Wasting of the small muscles of the hand

Frequency in survey: main focus of a short case in 4% of attempts at MRCP short cases. Additional feature in a further 11%.

Record

There is *wasting* (and weakness) of the *thenar* and *hypothenar* eminences and of the other small muscles of the hand so that *dorsal guttering* is seen. There is (may be) hyperextension at the metacarpophalangeal joints and flexion at the interphalangeal joints (due to the action of the long extensors of the fingers being unopposed by the lumbricals. In the advanced case a claw hand or *main-en-griffe* is produced).

Generalized wasting of the small muscles of the hand suggests a lesion affecting the lower motor neurones which originate at the level C8,T1 (unless there is arthropathy leading to disuse atrophy).

Causes

A lesion affecting the anterior horn cells at the level C8,T1 such as:

Motor neurone disease (?prominent fasciculation, spastic paraparesis, wasted fibrillating tongue, no sensory signs—p. 123)

Syringomyelia (fasciculation not prominent, ?dissociated sensory loss, burn scars, Horner's, nystagmus—p. 305)

Charcot–Marie–Tooth disease* (?distal wasting of the lower limb, pes cavus, etc.—p. 249)

Other causes are old polio, tumour, meningovascular syphilis, and cord compression.

A root lesion at the level C8,T1 such as:

Cervical spondylosis affecting the C8,T1 level (usually affects higher roots—C6,C7, and therefore significant wasting of the small muscles of the hand is uncommon—see p. 211; ?pyramidal signs in the legs, no signs above the level of the lesion, cervical collar)

Tumour at the C8,T1 level (e.g. neurofibroma).

A lesion damaging the brachial plexus (especially lower trunk and medial cord) such as:

Cervical rib (symptoms provoked by a particular posture or movement, e.g. sleeping on the limb, cleaning windows, etc.; ?supraclavicular bruit though Raynaud's and other vascular manifestations are rare in the presence of prominent neurological features)

Pancoast's tumour (?Horner's, clubbing, chest signs, lymph nodes, cachexia, etc.)

Damage caused by violent traction of arm (e.g. the patient who tried to stop himself falling from a tree by grabbing a passing branch; the same damage in obstetric practice produces Klumpke's paralysis).

Combined ulnar and median nerve lesions (see p. 129 and p. 333, respectively).

Arthritis leading to disuse atrophy† (wasting out of proportion to weakness).

Cachexia.

---

* It is not known whether the degenerative process in Charcot–Marie–Tooth disease originates in the distal axons, ventral nerve roots or in the anterior horn cells.
† E.g. Rheumatoid arthritis. The factors which may contribute to small muscle wasting in the hand in rheumatoid arthritis are disuse atrophy, vasculitis, peripheral neuropathy, mononeuritis multiplex and entrapment neuropathy (median nerve at wrist, ulnar at elbow, and branches—e.g. the deep palmar branch of the ulnar nerve damaged by subluxation of the carpal bones on the radius and ulna).

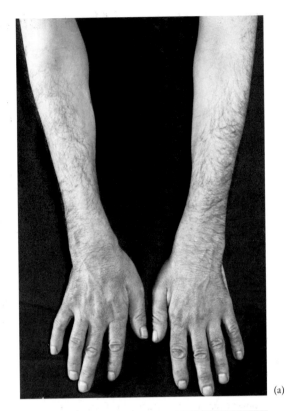

(a)

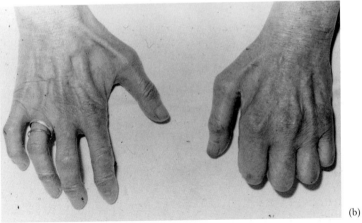

(b)

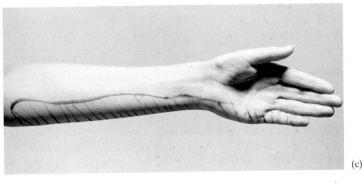

(c)

Fig. 3.45 (a) Charcot–Marie–Tooth disease. (b) Motor neurone disease. (c) Cervical rib.

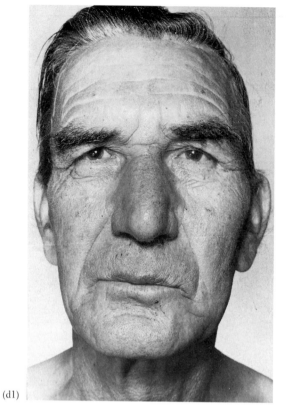

(d1)

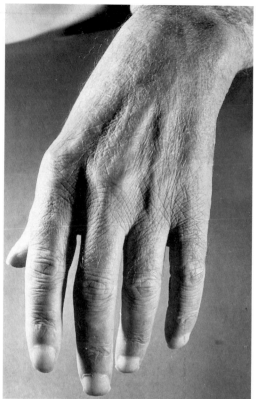

(d2)

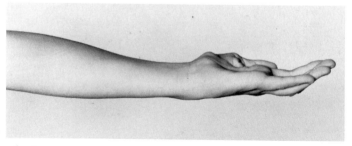

(e)

(f)

Fig. 3.45 (*continued*) (d1,2)
Pancoast's tumour (note left Horner's
syndrome and clubbing). (e)
Rheumatoid arthritis. (f) *Main-en-
griffe* (cervical rib).

46 / Generalized lymphadenopathy

Frequency in survey: main focus of a short case in 4% of attempts at MRCP short cases. Additional feature in a further 6%.

Record

There is generalized lymphadenopathy with/without . . . cm *splenomegaly* (or hepatosplenomegaly).

The likeliest causes would be a *lymphoreticular disorder* (Hodgkin's and non-Hodgkin's lymphoma, etc.) or *chronic lymphatic leukaemia*.

Other causes

Infectious mononucleosis* (?sore throat)
Sarcoidosis (?erythema nodosum or history of)
Tuberculosis (?ethnic origin, lung signs)
Brucellosis (?farm worker)
Toxoplasmosis* (glandular fever-like illness)
Cytomegalovirus* (glandular fever-like illness)
Thyrotoxicosis (?exophthalmos, goitre, tachycardia, etc.—p. 114)
Progressive generalized lymphadenopathy (HIV—365).

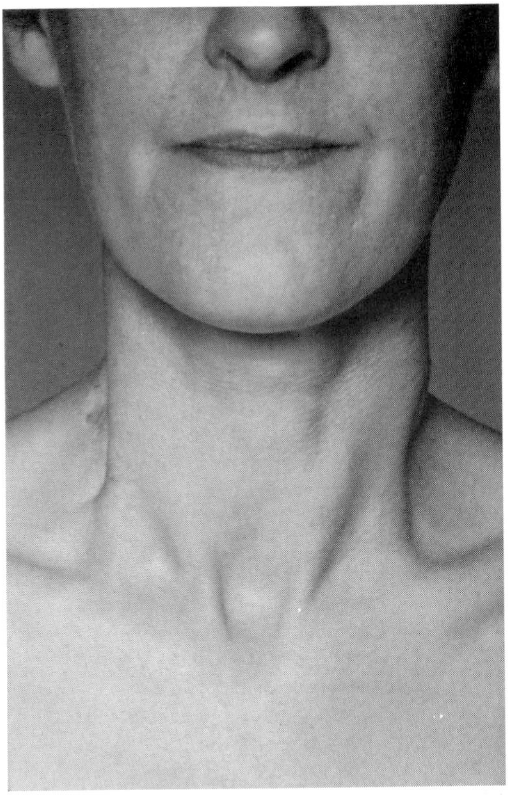

Fig. 3.46 A cervical lymph node seen from the end of the bed.

* Lymph nodes likely to be tender in acute infectious cases.

47 / Papilloedema

Frequency in survey: main focus of a short case in 3% of attempts at MRCP short cases. Additional feature in a further 2%.

Record

There is bilateral papilloedema* (search carefully for haemorrhages, exudates and AV nipping).

Possible causes

1 These include:

(a) *an intracranial space-occupying lesion* (?localizing neurological signs†)

(b) tumour (infratentorial more often than supratentorial)

(c) abscess (fever not always present, ?underlying middle ear infection, underlying suppuration elsewhere—e.g. bronchiectasis or empyema)

(d) haematoma.

2 *Malignant hypertension* (check blood pressure—haemorrhages and exudates are not always present; ?narrow tortuous arterioles that vary in calibre, AV nipping—p. 136).

3 *Benign intracranial hypertension*‡ (?obese female aged 15–45, no localizing neurological signs).

---

*The disc oedema of papillitis (disc usually pink due to hyperaemia) must be differentiated from developing papilloedema due to raised intracranial pressure. Papilloedema causes enlargement of the blindspot and constriction of the peripheral field, but visual acuity is unaffected. Papillitis (optic neuritis affecting the intraorbital portion of the optic nerve) causes central scotoma, diminished visual acuity, and sometimes tenderness and pain on eye movement during the acute attack. Furthermore, in papillitis there may be a pupillary reflex defect, loss of the central cup and cells may be present in the vitreous over the disc.

† VIth nerve palsy in the presence of papilloedema may be a false localizing sign due to raised intracranial pressure stretching the nerve during its long intracranial course. A localizing sign may occasionally be rapidly apparent in the case of contralateral optic atrophy—the *Foster–Kennedy syndrome* (a frontal tumour pressing on the optic nerve to cause atrophy and at the same time raising intracranial pressure to cause papilloedema in the other eye). It must be remembered that tumours in and around the frontal lobes can present simply with dementia in the absence of signs and symptoms of raised intracranial pressure (i.e. without papilloedema). A classic lesion to present in this manner is a subfrontal olfactory groove meningioma. These may grow to considerable size, initially causing only memory impairment and marked apathy. On examination and upon closer questioning there is usually a history of diminished or absent sense of smell. Loss of urinary control associated with dementia should be regarded as indicating organic pathology until proven otherwise. A much shorter history of dementia and urinary incontinence together with increasingly severe headache may indicate an underlying malignant glioma of the corpus callosum or of one or other frontal lobe.

‡ This syndrome (also called pseudotumour cerebri, serous meningitis or otitic hydrocephalus) is known to have occurred following middle ear infection which caused lateral sinus thrombosis. It may be that thrombosis of the venous sinuses is the aetiological factor in many other cases. The condition has been associated with the contraceptive pill, long-term tetracycline treatment for acne, corticosteroids (often reduction in dose during long-term therapy), head injury and times of female physiological hormone disturbance such as menarche, pregnancy and puerperium. The cerebrospinal fluid pressure is high, frequently above 300 mm, but the composition of the fluid is normal; the protein content is usually low normal, below 20 mg/dl.

The first sign of raised intracranial pressure is loss of venous pulsation, but recognition of this sign requires much practice and experience (see p. 19). If there is doubt about the normality of the disc, the presence of venous pulsation makes papilloedema and raised intracranial pressure unlikely.

Other causes of papilloedema

Meningitis (especially tuberculous)

Hypercapnoea (cyanosis, flapping tremor of the hands)

Central retinal vein thrombosis (sight affected, usually unilateral, dilated veins, widespread haemorrhages)

(Graves') Congestive ophthalmopathy (= malignant exophthalmos though exophthalmos is not always present; prominent eyes, eyelids and conjunctivae swollen and inflamed, marked ophthalmoplegia, often pain)

Cavernous sinus thrombosis (usually becomes bilateral, follows infection of orbit, nose and face; eyeball(s) protrudes, is painful, immobile and there is extreme venous congestion)

Hypoparathyroidism (tetany, epilepsy, cataracts, etc.)

Severe anaemia especially due to massive blood loss and leukaemia (there may be haemorrhages and cotton wool spots as well)

Guillain–Barré syndrome (papilloedema possibly due to impaired cerebrospinal fluid resorption because of the elevated protein content)

Paget's disease (large head, bowed tibiae)

Hurler's syndrome (dwarf, large head, coarse features, hepatosplenomegaly, heart murmurs)

Poisoning with vitamin A, lead, tetracyclines or naladixic acid

Ocular toxoplasmosis.

For colour photograph see p. 528.

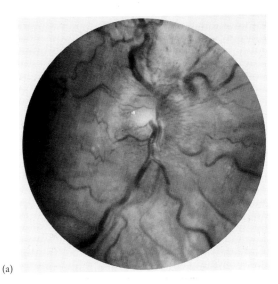

(a)

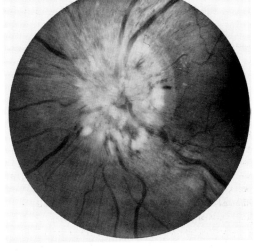

(b)

Fig. 3.47 (a,b) Papilloedema.

48 / Diabetic foot

Frequency in survey: main focus of a short case in 3% of attempts at MRCP short cases. Additional feature in a further 2%.

Record 1

There is an *ulcer* on the sole of the R/L foot (most commonly at the site of the pressure point under the head of the first metatarsal) and two of the toes have previously been amputated. There is thick *callous* formation over the pressure points of the feet, and the normal concavity of the transverse arch at the head of the metatarsals is lost. There is *loss* of *sensation* to light touch, vibration and pinprick in a *stocking distribution*. The feet are *cold*, the foot pulses are not palpable* and there is *loss of hair* on the lower legs which are *shiny*.

This patient has *peripheral neuropathy*, a *neuropathic ulcer* on the sole of his foot and evidence of *peripheral vascular disease*. It is likely that he has underlying diabetes mellitus (?fundi).

Factors which may contribute to the production of the diabetic foot lesions

Injury—always a provocative factor
Neuropathy—trivial injury is not noticed
Consequent formation of callosities at repeatedly traumatized pressure points
Small vessel disease
Large vessel disease producing ischaemia and gangrene of the foot
Increased susceptibility to infection
Maldistributed pressure and foot deformity leading to increased likelihood of friction and trauma.

From the list of the other causes of peripheral neuropathy (p. 134) **neuropathic ulcers** are particularly associated with
1 Tabes dorsalis (?facies, pupils, etc.—p. 381)
2 Leprosy
3 Porphyria (?vesicles, crusts—p. 368)
4 Amyloidosis
5 Progressive sensory neuropathy (both familial and cryptogenic)

and rarely as a late manifestation of
6 Charcot–Marie–Tooth disease (distal muscle wasting, pes cavus, etc.—p. 249).

Record 2 (Charcot's joint)

As relevant from *record 1* plus: the ankle joint is greatly *deformed* and *swollen*, and there is loud *crepitus* accompanying *movement* which is of an *abnormal range*.

This is a Charcot's joint (neuropathic arthropathy—gross osteoarthrosis and new bone formation from repeated minor trauma without the normal protective responses which accompany pain sensation; the joint is painlessly destroyed).

Main causes of a Charcot's joint

Diabetes mellitus (toes—common; ankles—rare)
Tabes dorsalis (especially hip and knee; —?facies, pupils, etc.)
Syringomyelia (elbow and shoulder; — ?Horner's, wasted hand muscles, dissociated sensory loss, etc.—p. 305)

---

* NB In the predominantly neuropathic foot the pulses may be present or even bounding, and the veins may be prominent —autonomic denervation opens up arteriovenous shunts; as a consequence blood passes down the arteries, through the shunts and back up the veins, missing out the nutrient capillaries on the way—this contributes to the poor healing.

Leprosy (important on a worldwide basis).

Other rare causes include yaws, progressive sensory neuropathy (familial and cryptogenic), other hereditary neuropathies (e.g. Charcot–Marie–Tooth), and neurofibromatosis (pressure on sensory nerve roots), though any cause of loss of sensation in a joint may render it liable to the development of a neuropathic arthropathy.

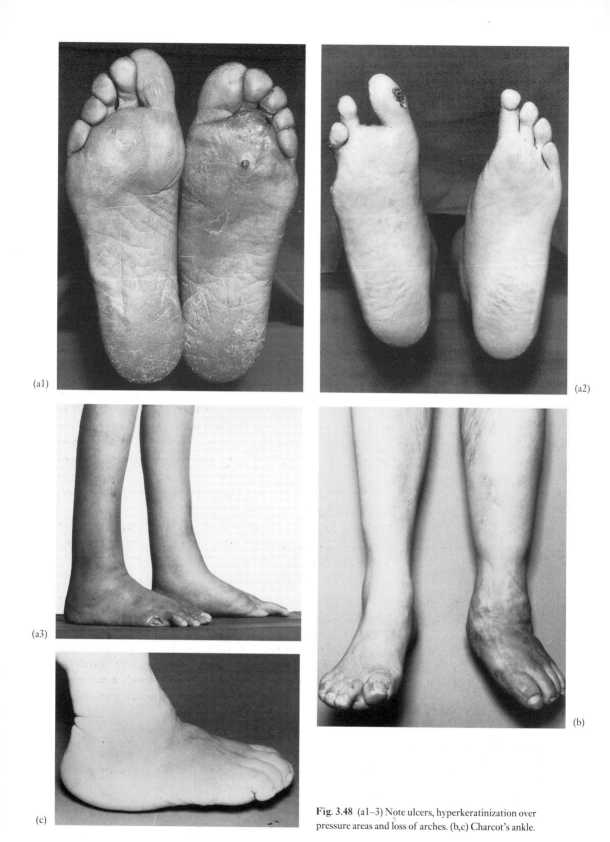

(a1)

(a2)

(a3)

(b)

(c)

Fig. 3.48 (a1–3) Note ulcers, hyperkeratinization over pressure areas and loss of arches. (b,c) Charcot's ankle.

49 / Nystagmus

Frequency in survey: main focus of a short case in 3% of attempts at MRCP short cases. Additional feature in a further 2%.

Survey note: in most cases nystagmus was cerebellar in origin—usually due to multiple sclerosis.

Record 1

There is nystagmus, greater on the R/L with the fast component to the same side. This suggests:

1 an ipsilateral cerebellar lesion (?cerebellar signs—p. 142)

or

2 a contralateral vestibular lesion (?vertical nystagmus, ?vertigo—see below). (Now, if allowed, *look for cerebellar signs*; occasionally there will be signs of a lesion in the brainstem, e.g. infarction—p. 438, syringobulbia*—p. 305.)

Record 2

The nystagmus is *ataxic* in that the *abducting eye has greater nystagmus* than the adducting eye.† With this there is dissociation of conjugate eye movements. There is (may be) a divergent strabismus at rest. On looking to the right, the right eye abducts normally, but there is *impairment of adduction*† of the left eye. On looking to the left, the left eye abducts normally but there is *impairment of adduction*† of the right eye (occasionally the reverse may occur with weakness of abduction on each side but adduction remains normal). When the abducting eye is covered, however, the medial movement of the other eye occurs normally.

The diagnosis is *internuclear ophthalmoplegia*. It suggests multiple sclerosis‡ with a lesion in the medial longitudinal fasciculus. (Now, if allowed, *look for cerebellar signs*, pyramidal signs, pale discs, etc.—pp. 142 and 433.)

Causes and types of nystagmus

A diagramatic representation of conjugate gaze and its various connections is depicted in Fig. 3.49. As can be seen from the multiplicity of these pathways a disorder within the end-organs (i.e. eye, labyrinth, semicircular canals), or in the medial longitudinal fasciculus anywhere through its long course, or in its nuclear connections (i.e. cerebellar, vestibular nuclei, etc.) can cause nystagmus. Nystagmus can be divided into:

Physiological nystagmus (a few brief jerks can occur in the normal eye at the extreme lateral gaze)

Ocular nystagmus (in patients with a congenital visual defect in one eye a pendular movement of

---

* As can be seen from the diagram, the medial longitudinal bundle extends into the spinal cord so that syringomyelia confined to the spinal cord, if extending above C5, may also cause nystagmus.

† The key sign of the internuclear ophthalmoplegia is the *failure of adduction*—the nystagmus is not essential.

‡ Internuclear ophthalmoplegia is highly characteristic of multiple sclerosis though rarely it may be caused by brainstem gliomas or vascular lesions, or Wernicke's encephalopathy (ocular palsy, nystagmus, loss of pupillary reflexes, ataxia, peripheral neuropathy, Korsakoff's psychosis or other disturbance of mentation; dramatic response to thiamine in the early stages).

the eye occurs while gazing straight — fixation nystagmus)

Vestibular nystagmus (see below)
Cerebellar nystagmus (*record* 1)
Ataxic nystagmus (*record* 2).

Vestibular nystagmus

This may arise in the periphery (labyrinth or vestibular nerve) or in the central vestibular nuclei and its connections.

Peripheral. The fast component is towards the contralateral side (except with an early irritative lesion when it can be on the side of the lesion) and the nystagmus is fatiguable — it becomes less and less intense on repetition of the test. The patient tends to be unsteady on the ipsilateral side (contralateral to the fast component) as can be revealed whilst assessing Romberg's test (the patient cannot stand on a narrow base even with the eyes open in this situation whereas the patient with sensory ataxia becomes more unsteady when the eyes are closed) and gait (tends to reel on the affected side). Cochlear function is usually affected (diminishes leading to deafness—e.g. Menière's syndrome) and the patient may have vertigo.

Causes of peripheral vestibular nystagmus:
Labyrinthitis (probably viral and self-limiting; nystagmus may be absent and only positional and provoked by movements of the head—often it can be elicited by bending the head backwards about 45° — the nystagmus, as well as the vertigo, may appear but fades with repeated testing)

Menière's syndrome (progressive deafness and tinnitus, with recurrent attacks of vertigo)

Acoustic neuroma (progressive tinnitus and nerve deafness; neighbouring nerves—Vth, VIth, VIIth may be involved and there may be cerebellar signs, etc.—p. 335)

Vestibular neuronitis (acute vertigo without deafness or tinnitus which usually improves within 48 h; full recovery may take weeks or months; may be viral).

Other causes include degenerative middle ear disease, hypertension and head injury.

Central. Lesions affecting vestibular nuclei (cerebrovascular accident, multiple sclerosis, encephalitis, tumours, syringobulbia, alcoholism,§ anticonvulsants, etc.) cause nystagmus which is spontaneous but may be brought on or increased by head movements. It is not adaptable and usually has a vertical component. *Downbeat nystagmus* with the eyes looking straight ahead is characteristic of Arnold–Chiari malformation.‖ Downbeat nystagmus on lateral gaze normally indicates a lesion at foramen magnum level (tumour, syringomyelia or cerebellar degeneration).

§ Acute alcohol toxicity may cause nystagmus. Nystagmus is also almost always present in Wernicke's encephalopathy. Paradoxically alcohol may reduce congenital nystagmus—a condition which may be gross but symptomless.
‖ *Arnold–Chiari malformation* may be asymptomatic until adult life when the patient gradually develops cerebellar symptoms and signs. There is cerebellar herniation through the foramen magnum. There may be coexisting syringomyelia of the cervical cord and medulla (p. 303). Commonly there is radiographic evidence of fusion of the cervical vertebrae, platybasia or basilar impression. MRI (CT may miss it) establishes the diagnosis when there are no coexisting bony abnormalities. Surgical intervention may benefit selected cases.

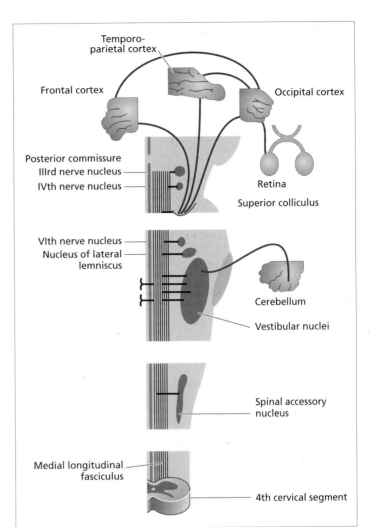

Fig. 3.49 Cortical, brainstem and peripheral control of conjugate gaze. The medial longitudinal bundle starts just below the posterior commissure and ends in the upper cervical spinal cord. During its long course it receives fibres from various nucleii (and the lateral pontine gaze centre) which are concerned with the control of conjugate gaze. Interruption in the cortical or midbrain connections often produces a disorder of conjugate gaze rather than nystagmus. Lesions in the brainstem or below result in nystagmus.

50 / Old choroiditis

Frequency in survey: 3% of attempts at MRCP short cases.

Invigilator's observation: easily confused with laser burn scars in the diabetic fundus.*

Record
There is evidence of old choroiditis in the . . . region of the R/L fundus.
or
In the . . . region of the R/L fundus there is a *patch of white** (or yellow or grey). It suggests exposed sclera due to atrophy of the choroidoretina secondary to old choroiditis. Together with this there are also scattered *pigmented patches* due to proliferation of the retinal pigment epithelium.

In most cases the cause of the choroiditis is unknown but *toxoplasmosis* is commonly implicated.

Other causes

Sarcoidosis (?lupus pernio, chest signs, etc.)

Tuberculosis (often inactive; ?ethnic origin, chest signs)

Syphilis (?tabetic facies and pupils, posterior column signs, extensor plantars, etc.)

Toxocara

Trauma.

For colour photograph see p. 529.

---

* Candidates sometimes call laser burns on the diabetic fundus (p. 65) old choroiditis, and old choroiditis laser burns, thus diagnosing old choroiditis as diabetic retinopathy. The confusion can be understood when one realizes that laser burn scars are, in a way, a form of old choroiditis. The matter is made worse because the patient with diabetic retinopathy may also happen to have old choroiditis (as diabetics are the main group of people having their fundi carefully examined on a large scale, patients with old choroiditis among them are readily detected). Laser burns can usually be distinguished by their more regular uniform appearance as in colour photograph A4 on p. 527.

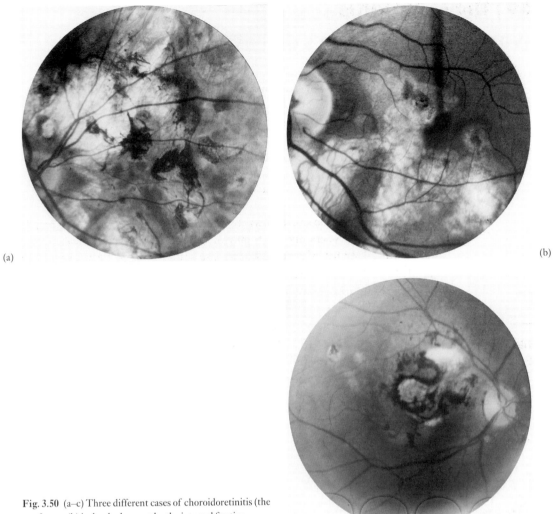

(a)

(b)

Fig. 3.50 (a–c) Three different cases of choroidoretinitis (the artefact on (b) is the shadow cast by the internal fixation device of the fundus camera).

(c)

51 / Neurofibromatosis (von Recklinghausen's disease)

Frequency in survey: main focus of a short case in 3% of attempts at MRCP short cases. Additional feature in a further 1%.

Survey note: occurred as either a spot diagnosis, with or without a mention of the associated features, or as a case with an associated nerve pressure effect (such as one with an ulnar nerve/T1 lesion).

Record

There are multiple *neurofibromata* and *café-au-lait spots* (normal person allowed up to five of the latter).
    The diagnosis is neurofibromatosis.*

or

There are multiple skin lesions: *sessile* and *pedunculated* cutaneous *fibromata*, as well as neurofibromata which are both *soft* and *firm*, *single* and *lobulated*, and felt both as mobile subcutaneous lumps† and *nodules* along the course of peripheral nerves. There are *café-au-lait* spots (especially in the axillae—axillary freckling).
    The diagnosis is neurofibromatosis.*

Autosomal dominant.
The condition is usually asymptomatic.

Complications

Kyphoscoliosis
Pressure effects of the neurofibromata on peripheral nerves and cranial nerves, especially:
  (a) acoustic neuroma (?Vth, VIth, VIIth, VIIIth nerve lesions, nystagmus and cerebellar signs; may be bilateral—p. 335)*
  (b) Vth nerve neuroma
Spinal nerve root involvement which may cause
  (a) cord compression
  (b) muscle wasting
  (c) sensory loss (Charcot's joints may occur)
Sarcomatous or other malignant change (5–16%)
Lung cysts (honeycomb lung)
Pseudoarthrosis and other orthopaedic abnormalities
Plexiform neuroma.‡

Other intracranial tumours which can occur in this condition are:
Gliomata (optic nerve and chiasma; cerebral)
Meningiomata*
Medulloblastomata.

---

* The phakomatoses or neurocutaneous syndromes are characterized by disordered growth of neurocutaneous tissues. More than 20 syndromes have been described the most important of which are *neurofibromatosis 1 (von Recklinghausen's*—chromosome 17), neurofibromatosis 2 (chromosome 22), tuberous sclerosis (p. 308) and Sturge–Weber disease (p. 193). *Neurofibromatosis 2*, often called *central neurofibromatosis*, is rare and characterized by bilateral acoustic neuromata and often other intracranial tumours such as meningiomata or ependymomata. A few *café-au-lait* spots are present in about 40% of cases. At-risk family members should be screened regularly with hearing tests, etc.

† Neurofibromatosis should not be confused with lipomatosis with its characteristic soft subcutaneous lumps. In Dercum's disease (usually middle-aged females) subcutaneous lipomata may be painful and associated with marked obesity.

‡ An entire nerve trunk and all its branches are involved in diffuse neurofibromatosis with associated overgrowth of overlying tissues leading to gross deformities (temporal and frontal scalp are favourite sites but it may occur anywhere); may grow to lemon or even melon size.

Other features of neurofibromatosis

An association with phaeochromocytoma — 5% of
  cases (?blood pressure)
Nodules of the iris

Hamartomata of the retina
Rib notching.

For colour photograph see p. 539.

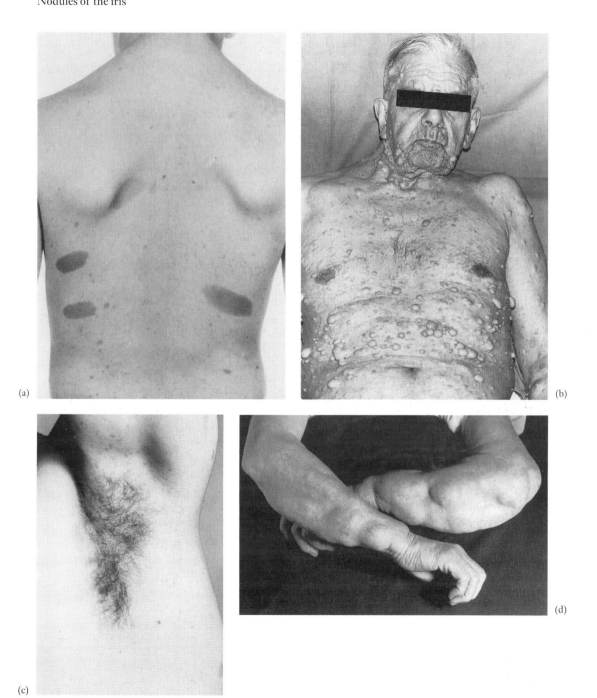

(a)

(b)

(c)

(d)

Fig. 3.51 (a) *Café-au-lait* spots. (b) Gross neurofibromatosis.
(c) Axillary freckling. (d) Lipomatosis.

52 / Erythema nodosum

Frequency in survey: 3% of attempts at MRCP short cases.

Survey note: this usually occurs as a spot diagnosis followed by questions about the possible causes. Histology was asked for on one occasion.

Record

There are in this (usually) female patient *raised* (become flat with healing) *red* (pass through the changes of a *bruise* with healing), *tender* lesions 2–6 cm in diameter on the *shins* (and occasionally thighs and upper limbs).

The diagnosis is erythema nodosum (?fever, arthralgia).

Possible causes

1 Acute sarcoidosis (bilateral hilar lymphadenopathy; fever, arthralgia, palpable cervical and axillary lymph nodes, mild iridocyclitis)
2 Streptococcal infection (e.g. throat)
3 Rheumatic fever (tachycardia, murmur, nodules, etc.)
4 Primary tuberculosis (?ethnic origin, chest signs, etc.)
5 Drugs (sulphonamides, penicillin, oral contraceptives, codeine, salicylates, barbiturates).

Other causes

Pregnancy
Ulcerative colitis
Crohn's disease
Yersinia enterocolitis
Malignancies (lymphoma and leukaemia)
Syphilis
Leprosy (important cause on a worldwide basis)
Tinea and other fungal infections
Coccidioidomycosis
Toxoplasmosis
Lymphogranuloma venereum
Behçet's disease (orogenital ulceration, iridocyclitis, etc.)
Idiopathic.

Histology

Perivascular mixed cell infiltrate followed by giant cell formation. There is oedema and a variable amount of extravascular blood. The inflammation spreads into the subcutaneous fat.
or
In a nutshell: subcutaneous inflammatory changes which are vasculitic in origin.

For colour photograph see p. 538.

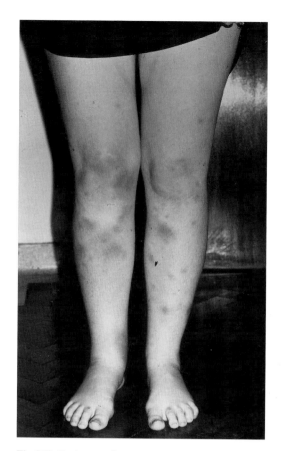

Fig. 3.52 Erythema nodosum.

53 / Horner's syndrome

Frequency in survey: main focus of a short case in 3% of attempts at MRCP short cases. Additional feature in a further 1%.

Record

There is *miosis,** *enophthalmos* and slight *ptosis* on the R/L side (the other features are ipsilateral *anhydrosis* and vasodilatation of the head and neck).

This is a R/L sided Horner's syndrome—now examine the *neck* (scars, nodes, aneurysms), *hands* (wasting of the small muscles) and *chest* (ipsilateral apical signs).

Causes of Horner's syndrome

1 Neck surgery or trauma (?scars)
2 Carotid and aortic aneurysms
3 Brainstem vascular disease (e.g. Wallenberg's syndrome†)
4 Pancoast's syndrome (?wasting of ipsilateral small muscles of the hand, T1 and sometimes C7/C8 sensory loss and pain, clubbing, tracheal deviation, lymph nodes, ipsilateral apical signs)
5 Enlarged cervical lymph nodes especially malignant (?evidence of primary)
6 Idiopathic (common in neurological practice)
7 Syringomyelia (?bilateral wasting of the small muscles of the hand, dissociated sensory loss, scarred hands, bulbar palsy, pyramidal signs, nystagmus—p. 305)
8 Brainstem demyelination (?nystagmus, cerebellar signs, pyramidal signs, pale discs, etc.).

The syndrome can be caused by any other lesion in the sympathetic nervous system as it travels from the sympathetic nucleus, down through the brainstem to the cord, out of the cord at C8,T1,T2, to the sympathetic chain, stellate ganglion and carotid sympathetic plexus (see Fig. 3.53b). Some cases of Horner's are idiopathic (usually females).

---

* NB Argyll Robertson pupils in neurosyphilis are usually bilateral, irregular and very small.
† Ipsilateral Vth, IXth, Xth, XIth nerve lesions, cerebellar ataxia and nystagmus. Contralateral pain and temperature loss (see p. 438).

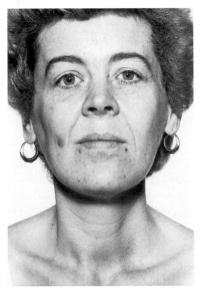

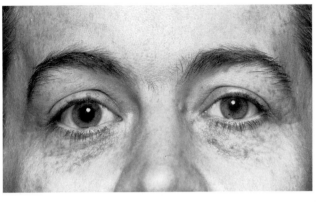

(a2)

(a1)

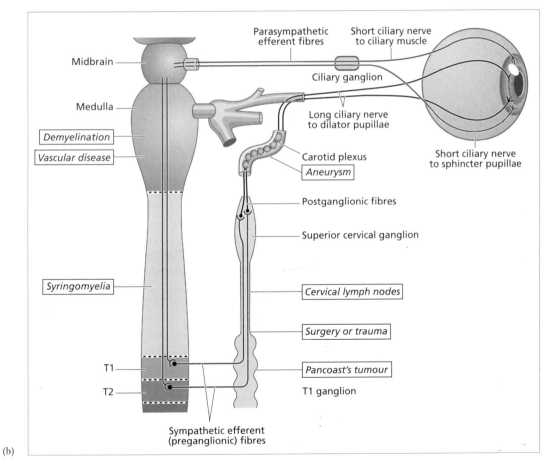

(b)

Fig. 3.53 (a1,2) Left Horner's syndrome (note the scar over the left clavicle). (b) Sympathetic and parasympathetic nerve supply to dilator and sphincter pupillae. The diagram shows the sympathetic pathway and the sites where it may be interrupted to produce Horner's syndrome. (Pathways diagram adapted from *Gray's Anatomy of the Human Body* by kind permission of the publisher, Lea & Febiger.)

54 / Old polio

Frequency in survey: main focus of a short case in 3% of attempts at MRCP short cases. Additional feature in a further 1%.

Record

The R/L leg is *short, wasted, weak* and *flaccid* with *reduced (or absent) reflexes* and a normal plantar response. There is *no sensory defect*. The disparity in the length of the limbs suggests growth impairment in the affected limb since early childhood. The complete absence of sensory and pyramidal signs point to a condition affecting only lower motor neurones.*

The diagnosis is old polio affecting the R/L leg.

If you see one limb smaller than the other a possible differential diagnosis to consider is infantile hemiplegia. In this there is usually hemismallness of the whole of that side of the body and the neurological signs will reflect a contralateral hemisphere lesion (i.e. upper motor neurone).

---

*Fasciculation is only occasionally seen in old polio. Very rarely patients with old polio for many years develop a progressive wasting disease (with prominent fasciculation) which is indistinguishable from progressive muscular atrophy motor neurone disease or chronic asymmetrical spinal muscular atrophy (see p. 123).

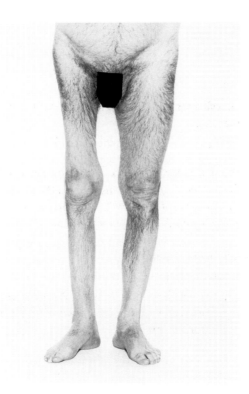

Fig. 3.54 Generalized wasting of the right lower limb due to old poliomyelitis.

55 / Ankylosing spondylitis

Frequency in survey: 3% of attempts at MRCP short cases.

Survey note: candidates were asked to examine either the chest, the back, the neck, to watch the patient walk, or to watch the patient 'look at the ceiling'. One-third of candidates made the point that the diagnosis was not apparent with the patient lying down.

Record

There is (in this male patient) *loss of lumbar lordosis* and *fixed kyphosis* which is compensated for by extension of the cervical spine (to attempt to keep the visual axis horizontal) producing a *stooped*, 'question mark' posture. When I ask the patient to turn his head to look to the side his whole body turns as a block (the spine being rigid with little movement). *Chest expansion* is *reduced*; the patient breathes by increased diaphragmatic excursion which is the cause of the *prominent abdomen*.

The diagnosis is ankylosing spondylitis. (If allowed, look at the *eyes* — iritis, listen to the *heart* — aortic incompetence, and examine the *chest* — apical fibrosis).

Ratio of males to females is 8:1.

Complications and extra-articular manifestations

Iritis — 30% (acute, deep aching pain, redness, photophobia, miosis, sluggish pupillary reflex, circumcorneal conjunctival injection; may result in synechiae or cataracts)

Aortitis — 4% (?collapsing pulse and early diastolic murmur of aortic incompetence; ascending aortic aneurysm)

Apical fibrosis — rare (?apical inspiratory crackles; probably secondary to diminished apical ventilation; there may be calcification and cavitation; may get secondary aspergillus infection)

Cardiac conduction defects — 10% (usually AV block; other cardiac abnormalities may occur — pericarditis and cardiomyopathy)

Neurological (atlantoaxial dislocation or traumatic fracture of a rigid spine may injure the spinal cord — tetra/paraplegia; involvement of the sacral nerves at the sacroiliac joints may cause sciatica; rarely cauda equina involvement can cause urinary or rectal sphincter incompetence)

Secondary amyloidosis (kidneys, adrenals, liver — ?hepatomegaly).

Other features

There is a strong (87%) association with HLA-B27. There is a familial tendency; 50% of relatives are HLA-B27 and 9% have sacroiliitis which may be symptomless.* Ankylosing spondylitis usually starts before the age of 45.† It may present as an asymmetrical peripheral arthritis usually of large, weight-bearing joints; the small joints of the hands and feet are only rarely involved. It commonly presents with low back pain:

Ankylosing spondylitis — pain worse on waking, eases with exercise

Compared with

---

*The disease is more severe in sporadic cases (about 80%) than in the familial form (20%). Sibling pairs concordant for the disease tend to have disease of comparable severity.

† In the early stages, loss of lateral flexion of lumbar spine is usually the first sign of spinal involvement, followed by loss of lumbar lordosis.

Mechanical back pain — no pain on waking; pain brought on by exercise.

In the *'heels, hips, occiput'* test the patient is asked to demonstrate that he can put all three against a wall at once. *Schober's test* refers to the normal 10 cm excursion of two points 5 cm apart when the patient bends forward.

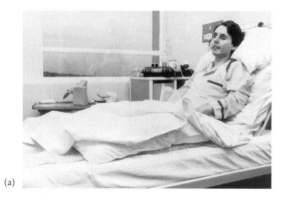
(a)

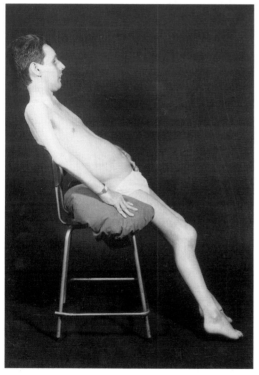
(b)

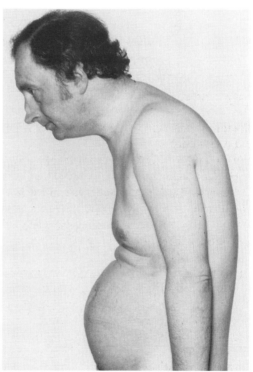
(c)

Fig. 3.55 (a) The ankylosing spondylitis is less obvious when reclining in bed. (b) In the same patient as (a), a rigid and immobile spine was revealed by his attempt at sitting up (note the generalized involvement of the joints in this severe case). (c) Patient attempting to look straight ahead (note the kyphosis, loss of lumbar lordosis and protuberant abdomen).

Frequency in survey: main focus of a short case in 3% of attempts at MRCP short cases. Additional feature in a further 3%.

Survey note: relative frequencies in the survey: cerebellar ataxia 45%, spastic paraplegia 27%, sensory ataxia 9%, Parkinson's disease 9% and Charcot–Marie–Tooth (steppage gait) 9%. Neither hemiplegia, waddling gait nor gait apraxia occurred in our survey.

Record 1

The gait is *wide-based* and the arms are held wide (both upper and lower limbs tend to tremble and shake). The patient is *ataxic* and tends to fall to the R/L, especially during the *heel-to-toe* test which he is unable to perform. Romberg's test is negative.

This suggests *cerebellar disease* which is predominantly R/L sided. (Now, if allowed, examine for other cerebellar signs: finger–nose, rapid alternate motion, nystagmus, staccato dysarthria, etc.—p. 142.)

Possible causes

1 Demyelinating disease (?pale discs, pyramidal signs, etc.—p. 433)
2 Tumour (primary or secondary—?evidence of primary—e.g. bronchus, breast, etc.)
3 Non-metastatic syndrome of malignancy (?evidence of primary especially bronchus—clubbing, cachexia, etc.)
4 Alcoholic cerebellar degeneration
5 Other cerebellar degenerations (?pes cavus, kyphoscoliosis, absent ankle jerks and extensor plantars, etc. of Friedreich's ataxia).

Record 2

The patient has a *stiff*, awkward 'scissors' or 'wading through mud' gait.

This suggests *spastic paraplegia*. (Now, if allowed, examine tone, reflexes, plantars, sensation, etc.—p. 102.)

Possible causes

1 Demyelinating disease (?impaired rapid alternate motion in arms, pale discs, etc.—p. 433)
2 Cord compression (?sensory level with no signs above)
3 Hereditary spastic paraplegia (rare)
4 Cerebral diplegia (rare).

Record 3

The gait is ataxic and *stamping* (his feet tend to 'throw'; both the heels and the toes slap on the ground). The patient walks on a wide base, *watching his feet and the ground* (to some extent he can compensate for lack of sensory information from the muscles and joints by visual attention). He has difficulty walking heel to toe and the ataxia becomes much worse when he closes his eyes; *Romberg's* test is *positive*.

He has *sensory ataxia* (now look for Argyll Robertson pupils and for clinical anaemia).

Possible causes

1 Subacute combined degeneration of the cord (?pyramidal signs, absent ankle jerks plus peripheral neuropathy; anaemia, spleen, etc.; no Argyll Robertson pupils—p. 314)
2 Tabes dorsalis (?facies, pupils, pyramidal signs if taboparesis, etc.—p. 381)
3 Cervical myelopathy (?mid-cervical reflex pattern in the arms; pyramidal signs in legs—p. 211)
4 Diabetic pseudotabes (?fundi)
5 Friedreich's ataxia (pes cavus, scoliosis, cerebellar signs, etc.—p. 234)
6 Demyelinating disease (ataxia in multiple sclerosis is usually mainly cerebellar).

Record 4

This (depressed, expressionless, unblinking and stiff) patient *stoops* and his gait, initially *hesitant*, is *shuffling* and has lost its spring. The *arms* are held flexed and *do not swing*. The hands show a *pill-rolling tremor*. His gait is *festinant*, i.e. he appears to be continually about to fall forward as if chasing his own centre of gravity.

He has *Parkinson's disease*.* (Now examine the wrists for cog-wheel rigidity, elbows for lead-pipe rigidity, and for the glabellar tap sign, etc.—p. 148.)

Record 5

The patient has a *steppage* gait. He lifts his R/L foot high to avoid scraping the toe because he has a R/L *foot-drop*. He is unable to walk on his R/L heel.

Possible causes

1 Lateral popliteal nerve palsy (?evidence of injury just below and lateral to the knee—p. 343)
2 Charcot–Marie–Tooth disease (?pes cavus, atrophy which stops abruptly part of the way up the leg, wasting of the small muscles of the hand, palpable lateral popliteal ± ulnar nerve—p. 249)
3 Old polio (?affected leg short as polio in childhood—p. 182)
4 Heavy metal poisoning such as lead (rare).

Record 6

The R/L leg is stiff and with each step he tilts the pelvis to the other side trying to keep the toe off the ground; the R/L leg describes a *semicircle* with the toe scraping the floor and the forefoot flops to the ground before the heel. The R/L arm is flexed and held tightly to his side and his fist is clenched.†

The patient has a *hemiplegic gait*.

Record 7

The patient has a lumbar lordosis and walks on a

---

* In the mild case, tell-tale signs are (i) the lesser swing of one arm compared to the other; (ii) the tremor which is often unilateral.

† Should not be seen these days with good physiotherapy care!

wide base with a *waddling gait*, his trunk moving from side to side and his pelvis dropping on each side as his leg leaves the ground. At each step his toes touch the ground before his heel. (This is a description of the typical gait of a patient with Duchenne muscular dystrophy — the commonest cause of a waddling gait. Other conditions causing wasting or weakness of the proximal lower limb and pelvic girdle muscles also cause it — e.g. polymyositis, rickets/osteomalacia.)

Record 8

The patient (an elderly person) walks with a broad-based gait, taking short steps and placing his feet flat on the ground like a person 'walking on ice'. (There is a tendency to retropulsion which increases the danger of falling.) The patient cannot hop on one foot.

This is *gait apraxia* (a common but little recognized disorder of the elderly; frontal lobe signs including dementia and grasp and suck reflexes will confirm the diagnosis). The commonest cause is a degenerative process similar to Alzheimer's disease. Other causes include subdural haematoma, tumour, normal pressure hydrocephalus, or a lacunar state. (Treatments include: small doses of L-dopa, mild stimulants, balancing exercises, use of a cane, daily walking.)

57 / Irregular pulse

Frequency in survey: main focus of a short case in 3% of attempts at MRCP short cases. Additional feature in at least a further 22%.

Survey note: though an irregular pulse was usually encountered in the examination as a feature in the common valvular short cases, occasionally it was itself the main focus of a short case. This was often because the patient had a goitre.

Record

The pulse is . . . /min and *irregularly irregular* in rate and volume suggesting controlled* (or uncontrolled if rate fast) atrial fibrillation. Now look at the *neck* (goitre), *eyes* (exophthalmos), *face* (mitral facies, hypothyroidism,† or hemiplegia due to an embolus) and *chest* (thoracotomy scar).‡

Differential diagnosis

The differentiation of an irregular pulse due to controlled atrial fibrillation from that of multiple extrasystoles, will depend upon the observation that only in atrial fibrillation do long pauses occur in groups of two or more (with ectopic beats the compensatory pause follows a short pause because the ectopic is premature). Furthermore, exercise may abolish extrasystoles but worsen the irregularity of atrial fibrillation. Atrial fibrillation can be difficult to distinguish from atrial flutter with variable block, from multiple atrial ectopics due to a shifting pacemaker, and sometimes from paroxysmal atrial tachy-cardia with block. Only in atrial fibrillation is the rhythm truly *chaotic*.

Causes of atrial fibrillation

Ischaemic heart disease (especially myocardial infarction)
Rheumatic heart disease
Hypertensive heart disease
Thyrotoxicosis
Cardiomyopathy§
Acute infections (especially lung)
Constrictive pericarditis.

---

*Though controlled atrial fibrillation may sometimes feel regular initially, if you concentrate there is a definite irregular variation in beat-to-beat time interval (NB experience 89, p. 459).

† Previously treated Graves' disease now on inadequate thyroxine replacement—pulse rate slow, ankle jerk relaxation slow, etc.

‡ If allowed follow up any positive findings from this *visual survey* by appropriate examination of the relevant system. If there is no visible abnormality proceed, if allowed, to examine the heart, the neck for a goitre, and thyroid status.

§ Though in most patients with cardiomyopathy no cause can be found ('idiopathic'), sometimes the causal disorder can be identified. Some of the usual causes can be grouped as follows:

1 Toxic (alcohol, adriamycin, cyclophosphamide, emetine, corticosteroids, lithium, phenothiazines, etc.)

2 Metabolic (thiamine deficiency, kwashiorkor, pellagra, obesity, porphyria, uraemia, electrolyte imbalance)
3 Endocrine (thyrotoxicosis, acromegaly, myxoedema, Cushing's, diabetes mellitus)
4 Collagen diseases (SLE, polyarteritis nodosa, etc.)
5 Infiltrative (amyloidosis, haemochromatosis, neoplastic, glycogen storage disease, sarcoidosis, mucopolysaccharidosis, Gaucher's disease, Whipple's disease)
6 Infective (viral, rickettsial, mycobacterial)
7 Genetic (hypertrophic obstructive cardiomyopathy, muscular dystrophies)
8 Fibroplastic (endomyocardial fibrosis, Löffler's endocarditis, carcinoid)
9 Miscellaneous (ischaemic heart disease, postpartum).

58 / Single palpable kidney

Frequency in survey: main focus of a short case in 3% of attempts at MRCP short cases. Additional feature in a further 3%.

Record
There is a mass (describe consistency, edges, size, etc.) on the R/L side* of the abdomen in the mid-zone. It is *bimanually ballotable*, I can *get above it*, and the percussion note is *resonant* over it.

It is, therefore, likely to be renal in origin (check for the pale, brownish-yellow tinge of uraemia, dialysis fistula/shunt/scars, etc.).

Possible causes
1 Polycystic disease (p. 86) with only one kidney palpable
2 Carcinoma (?weight loss, evidence of secondaries, anaemia, polycythaemia, pyrexia)
3 Hydronephrosis
4 Hypertrophy of a single functioning kidney (unilateral renal agenesis may predispose in the long term to proteinuria, hypertension and glomerular sclerosis).

*NB A palpable right kidney may be normal in a thin person.

59 / Ascites

Frequency in survey: main focus of a short case in 3% of attempts at MRCP short cases. Additional feature in a further 5%.

Survey note: occurred in the examination (i) as part of cirrhosis; (ii) on its own without a clearly defined underlying cause, in which case it was the main focus and possible causes were often discussed; and (iii) in association with an obvious mass or the irregular liver of malignancy.

Record

There is *generalized swelling* of the abdomen and the umbilicus is *everted*. The flanks are *stony dull* to percussion but the centre is resonant (floating, gas-filled bowel). The dullness is *shifting* and a *fluid thrill* can be demonstrated (in tense, large ascites).

This is ascites.

Usual causes

1 Cirrhosis with portal hypertension (?hepatomegaly, icterus, spider naevi, leuconychia, etc.—p. 84)
2 Intra-abdominal malignancy (especially ovarian and gastrointestinal — ?hard knobbly liver, mass, cachexia, nodes, e.g. Troisier's sign)
3 Congestive cardiac failue (?JVP↑, ankle and sacral oedema, hepatomegaly (pulsatile if tricuspid incompetence), large heart, tachycardia, *S3* or signs of the cardiac lesion).

Other causes

Nephrotic syndrome (?young, underlying diabetes (fundi), evidence of chronic disease underlying amyloid, evidence of collagen disease, etc. — p. 322)

Other causes of hypoalbuminaemia (e.g. malabsorption)

Tuberculous peritonitis* (?ethnic origin, chest signs)

Constrictive pericarditis (JVP raised, abrupt *x* and *y* descent, loud early *S3* ('pericardial knock') though heart sounds often normal, slight 'paradoxical' pulse, *no signs in lung fields*; chest X-ray may show calcified pericardium; rare but important as response to treatment may be dramatic)

Budd–Chiari syndrome (ascites develops rapidly with pain, icterus but no signs of chronic liver disease, smoothly enlarged tender liver; causes include tumour infiltration, oral contraceptives, polycythaemia rubra vera, ulcerative colitis and severe dehydration)

Myxoedema (?facies, ankle jerks, etc.—very rare)

Meigs' syndrome (ovarian fibroma — important as easily correctable by surgery)

Pancreatic disease

Chylous ascites (due to lymphatic obstruction — milky fluid).

---

* NB Tuberculous peritonitis may attack debilitated alcoholics. Therefore it should always be considered when ascites is present in a cirrhotic. Fever or abdominal pain are suggestive but may not be present. Examination of the ascitic fluid may help—an exudative protein content ($> 25\,g\,l^{-1}$) with lymphocytes is also suggestive. Staining of the fluid for acid–fast bacilli (AFB) is rarely positive and culture only positive in somewhat less than 50%. Diagnostic procedures include peritonoscopy (bowel adhesions may cause difficulty) and open peritoneal biopsy.

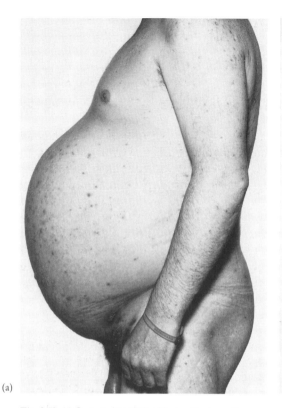
(a)

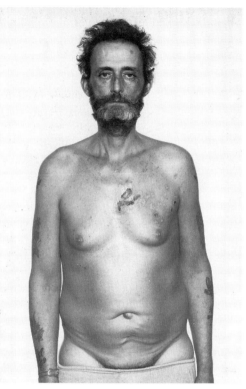
(b)

Fig. 3.59 (a) Gross ascites. (b) Residual ascites in another patient on treatment with diuretics (see also p. 85).

Frequency in survey: 3% of attempts at MRCP short cases.

Survey note: patients with unilateral and bilateral lesions were seen. One case had buphthalmos. There was discussion on the skull X-ray appearance including the site of calcification and, on one occasion, on temporal lobe epilepsy.

Record

There is a *port-wine stain* (capillary haemangioma) involving the area supplied by the first (and/or second) division of the trigeminal nerve on the R/L side. There may be an associated ipsilateral intracranial capillary haemangioma* of the pia arachnoid with *tramline calcification* (which outlines the cortical mantle in an undulating manner) on skull X-ray and a history of *epilepsy*, in which case the diagnosis would be Sturge–Weber syndrome.†

There may be a genetic predisposition.

Congenital abnormalities may be found in the eye on the affected side:
Glaucoma (blindness frequent)
Strabismus
Buphthalmos or ox eye
Angiomata of the choroid
Optic atrophy.

If the port-wine stain is in the area supplied by the first division of the trigeminal nerve the intracranial lesion is often in the occipital lobe. A facial naevus is more commonly associated with involvement of parietal and frontal lobes. The calcification seen on skull X-ray is in the cortical capillaries. The capillary haemangioma does not contain large vessels and does not fill on arteriography. The underlying brain damage is a rare cause of infantile hemiplegia (?hemismallness) and mental retardation as well as epilepsy.

For colour photograph see p. 533.

---

* Rare association with port-wine stain in real life but common in the examination!

† A phakomatosis, see footnote, p. 176.

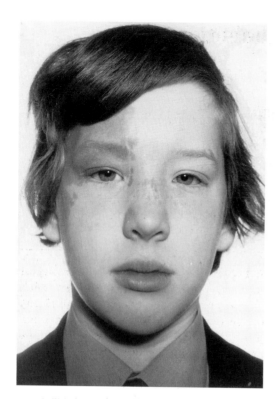

Fig. 3.60 Sturge–Weber syndrome (note strabismus).

61 / Necrobiosis lipoidica diabeticorum

Frequency in survey: 3% of attempts at MRCP short cases.

Record

There are *sharply demarcated*, coalescing *oval plaques* on the *shins* (occasionally arms and elsewhere) of this lady (usually a female aged <40). The lesions have a *shiny atrophic surface*, with characteristic *waxy yellow centres* and *brownish-red edges*. There is (usually) telangiectasia over the surface.

The diagnosis is necrobiosis lipoidica diabeticorum.

It is rare, usually associated with diabetes, but can occur in the prediabetic and on its own. It may have to be differentiated from granuloma annulare, from nodular vasculitis when small, and from localized scleroderma or sarcoidosis when larger.

The lesions may ulcerate. Opinions vary as to whether good diabetic control can improve healing, but this should be tried. Gradual healing, with scarring, occurs over a period of years. Steroids (topical or local injection) administered cautiously (to avoid local atrophy) may help. Severe cases can be treated by excision and skin grafting. The histology varies, some containing large amounts of lipid, some not. There is necrosis of collagen, surrounded by palisades of granulomatous epithelioid cells, and the aetiology is obscure.

Granuloma annulare (did not occur in original survey): pale or flesh-coloured papules coalescing in rings of usually 1–3 cm diameter especially on the backs of the hands and fingers. Blanching by pressure reveals a characteristic beaded ring of white dermal patches. It is sometimes associated with diabetes especially when the lesions are extensive and atypical. The histology is almost identical to necrobiosis lipoidica diabeticorum. The lesions regress spontaneously.

Diabetic dermopathy (did not occur in original survey): Atrophic pigmented patches (start as dull red oval papules; sometimes with a small blister) occurring mostly on the shins of diabetics. It has been suggested that they are precipitated by trauma in association with neuropathy.

Other skin lesions in diabetics

Infective (bacterial — boils, etc.; and fungal — candidiasis)

Foot/leg ulcers (ischaemic and neuropathic)

Vitiligo (?other associated organ-specific autoimmune disease—p. 279)

Fat atrophy (very rare with highly purified insulins)

Fat hypertrophy (recurrent injection of insulin into the same site)

Xanthomata (associated hyperlipidaemia—may disappear with control of diabetes as this causes improvement in the hyperlipidaemia—p. 218)

Insulin allergy (immediate and delayed; though less likely this can even occur in patients on human insulin given subcutaneously)

Sulphonylurea allergy (erythema multiforme, phototoxic and other eruptions)

Acanthosis nigricans (see p. 419)

Peripheral anhydrosis (due to autonomic neuropathy)

Chlorpropamide alcohol flush.

For colour photographs see pp. 530 and 540.

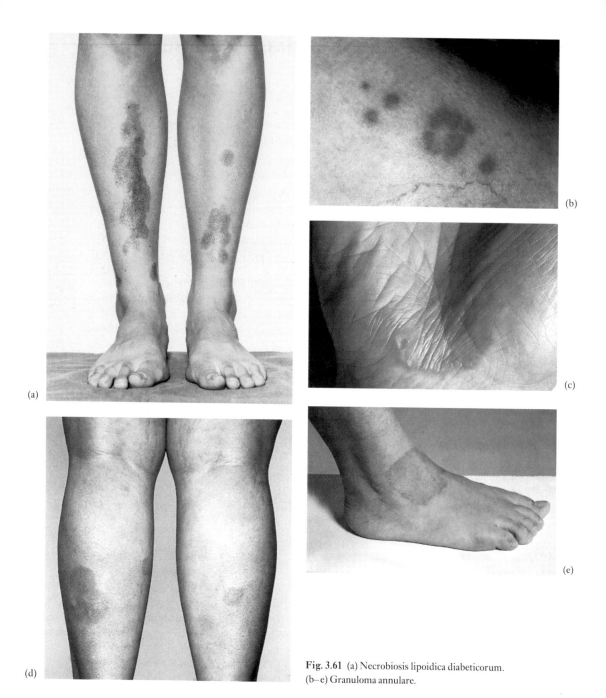

(a)

(b)

(c)

(d)

(e)

Fig. 3.61 (a) Necrobiosis lipoidica diabeticorum.
(b–e) Granuloma annulare.

62 / Ventricular septal defect

Frequency in survey: main focus of a short case in 3% of attempts at MRCP short cases. Additional feature in a further 1%.

Survey note: youthfulness of patient sometimes a clue to the diagnosis.

Record

The pulse is regular (give rate) and the venous pressure is not raised. The apex beat is (may be) palpable half-way between the midclavicular line and the anterior axillary line, and there is a *left parasternal heave* (there may be a systolic thrill). There is a *pansystolic murmur* at the lower left sternal edge which is also audible at the apex. (The pulmonary second sound may be loud due to pulmonary hypertension and there may be an early diastolic murmur of secondary pulmonary incompetence.)

The diagnosis is ventricular septal defect.

Other features of ventricular septal defect

Maladie de Roger (small haemodynamically insignificant hole, loud murmur, normal heart size, etc.; tends to close spontaneously)

Development of Eisenmenger's complex (p. 205) if a significant defect is left untreated

Susceptibility to subacute bacterial endocarditis (defects of all sizes—NB chemoprophylaxis)

Association with aortic incompetence in 5% of cases (10% in Japan)

Possibility of a mitral mid-diastolic flow murmur if shunt is large

May occur following acute myocardial infarction with septal rupture

Sometimes associated with Down's syndrome and Turner's syndrome.

63 / Lower motor neurone VIIth nerve palsy

Frequency in survey: 3% of attempts at MRCP short cases.

Record
On the R/L side there is *paralysis* of the *upper* and lower face*, so that the *eye cannot be closed* (or it can easily be opened by the examiner); the eyeball turns up on attempted closure (*Bell's phenomenon*) and the patient is unable to raise his R/L eyebrow. The corner of the *mouth droops*, the *nasolabial fold* is *smoothed out*, and the voluntary and involuntary (i.e. including emotional) movements of the mouth are paralysed on the R/L side (the lips may be drawn to the opposite side and the tongue may deviate as well—not necessarily hypoglossal involvement—see footnote, p. 106).

This is a R/L lower motor neurone VIIth nerve lesion (now check the ipsilateral ear for evidence of *herpes zoster*).

Causes of a lower motor neurone VIIth nerve lesion
1 Bell's palsy†
2 Ramsay Hunt syndrome (herpes zoster on the external auditory meatus and the geniculate ganglion—taste to the anterior two-thirds of the tongue is lost; there may be lesions on the fauces and palate).

Other differential diagnoses
Cerebellopontine angle compression (acoustic neuroma or meningioma; Vth, VIth, VIIth, VIIIth nerve palsy, cerebellar signs and loss of taste to the anterior two-thirds of the tongue—p. 335)

Parotid tumour (?palpable; taste not affected)

Trauma

A pontine lesion (e.g. multiple sclerosis, tumour or vascular lesion)

Middle ear disease (deafness)

The causes of mononeuritis multiplex (diabetes, polyarteritis nodosa and Churg–Strauss syndrome, rheumatoid, SLE, Wegener's, sarcoid, carcinoma, amyloid and leprosy).

Causes of bilateral lower motor neurone VIIth nerve paralysis‡
Guillain–Barré syndrome (occasionally only VIIth nerves affected)

Sarcoidosis (parotid gland enlargement not always present)

Bilateral Bell's palsy

Myasthenia gravis (?ptosis, variable strabismus, proximal muscle weakness, etc.—p. 269)

Congenital facial diplegia

Some forms of muscular dystrophy

Motor neurone disease (rarely)

Lyme disease (may be bilateral, alone or with signs of meningoencephalitis or peripheral radiculoneuropathy, knee effusion, Baker's cyst rupture, heart block, etc.).

---

* That is, including frontalis ('raise eyebrows'), corrugator superficialis ('frown') and orbicularis oculi ('close your eyes tight').
† In the mild case of Bell's palsy taste over the anterior two-thirds of the tongue is usually preserved, because the lesion is due to swelling of the nerve in the confined lower facial canal.

In cases with more extensive involvement this taste is lost and the patient may also show increased susceptibility to high-pitched or loud sounds (hyperacusis due to stapedius paralysis).
‡ Bilateral lower motor neurone VIIth nerve lesions are easily missed because there is no asymmetry.

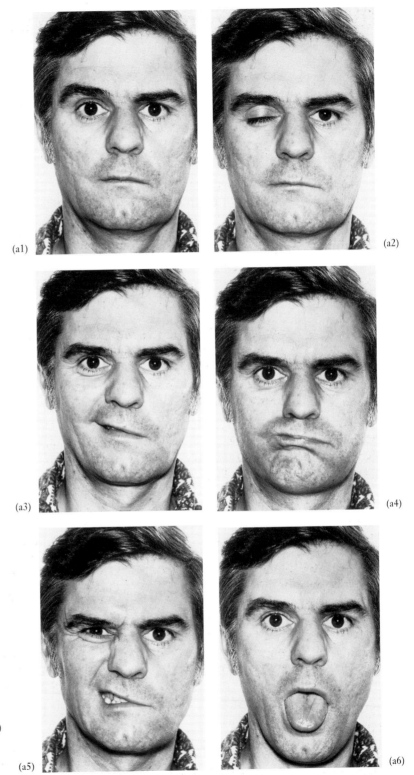

Fig. 3.63 (a) Left Bell's palsy:
(1) 'Look straight ahead'; (2)
'Close your eyes'; (3) 'Smile'; (4)
'Puff out your cheeks', (5)
'Show me your teeth'; (6) 'Put
out your tongue'.

(a1)   (a2)   (a3)   (a4)   (a5)   (a6)

The chorda tympani leaves the facial nerve in the middle ear to supply taste to the anterior two-thirds of the tongue. The superficial petrosal branch to supply the lachrymal glands, and the nerve to stapedius both leave higher in the facial canal than the chorda tympani. The level of the lesion in the facial canal can sometimes be assessed (very unlikely to be required in the examination) by assessing the relative involvement of these nerves.

Variation of the Ramsay Hunt syndrome Occasionally facial palsy is associated with trigeminal, occipital or cervical herpes with or without auditory involvement (see first person anecdote 40, p. 497). In some of these cases the geniculate ganglion may be spared—see p. 325.

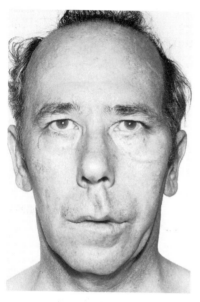
(b1)

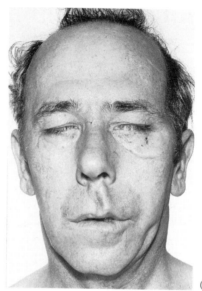
(b2)

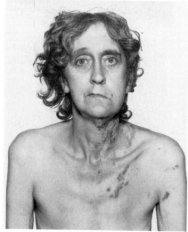
(c)

Fig. 3.63 (*continued*) (b1) Bilateral lower motor neurone VIIth nerve palsy (Guillain–Barré syndrome); (2) 'Close your eyes'. (c) Ramsay Hunt syndrome.

64 / Clubbing

Frequency in survey: main focus of a short case in 2% of attempts at MRCP short cases. Additional feature in a further 13%.

Record

There is finger clubbing* (*thickening of the nail bed*† with *loss of the obtuse angle* between the nail and the dorsum of the finger—becomes >180°‡; *increased curvature* of the nail bed—both side-to-side and lengthwise; increased *sponginess or fluctuation* of the nail bed; and sometimes, when there is marked swelling of the nail bed, the fingers may have a *drumstick appearance*).

Causes of clubbing

1 Carcinoma of the bronchus (the commonest cause—?nicotine staining, obvious weight loss with temporal dimples, lymph nodes, chest signs, evidence of secondaries, etc.—p. 145)

2 Fibrosing alveolitis (?basal crackles—p. 104)

3 Cyanotic congenital heart disease (?cyanosis, thoracotomy scars, Fallot's — p. 284, Eisenmenger's—p. 205)

4 Bronchiectasis (?productive cough, crepitations, etc.—p. 161)

5 Cirrhosis (?icterus, spider naevi, palmar erythema, Dupuytren's, xanthelasma—especially in primary biliary cirrhosis, hepatosplenomegaly, etc.—p. 69).

Other causes

Subacute bacterial endocarditis (heart murmur, fever, splenomegaly, petechiae, splinter haemorrhages, Osler's nodes, Janeway's lesions, Roth spots, etc.)

Empyema

Lung abscess

Crohn's disease

Ulcerative colitis

Asbestosis (especially with mesothelioma)

Thyroid acropachy (?exophthalmos, pretibial myxoedema, goitre, thyroid status, etc.—p. 114)

Hereditary (rare; dominant).

* Indisputable clubbing is one of the important fundamental clinical signs which, when present, have clear implications. Less clear-cut changes in the finger nails are susceptible to assessment which (even if dogmatic) may be very subjective. Such finger nails are best described as showing 'debatable clubbing' (in that physicians will disagree as to whether there are significant changes or not). Genuine 'debatable clubbing' occurring in the examination may cause trouble if you recognize it as such, but you are not sure what your examiners' opinion is. The safest course in a case of doubt is to use nail bed thickening as your guide and quote the nail angle rule in a way that cannot be argued with. For example:

'The appearance of the nails (e.g. increased curvature) is initially suggestive of clubbing, but the obtuse angle between the nail and the dorsum of the finger is preserved, and therefore by definition (loss of the angle being the "official" first sign) the diagnosis of definite clubbing cannot be accepted in this case'.

† Before palpating always inspect the fingers in profile for a slightly bulbous appearance due to thickening of the nail bed.

‡ *Shamroth's sign:* If you put the fingernails of the same fingers of each of your hands together, against each other, you will see a gap at their base between them. This gap may be lost when the angle is lost in finger clubbing.

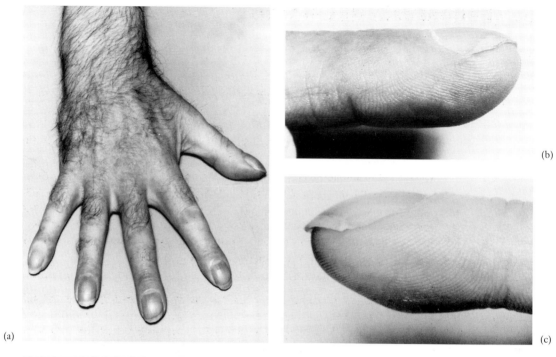

(a)

(b)

(c)

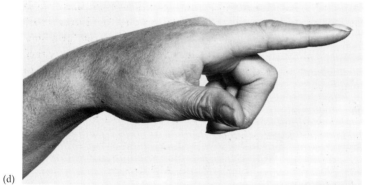

(d)

Fig. 3.64 (a) Clubbing (carcinoma of the bronchus). (b) Loss of the angle. (c) Thickening of the nail bed (early drumstick appearance—same patient as in (a)). (d) Clubbing and leuconychia (cirrhosis of the liver).

65 / Retinal vein thrombosis

Frequency in survey: 2% of attempts at MRCP short cases.

Record

The veins are *tortuous* and *engorged*. *Haemorrhages* are *scattered riotously* over the whole retina, irregular and superficial, like bundles of straw alongside the veins (*papilloedema* and *soft exudates* may also be seen).

The diagnosis is central retinal vein thrombosis. There may be *hypertension, hyperlipidaemia* or *diabetes mellitus* or there may be an underlying *hyperviscosity syndrome,** especially *Waldenström's macroglobulinaemia* (?lymphadenopathy, hepatosplenomegaly, bruising and purpura), but also occasionally *myeloma* (?urinary Bence-Jones protein) and *connective tissue disorders.*

The condition is commoner in eyes prone to simple glaucoma (which should, therefore, be excluded in the other eye), in the elderly arteriosclerotic, and the hypertensive, but may also arise in young adults (especially women). It causes incomplete loss of vision and improvement may be scant. About 3 months after the acute event 20% of cases lose the remaining sight in the affected eye because of an acute secondary glaucoma. This is due to new vessels on the iris root developing as a result of retinal hypoxia. Panretinal photocoagulation may decrease the risk of subsequent neovascular glaucoma. A less severe ophthalmoscopic appearance is encountered in younger patients when the terms *partial retinal vein occlusion* and *venous stasis retinopathy* are used; visual acuity in this situation is only slightly reduced and visual prognosis is good.

In thrombosis of a branch of the retinal vein (also occurred in our survey) the occlusion usually occurs at an arteriovenous crossing with the changes confined to the sector beyond this — haemorrhages and cotton-wool spots spread out in a wedge from the AV crossing. Any loss of sight† recovers and there is no secondary glaucoma. Branch retinal vein occlusion must be distinguished from *viral retinitis* which it resembles ophthalmoscopically (see p. 365). In view of the association with hypertension, hypertensive changes may be visible in the rest of the fundus (thin arterioles, AV nipping, etc.).

For colour photograph see p. 529.

* The symptoms and signs of a hyperviscosity syndrome are principally neurological due to sluggish cerebral circulation. Cardiac failure may occur in the elderly. Waldenström's macroglobulinaemia is the cause in 90% of hyperviscosity syndromes.

† Think of this diagnosis if you find a quadrantic field defect in one eye only.

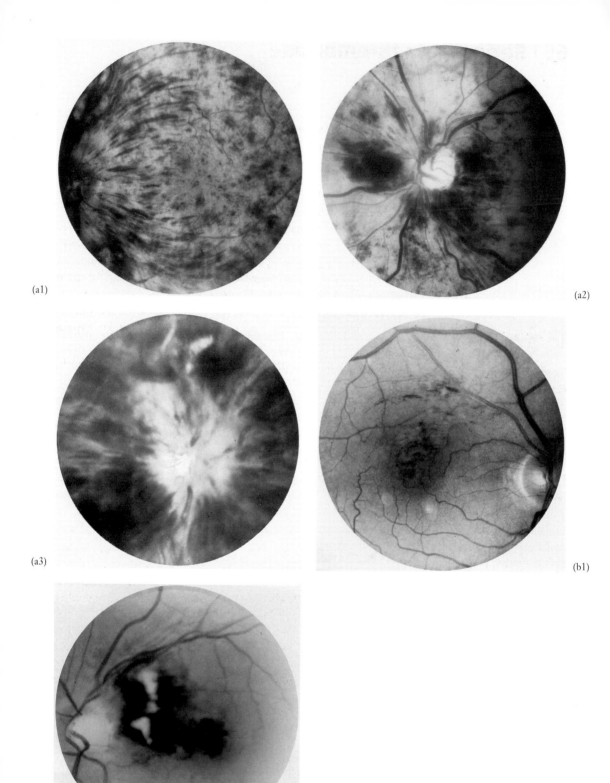

(a1)

(a2)

(a3)

(b1)

(b2)

Fig. 3.65 (a1–3) Three different cases of central retinal vein thrombosis. (b1,2) Two different cases of branch retinal vein thrombosis.

66 / Eisenmenger's syndrome

Frequency in survey: main focus of a short case in 2% of attempts at MRCP short casis. Additional feature in a further 1%.

Record

There is *central cyanosis* and *clubbing* of the fingers (may be only in the toes in patent ductus arteriosus). The pulse (give rate) is regular (and small in volume). A large *a* wave is (may be) seen in the venous pulse (due to forceful atrial contraction in the face of the right ventricular hypertrophy). There is a marked *left parasternal heave* and (often) a palpable (pulmonary) second heart sound. On auscultation (the signs of pulmonary hypertension are heard) the *second heart sound* is *loud*, there is (may be) a right ventricular fourth heart sound, (may be) a pulmonary early sys-tolic ejection click, (may be) an early diastolic murmur (dilated pulmonary artery leads to secondary pulmonary incompetence), and (may be) a pansystolic murmur (secondary tricuspid incompetence—*v* wave in JVP).

These findings suggest Eisenmenger's syndrome with pulmonary hyperten-sion leading to reversal of a left-to-right shunt.

Causes

1 Ventricular septal defect (VSD)* (single or closely split second heart sound because the right and left ventricular pressures are similar)
2 Atrial septal defect (fixed and wide splitting of the second sound)
3 Patent ductus arteriosus† (normal splitting of the second sound—*P2* follows *A2* and the split widens with inspiration; only the lower limbs are cyanosed—differen-tial cyanosis).

Once Eisenmenger's syndrome has developed it is too late (high mortality) for correction of the cardiac anomaly. A palliative procedure involving redirec-tion of the venous return has been successful in the presence of transposition of the great arteries, VSD and severe pulmonary vascular disease. Transplan-tation of heart and lungs is being tried because patients with irreversible changes within the pul-monary arterioles and progressive symptoms are at great risk of dying. Death commonly occurs between the ages of 20 and 40 years and is usually due to pulmonary infarction, right heart failure, dysrhythmias and, less often, infective endocarditis or cerebral abscess.

The absence of chest signs helps to differentiate Eisenmenger's syndrome from the cyanosis and pulmonary hypertension of cor pulmonale. The features which may be helpful in differentiating

---

*When due to a VSD it is termed Eisenmenger's complex. The classical pansystolic murmur of the VSD tends to disappear as the right and left ventricular pressures equalize. A pansystolic murmur in Eisenmenger's complex is more likely to be from tricuspid incompetence.

† Again the classical patent ductus arteriosus murmur tends to shorten to a soft systolic murmur, and then disappear as the pressures in the pulmonary artery and descending aorta equalize.

Table 3.66 The features which may be helpful in differentiating Eisenmenger's syndrome from the tetralogy of Fallot

	Eisenmenger's syndrome	Fallot's tetralogy
Pulmonary systolic thrill	Absent	Present
Pulmonary systolic murmur	Absent	Intense (unless such severe stenosis that no flow)
Right ventricle	Very hypertrophied	Hypertrophied
Chest X-ray	Large pulmonary arteries	Small pulmonary arteries

Eisenmenger's syndrome from Fallot's tetralogy (the commonest cause of central cyanosis in the adolescent or young adult) are shown in Table 3.66. Furthermore, the patient with Fallot's tetralogy in the examination may well have thoracotomy scars and a pulse which is weaker on the left than on the right, from a previous Blalock shunt operation (see p. 284).

67 / Crohn's disease

Frequency in survey: 2% of attempts at MRCP short cases.

Survey note: there were several different presentations: as a right iliac fossa mass, as multiple scars and sinuses on the abdomen, as perianal Crohn's disease and as Crohn's disease of the lips. In one-third of cases the clue was given that the patient had diarrhoea.

Record 1

The *multiple laparotomy scars* suggest a chronic, relapsing, abdominal condition which has led to crises requiring surgical intervention on several occasions. In view of the associated *fistula* formation, Crohn's disease is likely.

Record 2

The chronically *swollen lips* (granulomatous infiltration) and history of chronic diarrhoea are suggestive of Crohn's disease (examine inside the *mouth for ulcers* which vary in size).

Record 3

There is a (characteristic) *dusky blue discoloration* of the perianal skin. There are *oedematous skin tags* (which look soft but are very firm), there is *fissuring, ulceration* and *fistula* formation.

The diagnosis is perianal Crohn's disease (may antedate disease elsewhere in the bowel).

Record 4

Right iliac fossa mass—see p. 157.

Other physical signs in Crohn's disease

Fever
Anaemia (malabsorption, chronic disease and gastrointestinal blood loss)
Clubbing
Arthritis (including sacroiliitis)
Erythema nodosum (p. 178)
Pyoderma gangrenosum (p. 431)

Iritis
Ankle oedema (hypoproteinaemia).

Other causes of anal fistulae (rare)

Simple fistula from an abscess of an anal gland
Tuberculosis
Ulcerative colitis
Carcinoma of the rectum.

For colour photograph see p. 543.

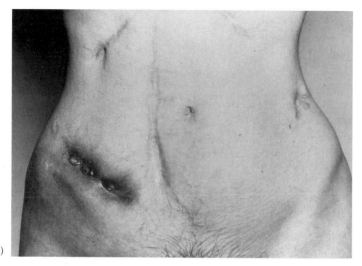

(a)

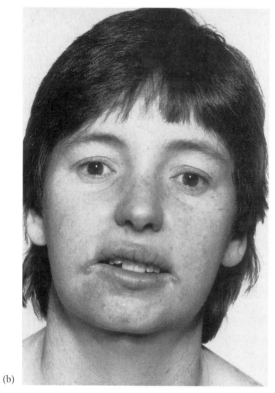

(b)

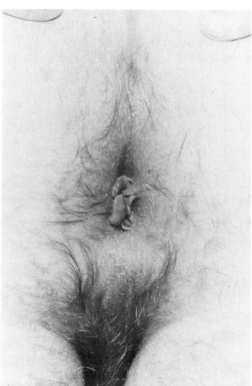

(c)

Fig. 3.67 (a) Multiple scars and fistulae. (b) Crohn's lips.
(c) Perianal lesions.

68 / Mitral valve prolapse

Frequency in survey: 2% of attempts at MRCP short cases.

Record

The pulse (in this well-looking patient) is regular (give rate) and the venous pressure is not raised. The apex beat is palpable in the fifth intercostal space in the mid-clavicular line. There are no heaves or thrills. On auscultation the heart sounds are normal but there is a *mid-systolic click** (which is usually but not always) followed by a late *systolic crescendo-decrescendo murmur* loudest at the left sternal edge (as the condition progresses the murmur develops the characteristics of mitral incompetence—p. 121).

These findings suggest mitral valve prolapse (floppy posterior mitral valve leaflet—echocardiography useful for confirmation).

The prolapse is increased by anything which decreases cardiac volume (standing position; Valsalva manoeuvre) and as a result the click and murmur occur earlier during systole and the murmur is prolonged. Increasing cardiac volume (squatting position, propranolol) has the reverse effect. Phonocardiography documents these effects well. Mitral valve prolapse (said to occur in 5–10% of the population,† more commonly in females) is usually asymptomatic but may be associated with atypical chest pain, palpitations, fatigue and dyspnoea. The symptoms may become worse once the patient knows there is a murmur. The prognosis is good† but complications can include infective endocarditis, atrial and ventricular dysrhythmias, worsening mitral incompetence, embolic phenomena (transient ischaemic attacks, amaurosis fugax, acute hemiplegia), rupture of the mitral valve (age-related degenerative changes) and sudden death. The condition may be familial and there may be a family history of sudden death. There is a serious risk of precipitating cardiac neurosis which may, at least in part, contribute to the association with atypical chest pain. There is often myxomatous degeneration of the mitral valve, deposition of acid mucopolysaccharide material and redundant valve tissue.

Causes and associations

Marfan's syndrome
Rheumatic heart disease
Polycystic kidney disease
Coronary artery disease
Congenital heart disease
Congestive cardiomyopathy
Hypertrophic obstructive cardiomyopathy
Myocarditis
Mitral valve surgery
Left atrial myxoma
Ehlers–Danlos syndrome
Osteogenesis imperfecta
Systemic lupus erythematosus

---

* The click is characteristic but easily missed if you have not heard one before. This may be because of the distraction of the murmur. Concentrate on listening for other sounds at different frequencies from the murmur and you will hear it.
† It may be that the clinically silent, echocardiographic mitral valve prolapse which is common in thin, young women is a variant of normal, distinct from the floppy valve or complication of chordal lengthening or rupture needing mitral valve replacement, which is commonest in elderly men. It seems likely that 'echo only' mitral valve prolapse carries a good prognosis whereas the complications are associated with the clinical variety. Since patients with auscultatory and echocardiographic evidence of mitral valve prolapse may be candidates for endocarditis, they should be recommended for antimicrobial prophylaxis before dental procedures, etc. This prophylaxis is only required if a murmur is audible. Click only patients have a very low incidence of subacute bacterial endocarditis.

Muscular dystrophy
Turner's syndrome
Athlete's heart
Primary mitral valve prolapse.

Other causes of a short systolic murmur audible at the apex should always be thought of and excluded. These are:

Trivial mitral incompetence (the usual cause — the murmur may not be pansystolic but there is no click)
Aortic stenosis/sclerosis (p. 104)
Hypertrophic obstructive cardiomyopathy (p. 436).

69 / Cervical myelopathy

Frequency in survey: main focus of a short case in 2% of attempts at MRCP short cases. Additional feature in a further 2%.

Survey note: cervical collar may be a clue.

Record

The legs (of this middle-aged or elderly patient) show *spastic weakness*,* the *tone* being *increased*, the *reflexes brisk* (?clonus) and the *plantar responses extensor*. *Vibration* and joint position senses are (may be) lost in the lower limbs (spinothalamic loss may also occur but is less common). In the upper limbs† there is (often asymmetrical) *inversion*‡ of the biceps and supinator jerks.

These features suggest cervical myelopathy as the cause of the spastic paraparesis. *Cervical spondylosis* is the commonest cause though a *spinal cord tumour* cannot be excluded clinically.

In the upper limbs there may be segmental muscle wasting and weakness particularly if there is an associated radiculopathy. Gross wasting of the small muscles of the hand due to cervical spondylosis is uncommon because the latter usually affects C5/6 or C6/7 and the small muscles are supplied by C8/T1. Mild wasting of the small muscles does sometimes occur probably due to vascular changes in the cord below the lesion.

There is often no sensory loss in the hand. Sometimes in the elderly a complaint of numb, useless hands may be accompanied by constant unpleasant parasthesiae and writhing ('sensory wandering' or 'pseudoathetosis') of the fingers when the eyes are closed. Position and vibration senses are lost in such hands.

Neck pain is surprisingly rare in cervical spondylosis causing cervical myelopathy, and sphincter function is seldom disturbed. Among patients with cervical spondylosis (which is very common) those with a narrow cervical canal are most likely to develop cervical myelopathy. Lhermitte's phenomenon may occur (see p. 314).

---

* In this condition signs often exceed symptoms and spasticity often exceeds weakness.
† The myelopathy hand sign may be present; see footnote, p. 40.
‡ When attempts are made to elicit the normal biceps and supinator tendon reflexes, there is a brisk finger flexion despite little or no response of the biceps and supinator jerks themselves. This is because the lower motor neurones and pyramidal tracts are damaged at the C5/6 level producing lower motor neurone signs at that level and upper motor neurone signs below. The combination of inverted biceps and supinator jerks (the C5/6 jerks) and a brisk triceps jerk (C7/8) is termed the 'mid-cervical reflex pattern'.

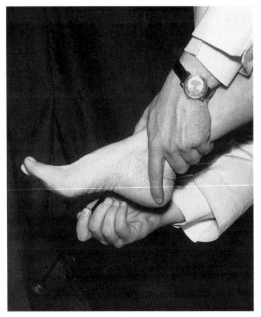

(a)

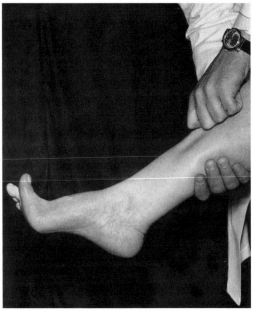

(b)

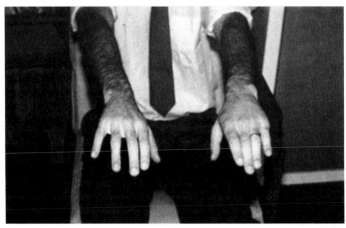

(c)

(d)

Fig. 3.69 (a) Babinski's sign.
(b) Oppenheim's sign (see p. 26).
(c) Pseudoathetosis. (d) The
myelopathy hand sign (in the right
arm).

Frequency in survey: 2% of attempts at MRCP short cases.

Record

The *pulse* is *collapsing* (may be normal if the duct is narrow and the 'run-off' from the aorta to the left pulmonary artery is small) in character, regular (give rate) and the venous pressure is not raised. The apex is *thrusting* in the anterior axillary line (may be normal if the ductus is small), and there is a *left parasternal heave*. On auscultation there is a continuous '*machinery*' *murmur** with systolic *accentuation* heard in the second left intercostal space near the sternal edge (but maximal 5–7.5 cm above or to the left of this, *beneath the clavicle*, and also *heard posteriorly*).

The diagnosis is patent ductus arteriosus.

Male to female ratio is 1 : 3.

The incidence is higher in patients born at a high altitude. Spontaneous closure is rare except in premature infants.

Other causes of a continuous murmur†
With collapsing pulse
Mitral incompetence and aortic incompetence
Ventricular septal defect and aortic incompetence.

Without collapsing pulse
Venous hum (common in normal children — maximal to the right of the sternum—diminishes or disappears when the child lies flat or when the right JVP is compressed)

Pulmonary arteriovenous fistula or shunt (e.g. Blalock).

Complications of patent ductus arteriosus
Infective endocarditis (infection of the ductus — even small ones; therefore closure is always recommended unless Eisenmenger's is already present)

Heart failure

Eisenmenger's syndrome (p. 205).

---

* The murmur seldom lasts for the whole of systole and diastole. It may occupy only the latter part of systole and the early part of diastole. Occasionally, particularly in young children, it may occur as a crescendo in late systole only.

† NB The murmur of patent ductus distinguishes itself by being loudest below the left clavicle. There should not usually be any diagnostic difficulty.

71 / Tricuspid incompetence

Frequency in survey: main focus of a short case in 2% of attempts at MRCP short cases. Additional feature in a further 2%.

Record

The JVP is elevated (say height*) and shows *giant v waves*† which oscillate the earlobe (if the venous pressure is high enough) and which are diagnostic of tricuspid incompetence. (Now, if allowed, examine the heart, respiratory system and abdomen.‡)

The commonest cause of tricuspid incompetence is *not* organic, but dilatation of the right ventricle and of the tricuspid valve ring due to right ventricular failure in conditions such as:

Mitral valve disease
Cor pulmonale
Eisenmenger's syndrome
Atrial septal defect
Right ventricular infarction
Primary pulmonary hypertension
Thyrotoxicosis.

Causes of primary tricuspid incompetence

Rheumatic heart disease (usually associated with tricuspid stenosis; almost invariably associated with other valvular disease — if there is pulmonary hypertension it may not be possible to differentiate organic from functional tricuspid incompetence on clinical grounds alone)

Infective endocarditis (especially intravenous drug addicts — recurrent septicaemia with pulmonary infiltrates should raise suspicion)

Congenital heart disease (e.g. Ebstein's anomaly)

Carcinoid syndrome (flushing, diarrhoea, hepatomegaly, sometimes asthma; fibrous plaques on the endothelial surface of the heart are associated with tricuspid incompetence and pulmonary stenosis)

Myxomatous change (may be associated with mitral valve prolapse or atrial septal defect)

Trauma.

---

* In centimetres vertically above the sternal angle, not the suprasternal notch or supraclavicular fossa. In tricuspid incompetence which is secondary to right ventricular dilatation, the venous pressure is usually of the order of 8–10 cm or more.

† These *v* waves are in fact *cv* waves because systole spans the time between *c* and *v* waves of the normal jugular pulse.

‡ In the *heart* you would expect to find the systolic murmur of tricuspid incompetence which may be louder on inspiration (Carvallo's sign) and augmented by the Müller manoeuvre (attempted inspiration against a closed glottis). There may be murmurs of associated or underlying disease of the heart valves, especially mitral. There may be a tricuspid diastolic murmur louder on inspiration and augmented by the Müller manoeuvre. This could be due to increased flow across the tricuspid valve or to concomitant tricuspid stenosis. In the *respiratory system* you would be looking for signs of the condition leading to underlying cor pulmonale. In the *abdomen* you may find forceful epigastric pulsations and hepatomegaly which is tender and pulsatile. In severe, long-standing tricuspid incompetence, ascites and signs of chronic liver disease (p. 84) can occur.

72 / Purpura

Frequency in survey: main focus of a short case in 2% of attempts at MRCP short cases. Additional feature in a further 3%.

Record

There is purpura.* Now look at the patient and note:

?*Age* ('senile purpura')

?*Cushingoid features* with thin skin (if present observe for features of underlying steroid-treated disease, e.g. asthma, rheumatoid arthritis, cryptogenic fibrosing alveolitis)

?*Rheumatoid arthritis* (phenylbutazone and gold as well as steroids)

?*Anaemia* (leukaemia, bone marrow aplasia or infiltration)

—as well as the distribution and type of purpura.

Causes of purpura can be divided into:

Thrombocytopenic purpura such as:

Idiopathic thrombocytopenic purpura (purpuric rash in a young female, ?spleen—may respond to steroids and/or splenectomy)

Marrow replacement by leukaemia (acute and chronic; ?spleen, nodes, liver, anaemia, oral and pharyngeal infection)

Marrow replacement by secondary malignancy (?cachexia, evidence of primary)

Marrow aplasia (idiopathic, secondary to drugs, hepatitis A or B).

Capillary defect (vascular; platelet count normal) such as:

Senile and steroid-induced purpura (purpura over loose skin areas)

Henoch–Schönlein purpura (children > adults; purpuric rash (a haemorrhagic vasculitis, sometimes papular) over the extensor surfaces of the limbs particularly at the ankles and on the buttocks; associated with arthritis of medium-sized joints, colicky abdominal pains, occasionally gastrointestinal bleeding and acute nephritis; see p. 327)

Coagulation deficiency such as:†

Haemophilia

Christmas disease

Anticoagulant therapy.

Other causes of purpura

Other drugs (e.g. sulphonamides, chloramphenicol, thiazides)

Hypersplenism (large spleen)

Von Willebrand's disease

Infective endocarditis (?heart murmur, splenomegaly, splinters, clubbing, Osler's nodes, etc.)

Systemic lupus erythematosus (?typical rash)

Polyarteritis nodosa (?arteritic lesions)

Osler–Weber–Rendu syndrome (p. 155)

---

* Purpura refers to a spontaneous extravasation of blood from the capillaries into the skin; petechiae = pin-head size, ecchymoses = large lesions.

† These conditions may cause ecchymoses rather than purpura.

Venous stasis (ankle and lower legs; obesity or vari-
    cose veins; accompanied by progressive pigmen-
    tation due to deposition of haemosiderin)
Scurvy (NB the neglected elderly patient with
    ecchymoses on the legs)
Paroxysmal nocturnal haemoglobinuria
Amyloidosis (periorbital purpura)
Uraemia (pale, brownish-yellow tinge to skin)
Disseminated intravascular coagulation
Thrombotic thrombocytopenic purpura
Haemolytic–uraemic syndrome
Paraproteinaemia
Meningitis (especially meningococcal)
Septicaemia (especially meningococcal)

Viral haemorrhagic fevers
Kaposi's sarcoma
Factitious purpura
Hereditary haemorrhagic telangiectasia (p. 155)
Ehlers–Danlos syndrome (p. 263)
Scarlet fever
Measles
Rubella
Glandular fever
Typhoid
Cyanotic congenital heart disease.

For colour photograph see p. 538.

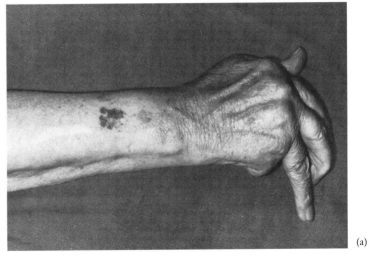

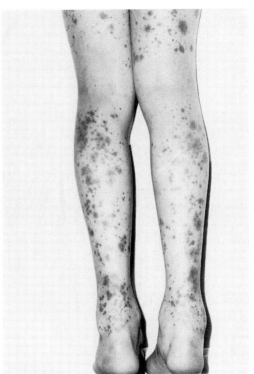

Fig. 3.72 (a) Purpura on forearm (note rheumatoid arthritis).
(b) Henoch–Schönlein purpura.

73 / Xanthomata

Frequency in survey: main focus of a short case in 2% of attempts at MRCP short cases. Additional feature in a further 2%.

Record 1

There are *tendon xanthomata* (?corneal arcus, xanthelasma) in the *extensor tendons* on the back of the *hand*, and on the *Achilles* and *patella* tendons.

They suggest *familial hypercholesterolaemia*. (In this condition raised and nodular *tuberous xanthomata* may also occur, usually symmetrically, over the *extensor aspects of the joints* and on the *buttocks*. They may be several millimetres to several centimetres in size.)

Record 2

There are (orange or) *yellow papules* (up to 5 mm in diameter) on the *extensor surfaces* particularly over the *joints*, on the *limbs* and on the *buttocks* and *back*. They are (sometimes) surrounded by a rim of erythema (and may be tender).

This is *eruptive xanthomatosis* (?lipaemia retinalis on fundoscopy. There is often abdominal pain and there is a risk of acute pancreatitis. It suggests severe *hypertriglyceridaemia* — plasma triglycerides of the order of 20–25 mmol l^{-1} — 'milky plasma' syndrome).*

Familial hypercholesterolaemia is associated with premature development of vascular disease. Familial hypertriglyceridaemia does not appear to be an important risk factor for atherosclerosis but equivalent hypertriglyceridaemia due to familial combined hyperlipidaemia† is associated with an increased risk.

Order of priorities in treating hyperlipidaemia‡

1 Identify and treat any causes of secondary hyperlipidaemia such as:

(a) diabetes mellitus (?fundi)
(b) alcoholism (may be the occult underlying cause of treatment failure)
(c) nephrotic syndrome (?generalized oedema)
(d) myxoedema (?facies, pulse, ankle jerks)
(e) cholestasis (?icterus)
(f) myelomatosis
(g) oral contraceptives

2 Dietary treatment for obesity
3 Dietary treatment for hyperlipidaemia
4 Lipid lowering drugs.§

* This level of hypertriglyceridaemia is usually due to overproduction of triglycerides occurring at the same time as hindrance of removal. For example, the coexistence of familial hypertriglyceridaemia (type IV), diabetes, and/or alcohol consumption. Treatment of the secondary cause usually leads to a dramatic reduction in triglyceride levels and greatly reduces the risk of acute pancreatitis which is the main threat of this condition.

† Affected family members show either a combined rise in plasma cholesterol and triglycerides, or hypercholesterolaemia alone, or hypertriglyceridaemia alone.
‡ NB the screening and treatment of families with hypercholesterolaemia.
§ There is increasing evidence that, by lowering cholesterol, statins reduce cardiovascular morbidity and mortality in patients at risk of cardiovascular disease.

Types of hyperlipidaemia simplified
Comparatively common
Type IIa (e.g. familial hypercholesterolaemia) — raised cholesterol only

Type IIb (e.g. familial combined hyperocholesterolaemia)—raised cholesterol and triglycerides

Type IV (e.g. familial hypertriglyceridaemia) — raised triglycerides.

Rare
Type I—raised chylomicrons

Type III—a defect in a particular step in lipid catabolism resulting in a rise in cholesterol and triglycerides to an equal extent

Type V—raised chylomicrons and triglycerides.

For colour photographs see p. 536.

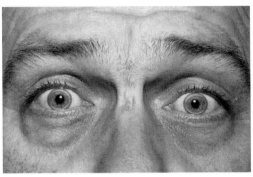

(a)

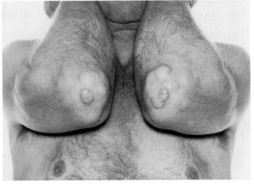

(b1)

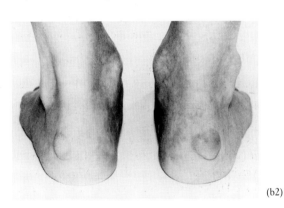

(b2)

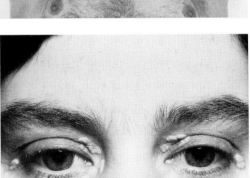

(c)

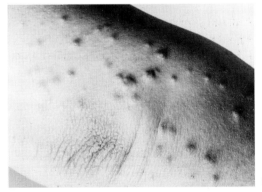

(d)

Fig. 3.73 (a) Arcus senilis. (b1,2) Elbows and Achilles of the same patient. (c) Xanthelasma. (d) Eruptive xanthomata.

74 / Drug-induced extrapyramidal syndrome

Frequency in survey: 2% of attempts at MRCP short cases.

Record

There are (in this ?elderly, chronic schizophrenic) stereotyped tic-like *orofacial dyskinesias* (involuntary movements) including *lip-smacking*, *chewing*, *pouting* and *grimacing*. There is (may be) *choreoathetosis* of the limbs and trunk.

The diagnosis is tardive dyskinesia.* (It is likely that the patient has been on sustained phenothiazine treatment for at least 6 months. The condition often persists when the drug is withdrawn, in which case tetrabenazine may help.)

Neuroleptics which may cause abnormal involuntary movements (by inhibiting dopamine function):

Phenothiazines (e.g. chlorpromazine)
Butyrophenones (e.g. haloperidol)
Substituted benzamides (e.g. metoclopramide)
Reserpine
Tetrabenazine.

Other neuroleptic-induced extrapyramidal adverse reactions (apart from tardive dyskinesia):

Acute dystonias (soon after starting the drug; e.g. oculogyric crises)
Akathisia (uncontrollable restlessness with an inner feeling of unease)
Parkinson's syndrome (indistinguishable from Parkinson's disease though tremor less common; tends to respond to anticholinergics rather than L-dopa).

---

* Called tardive (late) because it does not appear until at least 3 months, or more often a year, after the start or withdrawal of long-term treatment with neuroleptic drugs. This distinguishes tardive dyskinesia from acute dystonias and parkinsonism which develop early. The latter respond to anticholinergic drugs, while tardive dyskinesia responds poorly, or not at all.

75 / Bilateral parotid enlargement/ Mikulicz's syndrome

Frequency in survey: 2% of attempts at MRCP short cases.

Survey note: all patients with sicca symptoms (dry eyes and dry mouth) in our survey had parotid enlargement.

Record

There is *bilateral parotid enlargement*.* The conjunctivae are injected (the patient complains of *gritty eyes*—the dry eyes of keratoconjunctivitis sicca) and the tongue (touch it) is dry (or the patient complains of a *dry mouth*).

This is Mikulicz's syndrome (diffuse swelling of lachrymal and salivary glands) which is most likely to be produced by:

1 Sarcoidosis (?lupus pernio, chest signs) but may also be caused by
2 Lymphoma (?lymph nodes, hepatosplenomegaly — both signs, of course, may also occur in sarcoid)
3 Leukaemia (?pallor, hepatosplenomegaly).

Reduction in tear secretion can be demonstrated with *Schirmer's test* in which a 5 mm wide strip of filter paper is folded 3 mm from one end and hooked into the lower conjunctival sac. Normal tear secretion moistens more than 15 mm of strip within 5 min.

Secondary Sjögren's syndrome (*Mikulicz's disease*) is the triad of dry mouth (xerostomia), keratoconjunctivitis sicca and a connective tissue disease —most commonly rheumatoid arthritis (50%) but also including autoimmune liver disease and fibrosing alveolitis. Bronchial, pancreatic and vaginal secretions may also be diminished. The lachrymal and salivary glands are not swollen as in *Mikulicz's syndrome* (the issue is complicated, though, by the fact that there is a high incidence of lymphoma in Sjögren's syndrome!).

Primary Sjögren's syndrome (30%) does not have the associated connective tissue disease. It is sometimes referred to as the *sicca syndrome*.

* Painless parotid enlargement can also occur in bulimia nervosa.

76 / Primary biliary cirrhosis

Frequency in survey: 2% of attempts at MRCP short cases.

Record

This middle-aged lady is *icteric* (may not be) with *pigmentation* of the skin. There are *excoriations* (due to scratching) and she has *xanthelasma* (other xanthomas frequently occur over joints, skin folds and at sites of trauma). The liver is enlarged . . . cm (may be very large; there may be splenomegaly).

The clinical diagnosis is primary biliary cirrhosis (there may be *clubbing*). The scratch marks are due to *pruritus* (the predominant presenting symptom).

HLA phenotypes B8 and C4B2 = threefold increase in risk

Serum antimitochondrial antibody positive in 95–99%

Smooth muscle antibody positive in 50%

Antinuclear factor positive in 20%.

Impaired biliary excretion of copper occurs with excessive copper deposition in the liver. This may not be an important factor in the pathogenesis of the progressive liver disease, but it can be helpful in the diagnosis—sometimes differentiation from chronic active hepatitis (25% have antimitochondrial antibody) can be difficult (clinically and histologically) and the issue can be resolved by staining the biopsy specimen for copper. Kayser–Fleischer rings occasionally occur. Penicillamine (immunological, anti-fibrotic, as well as chelating effects) has been used in advanced disease but there is no evidence that it improves survival. Immunosuppressive agents (including corticosteroids, azathioprine, methotrexate and cyclosporin A) and antifibrotics (e.g. colchicine) may have a small effect. Ursodeoxycholic acid improves serum biochemistry, decreases the rate of referral for liver transplantation and reduces pruritus, but no effect on histology or survival has yet been convincingly demonstrated. Supplements of fat-soluble vitamins, calcium and phosphate are given in view of malabsorption. The pruritus often responds to cholestyramine (taken before and after meals) though phenobarbitone, rifampicin, opiate antagonists (e.g. naloxone), or propofol may also help. Resistant pruritus responds to norethandrolone but this deepens jaundice. Physical intervention (bile diversion, haemoperfusion, charcoal column perfusion or plasmapheresis) may also help severe pruritus. Liver transplantation has been used successfully but there is increasing evidence that the disease may recur in the transplanted liver.

The patient is at risk of

Bleeding oesophageal varices

Steatorrhoea and malabsorption, leading to Osteomalacia.

Associated conditions*

Sjögren's syndrome

Systemic sclerosis

CRST syndrome

Rheumatoid arthritis

Hashimoto's thyroiditis

Renal tubular acidosis

Coeliac disease

Dermatomyositis.

---

* The incidental finding of a raised alkaline phosphatase in patients with the conditions on this list should raise the suspicion of an associated primary biliary cirrhosis.

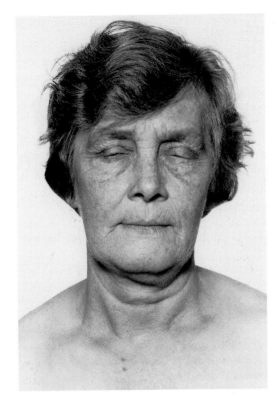

Fig. 3.76 Note xanthelasma, pigmentation and spider naevi.

77 / Lupus pernio

Frequency in survey: 2% of attempts at MRCP short cases.

Survey note: candidates often gave differential diagnoses such as SLE and rosacea before being led to the correct diagnosis. We suggest that candidates try to see real-life cases of all three conditions affecting the face before the examination so that they may recognize the differences.

Record

There is (in this female patient) a *diffuse*, livid, *purple–red infiltration* of the *nose* (and/or cheeks, ears, hands and feet).

The diagnosis is lupus pernio (usually associated with *chronic pulmonary sarcoidosis* which progresses to *fibrosis*; *chronic uveitis* and *bone cysts* in the phalanges are often present).

Other complications which may occur in chronic sarcoidosis

Facial palsy (may be bilateral; parotid enlargement not always present)

Peripheral neuropathy

Meningeal infiltrations and tumour-like deposits

Hypopituitarism and diabetes insipidus (granulomas extending from the meninges into the hypothalmus)

Hypercalcaemia and its nephropathy (probably hypersensitivity to vitamin D)

Mikulicz's syndrome (diffuse swelling of lachrymal and salivary glands by conditions such as sarcoidosis, lymphoma or leukaemia—p. 221)

Cardiomyopathy (clinical evidence rare; there may be arrythmias or heart block; cor pulmonale is more likely to be the cardiac consequence)

Chronic arthritis

Hypersplenism if sufficient splenomegaly

Infiltration of old scars by sarcoid tissue

Polymyositis (progressive muscle wasting).

Hepatic granulomata can be found in two-thirds of patients with sarcoidosis (symptoms rare). Sarcoidosis may affect most tissues.

For colour photograph see p. 531.

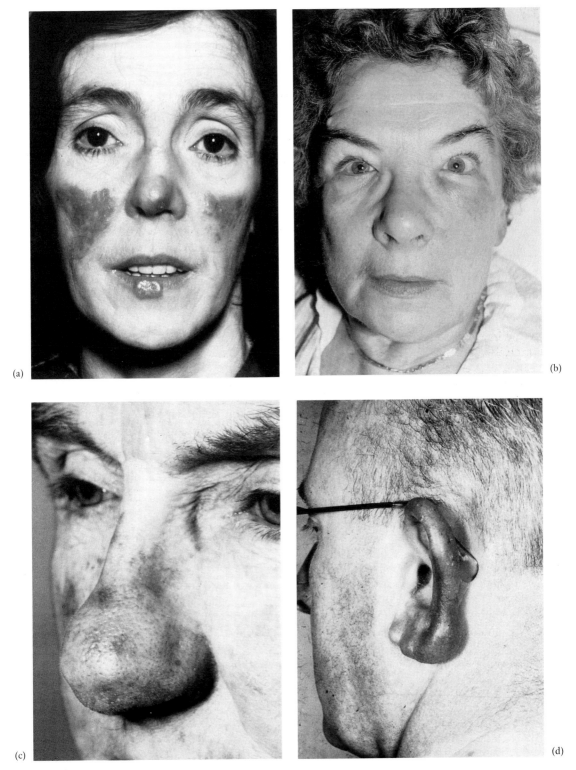

Fig. 3.77 (a) Lupus pernio on cheeks, nose and lip. (b) Lesions under the eyes especially on the left. (c) A close-up of lupus pernio on the nose. The treated case may just show a faint purplish discoloration on the end of the nose or cheeks. (d) Lupus pernio of the ear.

78 / Muscular dystrophy

Frequency in survey: 2% of attempts at MRCP short cases.

Survey note: all cases were of facioscapulohumeral except one possible case of limb-girdle type.

Record 1

The patient has a dull, unlined, expressionless face (*myopathic facies*) with lips that are (usually) open and slack. There is *wasting* of the *facial* and *limb-girdle muscles*, and the superior margins of the scapulae (viewed from the front) are (may be) visible above the clavicles. The movements of smiling, whistling and closing the eyes are impaired. There is *winging of the scapulae* (when the patient leans against a wall with arms extended). There is (may be) involvement of the trunk and legs (anterior tibials may cause bilateral foot-drop) now or in the future.

The diagnosis is *facioscapulohumeral* (Landouzy–Déjérine) muscular dystrophy* (autosomal dominant, course variable but usually relatively benign).

Record 2

There is *limb-girdle wasting* and *weakness* which affects some groups of muscles more than others (e.g. deltoid and spinati usually spared), and the *face* is *spared*. There is (not uncommonly) enlargement of the calf muscles.

These features suggest *limb-girdle* (Erb) muscular dystrophy (autosomal recessive, both sexes affected equally, more benign if the upper limb is involved first, usually begins in the second or third decade, sometimes arrests but usually patients are severely disabled within 20 years of onset).

Other muscular dystrophies

Duchenne or pseudohypertrophic — X-linked, severe, onset age 3–4 years, initially enlargement of calves, buttocks and infraspinati (this disappears later) while other muscles (especially the proximal lower limb) waste; waddling lordotic gait; usually confined to wheelchair by age of 10 years; cardiac muscle involved; face spared; death from respiratory infection and/or cardiac failure commonly at about age of 20

Benign X-linked (Becker) muscular dystrophy — similar to Duchenne but much less severe — onset 5–25 years; confined to wheelchair 25 years later

Distal muscular dystrophy—dominant; most cases occur in Sweden—eventually spreads to proximal muscles unlike peroneal muscular atrophy (p. 249) with which it is most often confused

Ocular myopathy — sporadic or dominant — first ptosis, then ophthalmoplegia, face and neck muscles often mildly involved — see footnote, p. 345

---

* There may be an inflammatory component in the aetiology of facioscapulohumeral muscular dystrophy, as perivascular inflammation may be seen on muscle biopsy and *retinal microvascular abnormalities* (sparse and dilated (telangiectatic) peripheral retinal vessels which may leak causing exudate to track to the posterior pole with consequent retinal detachment and blindness) also characterize the disorder. *Sensorineural deafness* may occur but clinical cardiomyopathy is rare.

Oculopharyngeal muscular dystrophy†—similar to ocular myopathy but late onset and dysphagia prominent—often French–Canadian ancestry

Childhood muscular dystrophy with autosomal recessive inheritance—rare, similar to Duchenne but more benign and girls may be affected

Congenital muscular dystrophy — rare, hypotonia from birth, prognosis unfavourable.

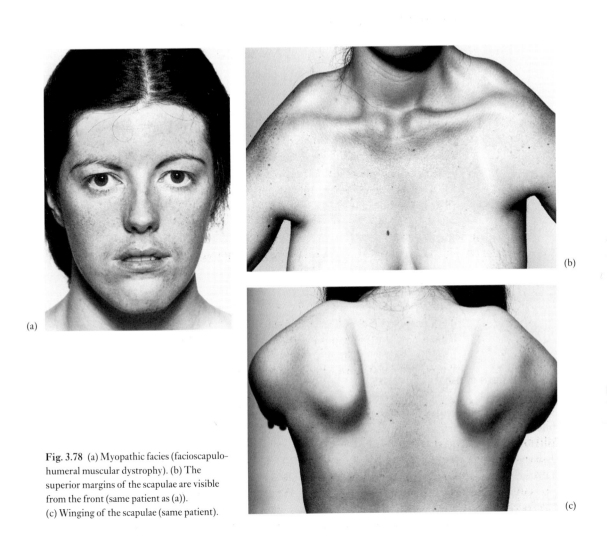

(a)

(b)

(c)

Fig. 3.78 (a) Myopathic facies (facioscapulo-humeral muscular dystrophy). (b) The superior margins of the scapulae are visible from the front (same patient as (a)). (c) Winging of the scapulae (same patient).

† Some patients with this syndrome have spinal muscular atrophy and some others have mitochondrial cytopathy; see footnote, p. 345.

79 / Prosthetic valves

Frequency in survey: main focus of a short case in 2% of attempts at MRCP short cases. Additional feature in a further 1%.

Survey note: both mitral and aortic prostheses occurred. Often leaking. There may also be murmurs from the unreplaced valve.

Record 1

There is a *midline sternotomy scar*. There is a *click at the first heart sound* (closing of the mitral prosthesis) and an *opening click* in diastole (this may occasionally be followed by a mid-diastolic flow murmur).

These clicks represent the opening and closing of a *mitral valve prosthesis*. (The pansystolic murmur ± signs of heart failure suggest it is leaking.)

Record 2

There is a *midline sternotomy scar*. The first heart sound is normal (unless there is accompanying mitral stenosis), and is followed by an *ejection click* (opening of the prosthesis), an *ejection systolic murmur* and a *click at* (as part of) *the second sound* (closing of the prosthesis).

These clicks suggest an *aortic valve prosthesis*. (The early diastolic murmur and collapsing pulse (?wide pulse pressure) suggest it is leaking.)

Complications of prosthetic valves

Thromboembolic disease (anticoagulants or anti-platelet agents reduce but do not abolish)

Infective endocarditis (always consider when leakage develops)

Leakage due to wear of the valve

Leakage due to inadequacy or infection (bacterial endocarditis) of valve siting

Near total or even total dehiscence of the valve from its siting (the valve will be seen to rock on X-ray screening when there is serious leakage)

Ball embolus (the ball of the Starr–Edwards valve)

Valve obstruction from thrombosis/fibrosis clogging up the valve mechanics

Haemolysis (aortic valve).

NB Porcine heterografts and cadavaric homografts do not cause clicks. They last on average 8–10 years and are therefore only used nowadays in the elderly.

Frequency in survey: 2% of attempts at MRCP short cases.

Survey note: often the differential diagnosis of Addison's/Nelson's was given and further differentiation was not required.

Record

There is *generalized pigmentation* (due to the direct action of ACTH causing increased melanin in the skin), which is more marked in the *skin creases* (e.g. palmar), in *scars* (especially more recent ones), in the *buccal mucosa* (look in the mouth), in the *nipples* and at *pressure points*.

This suggests Addison's disease or Nelson's syndrome (?temporal field defect, ?abdominal scar of bilateral adrenalectomy).

Patchy, almost symmetrical, areas of skin depigmentation surrounded by areas of increased pigmentation may occur due to vitiligo (15% of patients with idiopathic Addison's) which is one of the associated organ-specific autoimmune diseases. (For the others, which include autoimmune thyroiditis, diabetes mellitus, pernicious anaemia and hypoparathyroidism, see p. 279. Premature ovarian failure is particularly associated with Addison's disease.)

Common causes of primary hypoadrenalism

Autoimmune adrenalitis
Tuberculosis (?lung signs).

Other causes of primary hypoadrenalism

Bilateral adrenalectomy (malignant disease, e.g. breast cancer; Cushing's syndrome)
Secondary deposits
Amyloidosis (hypoadrenalism preceded by nephrotic syndrome—see footnote, p. 114)
Haemochromatosis
Granulomatous disease (rarely sarcoidosis)
Fungal diseases (e.g. histoplasmosis)
Congenital adrenal hyperplasia*
Meningococcal and pseudomonal septicaemia
Adrenal haemorrhage (newborn especially breech delivery; patients on anticoagulants)

Adrenal vein thrombosis after trauma or adrenal venography.

Skin pigmentation is usually racial (including buccal pigmentation) or due to sun-tanning. Other causes of abnormal generalized pigmentation include:

Endocrine
ACTH therapy (e.g. asthma)
Cushing's disease (?facies, truncal obesity, striae, etc.—p. 231)
Thyrotoxicosis (?exophthalmos, goitre, etc.—p. 114)
Ectopic ACTH (especially oat-cell carcinoma).

Chronic debilitating disorders (also, like Addison's, associated with lassitude and weight loss)
Malignancy (including reticuloses and leukaemias)
Malabsorption syndromes
Chronic infections (especially tuberculosis)
Cirrhosis (?icterus, spider naevi, etc. — pp. 84 and 222)
Uraemia (pale, brownish yellow tinge to skin).

Pigments other than melanin such as
Haemochromatosis (slate-grey pigmentation, hepatosplenomegaly, etc.—p. 253)
Argyria
Chronic arsenic poisoning.

---

* Series of inherited defects in adrenocortical steroidogenesis (e.g. 21-hydroxylase deficiency). Homozygotes present neonatally with salt wasting, hypotension and ambiguous genitalia in females.

Drugs
Phenothiazines (blue–grey pigmentation)
Antimalarials (blue–grey pigmentation)
Amiodarone (grey pigmentation)
Cytotoxics
Minocycline (purple–blue pigmentation; may get

blue oral discoloration due to blue–black discoloration of alveolar bone and hard palate—'black-bone disease').

For colour photographs see p. 535.

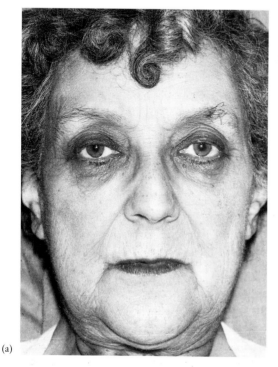

(a)

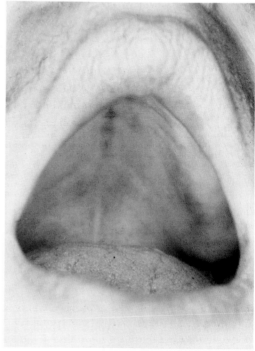

(b)

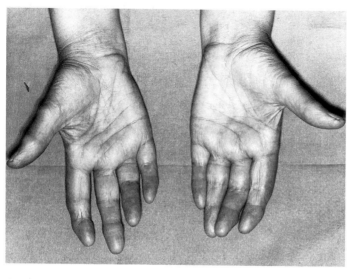

(c)

Fig. 3.80 (a–c) Addison's disease.

81 / Cushing's syndrome

Frequency in survey: main focus of a short case in 2% of attempts at MRCP short cases. Additional feature in a further 3%.

Survey note: almost all cases were secondary to therapeutic steroids — especially for asthma and rheumatoid arthritis, but also for cryptogenic fibrosing alveolitis and chronic active hepatitis, amongst others.

Record

The patient has a *moon face* with *acne* and *truncal obesity* with a *buffalo hump*. The skin is thin (demonstrate by raising a skinfold at the back of the patient's hand) and shows excessive bruising (*purpuric patches* — often at venesection sites), and there are purple *striae* on the abdomen (must be differentiated from the pale pink striae of obese adolescents and the stretch marks of pregnancy and simple obesity). She is *hirsute* with a *deep voice*. There is *proximal muscle weakness* (few patients with Cushing's syndrome can rise normally from the squatting position).

The diagnosis is Cushing's syndrome (?evidence of underlying steroid responsive inflammatory or immunological disorder).

Other features of Cushing's syndrome

Hypertension and peripheral oedema (salt retention)

Irregular menstruation

Impotence

Back pain (osteoporosis and vertebral collapse leading to kyphosis and loss of height)

Diabetes mellitus

Pigmentation (especially ectopic or exogenous ACTH)

Psychiatric disorder (commonly depressive illness).

Causes of Cushing's syndrome*

Therapeutic corticosteroids

Therapeutic ACTH

Cushing's disease—pituitary (basophilic or chromophobe pituitary adenoma) or hypothalamic lesion leading to excessive ACTH

Adrenocortical adenoma (occasionally part of *MEA type I* with one or more of: primary hyperparathyroidism, islet-cell tumour, pituitary tumour—see also p. 109†)

Adrenocortical carcinoma

Ectopic ACTH secreting non-endocrine tumours:

1 Oat-cell carcinoma of bronchus (weight loss, pigmentation, hypokalaemic alkalosis and oedema)

2 Bronchial adenoma

3 Carcinoid tumour (usually bronchial)

4 Carcinoma of pancreas

5 Non-teratomatous ovarian tumour.

For colour photographs see p. 536.

---

* When the syndrome is not iatrogenic, then in about 80% of affected adults the cause is Cushing's disease; whereas adrenal adenoma, carcinoma and ectopic ACTH syndrome contribute equally to the remaining 20%.

† The islet-cell tumour may secrete gastrin (Zollinger–Ellison syndrome) or insulin (insulinoma). The pituitary tumour may be eosinophilic (acromegaly) or a chromophobe adenoma which is non-secreting (bitemporal hemianopia, headaches, blindness, hypopituitarism and other pressure symptoms—tumour may become very large). Pituitary tumours may also secrete prolactin (impotence, amenorrhoea, galactorrhoea) or ACTH (Cushing's disease).

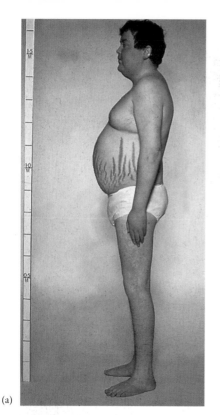

(a)

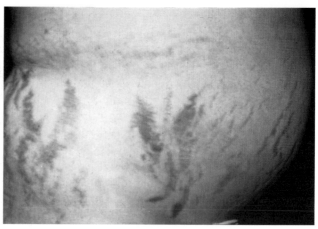

(b)

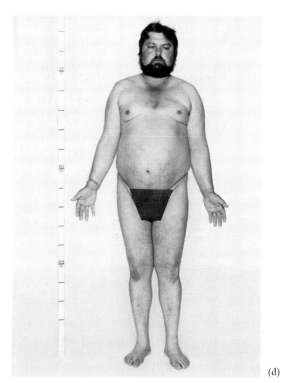

(c)

(d)

Fig. 3.81 (a) Cushing's syndrome. (b) Abdominal striae.
(c) Cushingoid facies (steroid therapy for cerebral lupus
erythematosus). (d) Truncal obesity (Cushing's disease).

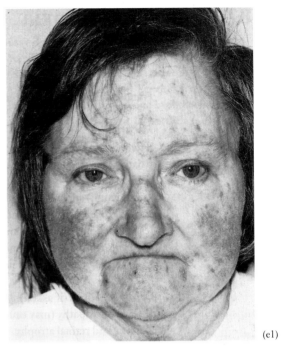

(e1)

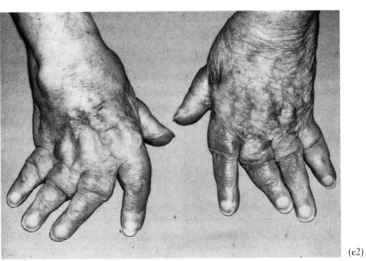

(e2)

Fig. 3.81 (*continued*) (e1,2)
Corticosteroid therapy in a patient
with rheumatoid arthritis.

cally affect the elbows, knees, hands and feet. The rash may be a punctate erythematous rash, palmar erythema, periungual erythema, or livedo reticularis (see pp. 265–6). Subcutaneous nodules may occur (5%) somewhat resembling those encountered in rheumatoid arthritis.

For colour photograph see p. 532.

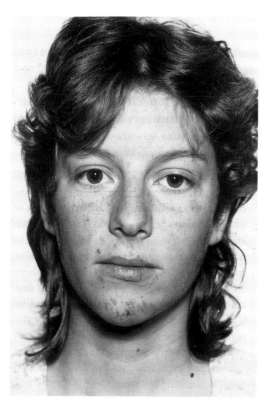

Fig. 3.84 Butterfly rash (see also p. 532).

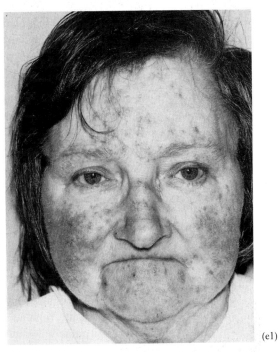

(e1)

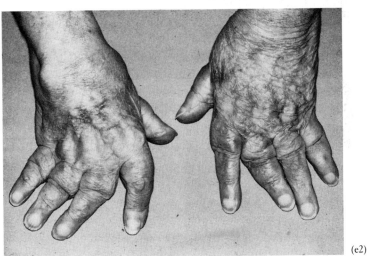

Fig. 3.81 (*continued*) (e1,2)
Corticosteroid therapy in a patient
with rheumatoid arthritis.

(e2)

Frequency in survey: 2% of attempts at MRCP short cases.

Record

There is *pes cavus*, *(kypho)scoliosis* and (may be) a deformed and high-arched palate. The patient is *ataxic* and clumsy with an *intention tremor* and his *head shakes*. There is *nystagmus* (often slow and coarse and observed before formal examination) and *dysarthria* (slow and slurred or scanning and explosive). There is (?gross) bilateral impairment of rapid alternate motion, finger–nose and heel–shin tests. Knee and *ankle jerks* are *absent* and the *plantar responses are extensor. Position and vibration* sense are diminished in the feet.

The diagnosis is Friedreich's ataxia.

Other features (if asked)

1 Cardiomyopathy (may cause sudden death)
2 Optic and retinal atrophy
3 Diabetes mellitus
4 Mild dementia.

The condition is one of the hereditary spinocerebellar degenerations. It is usually recessive but in some families it is dominant. The fully-fledged syndrome is rare among affected family members who more commonly show slight signs of abnormality in the lower limbs, chiefly pes cavus and absent reflexes (*formes fruste*).

The major classic ataxic conditions which may need to be differentiated from Friedreich's ataxia, particularly if the latter is mild and presents late, are multiple sclerosis and tabes dorsalis (rare). Typical features which may help to differentiate these conditions are shown in Table 3.82.

Table 3.82 Features which may help to differentiate the major ataxic conditions

	Friedreich's ataxia	Multiple sclerosis	Tabes dorsalis
Family history	Major	Minor	None
Onset before age 15	Usual	Rare	Rare
Knee and ankle jerks	Absent	Usually exaggerated	Absent
Spine	(Kypho)scoliosis	Normal	Normal
Feet shape	Pes cavus	Normal	Normal
Pupils	Normal	Normal	Argyll Robertson
Plantars	↑	↑	↓ or → (unless taboparesis)
Pain and deep pressure	Normal	Normal	Absent
Romberg's sign	±	−	+

Other conditions which may have features of Friedreich's ataxia (all are recessive)

Bassen–Kornzweig syndrome (abetalipoproteinaemia*) — steatorrhoea, acanthosis, pigmentary retinal degeneration and a spinocerebellar degeneration which resembles Friedreich's ataxia

Refsum's disease (elevated serum phytanic acid due to defective lipid α-oxidase) — pupillary abnormalities, optic atrophy, deafness, pigmentary retinal degeneration, cardiomyopathy, icthyosis and a Friedreich-like ataxia

Roussy–Lévy syndrome (this is a variant of type I hereditary motor and sensory neuropathy and its features are intermediate between Charcot–Marie–Tooth disease and Friedreich's ataxia) — ataxia, areflexia, pes cavus and kyphoscoliosis but absence of nystagmus, dysarthria, extensor plantar responses and posterior column signs.

---

* Low-density and very low-density lipoproteins (LDL, VLDL) and chylomicra are absent from the serum, cholesterol is very low and triglycerides are barely detectable.

83 / Peutz–Jeghers syndrome

Frequency in survey: 2% of attempts at MRCP short cases.

Record

There are (sparse or profuse) small brownish-black *pigmented macules* (2–5 mm) (lentigines) on the lips, around the *mouth* (and/or eyes or nose) and *buccal mucosa* (but never on the tongue). They are also (may be) seen on the hands and fingers.

This pigmentation (which tends to disappear in adult life) may be associated with *intestinal polyposis* (single or multiple polyps, which are *hamartomas*, may occur in small and large bowel) in which case the diagnosis would be Peutz–Jeghers syndrome.

Autosomal dominant.

Complications

Recurrent colicky abdominal pain
Intestinal obstruction or intussusception
Iron deficiency anaemia
Frank gastrointestinal haemorrhage
Malignant transformation (rare*).

Multiple polypectomy may be required for disabling symptoms but excision of bowel is to be avoided, if possible, as polyps may recur.

For colour photographs see pp. 534 and 535.

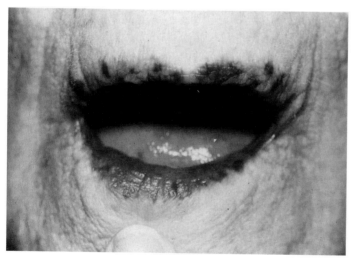

Fig. 3.83 Peutz–Jeghers syndrome.

* Cf. familial polyposis coli—adenomatous tumours in which malignant transformation is inevitable and for which premalignant treatment is colectomy, ileorectal anastomosis and fulgarization of remaining rectal polyps. This is followed by careful life-long 6-monthly follow-up with sigmoidoscopy and polyp fulgarization.

Frequency in survey: 2% of attempts at MRCP short cases.

Record

There is (in this *young female* patient) a *red, papular butterfly rash* on the face (and elsewhere — especially light exposed areas) with *scaling, follicular plugging** and *scarring*.

These features suggest lupus erythematosus (chronic discoid lupus erythematosus if only the skin is affected; SLE if there is evidence of multisystem involvement).

Discoid LE—males:females $= 1:2$.
SLE—males:females $= 1:9$.

Look for other features

Buccal mucosa (sharply defined whitish patches with red borders)

Scalp (scarring alopecia)

Hands and joints (arthritis; deformity may occur but usually mild; Raynaud's in 20%)

Skin (vasculitis—see below)

Lungs† (pleural effusions, or rarely crepitations from interstitial involvement)

Ankles (oedema — SLE is an important cause of nephrotic syndrome)

Heart (for pericardial friction rub, rarely pericardial effusion; cardiac enlargement or failure — myocarditis; or murmurs—Libman–Sachs endocarditis)

Proximal muscles (myalgia is common; polymyositis may occur)

Eyes (Sjögren's syndrome; fundal haemorrhages or white exudates called cytoid bodies; papilloedema)

Reticuloendothelial system (lymph nodes; splenomegaly)

Mucous membranes for pallor — anaemia is normochromic normocytic and/or haemolytic (Coombs' positive or negative); thrombocytopenia often occurs; haematological changes may antedate the other features of the disease by years

Hepatomegaly (chronic passive congestion — usually transient‡)

Urine (proteinuria and haematuria).

NB In SLE vasculitic rashes occur more commonly than the classic butterfly rash. They characteristi-

---

* Very close examination of the butterfly rash reveals that the scales in many areas appear as dots. These dots indicate where the follicle has been plugged by a scale. When the scales are removed (very unlikely to be required in the examination) and the undersurface is inspected, they clearly appear as tiny spicules projecting from the scaly mass. No other scaly condition produces this phenomenon. Healing of the discoid lesions occurs with atrophy, scarring (telangiectasia), hyperpigmentation or hypopigmentation (vitiligo).

† Drug-induced SLE involves the lungs more commonly and kidneys less commonly than classical SLE. The commonest (90%) drugs are hydralazine (slow acetylators), isoniazid, phenytoin and procainamide (rapid acetylators). Other drugs

include hydrochlorothiazide, oral contraceptives, penicillin, practotol, reserpine, streptomycin, sulphonamides, minocycline and tetracycline.

‡ Liver biopsy may be normal or show fatty infiltration and/or fibrosis. These manifestations in SLE should not be confused with the form of chronic active hepatitis, which often has a positive antinuclear factor, called 'lupoid hepatitis'. The liver biopsy in the latter shows an inflammatory infiltrate extending into the liver lobule, causing erosion of the limiting plate and piecemeal necrosis. Fibrous septa isolate rosettes of cells. Cirrhosis is usually present and eventually hepatic failure may develop.

cally affect the elbows, knees, hands and feet. The rash may be a punctate erythematous rash, palmar erythema, periungual erythema, or livedo reticularis (see pp. 265–6). Subcutaneous nodules may occur (5%) somewhat resembling those encountered in rheumatoid arthritis.

For colour photograph see p. 532.

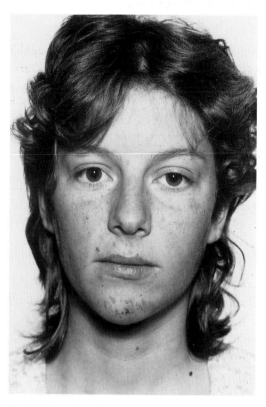

Fig. 3.84 Butterfly rash (see also p. 532).

85 / Superior vena cava obstruction

Frequency in survey: 2% of attempts at MRCP short cases.

Record

There is stridor. The face and upper extremities are *oedematous* (puffy) and *cyanosed*, and the eyes are *suffused*. The *superficial veins* over these areas are *dilated* and there is *fixed engorgement* of the *neck veins*. The undersurface of the tongue is covered with multiple venous angiomata. There is (may be) a radiation burn on the chest wall.

The diagnosis is superior vena cava obstruction, most likely due to carcinoma* of the bronchus, particularly small cell carcinoma (?lymph nodes, chest signs, clubbing, etc.—p. 145). It has been treated by radiotherapy.†

The patient may complain of headaches (may be severe on coughing), difficulty in breathing, dysphagia, dizziness or blackouts. Physical signs are frequently absent or minimal.

Other causes of superior vena cava obstruction

Lymphoma
Aortic aneurysm
Mediastinal fibrosis
Mediastinal goitre.

---

*The compression may either be by the tumour or by involved lymph nodes.
†Radiotherapy, or chemotherapy, is required urgently in this condition. A stent can sometimes be placed in the superior vena cava as a palliative procedure. Dexamethasone is also used.

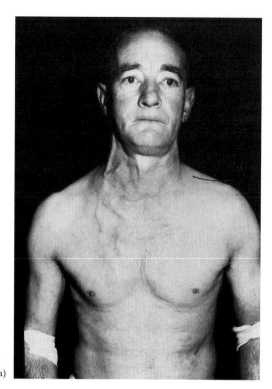

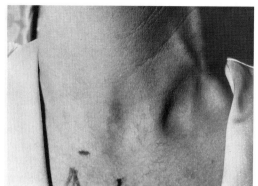

(b)

(a)

Fig. 3.85 (a,b) Superior vena cava obstruction. Note the
radiotherapy ink marks in (b).

86 / Vasculitis

Frequency in survey: main focus of a short case in 2% of attempts at MRCP short cases. Additional feature in a further 2%.

Record

There are (may be) small *nail-fold* and nail-edge *infarcts* (due to small vessel vasculitis affecting the terminal digital arteries—in severe cases there may be *digital gangrene*). There is (may be) a purpuric rash (macules, papules, nodules or pustules). There are (may be) chronic leg ulcers. There is (may be) a peripheral neuropathy (due to involvement of the vasa nervorum).

This patient has vasculitis (look for obvious signs of a cause, e.g. rheumatoid arthritis or SLE).

The term vasculitis refers to disorders involving the small vessels and larger arteries of the skin, either alone or in association with other organs (there is chronic inflammation in and around the vessel wall). This is usually caused by deposition of immunoglobulin and sustained by complement activation.

Other manifestations of vasculitis include nodular vasculitic lesions (e.g. erythema nodosum—p. 178), urticaria, erythema multiforme, and livedo reticularis (see p. 267).

Conditions associated with vasculitis

Rheumatoid arthritis (?hands, nodules, etc.—p. 73)

SLE (?rash, etc.—p. 237)

Polyarteritis nodosa* (medium and small arteries and adjacent veins—fever, hypertension, abdominal pain, mononeuritis multiplex, peripheral neuropathy, proteinuria, haematuria, renal failure, myocardial infarction)

Churg–Strauss syndrome (eosinophilic granulomatous vasculitis — similar to polyarteritis nodosa but asthma, eosinophilia, IgE elevation and pulmonary infiltrates are prominent; it may present as asthma)

Australia antigenaemia and vasculitis (a variant of polyarteritis nodosa)

Wegener's granulomatosis* (granulomatous ulceration of the upper and lower respiratory tract associated with generalized arteritis and glomerulitis)

Other connective tissue diseases (systemic sclerosis, etc.)

Drug reactions

Infective endocarditis

Mixed cryoglobulinaemia

Hypergammaglobulinaemia

Lymphoproliferative disorders

Henoch–Schönlein syndrome (children > adults; purpuric rash over the extensor surface of the limbs, particularly at the ankles and often on the buttocks; associated with arthritis of medium-sized joints, colicky abdominal pains, occasionally gastrointestinal bleeding and acute nephritis—p. 327)

Persistent urticaria (urticarial vasculitis)

Giant-cell arteritis (large and medium-sized vessels; elderly patients—headache, temporal artery tenderness, polymyalgia rheumatica — danger of blindness)

Behçet's disease (oral ulcers, uveitis, phlebitis, photosensitivity, spontaneous pustules)

Thromboangiitis obliterans — Buerger's disease (young man, nicotine staining, peripheral ischaemia, gangrene, migratory superficial thrombophlebitis; see also p. 316).

---

* Antineutrophil cytoplasmic antibodies (ANCA) occur in two staining patterns—cytoplasmic (cANCA) and perinuclear (pANCA). High titre cANCA strongly suggests necrotizing vasculitis of the Wegener's granulomatosis type. pANCA is particularly associated with microscopic polyarteritis nodosa.

Rheumatoid patients with vasculitis often have

Nodules
Circulating immune complexes
Cryoglobulins
Low complement levels
Rheumatoid factor
Antinuclear factor
Immunoglobulins and complement in the cutaneous lesions.

For colour photograph see p. 537.

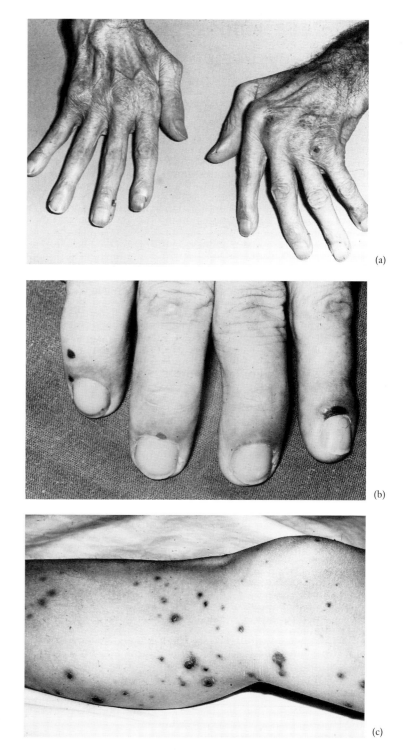

Fig. 3.86 (a) Rheumatoid arthritis.
(b) Nail-fold infarcts (rheumatoid
arthritis). (c) Vasculitis on the lower
limb.

87 / Deep venous thrombosis/ Baker's cyst/cellulitis

Frequency in survey: 2% of attempts at MRCP short cases.

Record 1

There is *unilateral* swelling of the R/L leg up to the knee joint which looks normal in appearance* (extension into the thigh suggests femoral or iliac vein thrombosis) associated with an erythematous or a cyanotic hue to the skin, and (feel gently) tenderness to palpation in the calf. The affected calf feels indurated† and is *warmer than the other leg*.

 The patient has a deep venous thrombosis.‡

Record 2

The R/L leg is *swollen, painful on movement* and *tender* on palpation. Both the knee joint and the upper, posterior compartment of the calf are swollen, and the normal contours of the joint are obscured by effusion (demonstrate the patellar tap—p. 297).§

 The diagnosis is a ruptured Baker's (popliteal) cyst (now check hands for rheumatoid arthritis—p. 73).‖

Record 3

There is an *erythematous, warm* swelling of the R/L leg. There are (may be) vesicles/bullae and crusts on the surface of the erythematous area (look for the portal of bacterial entry).¶ There is (may be) a puncture mark on the foot (say where exactly) perhaps caused by a thorn (or there may be fungal intertrigo of the feet with secondary bacterial infection).

 These features suggest cellulitis. There is (may be) *lymphangitis* (look for the reddish streaky lines running up the leg), and the inguinal lymph nodes are swollen and tender.

---

* If there was associated swelling of the knee it would bring ruptured popliteal cyst and disease of the joint (infection, gout and pseudogout) into the differential diagnosis.

† The calf in deep venous thrombosis feels bulky and indurated and moves *en mass* causing discomfort when gently swayed from side to side. This method is preferable to testing for the *Homan's sign* in which a sudden dorsiflexion of the corresponding foot can cause considerable pain. In the normal calf the muscle contours are clearly visible and a part of the muscle can be moved from side to side without pain or affecting the rest of the calf.

‡ The definitive diagnosis can usually be made by Doppler ultrasonography which is non-invasive, quick and less expensive than venography, though the latter remains the gold standard.

§ The popliteal cyst may rupture and dissect into the calf muscles causing pain and acute swelling involving the upper part of the calf. The cyst may cause compression of the popliteal vein leading to oedema of the entire leg.

‖ Ultrasound scanning has the advantage of being non-invasive but arthrography is the most definitive way to identify a popliteal cyst. The latter procedure also provides the opportunity for aspiration to rule out infection, gout and pseudogout.

¶ Group A streptococci and *Staphylococcus aureus* are the most commonly responsible organisms.

Record 4

The skin on the R/L leg is *swollen* and *erythematous with a sharply demarcated, irregular border* which is tender to touch, and has an 'orange-peel' epidermal surface. These features suggest erysipelas.**

The thrombophilia syndromes which predispose to deep venous thrombosis include:

Antiphospholipid syndrome (?livedo reticularis; see p. 266)

Resistance to activated protein C (up to 7% of population)

Deficiency of antithrombin III (up to 1/2000 of population)

Deficiency of protein C and protein S (vitamin K dependent factors that act together to neutralize factors V and VIII).

** Erysipelas is an acute infection of the skin and subcutaneous tissues casued by group A streptococci. It is most commonly seen on the face but may affect other parts of the body. The disease usually affects the two extremes of age.

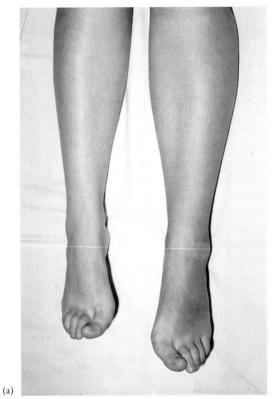

(a)

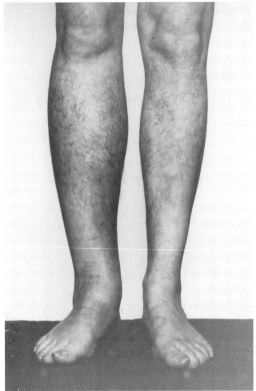

(b1)

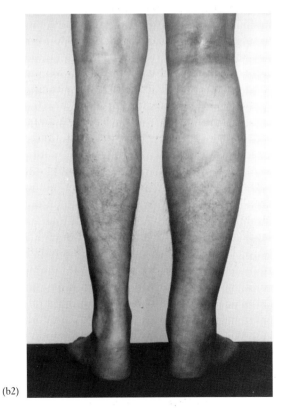

(b2)

Fig. 3.87 (a) Left deep venous thrombosis. (b1) Ruptured Baker's cyst; (2) posterior view.

88 / Cor pulmonale

Frequency in survey: 1% of attempts at MRCP short cases.

Record

The patient's fingers are *nicotine-stained* and there is *central cyanosis*. The pulse is regular, the *venous pressure is raised* (give height) with prominent small *a* waves and giant *v* waves (if there is secondary tricuspid incompetence), and there is *ankle* and *sacral oedema*. *Expiration is prolonged and noisy*. The *accessory muscles* of respiration are in use at rest, and there is a *tracheal tug*. The trachea is central, expansion is equal, the percussion note is resonant, and tactile fremitus and vocal resonance are normal. There is a *left parasternal heave* and a palpable second heart sound* (?pan-systolic murmur of tricuspid incompetence). There are (may be) widespread *expiratory rhonchi* and coarse inspiratory crepitations and the forced expiratory time (see p. 31) is 8 seconds. (There is no *flapping tremor* of the hands—if there were you would want to examine the fundi for papilloedema.)

These findings suggest cor pulmonale due to chronic bronchitis and emphysema. (Right heart failure is often precipitated by acute infection.)

The auscultatory cardiac signs of pulmonary hypertension, some of which may be audible,* are:
Loud pulmonary second sound
Pulmonary early systolic ejection click
Right ventricular fourth heart sound.

Causes of pulmonary heart disease

Chronic obstructive bronchitis (with or without emphysema; by far the commonest cause—p. 150)

Recurrent pulmonary emboli (signs of pulmonary hypertension without clinical evidence of other lung disease; ?deep venous thrombosis)

Primary pulmonary hypertension (signs of pulmonary hypertension without clinical evidence of other lung disease; usually a female)

Non-pulmonary causes of alveolar hypoventilation (kyphoscoliosis, obesity, neuromuscular weakness)

Pansystolic murmur of functional tricuspid incompetence (giant *v* waves)

Early diastolic murmur of functional pulmonary incompetence (Graham Steell murmur).

Lung diseases which only occasionally result in cor pulmonale including:

Progressive massive fibrosis (?coal dust tattoos on the skin; chronic bronchitis is the commonest cause of cor pulmonale in miners)

Bronchiectasis (especially cystic fibrosis; ?clubbing, cyanosis, full sputum pot, productive cough, crepitations—p. 161)

Cryptogenic fibrosing alveolitis (?clubbing, cyanosis, basal crackles—p. 103)

Systemic sclerosis (hands, facies—p. 96)

Sarcoidosis (?lupus pernio—p. 224)

Asthma (severe and chronic; may be missed if the reversibility is not checked in chronic small airways obstruction).

---

* These findings, which may be prominent in cor pulmonale due to other causes, may be difficult to elicit in cor pulmonale where a barrel-shaped chest and hyperinflation are present, and the heart is enfolded by over-inflated lungs.

Frequency in survey: 1% of attempts at MRCP short cases.

Record
There are *bright white*, streaky, irregular patches with frayed margins at the edge of the disc.

These are due to myelinated nerve fibres. They do not affect vision.

Normally the fibres of the optic nerve lose their myelin sheath as they enter the eye. Occasionally the sheath persists for some distance after the fibres leave the optic disc. If this phenomenon is extensive the disc and emerging vessels can be obscured.

For colour photograph see p. 529.

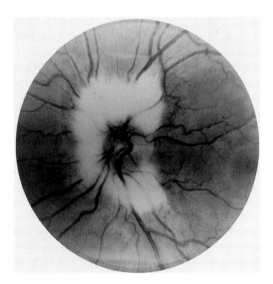

Fig. 3.89 Myelinated nerve fibres.

Frequency in survey: 1% of attempts at MRCP short cases.

Record

There is *distal wasting* of the *lower limb* muscles with relatively well-preserved thigh muscles.* The feet show *pes cavus* and clawing of the toes, and there is weakness of the extensors of the toes and feet. The *ankle jerks* are *absent* and the plantar reflexes show no response. There is only slight *distal involvement* of *superficial* modalities of *sensation* (though occasionally marked sensory loss may lead to digital trophic ulceration). The lateral popliteal (?and ulnar) nerves are palpable (in some families only). The patient has a *steppage gait* (bilateral foot-drop). There is (may be) *wasting of the small muscles of the hand*.

The diagnosis is peroneal muscular atrophy.†

Patterns of inheritance are variable.

The degree of disability in this condition is commonly surprisingly slight in spite of the remarkable deformities. Toe retraction and talipes equinovarus may occur and fasciculation (much less apparent than in motor neurone disease) is sometimes seen.

The degeneration is mainly in the motor nerves. It is sometimes also found in the dorsal roots and dorsal columns, and slight pyramidal tract degeneration is often seen (however, in classic cases extensor plantars are not found). The condition usually becomes arrested in mid-life. Other members of the patient's family may have a *formes fruste* and show just minor signs such as pes cavus and absent ankle jerks only.

---

* In classic descriptions, as the disease progresses, the wasting creeps very slowly up the limb, inch by inch, involving all muscles. According to the stage of the disease, the characteristic appearances have been described as 'stork' or 'spindle' legs, 'fat bottle' calves, and 'inverted champagne bottles'. The same process may occur in the arms; wasting of the small muscles of the hands is common with a tendency for the fingers to curl and the patient to have difficulty in straightening and abducting them. Classically, Charcot–Marie–Tooth wasting was described as stopping *abruptly* part of the way up the leg. In practice it is not usually so clear-cut and can be considered to be an example of neuromythology.

† Charcot–Marie–Tooth disease is now called *hereditary motor and sensory neuropathy* (HMSN) and is subdivided into HMSN type I (the hypertrophic form of Charcot–Marie–Tooth disease), HMSN type II (the neuronal form of Charcot–Marie–Tooth disease) and HMSN type III (previously called Déjérine–Scotas disease).

(a1)

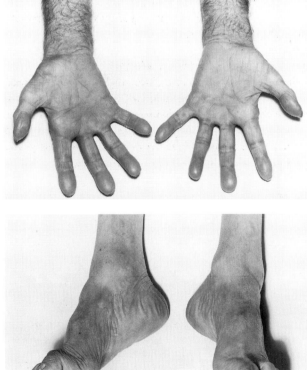

(a2)

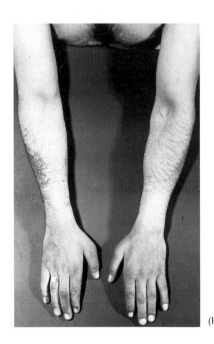

(b)

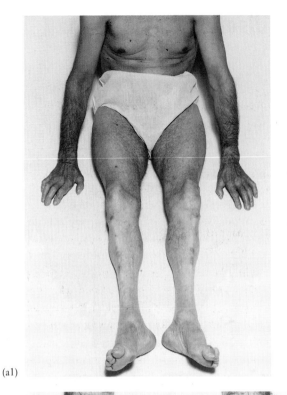

(a3)

Fig. 3.90 (a1–3) Note that the muscle wasting stops in the thighs, foot-drop, pes cavus, and wasting of the small muscles of the hand all in the same patient. (b) Distal wasting in the upper limbs.

91 / Cataracts

Frequency in survey: main focus of a short case in 1% of attempts at MRCP short cases. Additional feature in a further 4%.

Record

There are partial cataracts in both eyes (may be localized to the lens nucleus, or seen as flakes, dots or sector-shaped opacities within the lens periphery).

Commonest causes of cataract

1 Old age (usually nuclear, with a brownish discoloration, or of the cortical spoke variety)

2 Diabetic patients develop senile cataracts at younger ages than non-diabetics and this is the commonest type of cataract in diabetes. Rarely* a 'snowflake' (dot cortical opacities) cataract can develop in a young, poorly controlled diabetic, and progress rapidly to a mature cataract in months or even days (good control may halt and even reverse development).

Other causes of cataract in adults

Trauma

Chronic anterior uveitis

Hypoparathyroidism (Chvostek's and Trousseau's signs, tetany, paraesthesiae and cramps, ectodermal changes, moniliasis, mental retardation and psychiatric disturbances, papilloedema, epilepsy, bradykinetic-rigid syndrome)

Radiation (infra-red, ultraviolet, X-rays and possibly microwaves)

Dystrophia myotonica (?frontal balding, ptosis, sternomastoid wasting, myopathic facies, myotonia, etc.—p. 159)

Retinitis pigmentosa (including Refsum's, Laurence–Moon–Biedl—pp. 144 and 358)

Steroid therapy (10 mg prednisolone daily for more than 1 year)

Chlorpromazine (500 mg daily for 3 years or more)

Chloroquine.

Causes of cataracts in children

These include: perinatal hypoglycaemia, perinatal hypocalcaemia, maternal rubella, galactosaemia, galactokinase deficiency, genetically inherited, Down's syndrome (trisomy 21), Patau's syndrome (trisomy 13), Edward's syndrome (trisomy 18), Alport's syndrome, Lowe's syndrome.

---

* Rare with modern insulin therapy. A case was seen recently in an insulin-dependent patient who did not take insulin for prolonged periods for personal religious reasons.

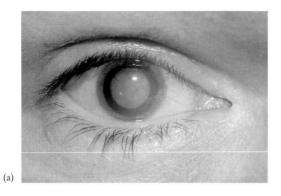

(a)

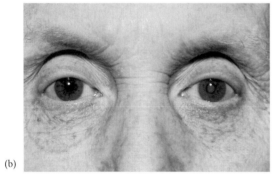

(b)

Fig. 3.91 (a) Cataract. (b) A cataract is seen in the left eye.

92 / Idiopathic haemochromatosis

Frequency in survey: 1% of attempts at MRCP short cases.

Record

There is (in this thin patient) *slate-grey pigmentation,** *decreased body hair* and *gynaecomastia* (and testicular atrophy*—iron deposition affecting hypothalamic–pituitary function). The *liver** is *enlarged* at . . . cm (in 95% of symptomatic patients; spleen is present in 50%).

The diagnosis is haemochromatosis.

Males > females.

In males it may present at any time in adult life. In females it usually presents after the menopause (physiological iron loss protects).

Autosomal recessive—association with HLA-A3. Gene on short arm of chromosome 6. A common genetic disorder—carrier rate about 1/10 in populations of Northern European origin. Homozygote rates vary between 1/200 and 1/600.

Other features which may be present

Spider naevi

Palmar erythema

Ascites

Jaundice

Diabetes mellitus* (not entirely due to iron deposition in the pancreas because insulin levels may be normal and there is a higher incidence of diabetes in relatives without iron overload; high incidence of insulin resistance and fat atrophy)

Arthropathy* (pseudogout—especially the second and third metacarpophalangeal joints, wrists, hips, and knees)

Cardiac involvement* (large heart, dysrhythmias, congestive cardiac failure; it is the presenting manifestation in 15%—sometimes young adults;

it may be *misdiagnosed* as idiopathic cardiomyopathy)

Hepatocellular carcinoma (develops in 33% of cirrhotic patients; it does not appear to occur if the disease is treated in the precirrhotic stage; hence the importance of *family screening*)

Addison's disease, hypothyroidism and hypoparathyroidism are exceedingly rare.

Treatment

Weekly *phlebotomy* (500 ml) until the haemoglobin concentration falls below $11 \, g \, dl^{-1}$ and the patient is marginally iron deficient (serum ferritin $< 10 \, \mu g \, l^{-1}$ —this usually takes 2 to 3 years), then maintenance phlebotomy to keep the serum iron and ferritin in the low normal range (about once every 3 months). When phlebotomy is initiated before cirrhosis develops, survival is normal. If anaemia and hypoproteinaemia preclude phlebotomy, *desferrioxamine* may be indicated. This is most practically administered by high dose subcutaneous infusion using a portable pump. *Ascorbic acid* given concurrently improves iron excretion.

NB Patients with alcoholic liver disease often have increased stainable iron on liver biopsy. These can

---

* The association of hepatomegaly, skin pigmentation, diabetes mellitus, heart disease, arthritis and evidence of hypogonadism should always suggest haemochromatosis. These days the precirrhotic condition is often diagnosed in young relatives by family screening. The diagnosis should be considered in any patient with unexplained hepatomegaly,

idiopathic cardiomyopathy, abnormal pigmentation or loss of libido (may antedate the other clinical manifestations of the disease). Ninety per cent of patients show bronzing of the skin due to excess melanin. In half, haemosiderin is also present, giving the skin the classic slate-grey appearance.

be divided into two groups: (i) mild to moderate increase in stainable iron but relatively normal body iron stores (< 3 g); and (ii) gross iron deposition and increased body iron stores. Phlebotomy may prolong survival in the latter (the majority of whom have idiopathic haemochromatosis) but not the former group.

Frequency in survey: main focus of a short case in 1% of attempts at MRCP short cases. Additional feature in many others (carcinoma of the bronchus and old tuberculosis—pp. 145 and 108).

Record

There is reduced movement of the R/L side of the chest. There is *dullness* to percussion over . . . (describe where) with *bronchial breathing*, *coarse crepitations*, *whispering pectoriloquy* and a *pleural friction rub*.

These features suggest consolidation (say where).

Commonest causes of consolidation

Bacterial pneumonia (pyrexia, purulent sputum, haemoptysis, breathlessness)

Carcinoma (with infection behind the tumour; ?clubbing, wasting, etc.—p. 145)

Pulmonary infarction (fever less prominent, sputum mucoid, occasionally haemoptysis and blood-stained pleural effusion).

94 / Coarctation of the aorta

Frequency in survey: main focus of a short case in 1% of attempts at MRCP short cases. Additional feature in a further 1%.

Record

The radial pulses (in this young adult with a well-developed upper torso) are regular, equal,* and of large volume (give rate). The *carotid pulsations* are *vigorous*,† and the JVP is not elevated (unless there is heart failure). The *femorals* are *delayed* and of *poor volume* (palpate the radial and femoral simultaneously). The *blood pressure* in the right arm is elevated at 190/110mmHg (it will be *low in the legs*). There are *visible arterial pulsations*‡ and *bruits* can be heard over and around the *scapula, anterior axilla* and over the *left sternal border* (internal mammary artery). The cardiac impulse is heaving but not displaced (unless in failure). Systolic *thrills* are palpable over the collaterals and suprasternally. There is a *systolic murmur* which is loudest at the level of the *fourth intercostal space posteriorly* (the level of the coarctation), but is also audible in the *second intercostal spaces* close to the sternum (the murmur—if present—of the associated bicuspid aortic valve is often obscured by that from the coarctation).§

These findings suggest a diagnosis of coarctation of the aorta.

Male to female ratio is 2:1.

Other features and associations of coarctation of the aorta

Rib notching* and poststenotic dilatation on chest X-ray

Bicuspid aortic valve in 25% (site of infective endocarditis and may lead to coexisting aortic incompetence; diagnosis can be made by echocardiography)

Berry aneurysms of the circle of Willis (may cause death even in corrected cases)

Ventricular septal defect (?pansystolic murmur, etc. —p. 197)

Patent ductus arteriosus (?machinery murmur, etc. —p. 213)

Turner's syndrome (check for features of Turner's if your patient is female—webbed neck, increased carrying angle, short stature, etc.—p. 352)

Marfan's syndrome (?tall, arachnodactyly, high arched palate, lens dislocation, etc.—p. 267)

High mortality after the age of forty. Hypertension may not be cured even in corrected cases (low perfusion of kidneys may involve the renin–angiotensin system).

Other causes of rib notching

Neurofibromatosis (multiple neuromata on the intercostal nerves)

Enlargement of nerves (amyloidosis, congenital hypertrophic polyneuropathy)

Inferior vena cava obstruction

Blalock shunt operation (left-sided unilateral rib notching)

Congenital.

---

* Rarely (2%) the coarctation is proximal to the origin of the left subclavian artery and the left arm pulses will be weaker than the right; rib notching will be unilateral and right sided.
† If you see vigorous carotid pulsations the likeliest cause is aortic incompetence (?collapsing pulse). The occasional patient, however, will have coarctation.

‡ Collaterals are best observed with the patient sitting up and leaning forward with the arms hanging by the side.
§ A continuous murmur in systole and diastole, arising from the dilated collaterals, may be heard over the back. An early diastolic murmur arising because of the dilated ascending aorta may be heard especially in older patients.

95 / Bulbar palsy

Frequency in survey: 1% of attempts at MRCP short cases.

Record

The *tongue* is *flaccid* and *fasciculating* (it is wasted, wrinkled, thrown into folds and increasingly motionless). The *speech is indistinct* (flaccid dysarthria), lacks modulations and has a *nasal twang*, and *palatal movement is absent*. There is (may be) saliva at the corners of the mouth (and while the patient talks he may be seen to pause periodically to gulp the secretions that have accumulated meanwhile in the pharynx; there may be dysphagia and nasal regurgitation).

This is bulbar palsy.

Possible causes

1 Motor neurone disease (?muscle fasciculation, absence of sensory signs, etc.— p. 123)
2 Syringobulbia (?nystagmus, Horner's, dissociated sensory loss, etc.—p. 305)
3 Guillain–Barré syndrome (?generalized including facial flaccid paralysis, absent reflexes, peripheral neuropathy or widespread sensory defect; monitor peak flow rate—p. 286)
4 Poliomyelitis
5 Subacute meningitis (carcinoma, lymphoma, etc.)
6 Neurosyphilis.

Frequency in survey: main focus of a short case in 1% of attempts at MRCP short cases. Additional feature in further 2%.

Survey note: often hemichorea associated with a hemiplegia.

Record

There are *brief, jerky, abrupt, irregular, quasi-purposeful, involuntary movements* (which never integrate into a coordinated act but may match it in complexity). The movements *flit* from one part of the body to another in a random sequence; they are *present at rest* and *accentuated by activity* (at rest the movements prevent the patient's relaxation and they interrupt and distort voluntary movement). The patient has a general air of restlessness. He is *unable* to keep his *tongue protruded* (it darts in and out). There is *abnormal posturing* of the *hands* in which the wrist is flexed and the fingers are hyperextended at the metacarpophalangeal joints. When the upper limbs are raised and extended there is *pronation of the forearm*.
   This is chorea.*

Causes of chorea

Sydenham's chorea (usually between age 5 and 15; ?heart murmur; one-third have a history of rheumatic fever; it may recur during pregnancy and when on the oral contraceptive pill)

Huntington's chorea (affects the lower limbs more often than the upper, producing a dancing sort of gait; chorea may precede dementia; onset age 35–50; family history)

Drug-induced chorea (e.g. neuroleptics, L-dopa)

Senile chorea (idiopathic orofacial dyskinesia; no dementia).

Other causes of chorea include epidemic encephalitis, the encephalopathies occurring with exanthema, idiopathic hypocalcaemia, thyrotoxicosis, SLE, carbon monoxide poisoning, and hereditary.

Causes of hemichorea/hemiballism†

Cerebrovascular accident† (?hemiplegia, homonymous hemianopia)

Intracerebral tumour (?pyramidal signs on the side of the chorea, papilloedema)

Trauma

Post-thalamotomy.

Other types of involuntary movement (dyskinesias)

Athetosis‡ (slow, coarse, irregular, writhing muscular distortion most commonly of the hands, feet and digits, though the face and tongue may be affected—many choreic and dystonic movements are indistinguishable from athetosis)

Dystonia‡ (sustained spasm of some portion of the

---

* In choreoathetosis (cerebral palsy, tumours involving the pallidum, vascular insufficiency, Wilson's disease, carbon monoxide poisoning, etc.) the movements mainly involve the upper limbs and cranial nerves (grimacing, writhing movements of the tongue, etc.). The hands are repeatedly brought in front of the chest shaped like cups with flexion at the metacarpophalangeal joints and extension at the interphalangeal joints.
† Hemiballism is wild irregular flinging or throwing movements of whole limbs on one side. Vascular lesions are

the commonest cause. The lesion is in the contralateral subthalamic nucleus. The ballistic movements often begin as the other neurological signs of the cerebrovascular accident start to clear (i.e. after an interval). They disappear during sleep. Though initially they may exhaust the patient, they usually die out gradually over 6–8 weeks.
‡ The common causes of the two closely linked dyskinesias, dystonia and athetosis, are drugs (neuroleptics, L-dopa) and post-hypoxia. There are many rare causes.

body; the movements are powerful and deforming, torticollis is a common example of torsion dystonia; lordosis and scoliosis may also be caused)

Myoclonus (rapid shock-like muscular jerks often repetitious and sometimes rhythmic — most common causes include epilepsy, essential (familial), physiological (sleep, exercise, anxiety), metabolic disorders (renal, respiratory or hepatic failure), subacute encephalitis)

Tremors (e.g. Parkinson's, anxiety, thyrotoxicosis, drugs (e.g. alcohol, caffeine, salbutamol), multiple sclerosis, spinocerebellar degeneration, cerebrovascular accident, essential/familial)

Tics.

Frequency in survey: main focus of a short case in 1% of attempts at MRCP short cases. Additional feature in at least a further 1%.

Survey note: the only dysarthria used as a short case in our survey was cerebellar (ataxic) dysarthria.

Record

There is dysarthria with *slurred*, *jerky* and *explosive* (slow, lalling, staccato, scanning) speech. (There may be inspiratory whoops indicating the lack of coordination between respiration and phonation).

This suggests cerebellar disease (?nystagmus, dysdiadochokinesis, finger–nose test, etc.—p. 142).

Other varieties of dysarthria

Spastic dysarthria

Conditions in which all or some of the articulatory parts are rigid or spastic:

Pseudobulbar palsy (indistinct, suppressed, without modulations, high-pitched, 'hot potato', 'Donald Duck' speech due to a tight, immobile tongue — ?bilateral spasticity with extensor plantars — p. 299)

Parkinson's disease (monotonous without accents or emphasis, somewhat slurred speech — ?expressionless unblinking face, glabellar tap sign, tremor, etc.—p. 148)

Dystrophia myotonica (slurred and suppressed speech—?ptosis, frontal balding, etc.—p. 159)

Huntington's chorea (slurred and monotonous — ?chorea, dementia)

General paresis of the insane — very rare (slurred, hesitant or feeble voice — ?dementia, vacant expression, trombone tremor of tongue, brisk reflexes, extensor plantars, etc.—p. 381).

Flaccid dysarthria

Bulbar palsy (nasal, decreased modulation, slurring of labial and lingual consonants — ?lingual atrophy, fasciculations, etc.—p. 257)

Paralysis of the VIIth, IXth, Xth or XIIth nerves (cerebrovascular accident).

Myopathic dysarthria

Myasthenia gravis (weak hoarse voice with a nasal quality, pitch unsustained, soft accents — ?ptosis, variable strabismus, facial and proximal muscle weakness all of which worsen with repetition, etc.— p. 269).

Variegated dysarthria

Hypothyroidism (low-pitched, catarrhal, hoarse, croaking, gutteral voice as if the tongue is too large for the mouth — ?facies, pulse, ankle jerks, etc.—p. 152)

Amyloidosis — large tongue (rolling and hollow, hardly modulated)

Multiple ulcers or thrush in the mouth (some parts of the speech indistinct)

Parotitis or temporomandibular arthritis (monotonous, suppressed, badly modulated).

98 / Dysphasia

Frequency in survey: main focus of a short case in 1% of attempts at MRCP short cases. Additional feature in a further 1%.

Survey note: where the type of dysphasia was reported by the candidate, it was always expressive.

Record 1

The patient's speech *lacks fluency*. He has *difficulty finding certain words* and sometimes produces the *wrong word* and makes grammatical errors. *Comprehension*, however, is *well preserved* (as are the higher cerebral functions and general intellect —the prognosis for eventual adaptation of the patient to his disability is good). His ability to repeat and to name objects is impaired.

The patient has Broca's (*expressive*, motor, non-fluent) *dysphasia* (?associated *right hemiplegia*). The brain damage causing this condition is believed to disconnect the dominant* inferior frontal gyrus (Broca's area).

Record 2

Though the patient *speaks fluently* (often rapidly) with normal intonation, his speech is completely *unintelligible*. He puts words together in the wrong order and mixes them with non-existent words† and phrases (*jargon dysphasia*). Attempts to repeat result in paraphasic† distortions and irrelevant insertions. *Comprehension* is severely *impaired* (and the patient may seem unaware of his dysphasia).

The patient has Wernicke's (*receptive*, fluent) *dysphasia* (?associated *homonymous visual field defect* and/or *sensory diminution* down the right side of the body). The brain damage causing this condition is believed to disconnect the posterior part of the dominant* superior temporal gyrus (Wernicke's area).

Record 3

The patient shows combined expressive and receptive dysphasia. There is marked disturbance in comprehension (and inability to read or write).

The patient has *global dysphasia*‡ (?dense right hemiplegia with sensory loss, homonymous visual field defect and general intellectual deterioration).

The common cause of this is infarction of the territory supplied by the left middle cerebral artery. The prognosis for recovery is poor.

Record 4

The patient has difficulty naming objects though he knows what they are (e.g. Hold up some keys: 'What

---

* The left hemisphere is dominant in right-handed and in 50% of left-handed people.

† **Paraphasia:** an incorrect syllable in a word (usually there is some phonemic relationship to the original word, e.g. 'tooth spooth' for 'toothbrush') or an incorrect word in a phrase (often with a semantic relationship to the correct word, e.g. 'hand' for 'foot').

Neologism: paraphasia with slight or no relationship to the original syllable/word.

‡ Global dysphasia is sometimes confused with Broca's dysphasia but the speech defects are severe in this condition affecting fluency, repetition, naming and comprehension. Some stereotypes may be preserved and the patient may be able to recite automatic sequences of prayer or popular songs (*speech automatism*).

is this?'—Patient does not answer. 'Is this a spoon?' — 'No'. 'Is it a pen?' — 'No'. 'Is it keys?' — 'Yes'). Despite this, comprehension and other aspects of speech production are relatively normal.

This is *nominal dysphasia* (uncommon in its pure form — usually part of a wider dysphasia). The underlying brain damage is believed to be in the most posterior part of the superior temporal gyrus and the adjacent inferior parietal lobule.

99 / Ehlers–Danlos syndrome

Frequency in survey: 1% of attempts at MRCP short cases.

Record

The patient (may be wearing glasses; myopia common) has *epicanthal folds*, a *flat nasal bridge* and prominent ears which point downwards. There is *hyperextensibility* of the skin which is *elastic* and *very thin*. There is evidence of *poor healing* with *thin scars* (the skin tears with minor injury, usually over the knees and elbows, producing *fish-mouth* wounds). *Purpura* is present and there are (commonly) *pseudotumours* over the knees and elbows (trauma→haematoma which organizes→fatty degeneration→calcification). The joints are (remarkably) *hyperextensible* and the patient has kyphoscoliosis, genu recurvatum and flat feet.

The diagnosis is Ehlers–Danlos syndrome.

There are at least seven distinct types which vary from mild to severe and show different patterns of inheritance (dominant, recessive, X-linked).

Complications

Bleeding (mostly from the gut)
Poor healing which makes surgery difficult
Recurrent dislocations of patellae, shoulders, hips, etc.
Recurrent hydrarthrosis
Repeated falls (poor control due to hypermobile joints)
Diaphragmatic herniae
Diverticula of the gastrointestinal and respiratory tracts
Spontaneous pneumothorax
Dissecting aneurysms
Spontaneous rupture of large arteries
Mitral valve prolapse (p. 209).

Other causes of hypermobile joints

Osteogenesis imperfecta* (p. 348)
Marfan's syndrome (tall, long bones, dislocated lens, etc.—p. 267)
Turner's syndrome (p. 352)
Noonan's syndrome (males and females; short stature, webbed neck, etc.—p. 352)
Down's syndrome (p. 337)
Pseudoxanthoma elasticum (p. 311)
Familial tendency in otherwise normal patients.

Cutis laxa: in this condition the skin may also be hyperextensible, but in contrast to Ehlers–Danlos syndrome it has decreased elasticity, and hangs in loose folds. Late in Ehlers–Danlos, the skin in localized areas may resemble that seen in cutis laxa.

*Blue sclerae often occur in Ehlers–Danlos also.

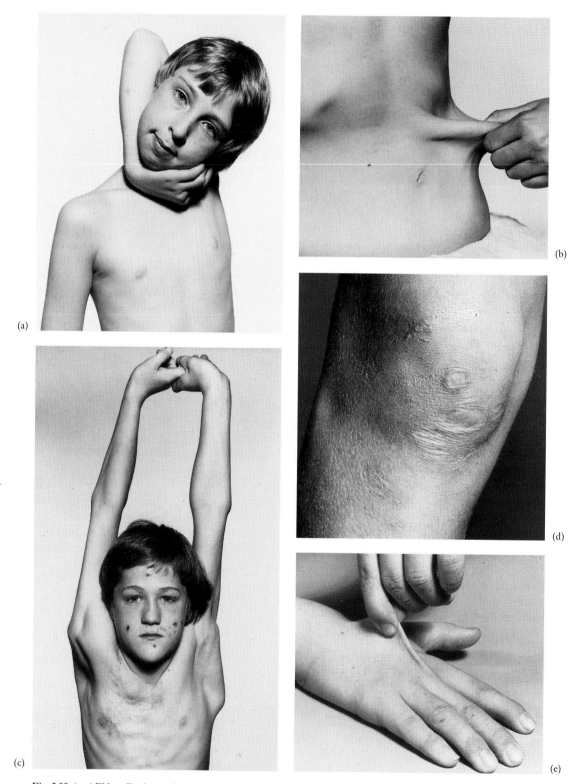

Fig. 3.99 (a–e) Ehlers–Danlos syndrome.

Frequency in survey: 1% of attempts at MRCP short cases.

Record

There is a *reticular pigmented* rash on the . . . (describe the site — usually lateral aspect of one *leg*).

It is characteristic of erythema ab igne.* (The patient obviously feels the cold. Look at the face and feel the pulse—?hypothyroidism.)

Other conditions which show a reticuloid pattern in the skin

Livedo reticularis (arborescent pattern of reddish-blue erythema or pigmentary change which may be associated with antiphospholipid antibody syndrome (APAS)†, collagen vascular disease — especially polyarteritis nodosa, cryoglobulinaemia, or a hyperviscosity syndrome)

Cutis marmorata (a physiological reaction to cold seen in 50% of normal children and many adults).

---

* Erythema ab igne is due to repeated infra-red heat injury. It can occur anywhere where heat is applied, e.g. on back or abdomen where a hot water bottle is used over a prolonged period in an attempt to alleviate pain. In long-standing cases, premalignant keratosis and squamous cell carcinoma can develop.

† A hypercoagulable condition leading to both venous and arterial occlusions. Lupus anticoagulant and anticardiolipin antibodies are the serological markers. Deep venous thrombosis, transient ischaemic attack, cerebrovascular accident, migraine, epilepsy and recurrent abortions may all be manifestations. Other arterial and venous thromboses may occur, as may heart valve disease. Sudden widespread organ failure may occur (catastrophic APAS). Sometimes, but not always, it may occur in the context of a connective tissue disease, particularly SLE. APAS (or APS) is also recognized as occurring as a primary condition (PAPS). APAS now tends to be referred to as *Hughes syndrome*.

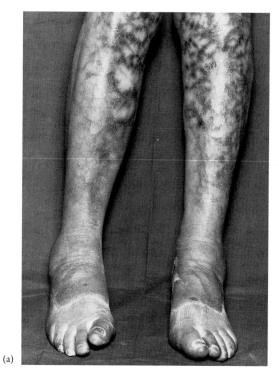
(a)

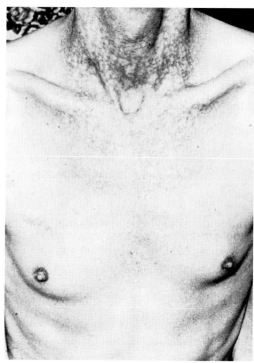
(b)

Fig. 3.100 (a) Erythema ab igne. (b) Livedo reticularis visible on the neck (SLE).

101 / Marfan's syndrome

Frequency in survey: 1% of attempts at MRCP short cases.

Record

The patient is *tall* with disproportionately *long extremities* (pubis–sole > pubis–vertex) and elongated fingers and toes (*arachnodactyly*). He has a *high-arched palate* (gothic), long narrow face and his span is greater than his height. His musculature is underdeveloped and hypotonic (and he may have a funnel or pigeon chest, pectus excavatum, kyphoscoliosis, flat feet, genu recurvatum, hyperextensibility of joints and recurrent dislocations). The tremor of the iris (*iridodonesis*) is evidence of *lens dislocation* (50–70% of patients; a slit lamp may be needed for detection in minor cases). He has (may have) a collapsing pulse (auscultate if allowed) suggestive of *aortic incompetence* (cystic necrosis of the aortic media leading to steadily progressive* dilatation of the aorta; aortic dissection can occur).

The diagnosis is Marfan's syndrome.

Autosomal dominant.
Defects in fibrillin (gene responsible is on the long arm of chromosome 15).

Other features which may occur in Marfan's syndrome

Heterochromia of the iris
Blue sclerae
Myopia
Undue liability to retinal detachment
Cystic disease of the lungs (tendency to spontaneous pneumothorax which is often recurrent and may be bilateral; other pulmonary manifestations are bullae, apical fibrosis, aspergilloma and bronchiectasis)
Mitral valve prolapse (p. 209 — common; severe mitral incompetence may occur)

Coarctation of the aorta
Bacterial endocarditis even on valves with only minor abnormalities
Inguinal or femoral herniae
Decreased subcutaneous fat
Miescher's elastoma (small nodules or papules in the skin of the neck)
Death due to cardiovascular component (average age is mid-forties).

NB *Homocystinuria* (autosomal recessive) may produce a similar clinical picture to Marfan's except in addition mental retardation, a malar flush and osteoporosis are common and ocular lens dislocation is downwards (in Marfan's it is upwards). Homocystine can be detected in the urine by the cyanide–nitroprusside test.

*Prophylactic β-blockade may slow the rate of aortic dilatation and reduce the development of aortic complications in some patients with Marfan's.

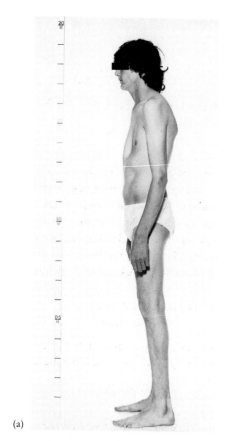

(a)

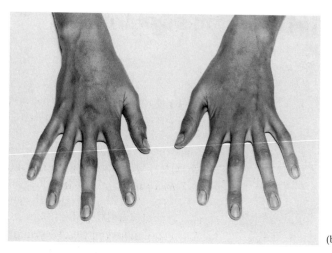

(b)

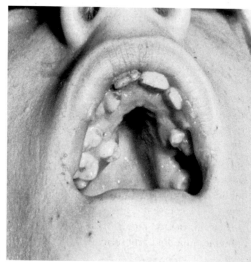

(c)

Fig. 3.101 (a–c) Marfan's syndrome.

Frequency in survey: main focus of a short case in 1% of attempts at MRCP short cases. Additional feature in a further 1%.

Record

There is *ptosis* (one or both sides) accentuated by upward gaze, *variable strabismus* (with *diplopia*) and when she tries to screw her eyes up tight, the eyelashes are not buried. The face shows a *lack of expression*, the mouth is slack and there is generalized *facial weakness*. The patient *snarls* when she tries to smile, she cannot whistle, and her *voice* is *weak* and *nasal* (if you ask the patient to count aloud, speech may become progressively less distinct and more nasal). There is *proximal muscle weakness*. Repetitive movements cause an increase in the muscle weakness (myasthenia = abnormal muscular fatiguability).

The diagnosis is myasthenia gravis. A Tensilon test will confirm it.

Male to female ratio is 1 : 2.

Other features of myasthenia gravis

Difficulty with swallowing, chewing and nasal regurgitation

Symptoms worsen as the day progresses

Tendon reflexes are normal or exaggerated (cf. Eaton–Lambert syndrome)

The *jaw-supporting sign*, if present, is pathognomonic—the patient puts her hand under her chin to support both the weak jaw and neck; may only become obvious after prolonged conversation

Antiacetylcholine receptor antibodies are present in 90%

In long-standing cases there may be an element of permanent irreversible myopathic change

Breathlessness is a sinister symptom requiring urgent attention (respiratory deterioration may develop rapidly and should be watched for by monitoring the peak flow rate)

Pathological changes are present in the thymus in 70–80% and some patients are improved by thymectomy; thymomata occur in 10–20% (mostly males) and give a worse prognosis.

Associated immune disorders include thyrotoxicosis (5% of patients), hypothyroidism, rheumatoid arthritis, diabetes mellitus, polymyositis, SLE, pernicious anaemia, Sjögren's syndrome, pemphigus and sarcoidosis.

Crisis

Signs of *cholinergic crisis* are collapse, confusion, abdominal pain and vomiting, sweating, salivation, lachrymation, miosis and pallor. The features which distinguish *myasthenic crisis* are response to edrophonium and absence of cholinergic phenomena. Occasionally it is exceptionally difficult to determine whether the collapsed myasthenic has been under- or over-treated. Temporary withdrawal of all drugs and assisted positive pressure respiration is then indicated.

Myasthenic crisis may be provoked by:

Infection

Emotional upset

Undue exertion*

Drugs (streptomycin, gentamicin, kanamycin, neomycin, viomycin, polymyxin, colistin, curare, quinine, quinidine, procainamide).

Eaton–Lambert syndrome (myasthenic-myopathic syndrome) is often associated with oat-cell carcinoma of the bronchus. There is proximal muscle wasting, weakness and fatiguability. Often,

* Childbirth requires careful management.

however, power is initially increased by brief exercise (reversed myasthenic effect). The tendon reflexes are depressed (but increased soon after activity). The electromyographic response to ulnar nerve stimulation shows a characteristic increase in amplitude (it declines in myasthenia gravis). Cholinergic drugs have no effect. Weakness and fatiguability may be greatly improved by guanidine hydrochloride.

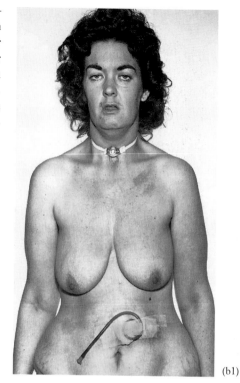

(b1)

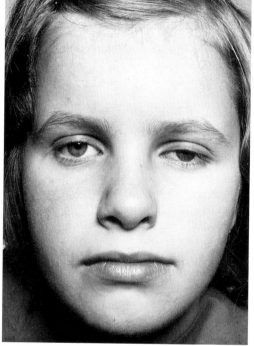

(a)

Fig. 3.102 (a) A mild case with unilateral ptosis. (b1,2) A severe case (note myasthenic facies, thymectomy scar, gastrostomy feeding tube and tracheostomy).

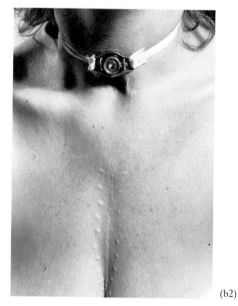

(b2)

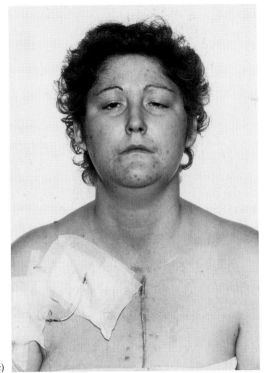
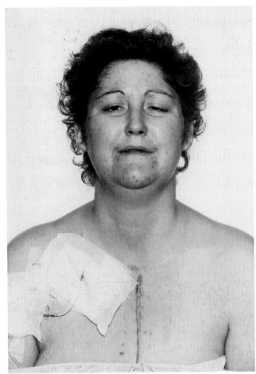

(c)

(d)

Fig. 3.102 (*continued*) (c) Myasthenic facies (note the subclavian line which was being used for plasmapherisis). (d) 'Smile'.

103 / Osteoarthrosis

Frequency in survey: 1% of attempts at MRCP short cases.

Record

There are *Heberden's nodes* present at the bases of the distal phalanges (and less commonly Bouchard's nodes at the proximal interphalangeal joints). There is a 'square hand' deformity due to subluxation of the base of the first metacarpal. There is swelling and deformity of the knee joints with development of varus (or valgus) deformity. There is crepitus in these joints. There is wasting and weakness of the quadriceps and glutei, and there is downward tilting of the pelvis when the patient stands on the affected leg (Trendelenberg's sign).

This patient has osteoarthrosis.

Complications

Pain

Deformity

Ankylosis

Entrapment of nerves (e.g. ulnar nerve palsy or carpal tunnel syndrome)

Cervical spondylosis.

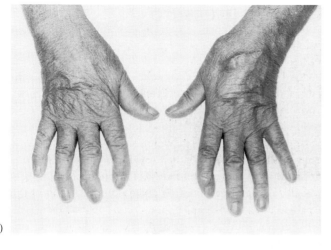

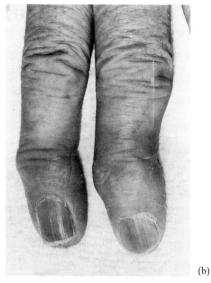

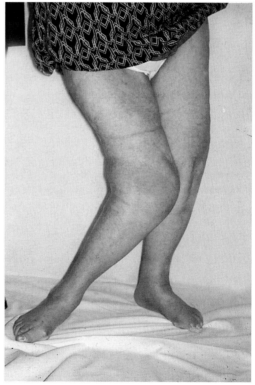

Fig. 3.103 (a,b) Note the square hand deformity, Heberden's nodes and lateral bending of the terminal digits.
(c) Osteoarthrosis of the knee joint with valgus deformity.

(a)

(b)

(c)

104 / Raised jugular venous pressure

Frequency in survey: main focus of a short case in 1% of attempts at MRCP short cases. Additional feature in many others.

Record

The JVP is elevated (measure) at . . . cm above the sternal angle (look for individual waves and time against the opposite carotid artery). The predominant wave is the systolic *v* wave which reaches the ear lobes. (If there is no oscillation of the blood column, sit the patient up to find the upper level. Make sure that there is no superior vena caval obstruction with the congestion of the face and neck, and prominent veins on the upper chest—p. 239). The carotid pulsation is irregularly irregular and the rhythm is atrial fibrillation (look for the evidence of congestive cardiac failure: ankle and sacral oedema, hepatomegaly, which may be pulsatile in tricuspid incompetence).

The large *v* wave suggests tricuspid incompetence either organic or due to congestive cardiac failure (see also p. 214).

Causes of a raised JVP (if venous obstruction is excluded)

Congestive cardiac failure (ischaemic heart disease, valvular heart disease, hypertensive heart disease, cardiomyopathy)

Cor pulmonale (?signs of chronic small airways obstruction, cyanosis, etc.—p. 247)

Pulmonary hypertension (large *a* wave in the JVP— primary (young females) and secondary to mitral valve disease or thrombo-obliterative disease)

Constrictive pericarditis (abrupt *x* and *y* descent, loud early *S3* ('pericardial knock') though heart sounds often normal, slight 'paradoxical' pulse, *no signs in the lungs*; chest X-ray may show calcified pericardium)

Large pericardial effusion (*x* descent, pulsus paradoxus, breathlessness, chest X-ray shows cardiomegaly, echocardiogram shows effusion).

105 / **Pretibial myxoedema**

Frequency in survey: main focus of a short case in 1% of attempts at MRCP short cases. Additional feature in a further 3%.

Record

There are *elevated symmetrical* skin lesions over the anterolateral aspects of the *shins* (may spread onto the feet; may affect other parts of the body, e.g. the face or the dorsa of the hands). The lesions are coarse, *purplish-red* (may be skin colour pink, or rarely, brown) in colour and raised with *well-defined* serpiginous *margins*. The skin is *shiny* and has an *orange peel appearance*. The hairs in the affected areas are coarse and the lesions are *tender* (and itch). The patient has *exophthalmos** (*?thyroid acropachy**) and is likely to have been rendered *euthyroid* (?pulse, etc.) by surgery (*?thyroidectomy scar*) or, more particularly, with *radioactive iodine*.

The diagnosis is pretibial myxoedema (occurs in about 5% of patients with Graves' disease).

The superficial layer of the skin is infiltrated with the mucopolysaccharide, hyaluronic acid. Biopsy scars of the area almost invariably develop keloid.

The latent interval between the treatment for hyperthyroidism and the clinical onset of pretibial myxoedema varies from 4 to 32 months with a mean time of 1 year.

Pretibial myxoedema in its most extreme form clinically resembles lymphoedema. It may be that mucin deposition in the dermis causes compression of the dermal lymphatics which results in dermal oedema and the clinical features of lymphoedema.

For colour photograph see p. 540.

---

* Pretibial myxoedema is almost always accompanied by exophthalmos. Thyroid acropachy (p. 116) is occasionally associated—diffuse thickening of distal extremities, subperiosteal new bone formation simulating clubbing of the digits. Exophthalmos has also been termed *infiltrative ophthalmopathy* and pretibial myxoedema, *infiltrative dermopathy*.

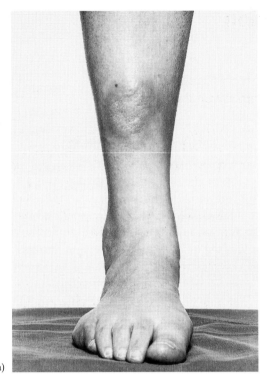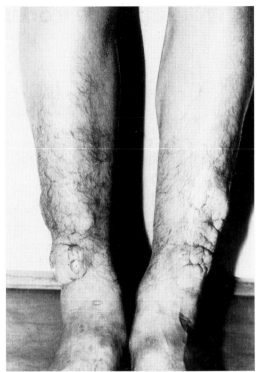

(a)
(b)

Fig. 3.105 (a,b) Pretibial myxoedema.

106 / Retinal artery occlusion

Frequency in survey: 1% of attempts at MRCP short cases.

Survey note: reported to have occurred as the underlying cause of optic atrophy with attenuated retinal arteries, and as a retinal artery branch occlusion causing a quadrantic field defect. No cherry-red spots were reported!

Record

The eye is blind, the *fundus* is *pale*, the *arterioles* are *thin* and *scanty* and there is a *cherry-red spot* at the macula (because the underlying choroidal circulation is intact).

The diagnosis is central retinal artery occlusion.

In the acute phase the whole fundus (except for the cherry-red spot) is milky white due to retinal oedema. By the time the retinal oedema has faded optic atrophy is generally apparent. The cherry-red spot is usually only seen for about 5–10 days. In retinal artery branch occlusion the fundoscopic appearances of thin arterioles and pale retina are limited to one area and there is a corresponding field defect (e.g. an inferior temporal field defect due to infarction of the superior nasal fundus).

The condition occurs most commonly in the elderly arteriosclerotic patient. It may be due to thrombosis, embolus (?carotid bruits, atrial fibrillation, heart murmurs) or spasm. Transient retinal artery occlusions associated with contralateral hemiparesis may occur from recurrent carotid emboli.

Occlusion of the central retinal artery may also follow giant-cell arteritis involving the arterioles around the optic disc (?headaches and temporal artery tenderness).

For colour photograph see p. 529.

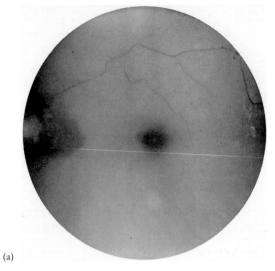
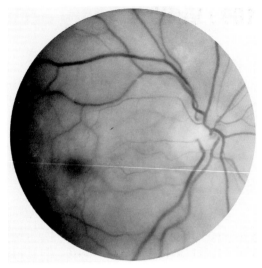

Fig. 3.106 (a,b) Retinal artery occlusion. Note macular cherry-red spots. The milky-white fundus due to retinal oedema is very pronounced in (a).

107 / Vitiligo

Frequency in survey: 1% of attempts at MRCP short cases.

Record

There are *areas* of *depigmentation* around the eyes, mouth, on the knees, and on the dorsum of the feet (the hands, axillae, groins and genitalia are the other commonly affected areas).

   The patient has vitiligo.

Sites subject to friction and trauma are often affected and Koebner's phenomenon (a lesion appearing at the site of skin damage) is common. Vitiligo is usually symmetrical but occasionally the depigmentation can be unilateral and follow the pattern of a dermatome. It is inherited as a dominant trait and individuals are usually otherwise healthy. Halo naevi (hypopigmented rings surrounding dark naevi), leucotrichia, premature greying of the hair and alopecia areata as well as vitiligo may all be associated with any of the **organ-specific autoimmune diseases:**

Myxoedema (?pulse, ankle jerks, facies—p. 152)
Hashimoto's disease (?goitre—p. 152)
Graves' disease (?exophthalmos, fidgety, goitre, tachychardia, etc.—p. 114)
Pernicious anaemia (?pallor, spleen, SACD—p. 375)
Atrophic gastritis associated with iron deficiency anaemia
Addison's disease (?buccal, skin crease, scar and general pigmentation, hypotension, etc.—p. 229)
Idiopathic hypoparathyroidism (Chvostek's and Trousseau's signs, tetany, paraesthesiae and cramps, cataracts, ectodermal changes, moniliasis, mental retardation, psychiatric disturbances, bradykinetic rigid syndrome, epilepsy)

Premature ovarian failure
Diabetes mellitus (?fundi)
Renal tubular acidosis
Fibrosing alveolitis (?basal crepitations—p. 103)
Chronic active hepatitis (?icterus, etc.)
Primary biliary cirrhosis (?xanthelasma, pigmentation, icterus, scratch marks, etc.—p. 222).

The organ-specific autoimmune diseases tend to occur in association with each other (*polyglandular autoimmune disease*) so that patients with one have an above normal chance of also developing another. Some patients are prone to extensive mucocutaneous candidiasis* (candidiasis-endocrinopathy syndrome) and from this two distinct syndromes emerge. The clinical features of the syndromes are compared in Table 3.107.

Vitiligo, the cutaneous marker of organ-specific autoimmune disease, may occur in the non-organ-specific autoimmune disease systemic sclerosis.† Other disorders associated with vitiligo are morphoea and malignant melanoma.

For colour photograph see p. 536.

---

* The mucocutaneous candidiasis is associated with hypergammaglobulinaemia, IgA deficiency and anergy to *Candida albicans*.
† Rarely there is an overlap between the organ-specific and non-organ-specific autoimmune diseases. Sjögren's syndrome occupies an intermediate position being associated with rheumatoid arthritis on the one hand and autoimmune thyroiditis on the other. Primary biliary cirrhosis is another condition which bridges the gap. It is associated with Sjögren's syndrome, Hashimoto's thyroiditis and renal tubular acidosis on the one hand, and systemic sclerosis, CRST syndrome, rheumatoid arthritis, coeliac disease, dermatomyositis and mixed connective tissue disease, on the other.

Table 3.107 Comparison of the clinical features of the major syndromes characterized by multiple endocrine gland hypofunction (from *Cecil's Textbook of Medicine*, 1992, 19th edn, p. 1389)

	Multiple endocrine deficiency syndrome (Schmidt's syndrome)	Polyglandular deficiency with mucocutaneous candidiasis
Hypoadrenalism	Common	Common
Hypothyroidism	Common	Rare
Diabetes mellitus (type I)	Common	Rare
Gonadal failure	Less common	Less common
Hypoparathyroidism	Rare	Common
Pituitary insufficiency	Rare	Rare
Autoantibodies to endocrine tissues and gastric parietal cells	Often present	Often present
Sex distribution	Strong female predominance	Female preponderance about 4 : 1
Inheritance	Usually 'sporadic', but susceptibility related to HLA haplotype and may be inherited as autosomal dominant	Generally inherited as autosomal recessive; no apparent HLA association; siblings characteristically affected
Time of onset	Usually becomes evident during adult life	Typically becomes evident during childhood preceded by chronic mucocutaneous moniliasis
Other associated 'autoimmune' diseases and characteristics	Pernicious anaemia; hyperthyroidism; coeliac disease; alopecia; vitiligo; myasthenia gravis; isolated red-cell aplasia	Pernicious anaemia; malabsorption; alopecia; vitiligo; IgA deficiency; hypergammaglobulinaemia; chronic active hepatitis; proliferative glomerulonephritis

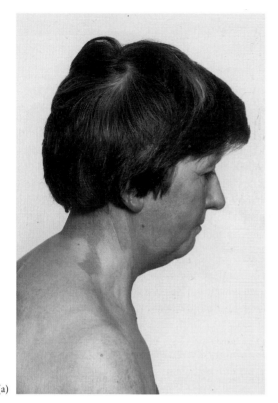

(a)

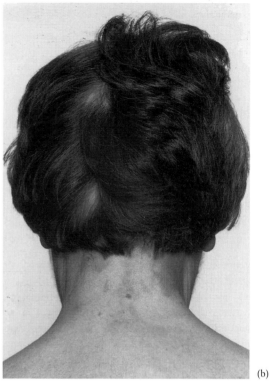

(b)

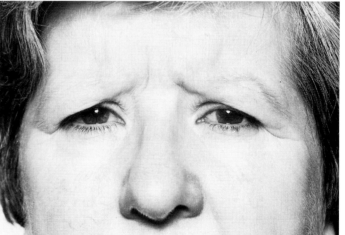

(c)

Fig. 3.107 (a–c) Note the areas of vitiligo and alopecia areata including loss of eyelashes (especially left upper lid) in this patient with diabetes mellitus.

Frequency in survey: 1% of attempts at MRCP short cases.

Record

There is *asymmetrical swelling* affecting the *small joints* of the *hands* and feet with *tophi* formation (in the periarticular tissues). These joints are (occasionally) severely *deformed*. There are tophi on the *helix* of the *ear* and in some of the tendon sheaths (especially the ulnar surface of forearm, olecranon bursa, the Achilles tendon, and other pressure points).

This patient has chronic tophaceous gout.

Chronic tophaceous gout results from recurrent acute attacks. Tophus formation is proportional to the severity and duration of the disease. However, patients with severe tophaceous disease appear to have milder and less frequent acute attacks than non-tophaceous patients. Large tophi may have areas of necrotic skin overlying them and may exude chalky or pasty material containing monosodium urate crystals. Sinuses may form. Tophi may resolve slowly with effective treatment of hyperuricaemia. Effective antihyperuricaemic therapy has reduced the incidence and severity of the tophaceous disease. A major complication is renal disease (urolithiasis, urate nephropathy). Carpal tunnel syndrome may occur.

Associations include obesity, type IV hyperlipidaemia and hypertension. These associations may be the cause of an association which has also been recognized between gout and two other conditions — diabetes mellitus and ischaemic heart disease.

Secondary hyperuricaemia may occur in many situations including:
Drugs: diuretics (especially thiazides), ethambutol, nicotinic acid, cyclosporin
Myeloproliferative and lymphoproliferative disorders (and other conditions with increased turnover of preformed purines)
Chronic renal failure
Alcoholism
Obesity.

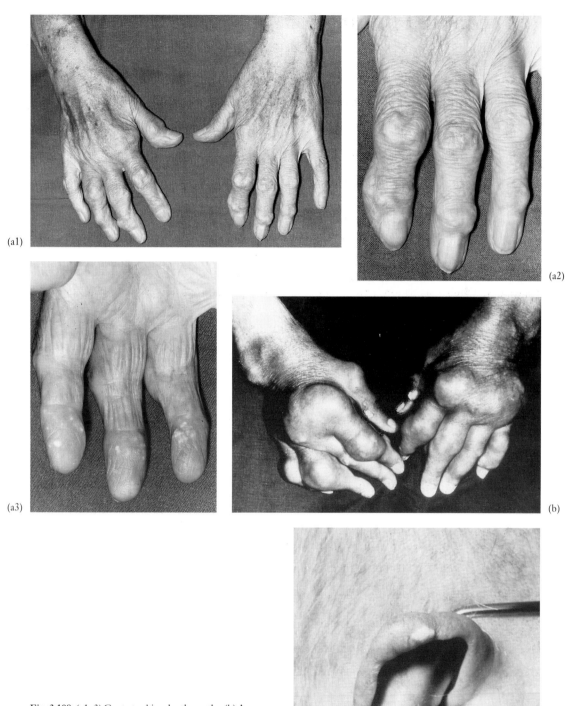

(a1)

(a2)

(a3)

(b)

(c)

Fig. 3.108 (a1–3) Gouty tophi and arthropathy. (b) An extreme case of tophaceous gout. (c) A tophus on the helix of the ear.

109 / Fallot's tetralogy with a Blalock shunt

Frequency in survey: 1% of attempts at MRCP short cases.

Survey note: the cases of Fallot's tetralogy in our survey all had a Blalock shunt.

Record

There is a thoracotomy scar. There is *central cyanosis* and *clubbing* of the fingers. The pulse is regular (give rate) and the *left pulse is weaker than the right*. The venous pressure is normal. The apex beat is (may be) palpable (say where), there is a *left parasternal heave and a systolic thrill* is palpable in the pulmonary area. There is a loud *ejection systolic murmur** (unless the stenosis is so severe that virtually no blood traverses it) in the *pulmonary area*.

It is likely that this patient has had a Blalock shunt† for Fallot's tetralogy (pulmonary stenosis, ventricular septal defect, right ventricular hypertrophy and overriding aorta).

The features which may be helpful in differentiating Fallot's tetralogy from Eisenmenger's are shown in Table 3.66 (p. 206).

---

*There may be a continuous murmur over the shunt (front or back of chest).

† Anastomosis of the subclavian artery to the pulmonary artery. This operation is not often performed nowadays as total correction on cardiopulmonary bypass is usually the treatment of choice.

110 / Slow pulse

Frequency in survey: main focus of a short case in 1% of attempts at MRCP short cases. Additional feature in a further 1%.

Record

The pulse rate is regular at 40/min (irregularly irregular pulse with beat-to-beat variation may be slow atrial fibrillation) and there is *no increase* in the rate on *standing* (complete heart block; mostly in older patients). The JVP is not elevated (unless there is heart failure) but just visible, and there is a complete dissociation of *a* and *v* waves with frequent *cannon waves* (flicking *a* waves occurring during ventricular systole).

This patient has complete heart block.

Other causes of bradycardia

Beta-blocker therapy: about 2% of patients receiving β-blockers have excessive bradycardia (heart rate increases by a few beats on standing and during exercise)

Slow atrial fibrillation: the patient may be on β-blockers and/or digoxin

Hypothyroidism (?facies, ankle jerks, etc.—p. 152)

Sino-atrial disease: bradycardia–tachycardia syndrome

Digitalis overdose.

Cardiac pacing

Most patients with complete heart block will benefit from a demand pacemaker (even asymptomatic patients with a heart rate < 40).

111 / Guillain–Barré syndrome (acute inflammatory demyelinating polyradiculopathy)

Frequency in survey: 1% of attempts at MRCP short cases.

Record

This (most commonly) young adult has a predominantly *motor neuropathy*. The weakness is more marked distally* and there is generalized *hyporeflexia*. There is a lower motor neurone *facial weakness* (often bilateral) and evidence of bulbar palsy. There is (may be) mild impairment of distal position and vibration perception and slight loss of pinprick sensation over the toes.† The patient has a tachycardia.‡

These features suggest Guillain–Barré syndrome (acute inflammatory demyelinating polyradiculopathy—AIDP).

Features of AIDP

Antecedent upper respiratory tract infection or gastrointestinal illness (e.g. *Campylobacter jejuni*) within 1 month in 60%§ of cases.

Bimodal age distribution — main peak in young adults, lesser peak in 45–64 year age group.

Cerebrospinal fluid protein usually normal during the first 3 days; it then steadily rises and may continue to rise even though recovery has begun; it may exceed $5 \, g \, l^{-1}$. A few mononuclear cells may be present in the cerebrospinal fluid ($< 10 \, mm^{-3}$).

Mortality is 5%. The apparently mild case may worsen rapidly and unpredictably. *Vital capacity* (peak flow rate measurement on its own is insufficient), blood gases, blood pressure and ability to cough and swallow should be closely monitored; if mechanical ventilation is anticipated from the results then it should be instituted early, before decompensation.

Paralysis is maximum within 1 week in more than 50% of cases and by 1 month in 90%. Recovery usually begins 2–4 weeks later.‖ Rate of recovery is variable, occasionally rapid even after quadraplegia. Eighty-five per cent of patients are ambulatory within 6 months. Residual peripheral nervous system damage in $> 50\%$.

Plasmapheresis in first 2 weeks shortens the clinical course and reduces morbidity. Intravenous immunoglobulin in the first 2 weeks is an alternative therapy that probably has equivalent efficacy to plasmapheresis.

Some patients present with rapid onset of symmetrical, multiple cranial nerve palsies, most notably bilateral facial palsy (polyneuritis cranials).

---

* Though the weakness classically begins in the distal lower limbs and spreads upwards (*ascending paralysis*) it may be more marked proximally or uniform throughout the limbs.
† The mild case may just have slight foot-drop which never progresses, while the severe case may have quadraplegia and inability to breathe, speak, swallow or close the eyes. The facial involvement helps to distinguish AIDP from other neuropathies except for that related to sarcoidosis. Complaints of numbness and paraesthesiae are common but are usually mild and transient and objective sensory loss is slight.
‡ Autonomic involvement is common with a relative tachycardia almost always present; orthostatic hypotension and hypertension are frequent and difficult to treat. Pupillary disturbances, neuroendocrine disturbance, peripheral pooling of blood, poor venous return and low cardiac output may all occur. *Sudden death* can occur following unexplained

fluctuations in blood pressure or cardiac dysrhythmias. Pharmacological interventions to control blood pressure are risky and should be avoided unless absolutely necessary. Patients who are unable to swallow or gag are given nasogastric feeding and should be sitting when food is given and for 30–60 min thereafter to reduce the risk of aspiration.
§ Predisposing factors that have been implicated include infectious mononucleosis, viral hepatitis, Epstein Barr virus, rabies, swine flu, HIV infection, surgery, pregnancy and malignancy (especially lymphoma).
‖ Pathologically, inflammatory cell infiltration followed by segmental demyelination is the hallmark, especially in spinal roots, limb girdle plexuses and proximal nerve trunks. Axons are relatively spared and blood vessels are normal. Within 2–3 weeks of onset, Schwann cell proliferation occurs as a prelude to remyelination and recovery.

Occasionally, there may be a combination of an external ophthalmoplegia, ataxia and areflexia (*Miller–Fisher syndrome*) associated with high cerebrospinal fluid protein and some motor weakness. Serum IgG antibodies to GQ1b ganglioside are found in acute phase sera of over 90% of Miller–Fisher syndrome patients. They disappear during recovery.

Most patients achieve good recovery from AIDP. The importance of fastidious supportive care during the acute stage cannot be overstressed.

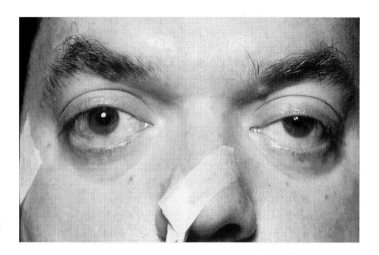

Fig. 3.111 External ophthalmoplegia in the Miller–Fisher syndrome.

Frequency in survey: 1% of attempts at MRCP short cases.

Survey note: some candidates had to discuss the chest X-ray of their pneumonectomy short case. It would usually show a 'white out' on one side, deviated trachea and compensatory hyperinflation on the other.

Record 1

There is a deformity of the chest with *flattening* on the R/L and a *thoracotomy scar* on that side. The trachea is *deviated* to the R/L and the apex beat is *displaced* in the same direction. On the R/L *expansion* is reduced, the percussion note is *dull* and the *breath sounds* are *diminished*. There is an area of bronchial breathing in the R/L upper zone (over the grossly deviated trachea).

These findings suggest a R/L pneumonectomy.

In the patient with lobectomy, as opposed to total pneumonectomy, the signs will be more confined. For example see *record* 2.

Record 2

There is a *deformity* of the chest with the left lower ribs *pulled in* and a left-sided *thoracotomy scar*. The *trachea* is central (may be displaced) but the *apex beat* is displaced to the left. The *percussion note is dull* over the left lower zone and *breath sounds* are *diminished* in this area.

These signs suggest a left lower lobectomy.

Surgical resection and the lung

Surgery has little role in the management of *small cell* carcinoma. In others, after a full assessment which includes clinical examination, lung function tests, bone and liver biochemistry, isotope bone scan, ultrasound or CT scan of the liver, mediastinal CT scan and, if necessary, mediastinoscopy, 25% of *non-small cell* lung cancers will be suitable for attempted surgical resection. The operative mortality for lobectomy is about 2–4% and this rises to about 6% for total pneumonectomy, which may be required if the tumour involves both divisions of a main bronchus or more than one lobe.

Surgical resection is often required for *solitary pulmonary nodules* of uncertain cause. The possibility of undiagnosed small cell cancer in this instance is not necessarily a reason for avoiding thoracotomy; resection of small cell lung cancer presenting as a solitary pulmonary nodule may have a 5-year survival comparable to that of other forms of nodular bronchogenic carcinoma treated surgically (approximately 25%).

Surgical resection is indicated in the treatment of *bronchiectasis* (p. 161) when other forms of treatment have failed to control symptoms, particularly if it is localized and if recurrent haemoptysis is present.

In the days before antituberculous chemotherapy, tuberculosis was sometimes treated surgically — p. 108.

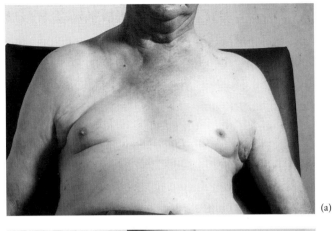

(a)

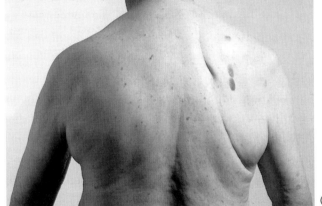

(b)

Fig. 3.112 (a) Deformity of the right chest
with flattening. (b) Right-sided thoracotomy
scar on the back.

113 / Obesity/pickwickian syndrome

Frequency in survey: main focus of a short case in 1% of attempts at MRCP short cases. Additional feature in many others.

Survey note: most cases revolved around features of the Pickwickian syndrome, though there was one case with an apronectomy scar and small testes in which Klinefelter's was suggested.

Record

The patient is *massively obese* and *cyanosed*. He has rapid and shallow breathing, his *venous pressure is elevated* and there is *ankle oedema*.

These features suggest *cor pulmonale* secondary to the extreme obesity—the Pickwickian syndrome.*

Respiratory problems associated with obesity

Severe obesity leads to increased demand for ventilation, increased breathing workload, respiratory muscle inefficiency, decreased functional reserve capacity and expiratory reserve volume. There is alveolar hypoventilation and reduced ventilatory sensitivity to CO_2. Peripheral lung units can close, resulting in a ventilation–perfusion mismatch. The overall result is chronic hypoxaemia with cyanosis and hypercapnia; the end-stage is the *pickwickian syndrome* in which nocturnal obstructive apnoea† and hypoventilation are so marked that the patient can only have undisturbed sleep when upright (more usually sitting than standing as in the original description!*), often in the daytime.

Pulmonary hypertension occurs, there are usually morning headaches and impotence and there may be polycythaemia. Eventually cardiac failure supervenes.

Sleep apnoea is very common in the severely obese. The most obese are not necessarily the most severely affected. It may be obstructive or central.† Day-time somnolence is common and is partly due to the hypoxia and partly from the continual disturbance of sleep at night—the patient tends to wake after each episode of sleep apnoea (cessation of breathing for 10 seconds or longer).

Body mass index (BMI) = weight (kg)/height (m)². As a rule of thumb, health risks increase as BMI increases above 25; however, BMI normally increases with age and one study found that the BMI associated with lowest mortality was approximately: 19.5 at age 20, 21 at age 30, 22.5 at age 40, 24.5 at age 50, nearly 26 at age 60 and 27.5 at age 70.

Body fat can be estimated by measuring skinfold thickness with callipers at the biceps, triceps, subscapular and suprailiac regions.

---

* The term is derived from the character in Charles Dickens *Pickwick Papers* and was first applied by Osler. The character, Joe, kept beating the door even after hearing a response from inside the room, because if he stopped, he would fall asleep standing on his feet! (See *American Journal of Medicine* 1956, **21**: 811–18 to read Dickens' wonderful description.)

† *Obstructive sleep apnoea*—the upper pharyngeal cavity collapses due to the negative intrathoracic pressure and the process is aided by a short neck, large accumulations of fat often in combination with micrognathia and enlarged tonsils. There are vigorous thoracoabdominal movements but no air

entry into the lungs. The obstruction leads to hypoventilation and hypoxia which somehow trigger apnoeic episodes making the hypoxia and hypercapnia worse. Weight loss and sometimes surgical removal of the obstructive tissues may help.

Central sleep apnoea—cessation of ventilatory drive from brain centres so that diaphragmatic excursions stop for periods of 10–30 seconds. There are no thoracoabdominal movements and there is no activity. It is not known why the obese are prone to this.

Adipocytes increase in size and then number as necessary to accommodate excess nutrient calories; but once formed, though they can decrease in size with weight loss, their total number does not decrease (the 'ratchet effect'). *Lipoprotein lipase* (LPL) generates free fatty acids (FFA) from circulating chylomicrons and VLDL and the FFA can then enter adipocytes. LPL activity is high in obese people and rises with initial weight loss and this may be a factor in the accelerated weight regain of many patients. Maintained weight loss, however, is associated with a decrease in LPL activity. Fat cells from the upper body are probably different in responsiveness to testosterone and oestrogens than lower body fat cells leading to:

Android fatness: fat distributed in upper body above the waist,

Gynaecoid fatness: fat predominantly in lower body —lower abdomen, buttocks, hips, thighs.

Android fatness carries a greater risk for hypertension, cardiovascular disease, hyperinsulinaemia, diabetes, gallbladder disease, stroke and a higher mortality than does gynaecoid fatness. Waist : hip (circumference) ratio greater than 0.85 for women and 1.0 for men is abnormal.

Other clinical manifestations of obesity

Insulin resistance (enlarged adipocytes less sensitive to the antilipolytic and lipogenic actions of insulin; decreased number of insulin receptors as well as postreceptor defect; liver and muscle also less sensitive to insulin; basal and stimulated hyperinsulinaemia results‡)

Diabetes mellitus (NIDDM approximately three times higher in the overweight; 85% of NIDDM patients in the USA are obese; though the development of NIDDM requires the appropriate genetic legacy, obesity by enhancing insulin resistance tends to unmask and exacerbate the underlying propensity)

Hypertension‡ (prevalence three times higher in the obese; mechanism is uncertain—hyperinsulinaemia‡ leading to increased tubular reabsorption of sodium may be a factor; weight loss by dieting lowers blood pressure even without dietary salt restriction)

Cardiovascular disease (in obesity increased blood volume, stroke volume, left ventricular end-diastolic volume, and filling pressure result in high cardiac output; this leads to left ventricular hypertrophy and dilatation, the former being exacerbated by hypertension; the result is greater risk of congestive heart failure and sudden death)

Lipid abnormalities (obesity is associated with low HDL cholesterol;‡ LDL may be elevated; hypertriglyceridaemia‡ is more prevalent, possibly because the insulin resistance and hyperinsulinaemia‡ cause increased hepatic production of triglycerides; the hypertriglyceridaemia tends to improve with weight loss; if a true genetic lipoprotein disorder coexists, more intensive therapy may be required)

Venous circulatory disease (severe obesity is often associated with varicose veins and venous stasis; congestive cardiac failure adds to the dependent oedema; increased propensity for thrombophlebitis and thromboembolism)

Cancer (obese women have a higher incidence of endometrial cancer, postmenopausal breast cancer, cancer of the gallbladder and of the biliary system; obese men have a higher mortality from cancer of the colon, rectum and prostate for unknown reasons)

Gastrointestinal disease (cholesterol gallstones leading to cholecystitis; obesity may be associated with fatty liver with modest abnormalities of liver function tests)

Arthritis (osteoarthritis due to excess stress placed on the joints of the lower extremities and back; multifactorial elevation in uric acid levels in the obese)

Skin (intertrigo in redundant folds of skin; fungal and yeast infections; *acanthosis nigricans*, which should always be looked for in obese patients, it may be associated with severe insulin resistance—p. 419)

Increased mortality (obesity itself may make an independent contribution to mortality, though

‡ NB Syndrome X (Reaven's syndrome). This refers to the clustering of insulin insensitivity, hyperinsulinaemia, varying degrees of glucose intolerance, hypertension, increased triglycerides and decreased HDL; a clustering which may predispose to vascular disease, in particular coronary artery disease. It is postulated that insulin insensitivity/ hyperinsulinaemia is the underlying factor.

the effect generally occurs through linkage with factors such as hypertension, diabetes and hyper-lipidaemia‡

Endocrine causes of obesity

(< 1% of obese patients)

Hypothyroidism (thickened and coarse facial features, dry skin, non-pitting swelling of subcutaneous tissues, hoarse voice, thinning hair, slow pulse, slow relaxing ankle jerks—p. 152)

Polycystic ovarian syndrome (hirsutism, oligo- or amenorrhoea, excess androgen production of ovarian origin, ultrasound scan may show the polycystic ovaries; patients with polycystic ovaries are often obese and insulin resistant)

Hypothalamic disease (damage to hypothalamic appetite systems and tracts by surgery, trauma, inflammation, craniopharyngioma or other tumours may lead to hyperphagic obesity)

Cushing's (truncal obesity, moon face, purple striae, proximal muscle weakness—p. 231).

Rare genetic diseases associated with obesity include

Prader–Willi syndrome (obesity may be massive, almond-shaped eyes, acromicria, mental retardation, diabetes, hypogonadism—p. 425)

Laurence–Moon–Bardet–Biedl syndrome (?retinitis pigmentosa, hypogonadism, dwarfism, mental retardation, polydactyly—p. 358)

Alström syndrome (see p. 358)

Cohen's syndrome (microcephaly, mental retardation, short stature, facial abnormalities and obesity)

Carpenter's syndrome (see p. 358)

Blount's disease (bowed legs, tibial torsion, obesity).

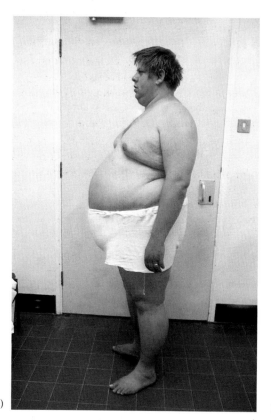

(a)

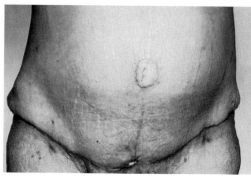

(b)

Fig. 3.113 (a) Pickwickian syndrome. (b) Apronectomy scar.

114 / Dermatomyositis

Frequency in survey: 0.9% of attempts at MRCP short cases.

Record

There is a *heliotrope* rash* around the *eyes* and the *backs* of the *hands*, especially around the *knuckles* (Gottron's papules) and *fingernails* (prominent nail-fold telangiectasia is characteristic). It is also present (may be) over the extensor surfaces of the elbows and knees. There is subcutaneous oedema (mainly around the eyes and due to a transient increase in capillary permeability). There is *proximal muscle weakness* and (may be) tenderness.

The diagnosis is dermatomyositis.

Male to female ratio is 2 : 1.

Other features of dermatomyositis

Features and associations similar to polymyositis (p. 329)

Association with malignancy (debatable—see footnote, p. 329)

Overlap with rheumatic fever, rheumatoid arthritis, scleroderma, lupus erythematosus and other connective tissue diseases may occur (steroid responsiveness more likely)

Signs of other connective tissue diseases commoner than in pure polymyositis

Dysphagia due to upper oesophageal involvement

Raynaud's and arthralgia are frequent

Subcutaneous and intramuscular calcifications may occur

Helpful investigations include serum muscle enzymes, urinary creatinine, EMG (fibrillation, polyphasic action potentials and in some patients high frequency bizarre repetitive discharges) and muscle biopsy. The erythrocyte sedimentation rate (ESR) is often normal despite active disease

The mainstay of treatment is steroids (initially in high doses). High dose intravenous immunoglobulin may be effective in refractory cases

May present with pseudohaematuria due to myoglobulinaemia

There is a juvenile form occurring in the first decade. Myopathy is severe, healing occurs with contractures and calcification in the skin and muscles, but Raynaud's is rare. There is no association with malignancy.

For colour photographs see p. 532.

---

* From the shrub *heliotropium* which has fragrant purple flowers. The characteristic rash is a purple/violet/lilac colour. The skin changes may be subtle and easily overlooked. The classical heliotrope rash is diagnostic of the condition and, though it is most commonly seen in the childhood form, it also occurs in the adult form. Other skin manifestations include *local and diffuse erythema, erythema nodosum-like lesions, eczema, exfoliating dermatitis, blisters and scaling* and *maculopapular eruptions*. The skin lesions may occasionally ulcerate.

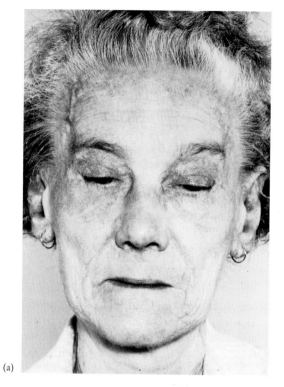

(a)

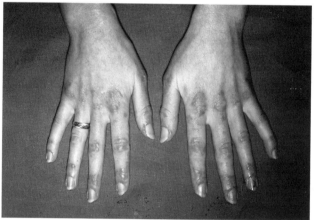

(b)

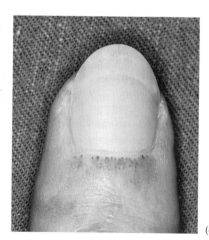

(c)

Fig. 3.114 (a) Note the characteristic distribution of the rash. (b) Gottron's papules. (c) Nail-fold telangiectasia is characteristic.

Frequency in survey: main focus of a short case in 0.9% of attempts at MRCP short cases. Additional feature in a further 0.6%.

Record

The patient's *skin* is *soft*, *wrinkled* and *pale* with a *yellow tint* (the pallor is due to a combination of lack of MSH (melanocyte-stimulating hormone) and anaemia—marrow hypofunction). The areolae of the breasts are (may be) depigmented. *Pubic*, *axillary*, *facial* and *body hair is reduced* (and the *genitals* and *breasts* are *atrophied*).

These features suggest hypopituitarism (now check for a bitemporal visual field defect).

With progressing hypopituitarism gonadotrophin secretion is usually impaired first, followed by growth hormone, TSH, ACTH* and antidiuretic hormone, in that order. With the onset of thyroid failure the features of hypothyroidism (p. 152) are superimposed on those in the above *record*. Lassitude, cold intolerance, dryness of skin and prolongation of the relaxation phase of the tendon reflexes occur though swelling of the subcutaneous tissues is usually less prominent. The insidious onset of asthenia, nausea, vomiting, postural hypotension, hypoglycaemia, collapse and coma mark progressive ACTH lack. Diabetes insipidus develops with lack of antidiuretic hormone, though impaired glomerular filtration caused by cortisol deficiency may mask the symptoms.

The main causes of adult panhypopituitarism (male to female ratio is 1:2) are:

Sheehan's syndrome (following severe obstetric haemorrhage or shock — much less common nowadays with good obstetric practice)

Pituitary tumour (especially chromophobe adenoma)

Craniopharyngioma

Pituitary granulomatous lesion (tuberculoma, sarcoidosis, Hand–Schüller–Christian disease, syphilitic gumma)

Iatrogenic (hypophysectomy, radiotherapy to sella or nasopharynx)

Head injury

Idiopathic.

The factors that lead to coma in hypopituitarism include hypoglycaemia, sodium depletion, water intoxication, cerebral anoxia, hypothyroidism, hypothermia and pressure on the midbrain or hypothalamus.

---

*Pituitary hypothyroidism may protect the patient from the effects of failing ACTH secretion. In this situation misdiagnosing the cause of hypothyroidism and waking the patient from hibernation with thyroxine alone may precipitate Addisonian crisis.

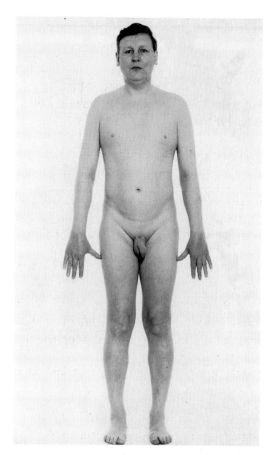

Fig. 3.115 Hypopituitarism (8 years after removal of pituitary adenoma).

Frequency in survey: main focus of a short case in 0.9% of attempts at MRCP short cases. Additional feature in a further 1.5%.

Survey note: half of the cases were due to rheumatoid arthritis.

Record

There is generalized *swelling* of the R/L *knee joint* obscuring the lateral dimples. The *patellar tap sign** is *positive* suggesting the presence of fluid in the synovial cavity. The swelling does not extend to the back in the popliteal fossa (always check).† The joint is *painful* to move and it is *warm*.

There is an *effusion* in the knee joint. (Now look at the hands for evidence of rheumatoid arthritis—p. 73.)

Causes of a swollen knee

Rheumatoid arthritis (the swelling may be due to synovial thickening—synovium palpable as boggy tissue around the joint margin)

Osteoarthritis (osteophytes on X-ray)

Rupture of a Baker's cyst (?rheumatoid arthritis— p. 244)

Pseudogout (calcified menisci; birefringent calcium pyrophosphate crystals; associated with a large variety of conditions including hyperparathyroidism, haemochromatosis, acromegaly, diabetes mellitus, Wilson's disease, hypothyroidism, alkaptonuria and gout; there are also idiopathic and hereditary varieties)

Septic arthritis (purulent fluid, organisms in a smear)

Gout (urate crystals)

Trauma

Charcot's knee (painless, ?tabes dorsalis—p. 381)

Haemarthrosis of haemophilia

Oedematous states (congestive cardiac failure, nephrotic syndrome).

---

* With one hand above the knee joint, exert pressure to drive fluid from the suprapatellar pouch into the knee joint proper. With the index finger of the other hand, depress the patella with a sharp jerky movement. If the patella rebounds this is definite evidence of fluid in the knee joint. The sign may not be positive if there is too much or too little fluid. To test for a small amount of fluid in the knee joint, displace fluid by depressing one of the obliterated hollows on either side of the ligamentum patellae. The hollow will slowly refill.

† Swelling in the popliteal fossa extending down to the upper third of the calf in cases of ruptured Baker's cyst—p. 244.

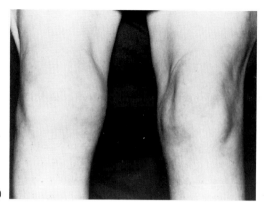 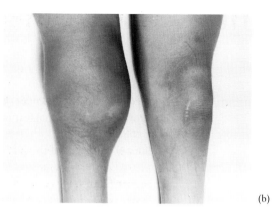

Fig. 3.116 (a) Osteoarthrosis with effusion of the knee joint.
(b) Charcot's knee (spina bifida).

117 / Pseudobulbar palsy

Frequency in survey: 0.9% of attempts at MRCP short cases.

Record

There is monotonous, slurred, high-pitched, 'Donald Duck' *dysarthria* and the patient *dribbles persistently* from the mouth (he has dysphagia and may have nasal regurgitation). He *cannot protrude his tongue* which lies on the floor of the mouth and is *small and tight. Palatal movement is absent*, the *jaw jerk* is *exaggerated* and he is *emotionally labile.*

The diagnosis is pseudobulbar palsy (?bilateral generalized spasticity and extensor plantar responses).

Commonest cause

Bilateral cerebrovascular accidents of the internal capsule.

Other causes

Multiple sclerosis
Motor neurone disease
High brainstem tumours
Head injury.

Frequency in survey: 0.9% of attempts at MRCP short cases.

Record 1

This middle-aged (or elderly) patient has flaccid *thin-roofed blisters* (usually over the axillae and trunk), which vary in size (usually 1–2 cm in diameter). Most of the blisters have *burst* leaving *red* and *exuding areas* (which are extremely tender). There are also (not always) red denuded patches in the *mouth* (the first site involved in up to 50%), *pharynx* and *eyes*.

The patient has pemphigus.

Record 2

This elderly patient has *tense blisters* varying in size from a few millimetres to a few centimetres in diameter involving . . . (describe where—usually it is the limbs but it can be widespread). There are also *reddened* and *urticarial* (sometimes eczematous) *patches* surrounding and separate from the blisters. There are no lesions in the mouth (they do occur but are uncommon).

The diagnosis is pemphigoid.

Pemphigus vulgaris: this condition occurs most commonly in Jewish people. The site of the blister is in the epidermis. Occasionally lesions may occur without initial blister formation. The mucous membranes never have blisters, only denuded patches. It is a progressive and fatal condition if not treated with corticosteroids in very high doses (initially 100–200 mg daily of prednisolone). Azathioprine may reduce the maintenance dose of steroid. It can be caused by penicillamine, phenylbutazone and rifampicin. There is an increased incidence in patients with thymoma and myasthenia gravis. *Acantholysis* is a characteristic histological feature. Nikolsky's sign* is invariably present. Immunofluorescence of biopsy shows intercellular immunoglobulins (usually IgG) and/or complement factor C3.

Pemphigoid: the site of the blisters is at the basement membrane between the epidermis and the dermis; therefore the blister is thicker and less likely to rupture than in pemphigus. Mucosal lesions are less common in pemphigoid. Though it is self-limiting (2 years) systemic steroids are usually given (initially 60–80 mg day⁻¹) and azathioprine may reduce the maintenance dose. It does not have a high mortality like pemphigus. It has been alleged that it is sometimes a manifestation of underlying malignancy but this point is not proven. Biopsy shows IgG and complement at the basement membrane zone.

Other bullous disorders

Dermatitis herpetiformis (groups of blisters on the elbows, knees and buttocks; associated with coeliac disease—p. 377)

Epidermolysis bullosa congenita (congenital blistering disorders usually of hands and feet; genetically determined; range from simple blisters to severe scarring with contractures; teeth and nails abnormal in some forms)

Epidermolysis bullosa acquisita (associated with inflammatory bowel disease, amyloidosis and internal malignancy)

* Firm pressure on apparently normal skin causes it to slide off. Nikolsky's sign may also occur in other severe bullous eruptions, such as toxic epidermal necrolysis.

Herpes gestationis (pregnancy or early puerperium, erythematous/urticarial lesions with blistering; no relation to herpes virus; resolves in a few weeks; may require steroids; recurs with increased severity in subsequent pregnancies)

Hailey–Hailey disease (benign familial pemphigus, onset age 10–30 years; unrelated to pemphigus).

For colour photograph see p. 533.

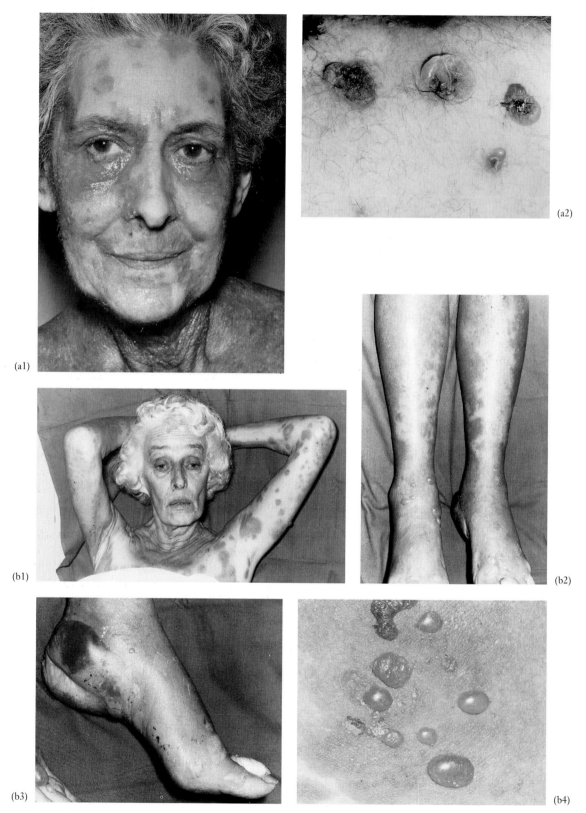

Fig. 3.118 (a1,2) Pemphigus. Note denuded areas and ruptured blisters. (b1–4) Pemphigoid. Note the tense blisters.

119 / Syringomyelia

Frequency in survey: 0.9% of attempts at MRCP short cases.

Record

This patient (with *kyphoscoliosis*) shows *wasting* and weakness of the *small muscles of the hands* (sometimes there is curling of the fingers), flattening of the muscles of the ulnar border of the forearm and the upper limb *reflexes are absent* (conspicuous fasciculation is uncommon). There is *dissociated sensory loss** over (one or both of) the upper limbs and the upper chest† and there are *scars* (from painless burns and cuts) on the hands. The lower limb reflexes are exaggerated and the plantars are extensor. A *Horner's syndrome* is (may be) present (involvement of sympathetic neurones especially at C8/T1).

These findings suggest syringomyelia (?*nystagmus*, which may occur with lesions from C5 upwards—i.e. involving the medial longitudinal bundle—see Fig. 3.49, p. 173).

Syringobulbia. Syrinxes may involve upper cervical and bulbar segments (usually an extension of syringomyelia but the syrinx may begin in the brainstem) and cause:

Nystagmus

Ataxia

Facial dissociated sensory loss (initially onion skin loss over the outer part of the face, from involvement of the lower part of the Vth nucleus in the cord, may occur before the syrinx reaches the medulla)

Bulbar palsy (wasted fasciculating tongue, palatal paralysis, nasal dysarthria, dysphagia, weakness of sternomastoids and trapezius from XIth nerve involvement, etc.—p. 257).

Trophic and vasomotor disturbances are common in syringomyelia, e.g.:

Areas of loss of, or excessive, sweating

La main succulente (ugly, cold, puffy, cyanosed hands with stumpy fingers and podgy soft palms)

Coarse, thickened skin over the hands with callosities over the knuckles and scars from old injuries

Slow healing and indolent ulceration of digits.

Charcot's joints may occur, usually at the elbow or shoulder. Tabes dorsalis (knees, hips) and diabetes mellitus (toes, ankles) are the other causes of Charcot's joints (see also p. 168).

Skeletal abnormalities which may be associated with syringomyelia:

(Kypho)scoliosis (mild, very common)

Short neck (e.g. fusion of the cervical vertebrae; Klippel–Feil syndrome—p. 385)

Asymmetrical thorax

Sternal depression or prominence

Cervical ribs (may cause diagnostic difficulty).

---

* Analgesia and thermoanaesthesia but light touch and proprioception intact. In the early stages cold stimuli may be perceived but not warm.

† Due to destruction by the syrinx of crossing axons carrying pain and temperature sensation. The area affected depends on the length of the syrinx—e.g. lower cervical and upper thoracic. Separate from this effect on crossing axons, the syrinx may also involve one or both spinothalamic tracts producing dissociated sensory loss in one or both lower limbs.

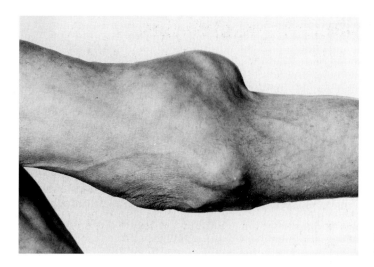

Fig. 3.119 Charcot's joint at the elbow.

Frequency in survey: 0.9% of attempts at MRCP short cases.

Record
The trachea in this Asian patient is central (may be deviated*) and the expansion is normal (may be reduced at the apex*). The percussion note is *dull* at the R/L apex with *diminished tactile fremitus*. There is *bronchial breathing* with *inspiratory crackles* over the area of dullness.

The diagnosis is R/L apical consolidation, with tuberculosis being a serious contender as the underlying cause.†

Principal varieties of tuberculosis
Primary pulmonary tuberculosis. The first infection with the tubercle bacillus (primary tuberculosis) usually includes involvement of the draining lymph node (the Ghon focus). All other tuberculosis lesions are regarded as postprimary and are not accompanied by major involvement of the draining lymph nodes (in Europeans), though sometimes in immigrants gross enlargement of the lymph nodes may be seen. *Erythema nodosum*, *phlyctenular conjunctivitis* and *pleural effusion* may accompany primary pulmonary tuberculosis.

Miliary tuberculosis. Acute dissemination of tubercle bacilli via the blood stream may occur, if the initial infection is an overwhelming one or the patient's defences are poor due to malnutrition, corticosteroid or immunosuppressive drug therapy, HIV or intercurrent disease. This condition should be borne in mind in at-risk groups (see below)

Tuberculous meningitis. May occur at any age but particularly common in small children as a complication of the primary infection.

Postprimary pulmonary tuberculosis. This form may arise either as direct progression of a primary lesion, reactivation of an old lesion, haematogenous spread or from contact with a patient with *open* (sputum-positive) tuberculosis. The predisposing factors for reactivation are malnutrition, poor and overcrowded housing conditions, silicosis and other occupational diseases, alcoholism and cigarette smoking, immunosuppressive drugs, and diseases associated with impaired cellular immunity (e.g. Hodgkin's disease, leukaemia, lymphoma, AIDS). Complications of postprimary pulmonary tuberculosis include *empyema*, *laryngitis*, *aspergillomata* (colonization of a cavity), *amyloidosis*, *tuberculosis of the organs* and *adult respiratory syndrome*.

Bone and joint tuberculosis. High rate in immigrants of Asian origin. Usually of haematogenous origin. The commonest site for skeletal tuberculosis is the spine followed by the weight-bearing joints. AFB may be obtained from synovial fluid or bone but diagnostic exploration may have to be undertaken. Patients with tuberculosis can also have a reactive arthritis known as *Poncet's disease*; this usually settles with control of the tuberculosis.

Urinary tract tuberculosis. Results from haematogenous spread to the kidney with subsequent spread down the ureteric tract. The patient may present with dysuria, nocturia, loin pain or may have pain-

---

* In the examination setting there are usually elicitable signs, even though in clinical practice one often encounters patients with pulmonary tuberculosis, sometimes with excessive radiological changes, who have no physical signs. The patient may have signs of fibrosis (e.g. deviated trachea), as seen in advanced cases, but the candidate should consider the diagnosis of pulmonary tuberculosis when there is only a dull percussion note, or a few crepitations at the apex of the lung.

† The differential diagnosis should include *carcinoma of the bronchus*, atypical pneumonia especially due to *Klebsiella pneumoniae*, pulmonary infarction and fungal infection.

less haematuria, though many patients with positive urine cultures are asymptomatic. A history of recurrent urinary tract infection or *pyuria with negative bacterial cultures* should be regarded with suspicion for urinary tract tuberculosis.

Genital tuberculosis. A large majority of patients have evidence of tuberculosis at extragenital sites. Females present with infertility, pelvic inflammatory disease or amenorrhoea. Adnexal masses are palpable on pelvic examination in about half the cases.

Tuberculous peritonitis. Usually haematogenous. Often associated with weight loss, abdominal pain and gross ascites. Diagnosis can be made at laparoscopy when the peritoneum studded with whitish granulomata can be seen. Peritoneal fluid is rarely positive for AFB by stained smear and even by culture is positive in somewhat less than 50% of cases. May occur in the alcoholic with cirrhosis (see footnote, p. 191).

Tuberculous lymphadenitis. Mostly seen in patients of Afro-Asian origin. The patient may present with painless swelling of cervical lymph glands, or sometimes with pyrexia and lymphadenopathy. Untreated swelling may form a 'cold' abscess or sinus.

Cutaneous tuberculosis. This may present in one of many ways including a *primary complex* (an ulcerating papule on the face), *miliary* tuberculosis (particularly in immunocompromised children), *verrucous* tuberculosis (warty lesions as an occupational hazard in patients working with infected material), *scrofuloderma* (breakdown of skin over a tuberculous focus), and *lupus vulgaris* (see p. 370).

At-risk groups

Contacts—should be screened by tuberculin testing and chest X-ray

Immigrants from the Asian subcontinent have a high notification rate

Inhabitants of some institutions—prisons, lodging houses, hostel dwellers and mental institutions

Nursing homes—outbreaks of tuberculosis among the elderly in nursing homes have been reported

Medical laboratory workers—the incidence is high among staff in hospital pathology departments

Other groups—doctors, dentists, hospital employees, schoolteachers and those carers who work with children are potentially exposed to the risks for contracting tuberculosis.

Treatment

Most patients can be treated at home. Segregation is required only for those patients who have smear-positive disease; they should be kept in hospital for the first 2 weeks of treatment. Treatment regimens should last for 6 months except in those who have tuberculous meningitis; they should be treated for 12 months.

Drug therapy should be given as combination tablets to aid compliance. The initial phase of 2 months should include three drugs (isoniazid, rifampicin and pyrazinamide). Ethambutol should be added if there is a risk of drug resistance. Treatment should be continued for 4 more months with rifampicin and isoniazid. Regular checks by nurses and health visitors are necessary to ensure compliance. The rifampicin in the combination tablets produces a pink/orange discoloration of the urine which will aid these checks.

121 / Rheumatoid lung

Frequency in survey: main focus of a short case in 0.9% of attempts at MRCP short cases. Additional feature in others.

Record

There is (may be) cyanosis (there may also be dyspnoea) and the principal finding in the chest is of *fine inspiratory crackles* (or crepitations — whichever term you prefer) on auscultation at both bases.

In view of the *rheumatoid* changes (p. 273) in the *hands* (there may also be clubbing) the likely diagnosis is fibrosing alveolitis associated with rheumatoid disease (rheumatoid lung).

Classical fibrosing alveolitis develops in 2%* of patients with rheumatoid arthritis and has a poor prognosis. It may progress to a honeycomb appearance on chest X-ray, bronchiectasis, chronic cough and progressive dyspnoea. Pulmonary function tests show reduced diffusion capacity, diminished compliance and a restrictive ventilatory pattern.

Gold, used in the therapy of rheumatoid arthritis, can also induce interstitial lung disease; it is indistinguishable from rheumatoid fibrosing alveolitis except that the gold-induced disease may reverse when the drug is discontinued.

Other pulmonary manifestations of rheumatoid disease

Pleural disease.† Though frequently found at autopsy, rheumatoid pleural disease is usually asymptomatic. The rheumatoid patient may have a pleural rub or pleural effusion but only occasionally would the latter be of sufficient size to cause respiratory limitation. The pleural fluid at diagnostic aspiration is never blood stained and often contains immune complexes and rheumatoid factor; it is high in protein (exudate) and lactate dehydrogenase and low in glucose, C3 and C4. The white count in the pleural fluid is variable but usually < 5000/μl.

Intrapulmonary nodules. Single or multiple radiological nodules may be seen in the lung parenchyma before or after the onset of arthritis. They are usually asymptomatic but may become infected and cavitate. As they have a predilection for the upper lobes and can cause haemoptysis, they can resemble tuberculosis or even carcinoma. They can rupture into the pleural space causing a pneumothorax. Massive confluent pulmonary nodules may be seen in rheumatoid lungs in association with pneumoconiosis (*Caplan's syndrome*).

Obliterative bronchiolitis. Rarely, small airway obstruction may develop into a necrotizing bronchiolitis, classically associated with dyspnoea, hyperinflation and a high-pitched expiratory wheeze or 'squawk' on auscultation. This complication may also result from therapy with gold or penicillamine.

Two other manifestations are *pulmonary arteritis* (reminiscent of polyarteritis nodosa) and *apical fibrobullous disease.*

---

*Though fibrosing alveolitis becomes overt in only 2% of patients, 25% of patients with rheumatoid arthritis show interstitial changes on chest X-ray and 50% have reduced diffusion capacity, suggesting that subclinical fibrosing alveolitis is common. There is no relationship between the extent of lung disease and the titre of rheumatoid factor.

† Though our surveys have not thrown up a case of pleural effusion and rheumatoid hands, it would nevertheless be worth a glance at the hands of a patient with a pleural effusion for possible rheumatoid changes as well as for the clubbing.

Frequency in survey: 0.9% of attempts at MRCP short cases.

Survey note: candidates were asked to look at the face; the clue was usually given that the patient had epilepsy or funny turns.

Record

There is a *papular*, *salmon-coloured* eruption on the centre of the face (over the *butterfly* area), especially in the *nasolabial* folds. The rash has the appearance of adenoma sebaceum (check for *ungual fibromata* and *shagreen patches*).

There may be a history of *epilepsy* and *mental deficiency** which together with *adenoma sebaceum* make up the triad associated with tuberous sclerosis (epiloia).

Tuberous sclerosis is a phakomatosis (see also footnote, p. 176). Autosomal dominant but 80% are sporadic due to new mutations. The gene is on the long arm of chromosome 11.

Hamartomata

Tuberous sclerosis is characterized by the development of hamartomata of the skin, central nervous system, kidneys, retina, heart, lungs and bone. Hamartomata consist of excessive overgrowth of mature, normal cells and tissues in an organ.

Skin lesions

A number of hamartomatous lesions of the skin are seen. The term *adenoma sebaceum* is a misnomer; the lesions are actually angiofibromata. They usually appear around the age of 4 and become more prominent after puberty. The leathery *shagreen patches* (flesh-coloured lumpy plaques which resemble studded leather) over the lower back and *ungual fibromata* (firm pink periungual papules which appear at puberty) growing out from the nail beds of the fingers and toes are seen in perhaps 40% of cases. *Hypopigmented macules* (in an oval or *mountain ash leaf* configuration, rounded at one end and tapered at the other), especially on the trunk or buttocks, are present from birth in *nearly all patients*;

they are easier to see in fair-skinned patients with a Wood's lamp. Intraoral fibromata are also seen and there may be increased pigmentation as manifest in bronzing of the skin and *café-au-lait* macules.

Other organs

Cerebral hemispheres contain multiple hamartomata or tubers (calcified lesions are well seen on CT scans but uncalcified ones may show up better on MRI). Epilepsy occurs in 80% of cases; it usually starts below the age of 5 and is often difficult to control. The diagnosis may be missed and subtle skin lesions should be sought even in adults presenting with epilepsy

Renal hamartomata (angiomyolipomata) in two-thirds of patients (may cause pain or bleeding). There may be polycystic kidneys

Retinal hamartomata[†] (phakomata), which appear yellow, in 50% (also occur in neurofibromatosis— p. 176)

Cardiac hamartomata (rhabdomyomata) in 30% (may cause dysrhythmias or congestive cardiac failure)

Cystic lung disease due to hamartomatous lesions composed of smooth muscle cells in 1% (mostly women over 20 years; may cause pneumothorax, breathlessness, cyanosis and cor pulmonale).

---

* May be mild or severe. One-third have normal, or even superior, intelligence.

† See also p. 422; optic disc drusen may also occur.

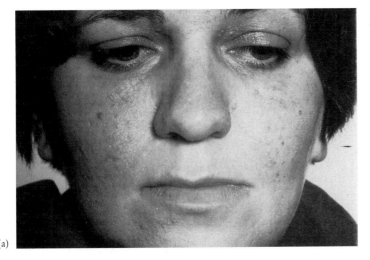
(a)

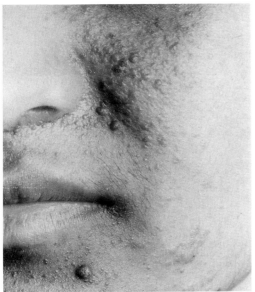
(b)

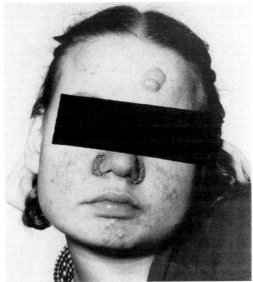
(c)

Fig. 3.122 (a) Angiofibroma papules in butterfly distribution. (b) Skin-coloured papules in the nasolabial fold. (c) Clusters of angiofibromata in the nasolabial folds.

123 / Proximal myopathy

Frequency in survey: 0.9% of attempts at MRCP short cases.

Record 1 (patient lying on a bed)
There is considerable *proximal muscular weakness* particularly in abduction at the shoulder joints and extension as well as flexion at the hip joints. The patient is *unable* to *sit up* with the upper limbs outstretched in front.
> This patient has a proximal myopathy.

Record 2 (patient sitting in a chair)
The patient has *proximal muscular weakness* in both *upper* and the *lower limb girdle groups*. I can overcome his abduction of the arms and he has considerable difficulty *standing up* from the chair. He is unable to *stand up from a squatting position*. (In both cases you should ask the examiners' permission to examine the gait.)
> This patient has a proximal myopathy.

Causes of proximal myopathy

Polymyalgia rheumatica — usually occurs over the age of 50 years, male to female ratio 1 : 3. The predominant features are fatigue, weight loss, proximal pain at rest and during movement and tenderness of the muscles. There is a sense of weakness but on careful testing muscle strength is found to be normal or nearly normal. ESR elevated. Closely related to temporal arteritis. Responds dramatically to corticosteroids

Cushing's syndrome (?moonface, acne, axial obesity, hirsutism, evidence of rheumatoid arthritis, etc. —p. 231)

Thyrotoxicosis (?eye signs, goitre, fidgety, tachycardia, etc.—p. 114); the proximal muscular weakness is particularly severe in upper limb muscles

Polymyositis (?tender muscles—p. 329)

Dermatomyositis (?heliotrope rash around the eyes, on the knuckles, the hands and over the knee joints, tender muscles, etc.—p. 293)

Drugs — alcohol, corticosteroids, amiodarone, chloroquine, β-blockers, lithium, isoniazid, labetalol, methadone, etc.

Carcinomatous myopathy—the muscular weakness may precede the neoplasia. The lower limb girdle is much more adversely affected than the upper limb girdle muscles. The onset is usually between the age of 50 and 60 years and men are more often affected than females. At times there may be many myasthenic features (Lambert–Eaton syndrome — p. 269) and the weakness is often improved after a short muscular contraction. The malignancy is often small cell carcinoma of the lung. The neurological symptoms may precede the neoplasia by 1–2 years

Osteomalacia (?ethnic origin—mostly females, waddling gait, bone pain—p. 393)

McArdle's syndrome (myophosphorylase deficiency; ?stiffness and cramps after exercise, exercising muscles feel hard, pain on movements)

Mitochondrial myopathy (a group of biochemical disorders involving the mitochondrial enzymes. Muscle biopsy may show 'ragged red fibres'. Typically there is slowly progressive weakness of limbs and/or external ocular (see footnote, p. 345) and other cranial muscles, abnormal fatiguability on sustained exertion, and lactic acidaemia on exertion or even at rest. Sometimes the myopathy is but one facet of a multisystem disease)

Endstage renal failure—(?uraemic facies).

124 / Pseudoxanthoma elasticum

Frequency in survey: 0.8% of attempts at MRCP short cases.

Record

There is *loose skin* mainly over the *neck, axillae, antecubital fossae* and *groins*, in which there are seen (1–3 mm) *yellow pseudoxanthomatous plaques* (there may be *redundant folds of lax skin*). There is a *'plucked chicken skin'* appearance because of the clear margins around the hair follicles.

This patient has pseudoxanthoma elasticum.

It is due to an inherited defect of elastin. There are four main types (two are recessive and two are dominant). An occlusive arteriopathy is the major cause of symptoms. Steroids should be avoided and the diagnosis is confirmed by skin biopsy.

Other features which may occur

Angioid streaks* in the retina (60% have eye changes)

Blue sclerae

Loose jointedness

Hypertension due to renovascular disease (50%)

Gastrointestinal (10%), genitourinary or respiratory haemorrhage

Coronary artery disease

Peripheral vascular disease (weak or absent pulses, claudication, often vascular calcification)

Mitral incompetence

Hypothyroidism (?due to involvement of thyroid vasculature).

For colour photographs see p. 542.

---

* The triad of skin lesions, angioid streaks of the retinae and vascular abnormalities is called the *Grönblad–Strandberg syndrome*. Other causes of angioid streaks (poorly defined, greyish streaks radiating across the fundus) include Ehlers–Danlos syndrome, Paget's disease of the bone and sickle-cell anaemia.

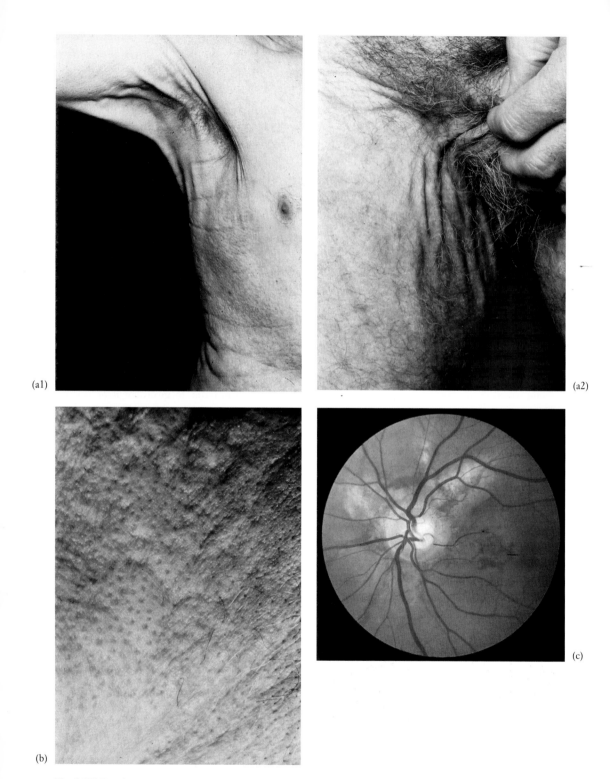

(a1)

(a2)

(b)

(c)

Fig. 3.124 Pseudoxanthoma elasticum (a1,2) note the loose skin. (b) Plucked chicken skin appearance. (c) Angioid streaks in the retina. There is a dark ring with irregular margins around the optic disc. Note a streak radiating outwards from it at 1 o'clock and another at 10 o'clock.

125 / Radiation burn on the chest

Frequency in survey: main focus of a short case in 0.8% of attempts at MRCP short cases. Additional feature in a further 4%.

Survey note: usually one of many physical signs in a patient with carcinoma of the bronchus (see experience 1, p. 447), sometimes causing superior vena cava obstruction. Rarely other intrathoracic malignancy. Occasionally the main focus of a short case.

Record

There is an area of *erythema* on the *chest* wall. The chest has been marked (radio-therapy *field markings* or 'Red Indian' marks) for deep X-ray therapy and this (or the signs of *intrathoracic malignancy*) suggests that it is due to a radiotherapy burn (see p. 145).

For colour photograph see p. 539.

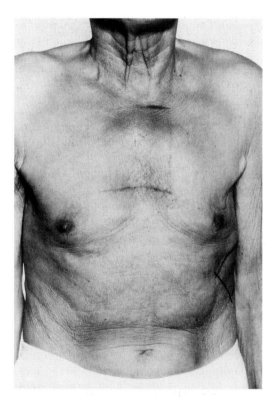

Fig. 3.125 Radiation burn between the two field marks over the chest, and marks over the left lower chest wall (carcinoma of the lung).

Frequency in survey: main focus of a short case in 0.8% of attempts at MRCP short cases. Additional feature in a further 0.4%.

Record

There is (in this patient who may complain of burning paraesthesiae in the feet) loss of *light touch*, *vibration* and *joint position* sensation over the feet (*stocking*, may also be *glove*), and *Romberg's* sign is positive. The legs are (may be) weak, and though the knee (may be brisk) and *ankle jerks* are *lost* (due to peripheral neuropathy) the *plantar responses are extensor*.

The pupils are normal, there are no cerebellar signs or pes cavus (p. 340) and though the patient is not (may not be) clinically anaemic* (having checked conjunctival mucous membranes) and the tongue and complexion are normal (glossitis and classical 'lemon yellow' pallor are now rarely seen in SACD), these findings suggest the diagnosis of subacute combined degeneration of the cord. (Findings in the abdomen might be splenomegaly, carcinoma of the stomach as this is commoner in pernicious anaemia, or a laparotomy scar from a previous gastrectomy.)

Though vitamin B_{12} neuropathy usually starts with peripheral neuropathy followed by posterior column signs, and signs of pyramidal disturbances are seldom marked in the early stages (progressive spasticity may occur), vitamin B_{12} deficiency should always be excluded in a patient in whom any of the following are unexplained:

Peripheral sensory neuropathy

Spinal cord disease

Optic atrophy (rare)

Dementia (frank dementia rare; progressive enfeeblement of intellect and memory, or episodes of confusion or paranoia may be seen; more commonly the patient is simply difficult and uncooperative).

Causes of severe vitamin B_{12} deficiency

Addisonian pernicious anaemia (NB associated organ-specific autoimmune diseases especially autoimmune thyroid disease, diabetes mellitus, Addison's, vitiligo and hypoparathyroidism—see also p. 279)

Partial or total gastrectomy

Stagnant loop syndrome

Ileal resection or Crohn's disease

Vegan diet

Fish tapeworm

Chronic tropical sprue

Congenital intrinsic factor deficiency.

Lhermittes phenomenon: the patient describes a 'tingling' or 'electric feeling' or 'funny sensation' which passes down his spine, and perhaps into lower limbs, when he bends his head forward.† The most common cause is multiple sclerosis but it can also occur in cervical cord tumour, cervical spondylosis and subacute combined degeneration of the cord.

---

* Though the patient may be anaemic, vitamin B_{12} neuropathy may develop without anaemia and with normal blood film and bone marrow (see p. 375). Serum vitamin B_{12} level may be required to confirm the diagnosis.

† A similar sensation provoked by neck *extension* is termed 'reversed Lhermittes phenomenon' and strongly suggests cervical spondylosis.

127 / Holmes–Adie–Moore syndrome

Frequency in survey: 0.8% of attempts at MRCP short cases.

Record

This young lady has a unilateral *dilated pupil* which *fails* (or almost fails) *to react to light*. There is no ptosis or diplopia and eye movements are otherwise normal (i.e. not IIIrd nerve palsy).

    The patient has a myotonic pupil. Her tendon reflexes may be lost (check if allowed).

If exposed to light for prolonged periods the pupil may constrict slowly. If then exposed to darkness for a long period it will again dilate very slowly. During accommodation–convergence, after a delay which may last several minutes, the abnormal pupil constricts slowly until it may become smaller than the normal pupil. The reaction to mydriatics is normal (Argyll Robertson pupil dilates poorly with mydriatics) and the pupil may be hyper-reactive to cholinergic substances.

The condition is usually chronic and symptomless but in some cases onset is acute with associated blurring of vision and photophobia. Syphilitic serology will be negative. Differential diagnosis from neurosyphilis may be difficult in the chronic stages of this disorder, when the pupil may be chronically constricted, and especially when both pupils are affected (bilateral involvement rare with Holmes–Adie pupils but invariable with syphilitic Argyll Robertson pupils—p. 330).

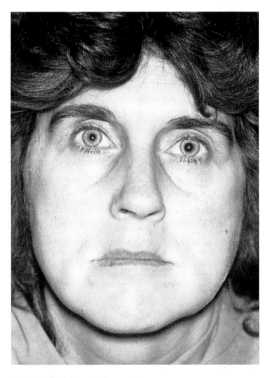

Fig. 3.127 Holmes–Adie pupil.

128 / Peripheral vascular disease

Frequency in survey: main focus of a short case in 0.8% of attempts at MRCP short cases. Additional feature in others.

Record

The lower leg(s) are pale (pregangrenous areas may be pink), the toes are bluish-red (there may be digital gangrene) and the *skin is atrophic* (may be stretched and *shiny*) and *hairless*. There are *no pulses** palpable below the femorals (if allowed, listen for a bruit) and the lower legs and feet are *cold* to touch. There is often asymmetry of signs.

These signs suggest peripheral vascular disease (?arcus senilis, ?xanthelasma, ?tendon xanthomata, ?nicotine-stained fingers, ?diabetes†).

Arteriosclerosis obliterans

This, the usual cause of peripheral vascular disease, is due to atheromatous plaques involving the intima of the arteries. As a rule there is superimposed thrombus formation. Degenerative changes occur in the media which frequently calcifies.† The superficial femoral artery is most commonly affected leading to calf claudication. The next most common sites are the popliteal and aortic bifurcation, the latter leading to:

Leriche's syndrome — claudication of low back, buttocks, thigh and calf; limb and buttock atrophy and pallor; impotence, weak or absent femoral pulses, systolic bruits over the lower abdomen and femorals; signs may be asymmetrical; may present as 'sciatica'.

Buerger's postural test

When the legs are lifted to 45° above the horizontal plane, cadaveric pallor develops if the arterial supply is poor. If, while the clinician supports the legs, the patient flexes and extends the ankles to the point of mild fatigue, this enhances the sign. The patient now sits with his feet lowered to the ground for 2–3 min and an impaired arterial supply is indicated by a ruddy, cyanotic hue which spreads over the affected foot (*Buerger's sign*). This sequence indicates occlusion of a major lower limb artery.

The ankle : arm Doppler pressure index uses a

Doppler ultrasonic flow probe to determine the ratio of the peak systolic pressure at the ankle to that in the arm. Symptoms are unlikely to be due to arterial disease if the index is above 0.8. Measurements made immediately after exercise give a good index of disease but are more difficult to perform reliably. In diabetic patients with calcified arteries† the test is unreliable as the pressure in the sphygmomanometer cuff may not reflect that in the artery.

Takayasu's disease†

This is an arteritis which affects chiefly, but not exclusively, young women from Japan and the Far East. It involves mainly the aortic arch and the large brachiocephalic arteries. Mononuclear cell infil-

---

* The patient with intermittent claudication may have few signs other than reduced or absent pulses in the affected limb. As the atheromatous disease advances, signs of ischaemia appear: low skin temperature, pallor or cyanosis, trophic changes including dry, scaly and shiny skin; the hair may disappear and the toenails can become brittle, ridged and deformed; ischaemic damage may cause persistent reddish or reddish-blue discoloration; ischaemic ulcers and gangrene may develop.

† Peripheral vascular disease in diabetic patients is more progressive, with greater involvement of the more distal vessels which are of smaller calibre; medial calcification is twice as common. See also p. 168.

‡ There were one or two anecdotes in our surveys to suggest that this may have appeared on rare occasions in the MRCP short cases.

trates and fibrous proliferation produce progressive narrowing of the lumen and reduced flow in the upper extremities and to the brain. It develops slowly so that although the pulses gradually vanish (hence the alternative name—*pulseless disease*), collateral circulation opens up allowing it to remain unnoticed for some time. Eventually the patient presents with symptoms such as fainting on turning the head suddenly or rising from supine to sitting, atrophy of the face, headaches, cataracts, optic atrophy, weakness and paraesthesiae of the upper extremities, hemiplegia and convulsions.

Buerger's disease (thromboangiitis obliterans)

An obstructive arterial disease with segmental inflammation and proliferative lesions in medium and small arteries§ and veins of limbs. Mostly affects young males aged 20–40 years, especially in Israel, the Orient and India. Patients are almost always moderate to heavy smokers; there may be an autoimmune mechanism triggered by tobacco products. Clinically the disease is characterized by ischaemia of the extremities§ and *migratory thrombophlebitis*. Raynaud's phenomonen (p. 350) is common. If the patient continues to smoke the disease will progress with increasing ischaemia leading to gangrene and amputation of the extremities which is required in a high percentage of patients.

For colour photograph see p. 540.

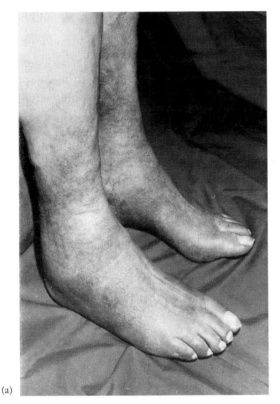

(a)

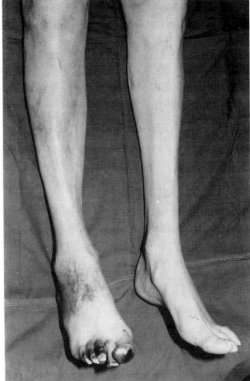

(b)

Fig. 3.128 (a) Peripheral vascular insufficiency.
(b) Peripheral vascular disease with gangrenous toes.

§ The features which distinguish this *thromboangiitis obliterans* from the common atheromatous arterial disease (*arteriosclerosis obliterans*), are the younger age of the patient, the relative sparing of larger arteries, the presence of migratory superficial thrombophlebitis, the increased involvement of the upper extremities, and more rapid progression. The diagnosis can be confirmed by biopsy of an early lesion showing a characteristic inflammatory and proliferative lesion on histology.

129 / Transplanted kidney

Frequency in survey: 0.8% of attempts at the MRCP short cases.

Survey note: although in real life the majority of patients who have a renal transplant have other causes, it is noteworthy that our surveys suggested that all the cases who appeared as MRCP short cases had polycystic kidney disease.

Record

There is fullness in the flanks and an impression of a swelling under the scar in the right iliac fossa. On palpation there are bilateral masses in the flanks which are bimanually ballotable and suggestive of *polycystic kidneys*. There is also an easily palpable rounded *mass under the scar in the right iliac fossa* which feels like a kidney.

I suspect this patient has had a renal transplant for renal failure due to polycystic kidney disease (p. 86).

Three most common diseases leading to referral for transplantation*

Diabetes mellitus with renal failure (transplantation offered earlier than in other forms of renal disease — post-transplant rehabilitation is more satisfactory if the damage due to other diabetic complications is minimal)

Hypertensive renal disease (incidence of end-stage renal failure not decreasing despite 'better' treatment of hypertension — reason not clear; occurs more often in the Afro-Caribbean than in the Caucasian patient)

Glomerulonephritis.

Diseases in which renal transplantation is a particular problem

Haemolytic-uraemic syndrome (disease can recur and cyclosporin can increase the risk of this; rapid graft failure may ensue)

Sickle-cell disease (increased incidence of sickle crises may result from the improved haematocrit)

Systemic sclerosis (post-transplant rehabilitation may be limited by the chronic vascular and gastrointestinal manifestations)

Focal glomerulosclerosis (recurrence within the graft is common)

Oxalosis (there may be severe recurrence of stone disease)

Cystinosis and Fabry's disease — p. 397 (continued disease activity).

---

* These three causes of end-stage renal failure account for 75% of referrals for renal transplantation.

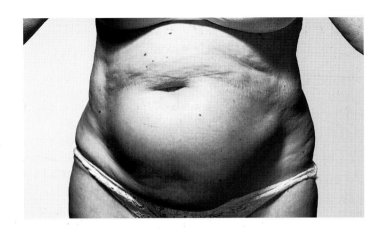

Fig. 3.129 Renal transplant in right iliac fossa.

Frequency in survey: 0.8% of attempts at MRCP short cases.

Survey note: usually the candidates were told that the patient had some difficulty with his vision, and they were asked to examine the visual fields. One candidate reported that he had found unilateral loss of the peripheral field and gave retinitis pigmentosa, extensive choriodoretinitis and diabetes mellitus with laser therapy as the possible causes, and the examiner told him that the patient had chronic glaucoma.

Record 1

There is unilateral R/L nasal visual field defect. This could be due to a space-occupying lesion compressing the lateral part of the optic chiasma* or it could be due to chronic simple glaucoma.* (Ask to examine the fundi.†)

Record 2

The visual fields are grossly constricted and the patient only has central vision (*tunnel vision*).

The most likely causes are retinitis pigmentosa, advanced chronic glaucoma or diffuse choroidoretinitis.

Several mass screening studies have shown a prevalence of 1–2% for glaucoma in the age group of more than 40 years; the greatest incidence of simple glaucoma being between 60 and 70 years. Heredity is an important predisposing factor in 13–25% of cases.

In the early stages a sickle-shaped extension of the blind spot may be demonstrated and some impairment of the nasal field may be apparent on the Bjerrum screen. As the condition progresses there is a contraction of the peripheral field leaving only the central vision intact.

The problem is often one of when to start treatment in a patient suspected of having chronic open angle glaucoma. In general, patients who have a raised intraocular pressure of 24mmHg or more, especially when it is persistent, those who have a family history of the disease, and those who are in their seventh decade should all be considered. Medical treatment consists of the instillation of miotics (e.g. pilocarpine, neostigmine, carbachol, etc.) in the eyes aiming to reduce the intraocular pressure to a normal level, and thereby to slow the progression of visual failure.

* The nasal field loss can be bilateral in chronic glaucoma but would not be bilateral with lateral chiasmal compression. The condition is insidious and asymptomatic in its early stages. It may be discovered accidentally when the vision of one eye is almost lost and of the other seriously impaired. The patient may need to change his/her presbyopic glasses frequently. There is usually accommodative failure. The patients find it difficult to see in a less illuminated room. Dark and light adaptation are slower than in normal subjects. Periodic eye examinations by an expert are advisable *for those who have a family history of glaucoma.*
† *Cupping of the disc* is an essential feature of chronic glaucoma. The sides of the disc are steep and the retinal vessels have the appearance of *being broken* off at the margin of the disc. The edges of the disc overhang and the course of the vessels, as they climb the sides of the cup, is hidden.

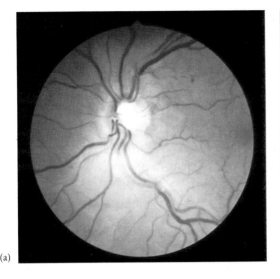

(a)

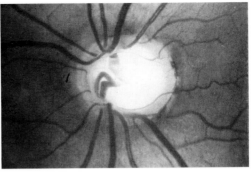

(b)

Fig. 3.130 (a) Early glaucoma. (b) Advanced glaucoma. Note large optic disc with sharply angulated vessels.

131 / Nephrotic syndrome

Frequency in survey: 0.7% of attempts at MRCP short cases.

Record

There is *extensive oedema* affecting the ankles, lower legs and periorbital tissues (especially in the morning) of this (may be young*) patient. The skin is pale (oedema in the skin). There are (may be) white bands across the nails (from chronic hypoalbuminaemia). There are (may be) bilateral *pleural effusions* and *ascites*.

This patient's extensive oedema could be due to nephrotic syndrome.†

Commonest cause

Glomerulonephritis (77% — usually minimal change in childhood but membranous in adults).

Other common causes in the UK

SLE (?characteristic rash, arthropathy, etc.—p. 237)
Diabetic nephropathy (?medic-alert bracelet, fundi)
Renal amyloidosis (usually secondary amyloidosis; ?evidence of rheumatoid arthritis or other chronic disease, etc.—see footnote, p. 69)
Renal vein thrombosis.

Malaria due to *Plasmodium malariae* is an important cause in areas where it is endemic. There are about 70 rare causes.

Investigations for nephrotic syndrome

Urine microscopy (?red cells, casts, lipid deposits)
24-h urinary protein

Urinary protein selectivity (clearance ratio of IgG to transferrin below 0.15 in minimal change disease, which carries a good prognosis)
Creatinine clearance (GFR — glomerular filtration rate)
Specific tests for the causal diseases (glucose, antinuclear factors, etc.)
Renal biopsy.

Complications

Thrombosis (deep venous, arterial, pulmonary, renal vein)
Malnutrition (high protein diet unless marked uraemia)
Atheroma and ischaemic heart disease (hypercholesterolaemia)
Infection.

---

* The oedema of the acute poststreptococcal glomerulonephritis (proteinuria, haematuria, oliguria, oedema, hypertension, renal failure) which mainly affects children and young adults, is usually due to salt and water retention. Only in a small proportion does heavier proteinuria leading to nephrotic syndrome develop.

† Defined as proteinuria >3.5 g per 1.75 m² of body surface per 24 h, hypoalbuminaemia and oedema. Hypercholesterolaemia is often present.

Frequency in survey: 0.7% of attempts at MRCP short cases.

Record

The patient has an *absent gag reflex* on the R/L side (and will have ipsilateral impaired taste over the posterior third of the tongue). *Palatal movements* on that side are *reduced* and the *uvula* is *drawn* to the *opposite side*. The R/L *sternomastoid* muscle is *wasted* and there is weakness in rotating the head to the opposite side. The *shoulder* is *flattened* and there is weakness of elevation of that shoulder.

There is therefore a lesion affecting the *IXth, Xth and XIth cranial nerves* on the R/L side.

This suggests a jugular foramen syndrome (to exclude a brainstem lesion* check carefully for evidence of ipsilateral wasting, fasciculation and deviation of the tongue — XIIth nerve, ipsilateral Horner's and, if allowed, for evidence of brainstem compression, e.g. spastic paraparesis).

An isolated lesion of the glossopharyngeal nerve is rare. It is usually damaged with the vagus and accessory nerves near the jugular foramen which all three nerves traverse (Fig. 3.132). A lesion inside the skull is more likely to cause a syndrome restricted to the IXth, Xth and XIth nerves only (syndrome of Vernet†). An internal lesion may cause brainstem compression.* A lesion outside the skull is more likely to involve the XIIth nerve as well (syndrome of Collet–Sicard†) — this nerve exits through the hypoglossal foramen near the external opening of the jugular foramen. An external lesion may also involve the cervical sympathetic* (syndrome of Villaret†). Other combinations of associated lower cranial lesions are vagus and accessory (syndrome of Schmidt†), and vagus, accessory and hypoglossal (syndrome of Hughlings Jackson†).

Causes of jugular foramen syndromes

Neurofibroma of IXth, Xth or XIIth nerves (especially left XIIth in young females)

Meningiomata

Epidermoid tumours (cholesteatomas)

Glomus or carotid body tumours

Metastases

Cerebellopontine angle lesions (p. 335 — may also extend down and involve the last four cranial nerves in numerical order)

Infection from the middle ear spreading into the posterior fossa

Granulomatous meningitis.

---

* Intrinsic brainstem disease may cause lower cranial nerve palsies and Horner's syndrome (e.g. pp. 303 and 438), but when the pathology is in the brainstem there is nearly always spinothalamic sensory loss on the opposite side of the body to the lesion.

† Though the age of such neurological eponyms is undoubtedly passing, their usage may still impress!

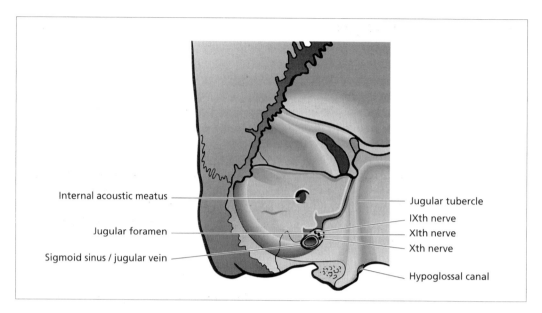

Internal acoustic meatus

Jugular foramen

Sigmoid sinus / jugular vein

Jugular tubercle

IXth nerve

XIth nerve

Xth nerve

Hypoglossal canal

Fig. 3.132 The posterior aspect of the posterior cranial fossa (after removal of the squamous part of the occipital bone) showing the jugular foramen and the nerves passing through it (note the position of the hypoglossal canal which conducts the XIIth nerve).

Frequency in survey: main focus of a short case in 0.7% of attempts at MRCP short cases. Additional feature in a further 2%.

Record

This elderly (or middle-aged) patient has a *vesicular rash* in the *area supplied by the . . . nerve* (say which/where).* The lesions are in *clusters* at different stages of development — the stages each cluster goes through is papule → vesicle → (pustule, sometimes haemorrhagic) → crusting → scar. The regional lymph nodes are enlarged.

The diagnosis is herpes zoster.

Complications

Cranial nerve palsy — especially facial nerve palsy which may occur not only with lesions of the external auditory meatus (Ramsay Hunt syndrome), but also with trigeminal zoster and zoster of the head, neck and mouth†

Peripheral motor palsy (lower motor neurone deficit from involvement of motor root — sometimes permanent)

Post-herpetic neuralgia (10%; commoner in the elderly; can be very severe and difficult to treat)

Eye damage (ophthalmic zoster)

Zoster sine herpete (typical pain, etc., but no rash — serological evidence confirms).

Other complications include visceral nerve involvement (pain or dysfunction in an organ), myelitis (transverse or ascending — rare), disseminated encephalitis (rare), cerebellar ataxia (rare) and diffuse polyneuritis (rare).

Generalized herpes zoster is usually associated with an underlying reticulosis (especially Hodgkin's), leukaemia, or carcinoma (especially bronchogenic).

For colour photograph see p. 533.

---

* The commonest is a thoracic dermatome. Cranial nerve involvement is next in frequency. The ophthalmic division of the trigeminal nerve is the commonest cranial nerve. With cranial nerve involvement there are often signs of meningeal irritation and sometimes mucous membranes are affected.

† In true Ramsay Hunt (see p. 198) the zoster is probably of the geniculate ganglion. In other cases there may be multiple cranial ganglia involvement (see anecdote 40, p. 497) and an associated localized encephalitis and neuronitis. Eighth nerve involvement (vertigo and deafness) is a particularly common association with facial palsy due to herpes zoster. Acyclovir given as soon as possible after the start of the infection is the treatment of choice.

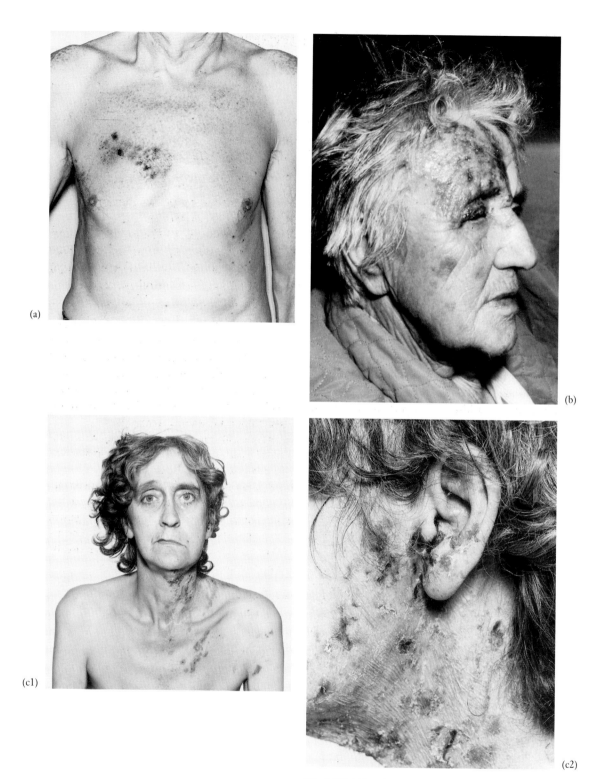

(a)

(b)

(c1)

(c2)

Fig. 3.133 (a) Involvement of a thoracic dermatome (probably T3). (b) Herpes zoster ophthalmicus. (c1,2) Ramsay Hunt syndrome.

134 / Henoch–Schönlein purpura

Frequency in survey: main focus of a short case in 0.7% of attempts at MRCP short cases. Additional feature in others.

Record

This patient (usually a male child or a young adult) has a *palpable purpuric rash* (initially macules which rapidly urticate and become purpuric and may go on to central necrosis) over the *extensor* surfaces of his *limbs* and *buttocks*.

The rash is typical of Henoch–Schönlein purpura. The patient may have other features of the Henoch–Schönlein syndrome—*polyarthralgia* (70%—large joints, usually knees and ankles), *bowel involvement* (25%—colic and haemorrhage) and *renal involvement* (30%—usually focal necrotizing glomerulonephritis).

The Henoch–Schönlein syndrome is also called *anaphylactoid purpura*.

Other features of Henoch–Schönlein syndrome

There may be a history of *recent infectious illness* (most commonly viral). Usually remits after 1 week but the cutaneous lesions may take several weeks to regress and the course is often punctuated by recurrent flare ups of the symptoms and/or signs

There may be a self-limiting hypertension

Polyarthralgia is common but frank arthritis is rare

Colicky abdominal pain may mimic an acute surgical abdomen

Patients may experience nausea, vomiting, diarrhoea, constipation and occasionally the passage of blood and mucus per rectum. *Intussusception* may occur rarely

Renal disease typically develops within 3 months of the onset of the other systemic manifestations of the Henoch–Schönlein syndrome. It is usually only a glomerulitis with microscopic haematuria and without any significant impairment of renal function. Renal failure is rare in children. Up to 25% of adults develop a severe crescentic lesion with rapidly progressive glomerulonephritis; nephrotic syndrome occurs in 50%

Patients usually recover spontaneously and completely. Corticosteroids may lead to symptomatic improvement

Involved tissues, including the skin, demonstrate vasculitis with IgA and complement deposition

IgA nephropathy (*Berger's disease*) is now regarded as a monosymptomatic form of the Henoch–Schönlein syndrome with mainfestations usually confined to the kidney.

For colour photograph see p. 537.

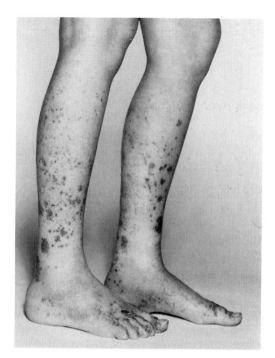

Fig. 3.134 Henoch–Schönlein purpura.

135 / Polymyositis

Frequency in survey: 0.6% of attempts at MRCP short cases.

Record

There is *symmetrical,** *proximal* muscle *weakness* (the patient may be unable to sit up from lying or stand up from squatting position) with associated muscle *wasting*. The muscles are *tender* (in 50% of cases—suggesting an inflammatory myopathy). The tendon reflexes are present though reduced.† There is (may be) dysphonia (and/or dysphagia) due to involvement of the bulbar muscles.

The diagnosis is polymyositis.

Male to female ratio is 1:2.

Features of polymyositis

A rash may occur (dermatomyositis—p. 293)

Features and associations similar to dermatomyositis (p. 293)

Association with malignancy‡

Onset of muscle weakness is usually insidious (with difficulty in running, climbing stairs, getting up from a chair, and combing hair)

Lower limb-girdle more often affected than shoulder-girdle

Ocular involvement is rare (if present, think of myasthenia gravis)

Respiratory muscle weakness can lead to respiratory failure—monitor peak flow rate and vital capacity

Cardiac muscle may be involved.

Other causes of proximal muscle weakness

(See also p. 310)

Carcinomatous neuromyopathy (including Eaton–Lambert syndrome—see p. 269)

Diabetic amyotrophy (?fundi, peripheral neuropathy)

Muscular dystrophies (?long-standing, familial — p. 226)

Dystrophia myotonica (?frontal balding, cataracts, myotonia, etc.—p. 159)

Alcoholism

Thyrotoxicosis (?eye signs, hypermobile, goitre, etc. —p. 114)

Corticosteroid treatment (?cushingoid facies, underlying disorder, etc.—p. 231)

Familial periodic paralysis

Osteomalacia

Hyperparathyroidism

Insulinoma.

Polymyalgia rheumatica is characterized by pain and stiffness of proximal muscles, especially shoulder girdle, in a patient who is usually elderly. The ESR is high. Significant objective weakness is not common. There is a relationship with temporal (giant cell) arteritis (see also p. 310).

---

* In general, if muscle weakness is symmetrical it suggests myopathic disease, and if asymmetrical neurogenic disease.

† If very reduced or absent it suggests underlying carcinoma causing polyneuropathy and polymyositis.

‡ Approximately 20% of adults with polymyositis or dermatomyositis also have cancer. Although this may seem higher than expected for the general population, there appears to be no significant difference in the frequency of malignancy when compared with appropriate age-matched control populations.

Frequency in survey: main focus of a short case in 0.5% of attempts at MRCP short cases. Additional feature in a further 0.4%.

Record

The pupils are *small* and *irregular* and react to *accommodation but not to light.**

The likely diagnosis is tabes dorsalis (?wrinkled forehead with ptosis, stamping ataxia, Romberg's test positive, loss of joint position and vibration sense, absent ankle jerks, Charcot's knee joint and aortic incompetence—p. 381).

The exact site of the lesion is not known. It is generally believed to be in the tectum of the midbrain proximal to the oculomotor nuclei. The classical Argyll Robertson pupil is very small. However, pupils affected by neurosyphilis are not always small and may even be dilated. They may be unequal in size. Though the signs may be more advanced in one eye than the other, pupillary abnormalities occurring in neurosyphilis are invariably bilateral. Argyll Robertson-like pupils occasionally occur in diabetes mellitus.

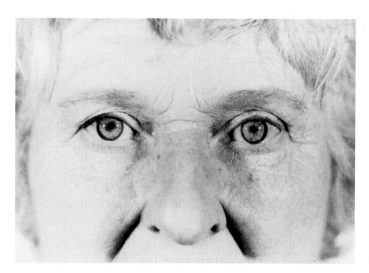

Fig. 3.136 Argyll Roberston pupils in a diabetic patient. Her serology was negative.

* The light reflex may become sluggish before it disappears, but the accommodation reflex is always brisker than the light.

137 / Congenital syphilis

Frequency in survey: 0.5% of attempts at MRCP short cases.

Record

There is flattening of the bridge of the nose (*saddle nose*), the superior maxilla is underdeveloped which makes the mandible appear prominent (*bull-dog jaw*), and there is frontal bossing. There are *rhagades* at the corners of the mouth and there are *Hutchinson's teeth* (widely spaced peg-shaped upper incisors with a crescentic notch at the cutting edge) and *Moon's molars* (dome-shaped deformity of the first lower molars with underdeveloped cusps). The *tibiae are sabre-shaped*.

The diagnosis is congenital syphilis.

Other manifestations of late congenital syphilis*

VIIIth nerve deafness

Clutton's joints (effusions into the knee joints with no pain or difficulty with joint movement)

Interstitial keratitis (acute attacks;† may eventually lead to corneal opacities—ground-glass appearance of cornea)

Old choroidoretinitis (peripheral and bilateral—'salt and pepper fundus')

Optic atrophy

Perforations of the palate or nasal septum

Collapse of the nasal cartilage.

---

* Early congenital syphilis in the first few months of life resembles severe secondary syphilis in the adult. Features include rhinitis, a mucocutaneous rash, osteochondritis, dactylitis, hepatosplenomegaly, lymphadenopathy, anaemia, jaundice, thrombocytopenia and leucocytosis. Nephrotic syndrome may occur.

† May be due to hypersensitivity. Corticosteroids may sometimes help.

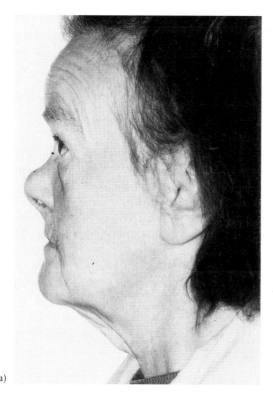

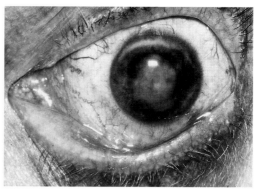

(b)

Fig. 3.137 Congenital syphilis. (a) Note the saddle nose.
(b) Interstitial keratitis has led to corneal opacification.

Frequency in survey: main focus of a short case in 0.5% of attempts at MRCP short cases. Additional feature in a further 0.8%.

Record

There is (in this ?stout, ?middle-aged lady who complains of pain, numbness or paraesthesiae in the palm and fingers which is particularly bad in the night*) *sensory loss* over the *palmar* aspects of the *first three and a half fingers* and *wasting of the thenar eminence*. There is weakness of *abduction, flexion* and *opposition of the thumb*.

The diagnosis is median nerve palsy. The non-involvement of the flexor muscles of the forearm (i.e. can flex distal interphalangeal joint of thumb) suggests that the cause is carpal tunnel syndrome (now check the facies for underlying *acromegaly* or *myxoedema*; underlying *rheumatoid arthritis* should be obvious). *Tinel's sign*† is positive to confirm this.

Though in early cases there may be no abnormal physical signs, usually some impairment of sensation over the affected fingers can be detected. Tenderness on compression of the nerve at the wrist† and thenar atrophy are relatively rare. If the story is characteristic the absence of physical signs should not deter one from advising treatment with intracarpal tunnel steroid injection or carpal tunnel decompression. Investigation with nerve conduction studies may be helpful in cases of doubt.

Causes of carpal tunnel syndrome

Idiopathic (almost entirely females, middle-aged, often obese; or younger women with excessive use of hands; may occur in males after unaccustomed hand use—e.g. house painting)

Pregnancy

Contraceptive pill

Myxoedema (?facies, hoarse croaking voice, pulse, ankle jerks, etc—p. 152)

Acromegaly (?facies, large spade-shaped hands, bitemporal hemianopia, etc.—p. 109)

Rheumatoid arthritis of the wrists (?spindling of the fingers, ulnar deviation, nodules, etc.—p. 73)

Osteoarthrosis of carpus (perhaps related to an old fracture)

Tuberculous tenosynovitis

Primary amyloidosis (?peripheral neuropathy, thick nerves, autonomic neuropathy; heart, joint and gut (rectal biopsy) involvement may occur—see also footnote, p. 134)

Tophaceous gout (p. 282).

---

* The nocturnal discomfort may be referred to the whole forearm with paraesthesiae extending beyond the cutaneous distribution of the median nerve in the hand. The sensory *signs* however, are confined to the classical median nerve distribution (Fig. 2.1, p. 23).

† *Tinel's sign* is tingling in the distribution of a nerve produced by percussion of that nerve. Percussion over the carpal tunnel sometimes produces a positive Tinel's sign in carpal tunnel syndrome. Other signs are *Phalen's sign* (the patient flexes both wrists for 60 seconds and this produces a prompt exacerbation of paraesthesia which is rapidly relieved when the flexion is discontinued) which is positive in half the patients, and the *tourniquet test* (a sphygmomanometer is pumped above systolic pressure for 2 min and this produces the paraesthesiae). Symptoms may sometimes be induced by *hyperextension* at the wrist.

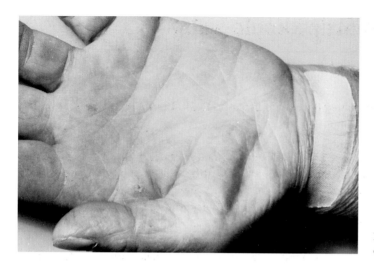

Fig. 3.138 Wasting of the thenar eminence.

139 / Cerebellopontine angle lesion

Frequency in survey: 0.5% of attempts at MRCP short cases.

Record

On the R/L side there is evidence of *Vth* (may be absent corneal reflex only), *VIth* (p. 114) and *VIIth cranial nerve impairment* (both may be minimal), *perceptive deafness* (*VIIIth* nerve—the patient usually has tinnitus but may complain of vague unsteadiness or giddiness*), and *cerebellar* impairment (may be slightly impaired rapid alternate motion of the hands only). There is *nystagmus* (again may be just a few beats intermittently; it may be cerebellar and/or vestibular in origin).

These findings suggest a lesion at the cerebellopontine angle, *acoustic neuroma†* being the commonest cause (X-ray for evidence of expansion of the internal auditory meatus — not always seen†). Meningioma can give a similar picture (normal auditory meatus on X-ray).

The IXth and Xth cranial nerves may be involved and dysphagia and dysphonia may occur. In severe cases, with large tumours, there may be signs of raised intracranial pressure (?papilloedema) in addition to ipsilateral cerebellar involvement.

---

* Rotational vertigo in acoustic neuroma seldom occurs in the discrete attacks that are found in Menière's syndrome.

† Acoustic neuromata may cause symptoms even if extremely small, if confined within the acoustic canal. They are much commoner than all other cranial nerve tumours. MRI scans accurately detect even very small acoustic neuromata. Patients with hearing loss developing in middle age should be considered to have acoustic neuroma until proved otherwise. Audiometry is suggestive but not diagnostic. Caloric testing almost always shows abnormalities but auditory evoked response is the most efficient physiological assessment. The cerebrospinal fluid protein is elevated (may be $>3\,\mathrm{g\,l^{-1}}$) but cerebrospinal fluid assessment should not usually be necessary and might be dangerous.

Frequency in survey: 0.5% of attempts at MRCP short cases.

Record

The pulse is regular (give rate) and of good volume. The jugular venous pressure is not raised. The apex beat is *not palpable on the left side*, but can be felt in the fifth *right* intercostal space in the mid-clavicular line.

   This patient has dextrocardia.* (If allowed, listen to the lung fields—Kartagener's syndrome—and feel the abdomen to see which side the liver is on—situs inversus.)

If situs inversus is present the patient is usually otherwise normal. Dextrocardia without situs inversus is usually associated with cardiac malformation. Dextrocardia may occur in Turner's syndrome.

Kartagener's syndrome: dextrocardia, bronchiectasis, situs inversus, infertility, dysplasia of frontal sinuses, sinusitis and otitis media. Patients have ciliary immotility.

---

* Consider the possibility of this diagnosis if you cannot feel the apex beat and then have difficulty hearing the heart sounds. As you gradually move the stethoscope towards the right side of the chest, they get louder.

141 / Down's syndrome

Frequency in survey: main focus of a short case in 0.5% of attempts at MRCP short cases. Additional feature in a further 0.6%.

Record

This short-statured patient has *low-set ears*, a *flattened nasal bridge*, *slanting eyes*, *epicanthus*, white *'Brushfield spots'* in the iris and a small *mouth which hangs open* revealing a large heavily fissured tongue. There is an over-rolled helix of each ear. There is a single *transverse palmar crease* (not pathognomonic) and a short inward curving little finger. The axial triradius is situated towards the centre of the palm (normally should be near the wrist). There is generalized hypotonia and hyper-extensibility of the joints.

The patient has Down's syndrome.

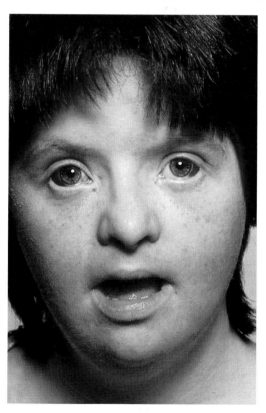

Trisomy 21 (occasionally translocation between 21 and 14).

Other features which may occur

Congenital heart lesions (septal defects, Fallot's tetralogy)

Lenticular opacities

Mental retardation which varies from very mild (author of an autobiography) to very severe

Dementia of Alzheimer type

Hypothyroidism.

Fig. 3.141 Down's syndrome.

Frequency in survey: main focus of a short case in 0.5% of attempts at MRCP short cases. Additional feature in a further 1.6%.

Survey note: all cases were due to either drugs or cirrhosis.

Record

There is gynaecomastia (it may be unilateral). This is confirmed on palpation by the presence of *increased glandular tissue*. Now look for signs of *cirrhosis, heart failure* (spironolactone), *atrial fibrillation* (digoxin), *clubbing and cachexia* (carcinoma of the lung), *absence of body hair* (hypogonadism, oestrogen therapy) or evidence of an *endocrine disorder*—see below.

There may be feminization of the nipples and tenderness of the breasts. Gynaecomastia must be differentiated from tumours of the breast and simple adiposity.

Causes of gynaecomastia

Pubertal (very common*—due to transient dominance of circulating oestradiol over testosterone)

Senile (normal rise in oestrogens and fall in androgens with age)

Cirrhosis of the liver (?stigmata—p. 84)

Thyrotoxicosis (?exophthalmos, goitre, etc.—p. 114)

Carcinoma of the lung (5% of patients; sometimes with hypertrophic pulmonary osteoarthropathy; hCG secreted by the tumour)

Carcinoma of the liver (hCG secreting)

Klinefelter's syndrome (47,XXY, small testes, mental deficiency, incomplete virilization, raised LH and FSH)

Pituitary disease,† i.e. acromegaly, hypopituitarism (?visual field defect)

Isolated gonadotrophin deficiency (e.g. Kallman's syndrome — hypogonadotrophic hypogonadism and anosmia, often with harelip or cleft palate)

Testicular tumours (due to hCG secretion, oestrogen secretion or excess aromatase activity in the tumour tissue)

Addison's disease (?pigmentation—buccal and scar; —p. 126)

Adrenal carcinoma

Testicular feminization (androgen insensitivity)

Drug-induced:‡
  (a) oestrogen therapy (carcinoma of the prostate)
  (b) digoxin
  (c) griseofulvin
  (d) alkylating agents (cause testicular damage)
  (e) antiandrogens (including cyproterone acetate, spironolactone, ketoconazole, metronidazole and cimetidine)

Other drugs include phenothiazines, reserpine, tricyclics, methyldopa, isoniazid, amphetamines, aromatizable androgens, anabolic steroids, penicillamine, captopril, calcium channel blockers, diazepam, marijuana and heroin.

---

* Thirty-nine per cent of 1855 adolescent boys of different ages at one boy scout camp though other surveys have found it less common.
† NB Prolactin excess in the absence of oestrogens produces galactorrhoea rather than gynaecomastia.

‡ The letters of the word MADRAS form a useful mnemonic: methyldopa, aldactone, digoxin, reserpine, alkylating agents, stilboestrol.

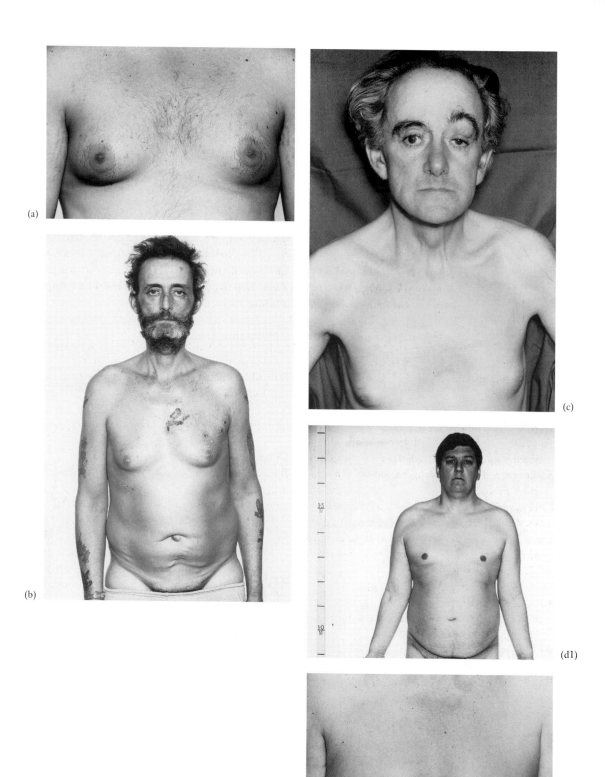

Fig. 3.142 (a) Bilateral benign gynaecomastia. (b) Chronic
liver disease. (c) Carcinoma of the lung (note left Horner's
syndrome). (d1,2) Hypogonadism. (2) is a close-up view of
the same patient as (1).

143 / Absent ankle jerks and extensor plantars

Frequency in survey: main focus of a short case in 0.5% of attempts at MRCP short cases. Additional feature in a further 1%.

Record

The knee and *ankle jerks are absent* and the *plantar responses are extensor.*

Possible causes

1 Subacute combined degeneration of the cord (?posterior column signs, positive Romberg's sign, clinical anaemia, splenomegaly, etc.—p. 314)

2 Syphilitic taboparesis (?Argyll Robertson pupils, ptosis and wrinkled forehead, posterior column signs, positive Romberg's sign, etc.—p. 381)

3 Multisystem degeneration, e.g. Friedreich's ataxia (?pes cavus, (kypho-)scoliosis, nystagmus, cerebellar ataxia, scanning speech, etc.—p. 234)

4 Motor neurone disease (?fasciculation, absence of sensory signs, etc.—p. 123)

5 Common conditions in combination* (e.g. an elderly person with diabetes and cervical myelopathy—see experience 61, p. 456—or cervical and lumbar spondylosis causing a mixture of upper and lower motor neurone signs in the legs).

---

* Whilst the above order in which the possible causes are listed represents the traditional order in which the conditions are presented, in practice number 5 is by far the commonest.

144 / Lichen planus

Frequency in survey: 0.5% of attempts at MRCP short cases.

Record

This young (or middle-aged) patient has *flat-topped*, *polygonal*, shiny, slightly scaly, violaceous *papules* on the wrists (and other flexor surfaces usually, though it may affect any part of the skin). Fine white streaks (*Wickham's striae*) are seen on the surface of the lesions. The *Koebner phenomenon* is present (i.e. lesions appear in a linear pattern along a scratch mark). There are also lesions in the *buccal mucosa* (in 50% of cases—white, lacy pattern).

This patient has lichen planus (itching is usual and may be quite severe).

Male to female ratio is 1 : 1.

Lichen planus usually resolves in 6–24 months but it may recur. Steroids (systemic, local or intralesional) may be required if pruritus is severe and in the hypertrophic variety (see below). Certain drugs such as thiazides, phenothiazines, gold, quinidine and antimalarials can cause lichen planus-like, generalized eruptions. Some patients with graft-versus-host disease develop a skin reaction that closely resembles lichen planus. There may be aetiological clues in this.

Other sites for lichen planus

Scalp (atrophy of the skin with patchy, permanent alopecia)

Nails (dystrophy of nail plate with longitudinal streaking of the nail; if it is severe there may be complete loss of the nail plate)

Palms and soles.

Other forms

Hypertrophic lichen planus (plaque-like lesions with a thick, warty surface on the front of the legs)

Erosive lichen planus (mouth)

Bullous lichen planus.

For colour photographs see p. 536.

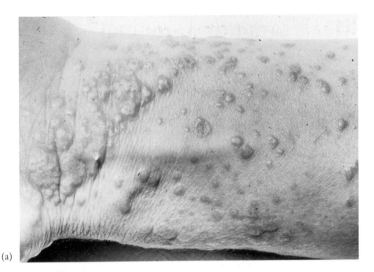

(a)

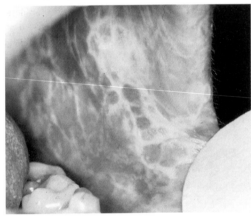

(b)

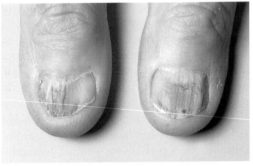

(c)

Fig. 3.144 (a) Lichen planus of the wrist. (b) The left buccal mucosa is exposed to show the characteristic lacy, white pattern. (c) Pterygium of the nail—lichen planus.

145 / Lateral popliteal (common peroneal) nerve palsy

Frequency in survey: 0.5% of attempts at MRCP short cases.

Record

There is *wasting* of the *anterior tibial* and *peroneal* group of *muscles*, the patient *cannot dorsiflex* or *evert* the R/L foot, and there is *impairment* of *sensation* over the *outer side* of the *calf*. He cannot stand on the R/L heel and the gait is altered as a result of *foot-drop* (there is an audible 'clop' of the foot as he walks).

The diagnosis is lateral popliteal (common peroneal) nerve palsy.

Injury to the nerve is usually at the head of the fibula where it can be involved in fractures or compressed by splints, tourniquets or bandages. Some individuals are particularly susceptible to temporary pressure palsy of this nerve (and in some cases other nerves such as the radial and ulnar as well), experiencing symptoms induced by crossing knees, squatting (strawberry picker's palsy) or unusual physical activity.

The nerve has two branches—the superficial and deep peroneal nerves. The superficial supplies sensation to the lateral calf and dorsum of the foot supplying the peroneus longus and brevis muscles. The deep branch supplies sensation to a triangular area of skin between the first and second toes dorsally and it innervates the anterior tibial muscles, the long extensors of the toes and the peroneus tertius muscle.

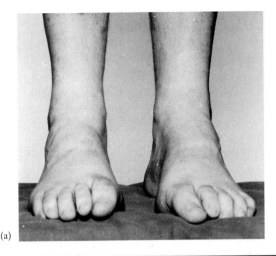

(a)

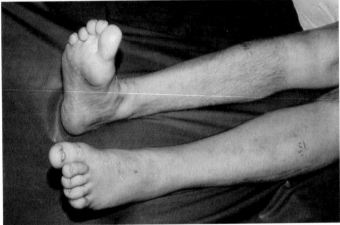

(b)

Fig. 3.145 (a) Right common peroneal nerve palsy. Note failure of eversion. (b) Left common peroneal nerve palsy. Note failure of eversion and dorsiflexion on the left side.

Frequency in survey: main focus of a short case in 0.5% of attempts at MRCP short cases. Additional feature in at least a further 5%.

Record 1

There is *unilateral* ptosis.*

Possible causes

1 Third nerve palsy (?dilated ipsilateral pupil, divergent strabismus, etc.—p. 117)
2 Horner's syndrome (?ipsilateral small pupil, etc.—p. 180)
3 Myasthenia gravis (may be the only sign of this condition; ?induced or worsened by upward gaze; variable strabismus, facial and proximal muscle weakness, weak nasal voice, all of which may worsen with repetition, etc.—p. 269)
4 Congenital/idiopathic† (may increase with age; there may be an associated superior rectus palsy)
5 Dystrophia myotonica (usually bilateral).

Record 2

There is *bilateral* ptosis.*

Possible causes

1 Myasthenia gravis
2 Dystrophia myotonica (?myopathic facies, frontal balding, wasting of facial muscles and sternomastoids, cataracts, myotonia, etc.—p. 159)
3 Tabes dorsalis (?Argyll Robertson pupils, etc.—p. 381)
4 Congenital† (may increase with age)
5 Bilateral Horner's (e.g. syringomyelia—?wasting of small muscles of the hand, dissociated sensory loss, scars, extensor plantars, etc.—p. 303)
6 Ocular myopathy‡ (?absence of soft tissue in the lids and periorbital region, ophthalmoplegia, mild facial and neck weakness)
7 Oculopharangeal muscular dystrophy‡ (similar to ocular myopathy but late onset and dysphagia prominent).

---

* NB Overaction of frontalis with wrinkling of the forehead tends to be associated with ptosis due to non-myopathic conditions.

† The Tensilon test should be negative before this diagnosis is accepted.

‡ Many of the ocular myopathies are associated with characteristic morphological features ('ragged red fibres') and mitochondrial myopathy and are now referred to as chronic progressive external ophthalmoplegia (CPEO). The disorder lies in the cytochromes and the conditions are sometimes termed the mitochondrial cytopathies. Ocular myopathy and oculopharangeal muscular dystrophy may be manifestations of the same condition.

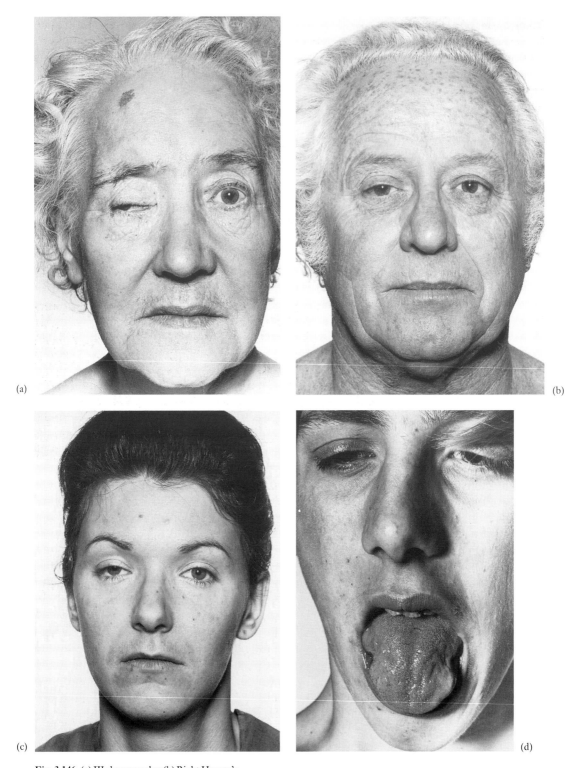

Fig. 3.146 (a) IIIrd nerve palsy. (b) Right Horner's syndrome. (c) Myasthenia gravis. (d) Dystrophia myotonica.

Other causes of ptosis

Pseudoptosis (following recurrent inflammation or extreme thinning of lids after repeated angioneurotic oedema)

Voluntary ptosis (to suppress diplopia)

Apraxia of the eyelids (the patient may need to pull down the lower eyelids, tilt back the head or open the mouth to enable the eyes to be opened; there is usually evidence of basal ganglia involvement).

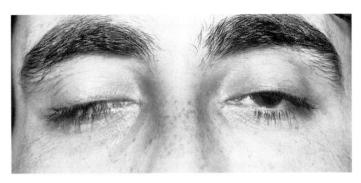

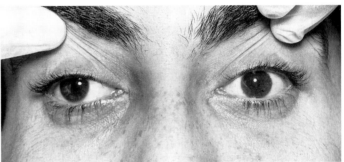

Fig. 3.146 (*continued*) (e) Ocular myopathy.

(e)

147 / Osteogenesis imperfecta

Frequency in survey: 0.5% of attempts at MRCP short cases.

Record

The *sclerae* are *slaty-blue*. (Look for evidence of *deformity* from poor fracture healing; ask the patient if he has been particularly prone to *fractures* in the past.)

The diagnosis is osteogenesis imperfecta (the patient may be deaf due to *otosclerosis*).

Osteogenesis imperfecta is due to defects in collagen. In the adult the diagnosis is likely to be the milder tarda type* (usually dominant). In this type the sclerae are more likely to be blue and the fragile bones of childhood become stronger after adolescence though they remain abnormal. The blueness is due to the thin sclerae allowing choroid pigment to show through. Though blue sclerae are not always present, some patients manifest only blue sclerae or otosclerosis without clinical bone disease. Deafness from otosclerosis does not usually develop before the third decade and may occur even later still. Laxity of ligaments, hypotonia of muscles and muscle wasting (partly disuse atrophy) are other features which may occur. Serum alkaline and acid phosphatases are often elevated and the urine often contains hydroxyproline, pyrophosphate and glycosoaminoglycans. Though no specific treatment is known, favourable responses to calcitonin have been reported. Osteogenesis imperfecta may be confused with idiopathic juvenile osteoporosis but in the latter condition osteoporosis is typically confined to the vertebral column, there is no family history of fractures and the sclerae are normal in colour.

Other conditions in which blue sclerae may occur

Marfan's syndrome (p. 267)
Ehlers–Danlos syndrome (p. 263)
Pseudoxanthoma elasticum (p. 311).

For colour photograph see p. 537.

---

*Other types are:
1 The severe prenatal type which causes intrauterine death or life for only a few days after birth
2 The severe type in which the baby survives but is extremely susceptible to fractures. The bones are soft as well as brittle and may therefore bow. Deformities are common and walking may induce fractures. Blue sclerae are less common.

Frequency in survey: 0.5% of attempts at MRCP short cases.

Record

The pulse is regular and the JVP is not elevated (prominent *a* wave in severe cases).* The cardiac apex is not palpable but there is (may be) a *left parasternal heave*. A *systolic thrill* is palpable over the left second and third interspaces. An *ejection click* and a *systolic murmur* (and maybe also a fourth heart sound) are heard over the *pulmonary area*. The murmur is louder during inspiration and radiates to the suprasternal notch. The second sound is (may be) split (the pulmonary component is soft).

The diagnosis is pulmonary stenosis.

Poststenotic dilatation of the pulmonary arteries may be seen on the chest X-ray and, in the severe case, right ventricular hypertrophy and diminution of pulmonary vascular markings. A minor degree of pulmonary stenosis is compatible with a normal life span. Surgical relief is required in symptomatic cases or if there is a gradient of more than 50 mmHg across the pulmonary valve. Balloon valvotomy is becoming the technique of choice in children and young adults, especially if the valve is not dysplasic. If treatment is delayed too long in severe pulmonary stenosis an irreversible fibrotic change can take place in the hypertrophied right ventricle.

* A patient with severe pulmonary stenosis may have cyanosis (check buccal mucosa) if the foramen ovale is unsealed and this may be intermittent.

149 / Raynaud's phenomenon

Frequency in survey: main focus of a short case in 0.5% of attempts at MRCP short cases. Additional feature in a further 2%.

Record

The *fingers* are *cold* and *cyanosed** with (may be) *atrophy* of the *finger pulps* (and in severe cases gangrene of the fingertips).

The patient is likely to have Raynaud's phenomenon (now look for features of underlying connective tissue diseases, especially systemic sclerosis).

Causes of Raynaud's phenomenon

1 Idiopathic Raynaud's disease* (common, especially young females, thumbs often spared, starts in childhood, usually benign)

2 Vibrating tools (e.g. pneumatic drills, polishing tools)

3 Systemic sclerosis (Raynaud's may be the first symptom; ?smooth, tight, shiny skin on the hands and face, typical mask-like facies, telangiectasia, etc.—p. 96)

4 Other connective tissue disorders (especially mixed connective tissue disease but also SLE, polymyositis, Sjögren's syndrome and rheumatoid arthritis)

5 Cervical rib (?supraclavicular bruit, ipsilateral diminished radial pulse especially during a Raynaud's attack, wasting of the small muscles of the hand and C8/T1 sensory impairment though neurological signs of cervical rib are often minimal if vascular signs are prominent).

Other causes

Cold agglutinins
Cryoglobulinaemia
Hypothyroidism
Heavy metal poisoning.

Women who develop toxaemia of pregnancy are more likely to have a history of Raynaud's disease (suggesting an abnormal vascular reactivity or unidentified humoral agent underlying both conditions).

For colour photograph see p. 538.

---

* In idiopathic Raynaud's disease the arteries show an exaggerated physiological response to cold and go into intense spasm to produce numb, dead-white fingers (p. 538). With rewarming the classical colour sequence is white to blue (cyanosis) then blue to red (rebound hyperaemia which is painful). The patient (usually with systemic sclerosis) in whom Raynaud's is discussed in the MRCP examination may have chronically impaired arterial circulation leading to cyanosis even in the warm hospital environment.

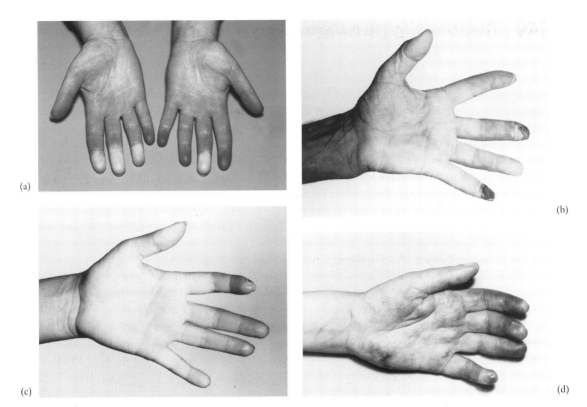

(a)

(b)

(c)

(d)

Fig. 3.149 (a) Raynaud's phenomenon. (b,c) Note gangrene of the fingertips. (d) Chronically impaired arterial circulation and atrophy of the finger pulps.

Frequency in survey: 0.5% of attempts at MRCP short cases.

Record

The patient (who probably presented with primary amenorrhoea) is *short* (usually less than 1.5 m) with a *short webbed neck** (only found in 54%) and shows *cubitus valgus* deformity. She has a *shield-like chest* (and may have widely separated nipples). The *nails are hypoplastic* and she has *short fourth metacarpals* (other metacarpals may also be short). The *hairline is low*, she has a *high-arched palate* and there are *numerous naevi*. The secondary sexual characteristics are underdeveloped (unless the patient has been treated with oestrogens).

The diagnosis is Turner's syndrome. (If allowed: examine the cardiovascular system — abnormal in 20%; especially coarctation of the aorta (p. 256) but also atrial septal defect (p. 430), ventricular septal defect (p. 197) and aortic stenosis (p. 112).)

The patient with Turner's syndrome is likely to have streak gonads and a chromosome constitution which is mostly 45,XO,† though mosaicism (XO,XX) does occur. Red–green colour blindness (an X-linked recessive character) occurs as frequently in Turner's as it does in normal males, and other X-linked conditions may occur.

Other features which sometimes occur

Lymphoedema
Genitourinary abnormality (e.g. horseshoe kidney)
Hypertelorism
Epicanthal fold
Mental retardation is rare
Strabismus
Ptosis
Intestinal telangiectasia
Premature osteoporosis
Premature ageing in appearance
Higher incidence of diabetes mellitus and Hashimoto's thyroiditis.

Noonan's syndrome: may affect both sexes. Females have Turner's phenotype but normal 46,XX, normal ovarian function and normal fertility. Noonan's are more likely to have right-sided cardiac lesions (especially pulmonary stenosis) whereas Turner's are more likely to have left-sided lesions. Mental retardation is frequent.

---

* A feature especially associated with cardiovascular abnormalities in this condition.
† Most 45,XO pregnancies end in spontaneous abortion.

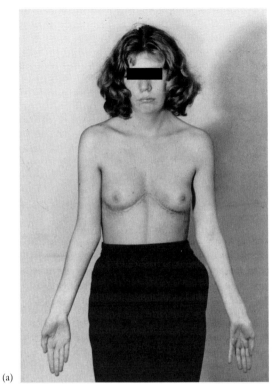

(a)

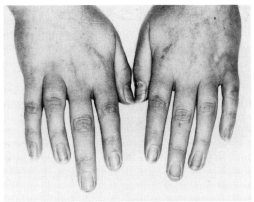

(b)

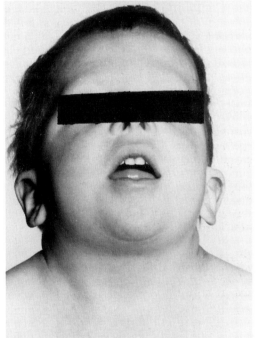

(c)

Fig. 3.150 (a) XO, XX mosaic. Note the webbed neck, increased carrying angle and scar under the breasts (special incision for atrial septal defect repair). (b) The hands of another patient showing short fourth metacarpal. (c) Noonan's syndrome.

151 / Mycosis fungoides

Frequency in survey: 0.5% of attempts at MRCP short cases.

Record
There are (in this middle-aged or elderly patient) erythematous, *well-defined thick-ened, indurated, scaly, plaque-like lesions* (which itch) over . . . (describe the site; can be on any part of the body). There are also (may be) raised ulcerated nodules.

The appearances are suggestive of mycosis fungoides (cutaneous lymphoma*).

Males > females.

Mycosis fungoides is a T-cell tumour of the skin* which usually shows no evidence of visceral involvement for several years. The initial lesions may be confused with psoriasis or eczema. They usually progress very slowly to nodules which may ulcerate. Diffuse exfoliative erythroderma may develop. Extracutaneous involvement (especially lung, liver and spleen) does not usually become manifest for many years (though it can be found in two-thirds of patients at autopsy). Lymph node involvement suggests the likelihood of further extracutaneous spread. Treatment includes steroids, cytotoxic agents, PUVA and radiotherapy.

Other reticuloses, for example Hodgkin's disease and leukaemia, may present as infiltrative papules or plaques in the skin diagnosed by skin biopsy.

For colour photograph see p. 537.

---

* Cutaneous T-cell lymphomata are lymphoproliferative disorders of helper T lymphocytes with an affinity for the skin in which atypical lymphocytes accumulate in clusters in the epidermis. They represent at least three types of lymphoma: mycosis fungoides, Sézary syndrome and adult T-cell lymphoma (HTLV-1 virus antibodies, hepatosplenomegaly, osteolytic bone lesions, *hypercalcaemia*).

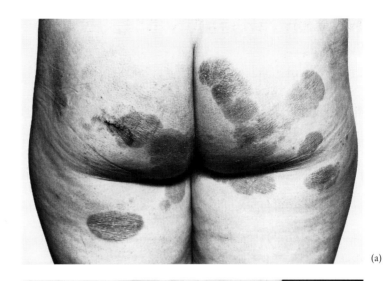

(a)

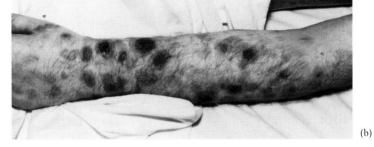

(b)

Fig. 3.151 (a) Early lesions of
mycosis fungoides showing well-
demarcated, scaly, atrophic,
erythematous patches. (b) Mycosis
fungoides showing early ulceration of
plaques.

Frequency in survey: 0.5% of attempts at MRCP short cases.

Record 1

There is an *indurated*, *poorly defined plaque* under the breast (may be anywhere on the trunk, face, axillae or perineum). The lesion is multicoloured with a central yellowish area, 2–5 cm in diameter (say how much), the surface is (may be) *smooth* and *shiny* with *no hair follicles* and *no sweat ducts*. There is (may be) a *lilac border* at one side of the plaque (diagnostic, if present). There is *hypoaesthesia* over the plaque which is adherent to deeper tissues. The plaque looks like a depressed area due to the *atrophy* of the *underlying tissue.**

The appearances are suggestive of localized scleroderma.

Record 2

There is a solitary indistinct induration over the trunk (say where). The area looks *discoloured* and *depressed* and there is (may be) telangiectasis.

This is probably a small patch of solitary, localized scleroderma.

Morphoea is also known as *localized or circumscribed scleroderma*. The aetiology is unknown but some patients with classical morphoea have sclerotic skin changes due to *Borrielia burgdorferi*.

Lichen sclerosus is a chronic atrophic disorder characterized by a *white* angular *well-defined* *indurated* plaque or plaques, which can usually be distinguished from morphoea by its characteristic clinical and histological features.

For colour photograph see p. 543.

---

* Deep involvement may be associated with *atrophy* of *muscles* and *bone*. There may be *scarring alopecia* on the scalp. A variant of morphoea, involving the frontoparietal scalp and face usually in a linear distribution, is rarely seen (*en coup de sabre*).

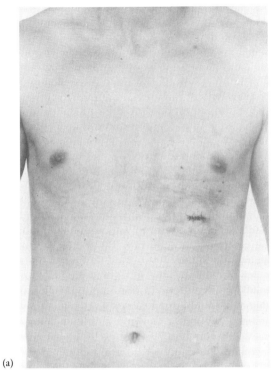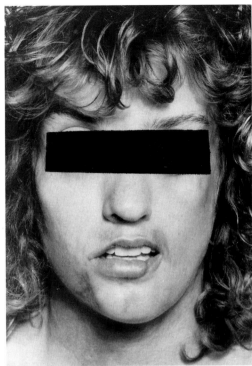

(a)

(b)

Fig. 3.152 (a) Morphoea—central pale area from which a biopsy has been taken. (b) Localized scleroderma of the lower lip.

Frequency in survey: 0.5% of attempts at MRCP short cases. Additional feature in others.

Record

On examination of the fundi of this *blind** patient, there is a pigmentary retinopathy suggestive of *retinitis pigmentosa*.* There is truncal *obesity*, *short stature* and *polydactyly*.†

These features suggest the diagnosis of the Laurence–Moon–Bardet–Biedl syndrome. (There is likely to be *mental retardation*† of variable severity, and *hypogonadism*†.)

Autosomal recessive

Renal structural and functional abnormalities are very common. Interstitial nephritis may lead to renal failure.

The 'splitters' and the 'lumpers'

Some investigators (the 'splitters') consider the Bardet–Biedl syndrome and the Laurence–Moon syndrome to be distinct; the Laurence–Moon syndrome being characterized by the absence of polydactyly and obesity and the presence of spastic paraparesis. Other investigators (the 'lumpers') believe these distinctions relate to variable expression of a single disorder.

Related disorders

Alström's syndrome: autosomal recessive; retinal dystrophy and obesity; blindness in early childhood; moderate deafness before the age of 10; diabetes mellitus and slowly progressive chronic nephropathy in early adulthood; *mental retardation and digital abnormalities do not occur*

Carpenter's syndrome (acrocephalopolysyndactyly): autosomal recessive; acrocephaly; syndactyly; characteristic facial appearance associated with obesity, mental retardation, hypogonadism and polydactyly of the feet. In view of the characteristic skeletal findings there should not be diagnostic difficulty.

---

* The retinal dystrophy of the Laurence–Moon–Bardet–Biedl syndrome is usually pigmentary. Total blindness usually occurs after the age of 30.

† Hypogonadism, mental retardation and polydactyly are less frequently found in females.

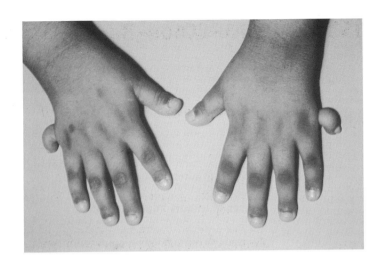

Fig. 3.153 Polydactyly.

154 / Short stature

Frequency in survey: 0.5% of attempts at MRCP short cases.

Record
The patient is abnormally short (?features of a major systemic disease or of one of the classic syndromes).

Causes of a short adult* include
Genetic
Familial (correlation between a patient's height and the mid-parental height of the parents)

Achondroplasia (?short limbs, relatively normal trunk, large head with bulging forehead and scooped nose)

*Turner's syndrome** (?webbed neck, cubitus valgus, short metacarpals, female phenotype, left-sided heart lesions—p. 352)

Noonan's syndrome (?triangular micrognathic facial appearance and posteriorly angulated low-set ears with a thick helix, webbed neck, shield-like chest, pectus excavatum, cubitus valgus, mental retardation, right-sided cardiovascular abnormalities—Fig. 3.150c, p. 353).

* The diagnoses in italics represent causes of short stature in adults that our surveys have shown have occurred in the MRCP with the short stature highlighted as a prominent feature. Short stature is a subject more commonly considered in childhood. Shortness which is out of keeping with parental height (familial) can usefully be considered as follows:

1 Child looks normal
(a) *Normal growth velocity*: constitutional delay in growth and adolescence (common; short throughout childhood; pubertal growth spurt delayed; bone age lags behind chronological age; patients usually attain normal height)
(b) *Low growth velocity*:

   Thin child (mostly due to a disease of a major system)
   Central nervous system (mental retardation)
   Cardiovascular system (congenital heart disease)
   Respiratory system (cystic fibrosis, asthma, tuberculosis)
   Gastrointestinal system (malabsorption, e.g. coeliacs, Crohn's)
   Renal system (chronic renal failure, renal tubular acidosis)

   Psychosocial problems (emotional deprivation; anorexia nervosa).

   Fat child (endocrine causes)
   Hypopituitarism
   Growth hormone deficiency
   Laron's syndrome (same phenotype as growth hormone deficiency but cause is somatomedin deficiency—resting growth hormone levels high; no response to growth hormone therapy)
   Hypothyroidism
   Cushing's
   Pseudohypoparathyroidism.

2 Child looks abnormal
(a) *Dysmorphic features*: recognizable syndrome (e.g. low birth weight, chromosomal abnormality)
(b) *Disproportionate short stature*
Short limbs (e.g. achondroplasia, hypochondroplasia, dyschondrosteosis, metaphyseal chondroplasia, multiple epiphyseal dysplasia)
Short back and limbs (e.g. metatrophic dwarf, spondyloepiphyseal dysplasia, mucopolysaccharidosis).

Nutritional or general diseases during childhood

Low birth weight and subsequent slow growth (some cases end up as short adults)

Congenital heart disease (?cyanosis, young adult)

Renal disease

Cystic fibrosis* (?clubbing, cyanosis, basal crackles, sputum pot, young person, p. 411)

Chronic infection

Collagenosis

Mental retardation

Coeliac disease

Rickets* (?lateral bowing of legs which is symmetrical, p. 393)

Diabetes.

Social

Severe emotional deprivation suppresses growth hormone release.

Endocrine problems during childhood

Isolated growth hormone deficiency

Panhypopituitarism

Hypothyroidism

Cushing's

Precocious puberty

Pseudohypoparathyroidism* (?round face, short neck, short metacarpals, decreased intelligence, subcutaneous calcifications, see also p. 362).

155 / Pseudohypoparathyroidism

Frequency in survey: 0.5% of attempts at MRCP short cases.

Record

The patient is *short* and *obese* with a *round* face (with frontal bossing of the skull) and a short neck. There is *shortening of the* (most often) fourth and fifth *metacarpals* (ask the patient to make a fist to demonstrate this) and, may be, metatarsals, as well as shortening and broadening of the distal phalanges. There are *subcutaneous calcifications.**

These features suggest the diagnosis of type 1a pseudohypoparathyroidism (Albright's† hereditary osteodystrophy).

Other features which may occur in Albright's hereditary osteodystrophy

Mental retardation (usually slight)
Hypothyroidism (without goitre)
Hypogonadism
Pseudopseudohypoparathyroidism‡ in first-degree relatives
Females affected twice as commonly as males
Parathyroid glands normal or hyperplastic
Usually presents early in life (mental deficiency, epilepsy or tetany)
Treatment is with vitamin D.

In pseudohypoparathyroidism there is target organ resistance to the action of parathyroid hormone. The defect occurs proximal to the formation of the second messenger, cyclic adenosine monophosphate (cAMP).§

Types of pseudohypoparathyroidism

Type 1a — appearance as described in the above *record*. Deficiency in the Gs protein that couples parathyroid hormone receptors to adenylcyclase, limits the normal cAMP production in response to parathyroid hormone as well as to other hormones such as TSH. As a result patients with type 1a pseudohypoparathyroidism have many abnormalities (e.g. *hypothyroidism, hypogonadism*)

as well as hypocalcaemia. The causative mutations in the gene encoding the Gs protein are inherited as *autosomal dominant*

Type 1b—appearance is normal. Gs protein normal —resistance limited to parathyroid hormone. A defective parathyroid hormone receptor is the postulated cause. Osteitis fibrosa cystica can occur in some subjects suggesting selective renal (but not skeletal) resistance to parathyroid hormone action; this *rare* combination has been called *pseudohypohyperparathyroidism*.

Other causes of hypoparathyroidism

Autoimmune (there may be an associated endocrine deficiency, most frequently Addison's disease, as

---

* Ectopic deposits of bone may develop in muscles, tendons, connective tissue and skin.
† Albright described pseudohypoparathyroidism as the first example of a hormone resistance disorder.
‡ Physical features of Albright's osteodystrophy without evidence of hormone resistance.

§ The diagnosis is suggested by the finding of an *elevated* parathyroid hormone in a patient with hypocalcaemia, hyperphosphataemia and normal renal function. Lack of urinary cAMP excretion in response to parathyroid hormone (commercially available 1–34 peptide) infusion confirms the parathyroid hormone resistance.

well as a T-cell defect predisposing to mucocutaneous candidiasis (p. 280); alopecia and vitiligo
may also be seen)
Surgical (incidence varies widely as a function of the
skill of the surgeon)
Iron deposition in parathyroids (e.g. repeated transfusions in thalassaemia)
Copper deposition in parathyroids (Wilson's
disease)
Failure of development of parathyroids (Di George
syndrome)

Idiopathic (inherited mutations in the parathyroid
hormone gene that prevent synthesis and secretion of parathyroid hormone)
Transient (hypomagnesaemia; transient suppression of normal parathyroids by a hyperparathy-
roid adenoma;‖ surgical injury to the parathyroids
is another postulated cause of transient postoper-
ative hypoparathyroidism).

‖ Though within a week the suppressed parathyroids should
be functioning again, the major cause of hypocalcaemia
following hyperparathyroidectomy is 'bone hunger'—with
removal of the high parathyroid hormone levels, the skeleton
rapidly takes in calcium. It may take weeks for the skeleton to
recover fully.

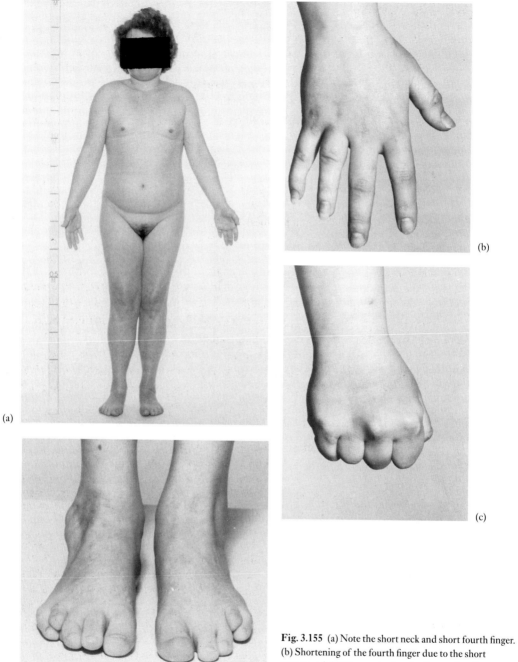

(a)

(b)

(c)

(d)

Fig. 3.155 (a) Note the short neck and short fourth finger.
(b) Shortening of the fourth finger due to the short
metacarpal. (c) Demonstrating the shorter fourth metacarpal.
(d) Short fourth toes due to the shorter metatarsals.

Frequency in survey: 0.5% of attempts at MRCP short cases.

Survey note: mostly Kaposi's sarcoma but cytomegalovirus choroidoretinitis occurred at least once.

Record 1

There are (may be numerous or solitary; may be firm, may be compressible) reddy-purple and bluish-brown macules, plaques and nodules (may appear initially as a dusky stain, especially about the toes).

The lesions are suggestive of Kaposi's sarcoma.

Record 2

The fundi show discrete areas of *white or yellow retinal opacification* with associated *haemorrhage* and *vascular sheathing* (the appearance resembles branch retinal vein occlusion—p. 203, but is distinguished because one eye often has multiple foci, and there is a tendency for both eyes to be affected).

The appearance (*'scrambled egg and tomato sauce'* and *'cottage cheese and jam'* are both terms that have been used to describe the typical appearance) is suggestive of cytomegalovirus choroidoretinitis in an *immunosuppressed patient*. The diagnosis could be substantiated by culture of throat and urine.

Kaposi's sarcoma classically occurs in four major clinical settings:
1 African Kaposi's (extremities)
2 Elderly Jewish or Mediterranean males (purplish on distal extremities; indolent course on distal extremities)
3 Immunodeficiency conditions (widespread, reddish-purple papules; rapidly progressive; may regress if immunosuppression discontinued)
4 AIDS (reddy-brown; wide distribution).

Features of Kaposi's sarcoma

May also occur in the viscera

May infiltrate the lymphatics of the leg leading to chronic oedema

Associated with cytomegalovirus on electron microscopy

May complicate treatment with immunosuppression for SLE or renal transplant

Especially affects homosexual men (most commonly fourth decade): smaller lesions than non-AIDS Kaposi's. May affect viscera first.

Natural history of HIV infection
Primary infection

Leads to transient fall in CD4$^+$ cells and may lead to opportunistic infection (usually oesophageal candidiasis) and an increase in cytotoxic CD8$^+$ T lymphocytes

Self-limiting (2–4 weeks), febrile myalgic illness often associated with oral and oesophageal ulceration, a maculopapular rash on the trunk and elsewhere, generalized lymphadenopathy (CD8$^+$ lymphocytes), 'aseptic meningitis-like' picture; conventional HIV antibody tests positive 2–6 weeks after onset of illness

Seroconversion at median of 2 months after exposure, 6 months in over 95%

At least 50% progress to severe immunodeficiency over a variable period—on average 10 years

After infection, despite immune response which results in approximately 1000-fold decrease in the amount of HIV, a slow but relentless destruction of CD4+ T lymphocytes occurs rendering the patient susceptible to opportunistic infections.

Early HIV disease (asymptomatic phase)

Attacks usually mild: generalized lymphadenopathy (B lymphocytes), irregular and unpredictable fevers, hypersensitivity reactions, reactivation or worsening of eczema, psoriasis or folliculitis. Polyclonal hypergammopathy (IgG, IgA) usual. CD8+ titre elevated; CD4+ normal. Less common features: thrombocytopaenia; vasculitis.

Intermediate stage (AIDS related complex)

Number of CD4+ lymphocytes starts to fall;* delayed type hypersensitivity to common antigens (*Trichophyton*, mumps, *Candida*, tetanus, tuberculin) lost

Increased susceptibility to pathogens not usually considered opportunistic (e.g. *Pneumococcus*, *Shigella*, *Salmonella*, *Haemophilus*) with more serious illness

Increased vaginal thrush, pelvic inflammatory disease, and cervical intraepithelial neoplasia (due to human papillomavirus infection)

Shingles more common

Kaposi's sarcoma at this stage or later.

Late phase HIV infection

Fall in CD4+ lymphocytes,* sometimes to zero, leads to profound immunodeficiency. CD8+ lymphocytes start to fall. Oral thrush common. Significant opportunistic infections depending on level of CD4+ count:

CD4+ level <300 cells μl^{-1}—reactivation of tuberculosis and syphilis

CD4+ level <200 cells μl^{-1} — Pneumocystis carinii pneumonia, cerebral toxoplasmosis, fungal infections (including cryptococcal meningitis)

CD4+ level <100 cells μl^{-1}—Mycobacterium avium

CD4+ level <50 cells μl^{-1}—cytomegalovirus retinitis, gastrointestinal disease.

In late phase HIV infection, direct HIV central nervous system involvement may occur (dementia, myelopathy); Kaposi's may be extensive and aggressive; high grade B-cell lymphomata are more likely to occur.

For colour photograph see p. 530.

---

*CD4+ count gives the most consistent predictive measure of the risk of progression. CD4+ < 250 cells μl^{-1} or CD4+ : CD8+ ratio < 0.3 indicates 2 : 3 chance of progression to AIDS in the next 2 years. Oral thrush and serum HIV p24 antigen are also predictors of progression.

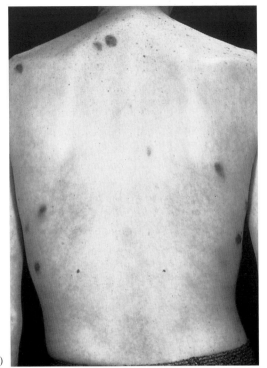

(a)

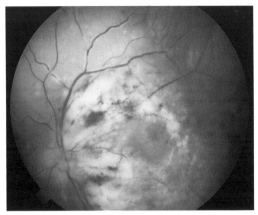

(b)

Fig. 3.156 (a) Kaposi's sarcoma. (b) Cytomegalovirus retinitis—'scrambled egg and tomato sauce'.

157 / Porphyria

Frequency in survey: 0.5% of attempts at MRCP short cases.

Survey note: only variegate porphyria and porphyria cutanea tarda have been reported as short cases in our surveys.

Record 1

There is *muscular weakness* in the upper and lower limbs particularly in the *proximal* groups. The *tendon reflexes* are *absent* (or diminished) and the plantars are flexor (or unresponsive). There are no sensory changes. The backs of the hands show *crusts*, *scarring*, areas of *fragility of the skin* and *blisters*.

These features suggest a diagnosis of variegate porphyria.*

Record 2

The skin on the backs of the hands shows *thin* and *traumatized areas*, *vesicles* and *bullae*, *crusts* and *scarring* and a few (say how many) *pearly white* to *yellow*, *subepidermal nodules* or *milia*, 1–5 mm in diameter, particularly over the knuckles. There are areas of hyperpigmentation with some patches of hypopigmentation, periorbital suffusion and *hypertrichosis* over the temples and cheeks. There is one crusted lesion on the pinna of the ear, presumably a remnant of a bulla.

The features of *cutaneous fragility*, *photosensitivity* and *bullous lesions* suggest a diagnosis of porphyria (possibly porphyria cutanea tarda†), though one has also to consider the possibility of a pseudoporphyria.‡ A complete clinical assessment and laboratory investigations are necessary for a more specific diagnosis.

Acute intermittent porphyria (the skin is not affected), *variegate porphyria** and *hereditary coproporphyria* (very rare) all exhibit acute episodes the clinical features of which may be abdominal pain, vomiting and constipation; peripheral neuropathy with weakness or paralysis; confusion and psychosis; tachycardia and hypertension.

Drugs and chemicals associated with the clinical

* *Variegate porphyria* has both the cutaneous changes of porphyria cutanea tarda and the systemic features of acute intermittent porphyria. The latter does not show photosensitivity or have any cutaneous changes.

† Virtually all patients with porphyria cutanea tarda have *excessive body iron stores* manifested as *increased serum iron and ferritin*. They excrete increased amounts of porphyrin into the urine, which can be demonstrated with a Wood's lamp as pinkish-red fluorescence. Freshly voided urine may look orange–red. A quick way to demonstrate orange–red fluorescence is by adding a few drops of 10% hydrochloric acid or acetic acid to the urine sample. A rapid screening test demonstrating excess porphobilinogen (PBG) in the urine can be done to diagnose acute intermittent porphyria. Freshly voided urine should be *exposed to sunlight* for several hours and a *deep red colour develops* which suggests that there is some excess PBG. Alternatively, a *few drops* of freshly voided *urine* are added to *2 ml* of *Ehrlich's reagent* and the urine forms a *cherry-red* colour suggesting the presence of PBG.

‡ The term *pseudoporphyria* is applied when patients clinically exhibit cutaneous manifestations of porphyria cutanea tarda without the characteristic abnormal porphyrin profile. The disorder may develop in association with certain drugs (frusemide, tetracycline, naproxen and pyridoxine), diabetes mellitus, and chronic renal failure on maintenance haemodialysis. In the initial stages the porphyrin levels in the urine, faeces and plasma may be normal in the last condition, but some studies have reported true porphyria cutanea tarda with excess porphyrins in dialysed patients.

expression of acute hepatic porphyria are ethyl alcohol, oestrogen hormones, hexachlorobenzene, chlorinated phenols, iron, etc. There is a long list of potentially hazardous drugs including barbiturates, carbamazepine, amphetamines, chloroquine, danazol, ethosuximide, frusemide, methyldopa, sulphonamides, rifampicin, hydralazine and valporic acid.

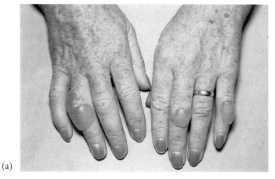 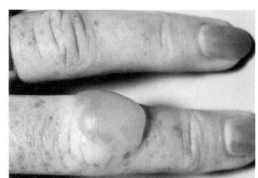

(a)   (b)

Fig. 3.157 (a,b) Porphyria cutanea tarda.

158 / Lupus vulgaris

Frequency in survey: 0.5% of attempts at MRCP short cases.

Record

There is a *reddish-brown flat plaque* with irregular edges of about 5 × 7 cm on the R/L side of the face.* The appearance is smooth (may be hyperkeratotic in later stages) and glistening but there is *fine scaling* over the middle (look for this). The *consistency is soft*† and there is some *scarring* (say where).

The characteristic appearance of this plaque with scarring and its soft consistency support the diagnosis of lupus vulgaris.‡

Lupus vulgaris is a progressive form of cutaneous tuberculosis occurring in a person with a moderate or high degree of immunity. A cool, moist dull climate (as in Northern Europe) seems to favour its development, but nowadays it is rare in Europe and the USA. Lupus vulgaris is disproportionately uncommon in Eastern countries where other forms of tuberculosis are frequently seen. Its clinical presentation falls into five general patterns:

Plaque form — starts as a tiny reddish-brown, flat plaque and extends gradually with little or no scarring. There may be excessive scaling which gives it a psoriasiform appearance. The edges often become thickened and hyperkeratotic

Ulcerative form — scarring and ulceration with crusts over the areas of necrosis are the major features of this type. The lesion erodes into deep tissues and cartilages producing deformities and contractures

Vegetating forms — ulcerates, sometimes quite rapidly, producing necrosis but there is minimal scarring. Mucous membranes may be invaded. Response to chemotherapy is excellent

Tumour-like forms — these lesions are deeply infiltrating and stand out over the surface of the skin as a group of soft, smooth nodules. Scaling and scarring are absent. In the 'myxomatous' form, large soft tumours occur, mostly on the ear lobes which become enlarged. The response to treatment may be poor

Papular and nodular forms — this is often the disseminated variety and multiple papular and nodular lesions may occur on the body ('miliary lupus'). The papulonodular lesions may be confined to the face and resemble acne.

Treatment

Standard antituberculous therapy should be given.

---

* The lesion commonly appears on normal skin of the head and neck in about 80% of the cases in Europe. The face, particularly around the nose, is the area of predilection. The arms and legs are sometimes involved but the trunk is often spared. In India the face is affected less frequently than the buttocks and trunk.

† The lesions of lupus vulgaris are soft and this, together with the associated scarring, is the main feature that distinguishes it from the lupus pernio of sarcoidosis. If the lesion is probed, the instrument breaks through the overlying epidermis. Diascopy (i.e. looking at a glass slide pressed against the lesion) reveals an '*apple-jelly*' (yellowish-brown) colour of the infiltrate.

‡ In the early stage (i.e. a small plaque/nodule on the face), lupus vulgaris may be confused with lymphocytoma, lupus pernio†, juvenile melanoma, lupus erythematosus and a 'port-wine' stain. Of these lupus pernio and lymphocytoma are the two conditions which may have solitary lesions on the face without any other manifestations and may present a diagnostic problem. Lymphocytoma cutis is often a red, even violaceous, nodule with an indurated centre. Lupus pernio (p. 224) is usually a purple-red induration of the skin. On diascopy these lesions look a pale, brownish-red colour.

Despite long periods of indolence, the natural course of an untreated lesion is inexorably progressive. The older the patient, the more rapid is the spread of the lesion. Spontaneous resolution may occur but leaves contractures, scars and mutilation.

For colour photograph see p. 534.

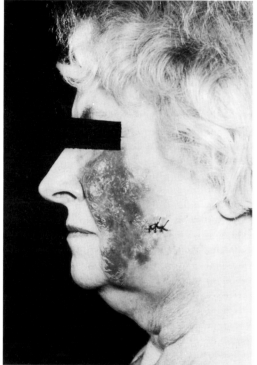

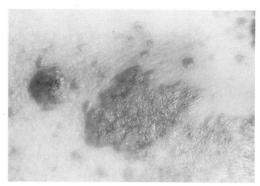

(a)

(b)

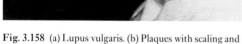

Fig. 3.158 (a) Lupus vulgaris. (b) Plaques with scaling and irregular edges.

159 / Cannon waves

Frequency in survey: 0.5% of attempts at MRCP short cases.

Survey note: one candidate was asked to examine the heart only, another was asked to look at the patient's neck and then examine the heart, and a third was asked to take the patient's pulse.

Record

There are sharp *a* waves* (cannon waves*) visible in this patient's jugular veins. (Feel the carotid pulse on the opposite side). These waves occur irregularly even though the pulse is regular but slow at 48 beats min^{-1}.

As the waves are irregular and the pulse is slow the explanation is that this patient has complete heart block. (The patient may have a demand pace-maker and it will be felt as a solid, mobile mass below the right clavicle. He/she may have been admitted for changing the defunct unit).

If allowed to auscultate you will hear an S1 of variable intensity; the sound coinciding with the cannon wave will be soft.

Causes of cannon waves

Regular cannon waves — nodal rhythm, paroxysmal nodal tachycardia, partial heart block with very long PR interval

Irregular cannon waves — complete heart block, multiple ectopic beats.

---

* Candidates who have never seen cannon waves have been known to confuse them with giant *v* waves (p. 214). Cannon waves are seen like sharp flicks and are quite characteristic in appearance. You should attempt to see some in the pace-maker clinic of a cardiology unit. Cannon waves are giant *a* waves and these occur whenever the right atrium contracts against a closed tricuspid valve, and the whole of the energy released by the right atrial contraction is transmitted to the JVP, as forward flow is impossible (the ECG complex associated with a cannon wave shows that the P wave falls between the end of the QRS and the T wave or at the end of the T wave).

160 / Polycythaemia rubra vera

Frequency in survey: 0.5% of attempts at MRCP short cases.

Record

This patient has *facial plethora* and a *dusky cyanosis* of the face, hands, feet and (look at the lips and ask the patient to protrude his/her tongue) mucous membranes. There are (may be) ecchymoses (spontaneous bruising) and *scratch marks* (pruritus). (Ask the patient's permission to gently pull down the lower eyelids.) The conjunctival vessels are markedly engorged. (If allowed, look at the fundi for markedly dilated retinal veins, and ask to feel the abdomen for splenomegaly* and to take the blood pressure which may be raised.)

These features suggest a diagnosis of polycythaemia rubra vera.

The characteristic laboratory findings reveal the consequences of increased bone marrow activity. Typically, the red cell, white cell and platelet counts are elevated. The haemoglobin and the haematocrit are raised. The mean corpuscular volume is reduced suggestive of iron deficiency erythropoiesis. Being a primarily malignant disorder, red cell proliferation continues until the iron stores are exhausted giving an iron deficiency picture with a high haemoglobin level.

Causes of secondary polycythaemia
Physiologically appropriate increased erythropoietin production

Arterial hypoxaemia — chronic pulmonary disease, right-to-left shunt, pickwickian syndrome (p. 290), etc.

Abnormal release of oxygen from haemoglobin — congenitally decreased red cell 2,3-diphosphoglycerate (DPG), smokers—carboxyhaemoglobinaemia

Interference with tissue oxygen metabolism—cobalt poisoning.

Physiologically inappropriate erythropoietin production

Neoplasms—renal, adrenal, hepatocellular, ovarian, cerebellar, haemangioblastoma, phaeochromocytoma, etc.

Non-neoplastic renal disease—cysts, hydronephrosis.

---

* Splenomegaly occurs in over 70% of patients and hepatomegaly may be present in about 40% of patients.

161 / Asteroid hyalosis

Frequency in survey: 0.4% of attempts at MRCP short cases.

Record

With the ophthalmoscope focused in front of the retina, the vitreous is seen to be filled with a *myriad* of *tiny*, *white*, discrete, shiny *opacities*, like a galaxy of stars. The diagnosis is asteroid hyalosis.

Asteroid hyalosis is usually diagnosed in patients aged between 60 and 65 years. It may be more common in males. It is *unilateral* in the majority of patients. Biomicroscopically there are *white* bodies of *oval* shape and varying size that are adherent to the framework of the vitreous gel. The opacities consist mainly of *calcium soaps*. Visual function is not disturbed and patients are unaware of the bodies which may be scattered throughout the entire vitreous cavity or may be accumulated in one part of it. Although it has been suggested by some authors that this condition is related to diabetes (approximately 30% of patients with asteroid hyalosis have diabetes), it is now generally agreed that the two are probably not connected. It probably reflects the fact that diabetic patients have their eyes looked into

more than others. It has also been suggested that the incidence of hypercholesterolaemia is higher and that of posterior vitreous detachment lower than expected for the age group concerned.

Synchysis scintillans appears to be rarer than asteroid hyalosis. Most descriptions relate it to injury or inflammation involving the vitreous cavity. In contrast to asteroid hyalosis it is usually *bilateral* and the opacities, which are *cholesterol crystals*, appear more *golden*. The opacities do not appear to be attached to the collagen fibrils and float freely in the vitreous fluid with ocular motion; they settle together at the bottom of the vitreous when the eye ceases to move. They have a *flat*, *angular*, *crystalline* appearance in contrast to the white spheres of asteroid hyalosis.

162 / Pernicious anaemia

Frequency in survey: 0.4% of attempts at MRCP short cases.

Record

The patient has *pallor* (may be a pale lemon yellow tinge), a *smooth tongue** and *angular stomatitis.** *Vitiligo*† is (may be) present.

The likely diagnosis is pernicious anaemia (splenomegaly and pyrexia‡ may both occur).

Other general clinical features of megaloblastic anaemias*

Gastrointestinal symptoms
Weight loss
Hyperpigmentation
Infertility
Orthostatic hypotension.

Haematological abnormalities associated with megaloblastic anaemias*

Anaemia
Reticulocytopenia
Macrocytosis
Neutropenia
Thrombocytopenia
Neutrophil hypersegmentation
Poikilocytosis
Anisocytosis
Raised lactate dehydrogenase
Raised bilirubin
Raised serum iron
Decreased haptoglobin
Hypercellular bone marrow with megaloblastic morphology, giant bands and metamyelocytes.

Neuropsychiatric abnormalities associated with vitamin B_{12} deficiency

(See also p. 314)
Paraesthesiae
Peripheral neuropathy (absent ankle jerks; impaired touch and pain perception; impaired vibration sense and joint position sense (may be Romberg's positive) may also be due to dorsal column involvement)
Ataxia (posterior column involvement; ?joint position sense; ?Romberg's)
Decreased reflexes (peripheral neuropathy—pp. 134 and 314)
Increased reflexes (pyramidal tract involvement — pp. 102 and 314)
Spasticity (pyramidal tract involvement)
Weakness
Dementia (memory loss, disorientation, obtundation)
Incontinence (urinary or faecal)
Impotence
Optic atrophy
Abnormal smell or taste
Lhermitte's phenomenon (p. 314)

---

* Most patients with folate or vitamin B_{12} deficiency do not have many of the features listed. Even anaemia and raised mean corpuscular volume may be absent in a patient with otherwise severe folate or vitamin B_{12} deficiency; in one prospective study of patients with vitamin B_{12} deficiency, 44% did not have anaemia, 36% had a mean corpuscular volume equal to or less than 100, 86% had a normal white cell count, 79% a normal platelet count, 33% had a normal peripheral blood film, 43% had a normal lactate dehydrogenase and 83% a normal bilirubin.

† The cutaneous marker of organ-specific autoimmune diseases (p. 114) creates the suspicion of Addisonian pernicious anaemia rather than any other cause of megaloblastic anaemia leading to pallor and a smooth tongue.
‡ Why were you not previously aware that untreated pernicious anaemia may be associated with fever? Perhaps it should be called *hypo-cyanocobalimic fever?*—see Appendix 5, p. 525.

Psychiatric abnormalities (depression, paranoia, listlessness, acute confusional state, hallucinations, delusions, insomnia, apprehensiveness, psychosis, slow mentation, paraphrenia, mania, panic attacks, suicide).

Causes of megaloblastic anaemia
Vitamin B$_{12}$ deficiency
Decreased ingestion (poor diet, lack of animal products, strict vegetarianism)

Impaired absorption

(a) failure of release of B$_{12}$ from food protein (old age; partial gastrectomy)

(b) intrinsic factor deficiency (pernicious anaemia; total gastrectomy; destruction of gastric mucosa by caustics; congenital abnormality or absence of intrinsic factor)

(c) chronic pancreatic disease

(d) competitive parasites (bacteria in bowel diverticula, blind loops, fish tapeworm)

(e) intrinsic intestinal disease (ileal resection, Crohn's disease, radiation ileitis; tropical sprue, coeliac disease; infiltrative intestinal disease such as lymphoma or scleroderma; drug-induced malabsorption; congenital selective malabsorption — Imerslund–Grasbeck syndrome)

Impaired utilization (congenital enzyme deficiencies; lack of transcobalamin II; nitrous oxide administration).

Folate deficiency
Decreased ingestion (poor diet, lack of vegetables; alcoholism; infancy)

Impaired absorption (intestinal short circuits; tropical sprue, coeliac disease; drugs such as anticonvulsants and sulphasalazine; congenital malabsorption)

Impaired utilization (folic acid antagonists such as methotrexate, triamterene, trimethroprim, pyrimethamine, ethanol; congenital enzyme deficiencies)

Increased requirement (pregnancy, infancy, hyperthyroidism, chronic haemolytic disease, neoplastic disease, exfoliative skin disease)

Increased loss (haemodialysis).

Drugs—metabolic inhibitors
Purine synthesis (methotrexate, 6-mercaptopurine, 6-thioguanine, azathioprine)

Pyrimidine synthesis (methotrexate, 5-fluorouracil)

Deoxyribonucleotide synthesis (hydroxyurea, cytosine arabinoside).

Miscellaneous
Inborn errors (e.g. Lesch–Nyhan syndrome, hereditary orotic aciduria)

Unexplained disorders (pyridoxine responsive megaloblastic anaemia, thiamine responsive megaloblastic anaemia, some cases of myelodysplastic syndrome, some cases of acute myelogenous leukaemia)

163 / Dermatitis herpetiformis

Frequency in survey: 0.3% of attempts at MRCP short cases.

Record

This middle-aged (or elderly) patient has *groups* of *erythematous papules* and *excoriations* on the *elbows, knees, buttocks, scalp, upper back* and at *pressure points* (very occasionally it is generalized). There are (may be) *vesicles* which have (usually) a raised, reddened background (vesicles may be present but have usually been ruptured by scratching—the lesions are intensely *pruritic*).

The diagnosis is dermatitis herpetiformis and this is nearly always associated with a gluten-sensitive enteropathy* (*coeliac disease*).

Male to female ratio is 2:1.
About 85% of patients are HLA-B8/DRw3.

Dermatitis herpetiformis can occur at any stage of adult life (rare in childhood). Once developed it is persistent. It is treated with a gluten-free diet and/or dapsone (side-effects include rashes, haemolysis and agranulocytosis). The differential diagnosis is from pemphigus, pemphigoid and other bullous disorders (p. 300) and from scabies. Involve-ment of the oral mucosa is uncommon. There may be a higher incidence of developing malignancies than in the general population.

Histology — subepidermal blister with micro-abscesses at dermal papillae.

Direct immunofluorescence (diagnostic) — IgA deposit at basement membrane (dermal papillae).

For colour photograph see p. 537.

---

* There may not be overt symptoms of malabsorption.

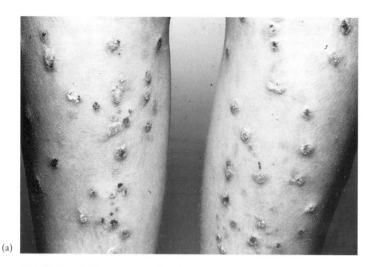

(a)

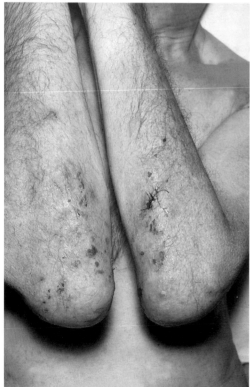

(b)

Fig. 3.163 (a) Dermatitis herpetiformis. (b) Grouped lesions.

164 / Urticaria pigmentosa (mastocytosis)

Frequency in survey: 0.3% of attempts at MRCP short cases.

Record

There are *multiple*, small, discrete, round (or oval), reddish-brown (or yellowish-brown) *pigmented macules* (and/or papules). After *friction, urticarial weals* develop (due to histamine release from the mast cells—*Darier's sign*).

The diagnosis is urticaria pigmentosa.

The adult variety is thought to be a form of reticulosis. If involvement is extensive, a hot bath followed by vigorous drying may lead to flushing, hypotension, bronchospasm and diarrhoea. In a minority, systemic involvement may occur with involvement of the liver, spleen and bone marrow. Bowel involvement may lead to malabsorption. A small percentage of patients develop leukaemia which can be, but is not usually, mast cell leukaemia.

For colour photographs see p. 539.

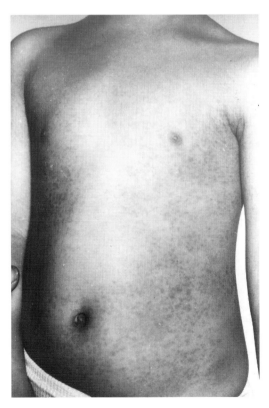

Fig. 3.164 Discrete pigmented macules.

165 / Pneumothorax

Frequency in survey: 0.3% of attempts at MRCP short cases.

Record

The R/L *side* of the chest (of this tall, thin, young adult male — old patients are usually bronchitic) *expands poorly* compared with the other side. Though the *percussion note* on the R/L side is *hyper-resonant*, the tactile fremitus, vocal resonance and *breath sounds* are all *diminished* (large pneumothorax of one side may push the *trachea* and apex beat to the opposite side).

These findings suggest a pneumothorax of the R/L side.

Male to female ratio is 6:1.

A 'crunching' sound in keeping with the heart beat may be heard when the pneumothorax is small.

Treatment is not required in a healthy individual with a small pneumothorax (i.e. if only a quarter of one side is affected). Drainage is indicated for:

Larger pneumothorax associated with dyspnoea, increasing in size or not resolving after 1 week

Tension pneumothorax

Pneumothorax complicating underlying severe chronic bronchitis with emphysema

Pneumothorax exacerbating acute severe asthma (hence chest X-ray mandatory in acute severe asthma).

When drainage is indicated, simple aspiration (with a plastic cannula, syringe and three-way tap so that aspirated air can be voided) should usually be attempted before resorting to intercostal drainage via a tube attached to an underwater seal. Tension pneumothorax should be released urgently by stabbing an intravenous cannula through the chest wall at the second intercostal space, mid-clavicular line, pending the insertion of an intercostal drain.

Recurrent spontaneous pneumothorax is treated by obliteration of the pleural space (pleurectomy; application of irritating substances into the pleural cavity; scarification of the pleura followed by intrapleural suction).

Causes of pneumothorax

Traumatic

Penetrating chest wounds

Iatrogenic (chest aspiration, intercostal nerve block, subclavian cannulation, transbronchial biopsy, needle aspiration lung biopsy, positive pressure ventilation)

Chest compression injury (including external cardiac massage).

Spontaneous

Primary (a common cause in young men*)

Secondary

  chronic obstructive pulmonary disease
  asthma
  congenital cysts and bullae
  pleural malignancy
  rheumatoid lung disease (p. 73)
  bacterial pneumonia (p. 78)
  tuberculosis
  cystic fibrosis (p. 411)
  tuberous sclerosis (p. 308)
  endometriosis of the pleura
  Marfan's syndrome (p. 267)
  sarcoidosis
  histiocytosis X
  whooping cough
  oesophageal rupture
  Pneumocystis carinii pneumonia.

---

* The risk of a second pneumothorax in a young adult following first episode is of the order of 25%. After a second episode, the risk increases to the order of 50%.

Frequency in survey: main focus of a short case in 0.3% of attempts at MRCP short cases. Additional feature in a further 0.8%.

Record 1

There are (in this underweight patient who appears older than his years) *Argyll Robertson pupils* (p. 330). There is bilateral *ptosis* with *wrinkling* of the *forehead* due to compensatory overaction of the frontalis, there is loss of *vibration* and *joint position* sense, loss of *deep pain* in the Achilles tendon, hypotonia, *absent reflexes* and plantar responses; the gait is ataxic and *Romberg's* test is *positive*.

The diagnosis is *tabes dorsalis.** The patient may have *optic atrophy* (may antedate other manifestations; centre of vision may be the last to be affected) and is at risk of developing a *Charcot's* neuropathic hip, knee, or ankle joint.

Record 2

As appropriate from the above plus: the *plantars* are *extensor* (with or without other pyramidal signs and other signs of general paresis of the insane (GPI)—see below).

The diagnosis is *taboparesis*.

Other features of tabes dorsalis, though well known, are rarely seen now; features such as:

Wide-based, high, stepping gait

Zones of cutaneous analgesia with delayed perception of pain

Ligament laxity allowing extreme degrees of lower limb movement

Perforating foot ulcers

Lightening pains (a good reliable history is virtually pathognomonic and may antedate other symptoms)

Bladder insensitivity.

Other forms of neurosyphilis

GPI† (dementia which classically progresses to euphoria and delusions of grandeur though this is less common than simple dementia, epileptic fits, tremor of the hands, lips and tongue ('trombone' tremor), spastic paraparesis of cortical origin)

Meningovascular syphilis‡ (may present in a wide variety of ways including: isolated cranial nerve palsies especially IIIrd and VIth, cerebral or spinal stroke, meningism, epilepsy. Rare syndromes include meningomyelitis, pachymeningitis, acute transverse myelitis, Erb's spastic paraplegia, syphilitic amyotrophy which resembles motor neurone disease).

---

* Tabes dorsalis occurs 10–35 years after infection and the prognosis is poor. There is atrophy of the posterior nerve root and (probably secondary) degeneration of the posterior columns (lumbosacral and lower thoracic worst affected).

† GPI occurs 10–15 years after infection and the prognosis is good if it is treated before the development of cortical atrophy (initially the patient may present simply with a change of temperament, slight pupillary abnormalities and brisk reflexes). There is meningeal thickening and degeneration of the cerebral cortex (especially frontal).

‡ Meningovascular syphilis (only 3% of syphilitic patients) occurs in the first 4 years after infection and shows a good response to treatment except where cerebral or spinal cord infarction has occurred. Fibrosed meninges may nip cranial nerves and endarteritis may produce areas of ischaemic necrosis.

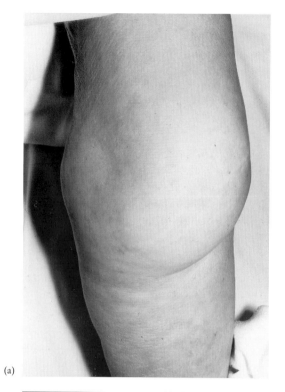

(a)

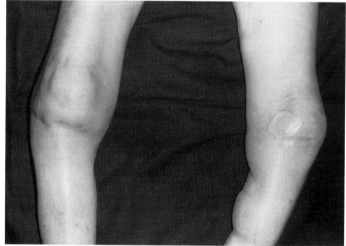

(b)

Fig. 3.166 (a,b) Charcot's knee joints.

167 / Tylosis

Frequency in survey: 0.3% of attempts at MRCP short cases.

Record

There is *diffuse, thick, yellowish hyperkeratosis* of the *palms* and (ask to see the feet) of the *soles*. The margins are delineated by a reddish line at the lateral border of the feet and at the wrist beyond which there is no hyperkeratosis. The areas are *moist* (*hyperhidrosis*) and there is (may be) evidence of dermatophyte infection.

The diagnosis is of diffuse palmoplantar keratoderma or tylosis.

Tylosis is transmitted through an autosomal dominant gene with high penetrance and occurs in all races. The condition is usually obvious by the age of 4. This is the commonest variety of hereditary palmoplantar keratoderma. Many associated disorders including *internal malignancy* (particularly of the oesophagus) have been reported, but sporadic cases occur commonly without any coexisting disorder.

For colour photograph see p. 539.

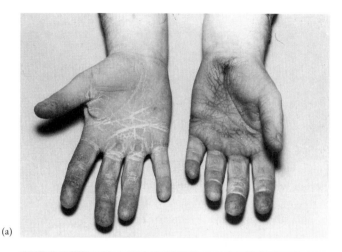

(a)

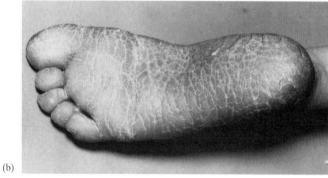

(b)

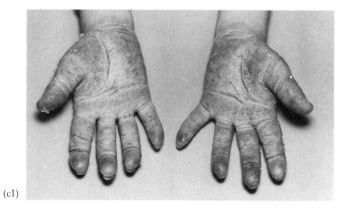

(c1)

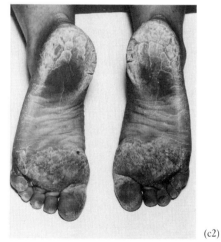

(c2)

Fig. 3.167 (a) Tylosis. (b) Tylosis—note the diffuse
hyperkeratotic areas. (c) Hyperkeratosis with secondary
fungal infection on (1) the palms and (2) the soles.

168 / Klippel–Feil syndrome

Frequency in survey: 0.3% of attempts at MRCP short cases.

Record

The patient has a *short neck*, with *limited rotation* of the head, a low hairline and a webbed neck.*

The limited rotation of the head suggests Klippel–Feil syndrome.

In Klippel–Feil syndrome the number of cervical vertebrae is reduced and two or more may be fused. This bony deformity leads to shortening of the neck, but this does not in itself cause neurological symptoms. There may, however, be neurological complications from coexisting anomalies of the central nervous system. Basilar impression and syringomyelia—p. 303—are problems which may be associated.

Other problems which may be associated

Hearing loss

Heart defects

Sprengel's deformity (upward displacement of the scapula)

Genitourinary anomalies (e.g. aplasia of the Müllerian structures).

---

* Webbing of the neck is usually associated with Turner's syndrome (short stature, increased carrying angle, shield-like chest, short metacarpals, amenorrhoea, coarctation of the aorta, p. 352) but is not pathognomonic. The limited rotation of the head is the pointer to the Klippel–Feil syndrome.

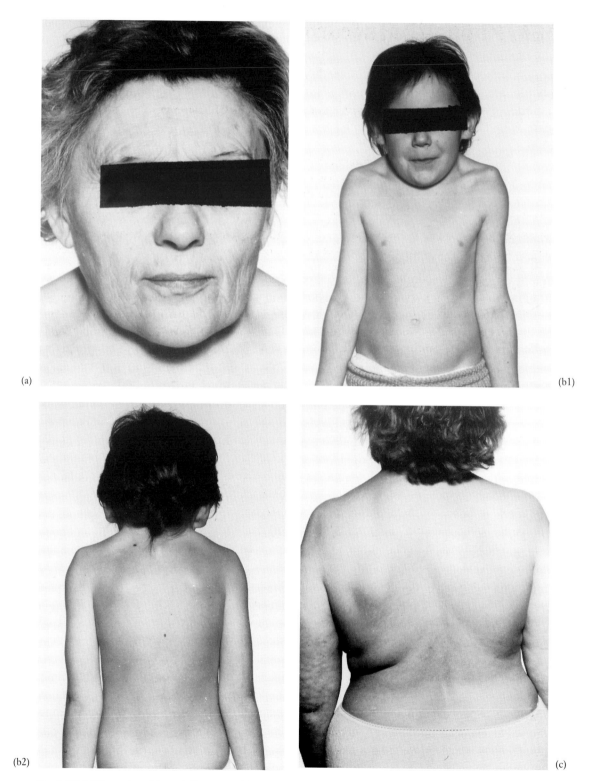

(a)

(b1)

(b2)

(c)

Fig. 3.168 (a) Shortening of the neck demonstrated by a reduced ear lobe to shoulder distance. (b) Note (1) webbed neck and (2) low hairline. (c) Scoliosis and low hairline resulting from deficiency of cervical vertebrae.

Frequency in survey: 0.3% of attempts at MRCP short cases.

Record

This *deaf* patient has a smooth, firm, symmetrical *goitre*.

In view of the combination of goitre and deafness one would have to consider the possibility of Pendred's syndrome.*

Congenital goitre (sporadic cretinism)

Goitrous infantile hypothyroidism is due to a defect in any of the steps of thyroid hormone synthesis (Fig. 3.169). Abnormalities that have been identified include defects in (i) iodide transport; (ii) organification of iodide (defect in the enzyme peroxidase); (iii) synthesis of thyroglobulin; (iv) thyroglobulin proteolysis; or (v) iodotyrosine deiodination. All the defects are rare. The most common is the *inability to organify iodine* due a defect in the enzyme peroxidase or to the synthesis of an abnormal thyroglobulin molecule. Large amounts of iodide accumulate in the thyroid and this can be demonstrated by the perchlorate discharge test. In some patients this defect is associated with an VIIIth nerve deafness and has the eponym *Pendred's syndrome*.

---

* Hearing impairment may be a manifestation of hypothyroidism *per se*, particularly in the elderly. In the adult with goitre and hypothyroidism, the hypothyroidism would be a much commoner cause of hearing impairment than Pendred's syndrome.

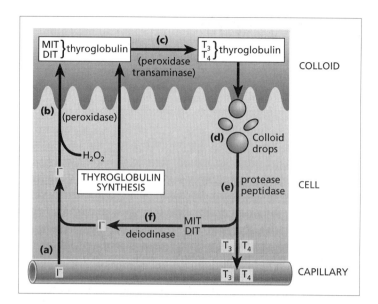

Fig. 3.169 Synthesis of thyroid hormones: inorganic iodide (I⁻) is concentrated in the thyroid follicles by active transport across the cell membrane (a) and then rapidly transferred across the cell into the colloid lumen. During this process, iodide is oxidized by peroxidase (b) and linked to tyrosine molecules to form monoiodotyrosines (MIT) and diiodotyrosines (DIT) within a large protein, thyroglobulin. These are then coupled by further enzyme action (c) to form thyroxine (T_4) and triiodothyronine (T_3) and, still linked to thyroglobulin, are reabsorbed into the follicular cells in colloid drops by endocytosis (d). T_4 and T_3 are then separated from the thyroglobulin by proteases (e) contained within lysozomes. Any uncoupled MIT and DIT are further deiodinated (f) to release tyrosine and iodide which may be available for recycling. T_4 and T_3 are then secreted into the circulation.

Frequency in survey: 0.3% of attempts at MRCP short cases.

Record

There are firm, well-demarcated round to oval papules, 0.5–1 mm in diameter, on the palms and (ask to see the feet) the soles of this patient. There are (may be) similar lesions on the trunk, face and the legs. Scattered among the papules are some macules. Both lesions are pinkish-brown, and many of the papules have some fine scaling in the centre.

The differential diagnosis lies between secondary syphilis, pityriasis rosea, a drug eruption (especially captopril), tinea versicolor, lichen planus and infectious mononucleosis.*

The characteristic maculopapular (sometimes pustular or vesicobullous) lesions with scaling and their predilection for the palms and soles favour the diagnosis of secondary syphilis.

Mucosal and other associated findings

Small, asymptomatic, flat-topped, round or oval, somewhat elevated macules and papules covered with a hyperkeratotic greyish membrane, occur on the oral or genital mucosa. There may be mucocutaneous papules (*split papules*) at the angles of the mouth. The patient may have lymphadenopathy (cervical, suboccipital, epitrochlear and axillary), splenomegaly or hepatosplenomegaly, periostitis of the long bones, diffuse pharyngitis and acute iritis. The diagnosis can be confirmed by dark-field examination and serology.

For colour photographs see p. 538.

---

* In *pityriasis rosea* there is often (about 80%) a bright red, 2–5 cm, *herald plaque*, and a fine scaling maculopapular rash is usually scattered on the trunk in a 'Christmas tree' distribution. A *drug eruption* will mimic any rash but generally tends to be distributed symmetrically over the trunk. *Tinea versicolor* is a chronic asymptomatic fungal infection of the *trunk* characterized by sharply marginated scaly macules which often take on a colour in contrast with the normal colour of the patient's skin. The flat-topped maculopapules of *lichen planus* (p. 341) may be mistaken for secondary syphilis but their predilection for the wrist and the presence of characteristic mucosal lesions should help make the diagnosis.

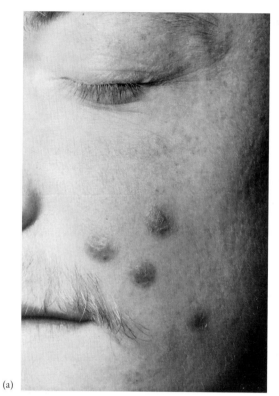
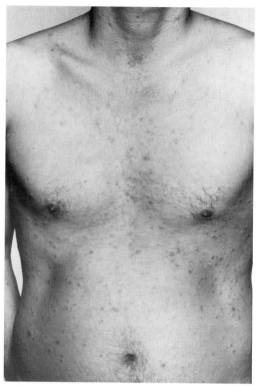

(a)

(b)

Fig. 3.170 (a) Round papules of secondary syphilis.
(b) Scattered papules and macules.

171 / Ectodermal dysplasia

Frequency in survey: 0.3% of attempts at MRCP short cases.

Record 1

The striking feature in this patient is *alopecia* with *sparse, dry, thin, spindly*, short hair. The *skin is dry* and finely wrinkled around the eyes. The nails are short, thin, ridged and brittle (ask the patient to show *his* teeth). The *incisors* and *canine teeth* are *underdeveloped, conical* and are *pointed*.

These features suggest that this patient has hypohidrotic ectodermal dysplasia.

Record 2

The *scalp hair* is *sparse, fine* and *brittle*. The eyebrows are (may be) absent. The *teeth* are *normal*. The *palms* and *soles* show diffuse *hyperkeratosis*. The *nails* are *short, thickened* and *discolored*. The *skin* feels *moist*.

The nail dystrophy and sparse hair with normal teeth and facial appearance suggest that this patient has hidrotic ectodermal dysplasia.

Ectodermal dysplasia is a congenital condition with one or more defects of hair, teeth, nails and sweating. Two main groups are identified. Hypohidrotic (or anhidrotic) ectodermal dysplasia is X-linked (over 90% of patients are males, but female carriers may show dental defects, sparse hair and reduced sweating) and characterized by partial or complete *absence* of *sweat glands, hypotrichosis* and *hypodontia*. In the complete form, the facial features are distinctive with prominent frontal ridges and chin, saddle-nose, sunken cheeks, thick lips, large ears and sparse hair. Absent or reduced sweating causes heat intolerance and affected individuals may present with unexplained fevers.

The *sweat glands* are *normal* in the other main group (hidrotic ectodermal dysplasia) which is transmitted as an autosomal dominant trait. This variety is characterized by *nail dystrophy, defects* of *the hair* and *keratoderma* of *palms* and *soles*.

For colour photograph see p. 530.

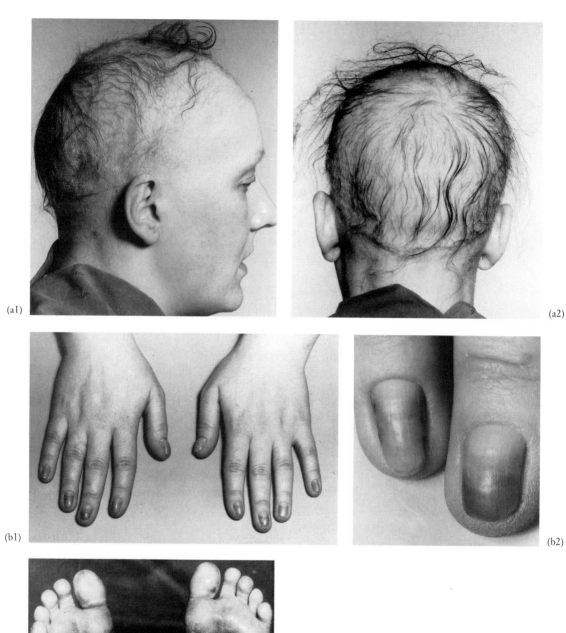

(a1)

(a2)

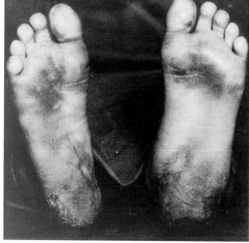

(b1)

(b2)

(c)

Fig. 3.171 (a1,2) Hydrotic ectodermal dysplasia showing alopecia with sparse, thin, spindly hair. (b1,2) Thin and excessively curved nails. (c) Diffuse hyperkeratosis.

172 / Old rickets

Frequency in survey: 0.3% of attempted MRCP short cases.

Record

The legs are *bilaterally and symmetrically curved laterally* in this *short-statured* patient. The bowing involves both the thighs (femurs) and the lower legs (tibiae). The curved areas are not warmer than the neighbouring areas, joints and feet.

The deformity is probably long standing* and the symmetrical appearance* suggests the diagnosis of old rickets. Although there are many causes of rickets and osteomalacia, the old age (may be 80 years or older) of this patient suggests that he/she may have suffered nutritional deprivation during childhood.†

Main causes of rickets and osteomalacia†

Decreased availability of vitamin D
   insufficient sunlight exposure
   low dietary intake
Malabsorption
   Billroth type II gastrectomy
   coeliac disease
   jejunoileal bypass
   regional enteritis
   pancreatic insufficiency
   biliary cirrhosis

Abnormal metabolism
   chronic renal failure
   liver disease
   X-linked hypophosphataemia
   renal tubular disorders
   anticonvulsants
   vitamin D-resistant rickets
Miscellaneous
   aluminium toxicity
   etidronate
   hypophosphatasia
   nephrotic syndrome (urinary loss)
   total parenteral nutrition.

---

* Unlike Paget's disease (p. 87) the deformity of old rickets is present from childhood. The bilateral involvement of the tibiae and the symmetrical appearance of the bowing are highly suggestive of old rickets. Bilateral Paget's disease of the legs is very rare and the deformity is very unlikely to be symmetrical.

† Bowing of the long bones results when poor exposure to sunlight and a low dietary intake of vitamin D occur during active skeletal growth, e.g. child refugees of the First and Second World Wars. Rickets with gross bony deformities is also seen in patients wtih *familial hypophosphataemia*, renal tubular disorders and in Asian immigrants of all ages.

‡ After closure of the epiphyses, vitamin D deficiency manifests as *osteomalacia*. Severe osteomalacia may present with bone pain, proximal muscle weakness, difficulty in climbing stairs and rising from chairs, and waddling gait. Pseudo-fractures (also known as Looser's zones or Milkman's fractures) on X-ray of pelvis, ribs, clavicles or lateral scapulae are pathognomonic of osteomalacia and rickets. However, osteomalacia is often diagnosed in relatively asymptomatic individuals. A raised alkaline phosphatase with low or low normal calcium should arouse suspicion. The level of vitamin D in the blood may be low, though elevation of serum parathyroid hormone level (secondary rise) is a more sensitive indicator.

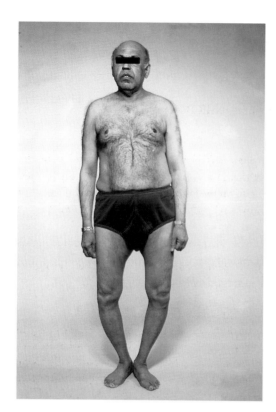

Fig. 3.172 Old rickets.

173 / Partial lipodystrophy

Frequency in survey: 0.3% of attempts at MRCP case studies.

Record

There is *loss of fat* in the *face* and *upper half* of the body.* The prominent muscles and inframaxillary dimples give the face a characteristic masculine appearance. There is (may be) hypertrophy of fat† on the lower half of the body.

This suggests the diagnosis of partial lipodystrophy, a condition which may be associated with *renal disease*.

Male to female ratio is 1:5.

Usually begins in children or young adults. A history of infection, frequently measles, has often been noted prior to onset.

Retinitis pigmentosa has been reported to occur in patients with partial lipodystrophy.

Association with renal disease

Patients with partial lipodystrophy often develop progressive mesangiocapillary glomerulonephritis and hypocomplementaemia. The prognosis depends on the severity of the renal disease.

Total lipoatrophy

Complete loss of subcutaneous fat* occurring in children or young adults. Associated with diabetes which may be difficult to treat because of extreme insulin resistance. Severe hepatic dysfunction may occur, sometimes with terminal liver failure.

---

* The lack of fat may give the appearance of emaciation, but closer inspection reveals that the muscles are not wasted, being well developed with clearly visible outlines beneath the skin. The whole appearance may give a false suggestion of virilization in females.

† The legs may be grossly fat and may give chronic discomfort.

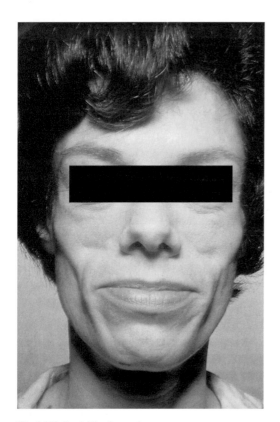

Fig. 3.173 Partial lipodystrophy.

174 / Fabry's disease

Frequency in survey: 0.3% of attempts at MRCP short cases.

Record

The *skin* is *dry* and *lax*, and there is (may be) *arthropathy* of the *terminal interphalangeal joints*. There is conjunctival injection with dilated and tortuous vessels. There are groups of *darkish-red* and *black telangiectatic macules* and *papules*, about 2–4mm in diameter, over the thigh (see p. 467) and around the umbilicus in this young man. The skin is somewhat roughened because of *hyperkeratosis*, and the *papules do not fade on pressure*.

These lesions are characteristic of the Anderson–Fabry's disease. The patient also has *superficial corneal dystrophy* (cornea verticillata) which is almost specific to this condition.*

Most cases of Fabry's disease occur in males and the female carriers are mostly symptomless. The cutaneous eruption first appears at or soon after puberty. The prognosis is usually grave with death occurring in the third or fourth decade from a *vascular accident* or *uraemia*. Patients are often mildly *hypertensive*, and there may be *varicose veins* and *stasis oedema*. *Albuminuria, haematuria* and *specific lipophages* may be seen in the urine resulting from lipid infiltration of the glomerular vessels.

Fabry's disease is also called *Anderson–Fabry's disease* and *angiokeratoma corporis diffusum*. It is a rare hereditary disorder (X-linked recessive) characterized by a *deficiency* of the *lysomal hydrolase α-galactosidase A*, resulting in the progressive deposition of uncleaved, neutral glycosphingolipids in the small blood vessels of the skin and viscera. The characteristic cutaneous eruption may be seen on the limbs, buttocks, around the umbilicus (periumbilical rosette), lower trunk and on the shaft of the penis.

For colour photograph see p. 539.

---

* Superficial corneal dystrophy is frequently present both in the affected patients as well as in female carriers. It is asymptomatic but of great diagnostic importance since the only other condition resembling it is *chloroquine keratopathy*.

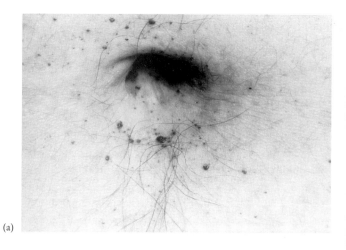
(a)

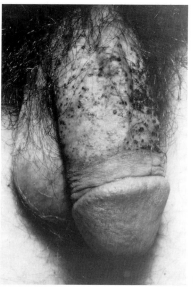
(b)

Fig. 3.174 (a) Fabry's disease. Groups of fleshy macules and papules around the umbilicus (periumbilical rosette). (b) Macules and papules with fine, keratotic crusts.

175 / Subclavian-steal syndrome

Frequency in survey: 0.3% of attempts at MRCP short cases.

Survey note: one candidate was told that the patient's arm got tired and that she felt faint whenever hanging out washing and he was asked what he would like to examine.

Record

The R/L arm (which gets easily tired on exercise) has a weaker pulse than the other side. The *tension* in the brachial artery (the ease with which the radial pulse can be obliterated by pressure in the brachial artery) is lower on the affected side and (ask to measure the blood pressure) the blood pressure is 100/70 compared with 140/80 in the normal side. There is a systolic bruit heard over the corresponding subclavian artery.

The features and the history suggest the subclavian-steal syndrome.

This rare syndrome occurs when there is stenosis of the subclavian artery near its origin, leading to a retrograde flow of blood down the ipsilateral vertebral artery, in order to supply the upper limb—subclavian steal. There is relative ischaemia of the arm during exercise. Symptoms are of cerebral ischaemia usually of vertebrobasilar insufficiency, e.g. vertigo, transient bilateral blindness, syncope, olfactory hallucination, diplopia and bilateral blurring of vision. Any combination of these symptoms may occur either spontaneously or after exercise in the affected arm.

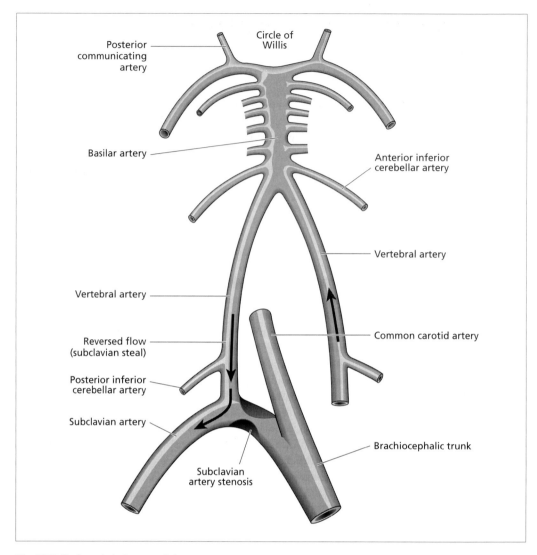

Posterior communicating artery

Circle of Willis

Basilar artery

Anterior inferior cerebellar artery

Vertebral artery

Vertebral artery

Reversed flow (subclavian steal)

Common carotid artery

Posterior inferior cerebellar artery

Subclavian artery

Brachiocephalic trunk

Subclavian artery stenosis

Fig. 3.175 Basilar–subclavian artery link.

176 / Reiter's syndrome/keratoderma blenorrhagica

Frequency in survey: 0.3% of attempts at MRCP short cases.

Record

On the *soles* of this patient's feet* and on the *palms* of his hands* there are *brownish-red macules* (early lesions), some *vesicopustules* (further developed lesions) and some crusted limpet-like masses of yellowish-brown scales (late lesions).

The appearances are those of keratoderma blenorrhagica.* If the patient has a history of *urethritis, conjunctivitis, arthritis, buccal ulceration* or *balanitis*, the combination would suggest the diagnosis of Reiter's syndrome.

The classic triad of Reiter's syndrome is urethritis, conjunctivitis and arthritis. However, it may manifest as a tetrad with the addition of buccal ulceration or balanitis to the triad; alternatively, only two of the cardinal features may be present. Classically arthropathy develops within 1 month of urethritis or *cervicitis*. However, it may follow either a dysenteric (e.g. *Shigella*) or venereal infection.

Other features which may occur

Uveitis

Balanitis may progress to *balanitis circinata* (scaling red patches evolve encircling the glans penis and within the groin)

Plantar fasciitis

Sausage-shaped digit is a typical manifestation of the arthropathy

Sacroiliitis†

Ascending spinal disease†

Plantar spurs on X-ray

Periosteal new bone formation on X-ray

Cardiac complications similar to ankylosing spondylitis as a late manifestation

HLA-B27 may predispose

Sex distribution difficult to define as the syndrome is diagnosed in women with difficulty because the urethritis and cervicitis are often clinically unapparent

Formes frustes of the syndrome (e.g. a woman with an inflammatory arthropathy of the knee, in association with HLA-B27, with or without uveitis, may have Reiter's syndrome)

High level of complement in synovial fluid (low level in rheumatoid arthritis)‡

About 80% of patients still have evidence of disease activity after 5 years.

For colour photograph see p. 541.

---

* At times Reiter's syndrome may be confused with psoriasis as pustular psoriasis on the palms and soles looks like keratodermic blenorrhagica. Psoriatic arthopathy is also a seronegative arthropathy with an HLA-B27 association. In severely affected Reiter's patients, the skin lesions may occur anywhere on the body. The toes and fingernails in Reiter's may be affected with thickening, ridging and opacity of the nails. The skin lesions of psoriasis and Reiter's are often indistinguishable clinically or histologically. In Reiter's the lesions are typically confined to the palms and soles and the presence of urethritis, iritis or conjunctivitis, balanitis,

asymptomatic lesions on the tongue and buccal mucosa, and occasionally diarrhoea should suggest the diagnosis.

† Occasionally the diagnosis of ankylosing spondylitis and Reiter's syndrome may be difficult to disentangle. The original urethritis of Reiter's may be forgotten or the patient with ankylosing spondylitis may happen to have an unrelated episode of urethritis.

‡ The high level in Reiter's reflects a non-specific inflammatory reaction whereas the low level in rheumatoid reflects immune-complex disease.

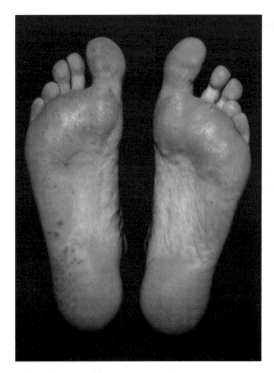

Fig. 3.176 Keratoderma blenorrhagica.

177 / Carcinoid syndrome

Frequency in survey: 0.3% of attempts at MRCP short cases.

Record

There is *cutaneous flushing*,* facial *telangiectasiae*, and the *liver* is *palpable* . . . cm below the right costal margin (may be irregular).

In view of the history of *diarrhoea*† these features are suggestive of the carcinoid syndrome.

Carcinoid tumours arise from enterochromaffin cells and are most commonly found in the appendix or rectum but these rarely give rise to the carcinoid syndrome. The actual carcinoid syndrome is produced by carcinoid tumours (usually ileal, but also from the stomach, bile duct, duodenum, pancreas, lung and gonads) which have metastasized to the liver, presumably because the metastatic tumour impedes hepatic clearance of mediators (including *serotonin (5–HT)*, bradykinin, histamine and tachykinins, as well as prostaglandins) released from the tumour. The flush is red initially but then becomes purple and commonly lasts only a few minutes but may continue for hours.* Frequent flushing may lead to telangiectasiae. During a flush the heart rate increases and the blood pressure falls.‡

Other features of carcinoid syndrome

Fibrotic lesions (probably due to chronic 5–HT excess):

Right-sided endocardial fibrosis (33% of patients; heart failure due to *pulmonary stenosis*,

tricuspid incompetence or both is less common but implies a poor prognosis)

Pleural, peritoneal and retroperitoneal fibroses

Bronchoconstriction (20% of patients; wheezing occurs during episodes of flushing and is probably not due to 5–HT)

Diagnosis confirmed by the finding of a very high urinary 5–HIAA

Somatostatin analogues and leucocyte interferon may both be beneficial in treatment.

Ectopic humoral syndromes in histological carcinoid tumours§

Cushing's syndrome (ACTH in bronchial carcinoid)

Dilutional hyponatraemia (antidiuretic hormone in bronchial carcinoid)

Gynaecomastia (hCG in gastric carcinoid)

Acromegaly (GHRH in foregut carcinoid)

Hypoglycaemia (insulin in pancreatic carcinoid).

For colour photograph see p. 534.

---

* Flushing tends to be more intense and longer lasting with bronchial carcinoids and more patchy (anywhere on the body) with gastric carcinoids. Headache commonly follows the flush. It may be precipitated by alcohol, food, stress, palpation of the liver, or it may follow administration of catecholamines, pentagastrin or reserpine. The mediator of the flush is uncertain and is probably not 5–HT. Conversely, the diarrhoea does seem to be mediated by 5–HT as it can be

reduced by inhibition of 5–HT synthesis. Nevertheless the diarrhoea is typically exacerbated during episodes of flushing.

† The examiner may mention this important fact in the history during the introductory remarks.

‡ Cf. pallor and hypertension with phaeochromocytoma.

§ Typically such patients do not have carcinoid syndrome.

Frequency in survey: 0.3% of attempts at MRCP short cases.

Record 1

The R/L leg (in this patient with normal intelligence, normal speech and no history of epilepsy) is slightly *shorter* and thinner than the L/R, its *reflexes* are *brisk* and the R/L *plantar* response is *extensor*.

These features suggest mild infantile hemiplegia affecting the R/L leg.

Record 2

There is (in this patient with epilepsy and mental retardation) marked *hypoplasia* of the R/L arm and leg, with *spasticity* and *contractures*, R/L *homonymous hemianopia* and R/L *ankle clonus* and *extensor plantar* response. There is *asymmetry of the trunk*, smaller on the R/L and diffuse impairment of sensation on the R/L. There is asymmetry of the skull, smaller on the L/R (the other side to the hemiplegia), *jaw clonus* and *spastic dysarthria* (there may be a squint, e.g. convergent on the L/R).

These features suggest severe infantile hemiplegia with spasticity affecting the R/L side.

Infantile hemiplegia results from a lesion which develops during the first year of life; only rarely is it from prenatal lesions or birth trauma. The hemiplegia may occur as a complication of an infective disorder such as pertussis, measles or scarlet fever; more commonly, however, there is no obvious predisposing cause and the hemiplegia is probably a manifestation of an encephalitis or toxic encephalopathy. There is an arrest of growth on the affected side and the hemiplegic limbs may be the site of spontaneous involuntary movements of either a choreic or athetoid character. Epilepsy is common with convulsions beginning on the affected side. The extent and severity of the hemiplegia and the degree of cerebral retardation depend on the extent of the original involvement of the cerebral cortex. In some cases the abnormality may be very slight—a smallness of a hand or foot, a thinness of a forearm or calf, a clumsiness of the fingers or contracture of the Achilles tendon. There may be just an imperceptible degree of general body asymmetry. Focal convulsions in an otherwise healthy child or adolescent should always raise the possibility of a minimal infantile hemiplegia. Only by careful scrutiny of the undressed patient as a whole will such slight asymmetry be detected.

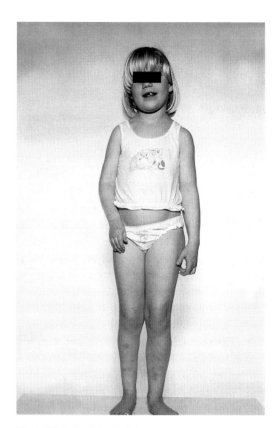

Fig. 3.178 Infantile hemiplegia. The right arm and leg are smaller than the left. The features continue into adulthood when the patient may then appear in the MRCP short cases.

179 / Pulmonary incompetence

Frequency in survey: 0.3% of attempts at MRCP short cases.

Record 1*

This patient has features of *mitral stenosis* (state them — p. 71) combined with evidence of *pulmonary hypertension* and *pulmonary incompetence* suggested by a *palpable second sound* in the pulmonary area, (*diastolic shock*) followed by an *early diastolic murmur*, which has a sharp whiffing quality, most loudly heard in the pulmonary area but radiating only for a few centimetres down the left sternal edge. There is also an early ejection systolic murmur audible over the pulmonary area.

The patient has a Graham Steell murmur complicating mitral stenosis with pulmonary hypertension.

Record 2*

This patient has *cyanosis* and a weak peripheral pulse. The JVP is *elevated* with both *a* and *v* waves being prominent. The apex beat is not palpable, but there is a strong right ventricular heave. The auscultatory signs are a *gallop of the fourth heart sound*, a *pansystolic murmur* over the tricuspid area (sometimes associated with a *thrill*), a *pulmonary ejection click*, grade 2/6 mid-systolic murmur over the pulmonary area and an *early diastolic murmur* heard over the same region. In addition she† also has ankle oedema.

These features suggest that she has *primary pulmonary hypertension* associated with pulmonary incompetence.

Record 3‡

The JVP is elevated with a large *v* wave reaching the right earlobe (there may be secondary *tricuspid incompetence*). There is a right ventricular lift but the apex beat is not palpable. There is a pansystolic murmur heard over the left third interspace and a high-pitched mid-diastolic murmur.§

The patient has pulmonary incompetence and tricuspid incompetence.

---

* The most likely scenario of a case where there is a focus on pulmonary incompetence is that of a patient who has established pulmonary hypertension and its associated features. Pulmonary hypertension results in dilatation of both the main pulmonary artery and the valve ring; the valve cusps do not close completely and a regurgitant murmur, known as the Graham Steell murmur, is produced. In some cases this becomes the focus of the examiners' attention and your record should take account of it.

† In primary pulmonary hypertension the ratio of males to females is 1 : 4.

‡ Rarely there may be a patient with a valvular pulmonary incompetence caused either by carcinoid (p. 403) involvement of the pulmonary valve or due to endocarditis (the patient may have been a drug addict). In patients with a valvular pulmonary incompetence there is unlikely to be any evidence of pulmonary hypertension. Other possible causes of valvular incompetence are congenital malformation or a previous surgical procedure.

§ The diastolic murmur of valvular pulmonary incompetence occurs after the delayed P_2 which is more like mid-diastolic than early diastolic in timing.

Causes of pulmonary hypertension

Hyperkinetic
    atrial septal defect
    ventricular septal defect
    patent ductus arteriosus
    aortopulmonary septal defect
Due to recurrent thromboembolism

Obliterative
    periarteritis nodosa
    schistosomiasis
Vasoconstrictive
    high altitude
    reactive due to mitral valve disease, left ventricular failure
    Eisenmenger group
Primary pulmonary hypertension.

Frequency in survey: 0.3% of attempts at MRCP short cases.

Survey note: some candidates were shown a pale adult of about 30 years of age and asked to examine the abdomen.

Record

This patient has *splenomegaly* (sometimes there may also be hepatomegaly), *pale skin* and conjunctivae* and *icteric sclerae.** The spleen is enlarged (say by how much) below the left costal edge (there may be a splenectomy scar† instead).

The underlying cause of this triad of jaundice, anaemia and splenomegaly may be haemolytic anaemia.‡

Causes of haemolytic anaemias

Hereditary haemolytic anaemias
  hereditary spherocytosis
  hereditary elliptocytosis
  thalassaemia
  sickle-cell anaemia
Acquired haemolytic anaemia
  acquired autoimmune haemolytic anaemia
  primary or idiopathic haemolytic anaemia

Secondary haemolytic anaemia
  lymphoproliferative disorders
  SLE
  chronic inflammatory disease (e.g. ulcerative colitis)
  drugs (e.g. methyldopa)
  infections (e.g. brucellosis, infectious mononucleosis, etc.)
  non-lymphoid neoplasms (e.g. ovarian tumours).

---

* Jaundice may be barely detectable or absent in some cases but anaemia is a regular feature of hereditary spherocytosis.
† Splenectomy is advisable in severe cases of hereditary spherocytosis and in mild cases with complications such as gallstones. Splenectomy removes a protective blood filtering bed and renders patients, especially the young ones, more vulnerable to infections. This tendency can be minimized, but not completely eliminated, by immunization with pneumococcal vaccines and careful attention to all infections.
‡ The other contender for this triad is a group of systemic conditions (e.g. infective endocarditis, SLE, pernicious anaemia, infectious mononucleosis, etc.). The absence of various stigmata of these and the presence of some of

hereditary spherocytosis (e.g. leg ulcers), the hint of a family history (autosomal dominant) from the examiner, and a relatively young age may give you enough confidence to suggest the diagnosis. However, the definitive diagnosis of this condition cannot be made without laboratory help (low mean corpuscular volume, high mean corpuscular haemoglobin concentration, spherocytosis on the blood film, increased osmotic fragility and, in most cases, a decreased spectrin content of the red cells). Anaemia, jaundice and splenomegaly are also present in other varieties of hereditary and acquired haemolytic anaemias. They may also, of course, occur together in chronic liver disease but then one would expect other diagnostic clues (p. 84).

181 / Juvenile chronic arthritis

Frequency in survey: 0.3% of attempts at MRCP short cases.

Record

This (febrile) *teenager* with painful joints (*polyserositis*) has an evanescent salmon-coloured *rash*, lymphadenopathy and hepatosplenomegaly.

These features are suggestive of Still's disease (juvenile chronic arthritis (JCA) of systemic onset).

Other features of Still's disease

Twenty per cent of patients with JCA

Rheumatoid factor and antinuclear antibodies not found

Usually a childhood disease but can begin at any age

Anaemia, leucocytosis and thrombocytosis common (can be confused with leukaemia or infection).

Other forms of JCA

Polyarticular onset

Forty per cent of patients with JCA

Female predominance

Usually seronegative* (if seropositive, HLA-DR4 common and follows a course similar to adult rheumatoid arthritis).

Pauciarticular onset

Forty per cent of patients with JCA.

Early age of onset and female preponderance

Antinuclear antibodies positive, rheumatoid factor negative

Risk of chronic iridocyclitis (prophylactic ophthalmological surveillance mandatory)

Arthritis usually resolves without deformity

HLA-DR5 and HLA-DRw8 associated.

Strong male predominance and later age of onset

Mostly HLA-DR27

Follows a course consistent with spondyloarthropathy.†

For colour photograph see p. 541.

---

* No HLA association except small subset with HLA-B27 who develop cervical spine fusion and less often sacroiliitis or ankylosing spondylitis.

† The seronegative spondyloarthritides are characterized by sacroiliac joint involvement, peripheral inflammatory arthropathy and the absence of rheumatoid factor. Pathological changes are concentrated around the *enthesis*—at sites of ligamentous insertions into bones (rather than the synovium). Changes may also develop in the eye, aortic valve, lung parenchyma and skin. Types include ankylosing spondylitis (p. 184), Reiter's syndrome (p. 401), psoriatic arthropathy (p. 90), enteropathic sacroiliitis (ulcerative colitis and Crohn's disease, p. 207), reactive arthritides (infections such as *Yersinia*, *Salmonella*, *Helicobacter*, *Campylobacter*), certain subsets of JCA, and perhaps a group of rarer disorders (Whipple's disorders, Behçet's syndrome and pustular arthro-osteitis).

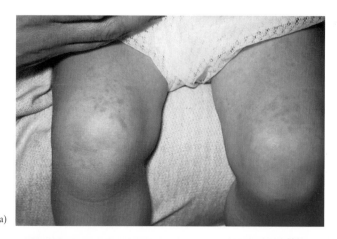

(a)

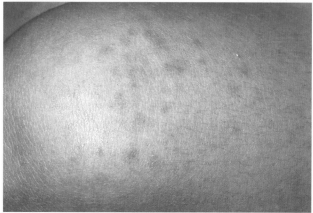

(b)

Fig. 3.181 Juvenile chronic arthritis. (a) Arthropathy affecting the knees. Note a crop of characteristic macular lesions. (b) Close-up view of the rash.

182 / Cystic fibrosis

Frequency in survey: 0.3% of attempts at MRCP short cases.

Record

This young patient (who is usually *underweight*, of *short stature* and rather pale, but may also be *breathless* and *cyanosed*) has *clubbing* of the fingers (often present) and a *productive cough* (there may be a *sputum pot* by the bed). There are (may be) *inspiratory clicks* and *expiratory wheeze* (heard with the unaided ear). There are *crepitations* over . . . (the area of bronchiectasis — state where). There is (may be) widespread *polyphonic expiratory wheeze*.

These features suggest *bronchiectasis* (p. 161) and a likely cause in this young patient suggest that the underlying disorder is cystic fibrosis. If so the patient is also likely to have *pancreatic insufficiency* and *malabsorption*.* The diagnosis can be confirmed by the *sweat sodium test*.†

Some patients have a well-developed *cor pulmonale* with *cyanosis, ankle oedema* and *right heart failure*.

Cystic fibrosis is a genetic disorder (autosomal recessive) and a child born to two heterozygote carriers has a 1/4 chance of having the disease. The disorder usually occurs in Caucasians; Africans and Asians are seldom affected.

---

* In most cases there is a history of frequent large foul stools which are difficult to flush down. These patients are underachievers in weight and height for their age; they have a good appetite, steatorrhoea and a protuberant abdomen. Hepatic symptoms are relatively uncommon but there may be *jaundice*. Sometimes there may be *portal hypertension*, glycosuria, biliary cirrhosis, cholelithiasis, intussusception and aspermia.

† A history of recurrent respiratory infections and of gastrointestinal symptoms, especially recurrent abdominal pain and faecal impaction, are highly suggestive of cystic fibrosis. The sodium and chloride levels are in excess of 70 mmol l^{-1} in the sweat, and these levels do not fall after the administration of aldosterone (o.1 mg kg^{-1}) for a week.

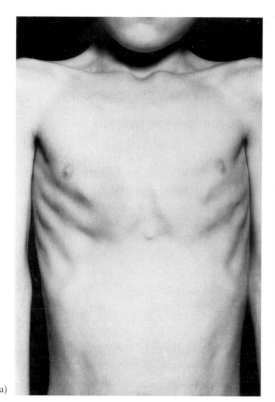

(a)

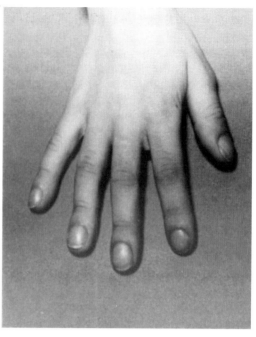

(b)

Fig. 3.182 (a) Hyperinflated rib cage with rib recession in an undernourished patient. (b) Clubbing of cyanosed fingers.

183 / Infective endocarditis

Frequency in survey: 0.3% of attempts at MRCP short cases.

Record

This patient has mitral incompetence* suggested by a pansystolic murmur over the precordium, radiating to the left axilla, a third heart sound, a dilated left ventricle with the point of maximum impulse in the left sixth intercostal space in the anterior axillary line, and a right ventricular lift. There are (may be) *splinter haemorrhages*, the conjunctivae are pale† and there is a *petechial haemorrhage* inside the right lower eyelid (look for the *cutaneous manifestations* elsewhere on the body). There is no clubbing‡ (ask to look for *splenomegaly* and for *Roth's spots*§).

There is an infusion line and I strongly suspect that this patient has infective endocarditis.

Cutaneous manifestations of bacterial endocarditis

Four lesions involving the *skin* and *its appendages* have traditionally been considered as the peripheral manifestations of subacute bacterial endocarditis: *petechiae, subungual ('splinter') haemorrhages, Osler nodes* and *Janeway lesions*. Since the advent of effective antibiotic therapy and early diagnosis in most cases, these signs have become less frequent in real life but, whenever available, would be presented in the MRCP clinical examination.

Petechiae are often present in the *conjunctivae*, on the skin of the *dorsum* of the *hands* and *feet*, the anterior chest and abdominal wall and on the oropharynx. Petechiae are common in both acute and subacute bacterial endocarditis but are not specific and may occur in *thrombocytopenia, scurvy, renal failure, bacteraemia* without endocarditis (e.g. *meningococcaemia*) and after *cardiopulmonary bypass* in the absence of infection (presumably due to fat microemboli).

Subungual (splinter) haemorrhages are more commonly seen after trauma and in *psoriasis* but they are common in both acute and subacute bacterial endocarditis.* A true splinter almost always occurs about 3–5 mm proximal to the free edge of the nail.

Osler nodes are small, raised, red to purple, *tender* lesions that are most often seen on the pulps of the fingers and toes. They may also be seen on the soles and palms. Osler nodes are not common, and they are almost always associated with a subacute rather than acute type of endocarditis.

Janeway lesions are small (1–4 mm in diameter), irregular, flat, erythematous, *non-tender macules* present most often on the palms, soles and around the ankles. They may appear on the tips of the fingers and toes and occasionally on the extremities and the trunk. These lesions *blanch on pressure*. They are not common, usually occur in acute rather than subacute bacterial endocarditis but seldom occur in bacteraemia without endocarditis and in the subacute variety.

---

* In the examination setting one usually expects a valvular lesion when asked to examine the heart of a patient with infective endocarditis. However, murmurs are not essential for this diagnosis.

† *Pallor* in a patient with a *valvular lesion* should alert the candidate to look for other circumstantial evidence (e.g. temperature chart, intravenous line) and cutaneous manifestations of subacute bacterial endocarditis.

‡ Clubbing is rare in endocarditis and only occurs in the subacute variety.

§ *Roth's spots* (infrequent; usually subacute variety) are seen on the retina as cotton-wool exudates, often surrounded by a haemorrhage. Histologically, these lesions are collections of lymphocytes in the nerve layer of the retina surrounded by oedema and/or haemorrhage. Roth's spots may occur in association with other infections.

Acute versus subacute bacterial endocarditis

Several important features distinguish acute from subacute bacterial endocarditis. The clinical course in *acute bacterial endocarditis* (commonest organism *Staphylococcus aureus*—50–70% of cases) is usually measured in *days*, the associated systemic illness is more severe and *early mortality higher*, the patient is more likely to suffer rapid destruction of the valve and more likely to have one or more focal collections outside the heart. Treatment in the acute variety should not be delayed until blood culture results are available. *Subacute bacterial endocarditis* (commonest organism *Streptococcus viridans*) may have a course measured in *weeks or months* with vague non-specific complaints of general malaise, anorexia, aches and pains, weakness and fatigue, low grade fevers and night sweats.

For colour photographs see p. 541.

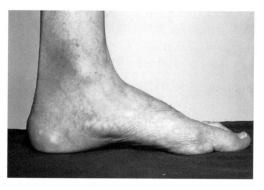

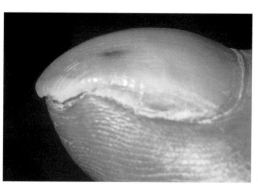

(a)

(b)

Fig. 3.183 (a) Janeway lesions above the ankle. (b) Splinter haemorrhage.

184 / Malignant melanoma

Frequency in survey: 0.3% of attempts at MRCP short cases.

Record

There is a *violaceous* (or darkish-brown/reddish-brown)* nodule with *variegated* appearance and *irregular edges* on this patient's leg (it may also be present on the trunk or face). It is about 8 mm in diameter (measure). The shape is asymmetrical (i.e. *one half unlike the other half*), it is unevenly pigmented* and it is elevated above the level of the skin.

These features suggest the diagnosis of a malignant melanoma.

Diagnosis

The North American approach to the diagnosis is to use the ABCDE mnemonic: A = *asymmetry*; B = *irregular border*; C = *colour variation*, mottled, haphazard shades of brown, black, grey and white; D = *a diameter more than 6 mm*; E = *elevated* above the skin. A seven-point check list is used in the UK consisting of three major (the first three) and four minor criteria: (i) change in size; (ii) change in shape; (iii) change in colour; (iv) diameter more than 7 mm; (v) the presence of inflammation; (vi) oozing or bleeding; and (vii) mild itch.

Cutaneous malignant melanomata

Superficial spreading melanoma: this variety appears mostly in the fourth or fifth decade on the trunk (mostly males) or legs (mostly females). Starts as a slightly elevated and hyperkeratotic, brown, pigmented lesion with well-defined but irregular margins. It may be present for years before it becomes invasive. Partial regression may cause central pigment loss while extension continues peripherally

Nodular melanoma: this usually occurs in the fifth or sixth decade and male:female ratio is 2:1. It presents as an elevated, dome-shaped or pedunculated nodule with reddish brown colour. There may be a varied red central area, with only a faint brown ring of melanin peripherally. Ulceration and bleeding occur frequently. This variety of malignant melanoma is frequently confused with a vascular lesion because of its rapid growth and paucity of melanin pigment. It carries a poor prognosis

Lentigo maligna melanoma: this occurs equally in males and females on sun-exposed areas, and tends to occur in the elderly. Most lesions occur on the face, commonly on the upper cheek or forehead. Initially, it is a flat, brown, stain-like lesion. This flatness with loss of skin markings is useful in distinguishing it from such lesions as actinic keratoses or seborrhoeic keratoses

Acral lentiginous melanoma (palmoplantar malignant melanoma): this represents 10% of all melanomata on white skin but almost 50% of all melanomata in Japan. The lesions are found mainly on the sole of the foot or the palm of the hand, and are characterized by a large, macular, lentiginous pigmented area around an invasive raised tumour

Desmoplastic melanoma: a rare variant of melanoma which may complicate any of the above, but is most commonly seen in lentigo maligna.

A pigmented naevus without any inflammation or granulation is unlikely to be mistaken for a malignant melanoma. The commonest errors occur with *benign pigmented lesions, seborrhoeic keratosis, pigmented angiomata* and *basal cell carcinoma*. In

---

*There is usually an array of colours in a gradation of red, grey or blue and mixed with brown or black. The colour may vary from one part to the other, and from the centre to the periphery, of the tumour.

general *any change* in a *pigmented lesion* in an adult between 20 and 40 years of age should be regarded with suspicion, and any *unusual pigmented lesion* on the lower leg of a female should be examined care- fully. The correct diagnosis can be made on excision biopsy.

For colour photograph see p. 543.

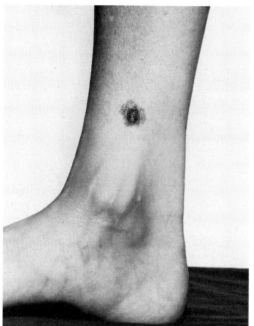

(a1)

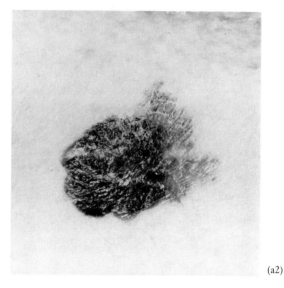

(a2)

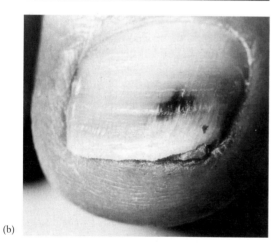

(b)

Fig. 3.184 (a1) Malignant melanoma. Note the variegated appearance and irregular edge. (2) Irregular edge with variegated surface. (b) Subungual melanoma.

185 / Leg oedema

Frequency in survey: main focus of a short case in 0.3% of attempts at MRCP short cases. Additional feature in many others.

Record 1

There is *swelling* of the lower limbs which *pits on pressure*. The patient is (may be) breathless at rest, the *venous pressure is raised* and oscillating the ear lobe and there is *sacral oedema*.

These features suggest the ankle oedema is due to congestive cardiac failure (now consider offering to extend the examination to look for features of the cardiac and/or pulmonary disease and hepatomegaly).

Record 2

This *elderly* female (or male) has bilateral lower limb oedema (check for pitting) up to the mid-calf (look for the presence of a walking aid, engorged jugular veins and, if allowed, sacral oedema).

Her *zimmer frame* suggests a degree of poor mobility and, in the absence of any other signs of cardiovascular disease, it is likely to be dependent oedema though the patient may be on some *salt-retaining drugs* such as steroids or non-steroidal anti-inflammatory agents.

Causes of leg oedema

Local causes

Dependent oedema

Venous disorders (chronic venous insufficiency) — pigmentation, induration and inflammation (lipodermatosclerosis)

Occlusion of a large vein
   phlebothrombosis—*unilateral*, see p. 244
   extrinsic compression

Popliteal (Baker's) cyst—*unilateral*, see p. 244

Cellulitis—*unilateral*, see p. 244

Lymphoedema — non-pitting, thickened and indurated skin ('pigskin'). May be idiopathic or secondary to proximal lymphatic obstruction (metastatic carcinoma, surgical removal of the regional lymph nodes, irradiation or chronic infection)

Gastrocnemius rupture — swelling and ecchymosis around the ankle joint and foot

Lipomatosis — in some cases of obesity the fat may be preferentially deposited in the lower limbs.

Systemic causes

Congestive cardiac failure

Hypoproteinaemia — nephrotic syndrome, liver cirrhosis, Kwashiorkor, protein-losing enteropathy

Hypo- and hyperthyroidism

Drugs — corticosteroids, non-steroidal anti-inflammatory drugs, vasodilators.

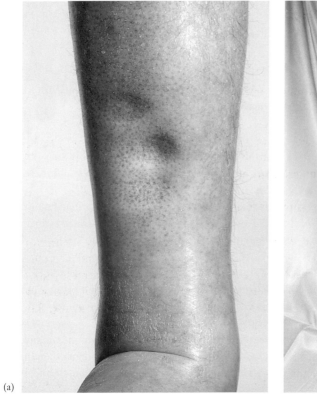

(a)

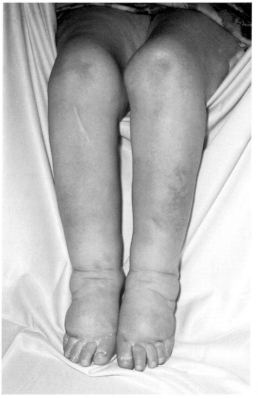

(b)

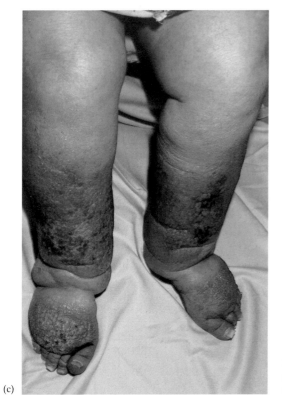

(c)

Fig. 3.185 (a) Oedema which has pitted with finger pressure. (b) Bilateral leg oedema in an elderly patient. (c) Lymphoedema of the legs.

186 / Acanthosis nigricans

Frequency in survey: 0.3% of attempts at MRCP short cases.

Record
There is a soft, *velvety*, verrucous, *brown* hyperpigmentation of the body folds, especially those of the *neck*, *axillae* and groin.

The diagnosis is acanthosis nigricans.

Patient age under 40 years (most common)
Associated with

*Obesity** and *insulin resistance* (high insulin levels, there may be glucose intolerance or frank diabetes, though glucose tolerance may be normal, depending on the severity of the insulin resistance; rarely insulin receptor antibodies are found)

Endocrinopathies (it is said that it may also be associated with a variety of endocrinopathies such as Cushing's disease, acromegaly, polycystic ovaries, hypothyroidism and hyperthyroidism)

May be familial.

Patient age over 40 years
May indicate

Underlying malignancy (usually adenocarcinoma especially of the *stomach*, gastrointestinal tract and uterus; less commonly, ovary, prostate, breast and lung; rarely lymphomata. Involvement of the tongue and oral mucosa highly suggestive of malignancy. Acanthosis nigricans may appear before the malignant neoplasm becomes manifest in 20% of cases. May regress with response to therapy for the tumour and worsen again with reactivation of the tumour raising the possibility of a humoral secretion from the tumour as the cause of the skin lesion).

Other cutaneous manifestations of malignancy
Non-genetic
Paget's disease of the breast (underlying intraductal mammary carcinoma)

Stewart–Treves syndrome (angiomatous, livid or dusky-red blebs and nodules exuding fluid indicating lymphangiosarcoma as a complication of chronic lymphoedema, especially after radical mastectomy)

Dermatomyositis (heliotrope rash around eyes and backs of hands, proximal muscle weakness — but see footnote, p. 329)

The Leser–Trélat sign (sudden appearance and growth of multiple seborrhoeic keratoses in the elderly may be a sign of underlying malignancy; however there is increasing doubt about this nowadays. Multiple seborrhoeic keratoses are very common in the elderly and one needs to exercise caution in chasing internal malignancy in everyone with multiple seborrhoeic keratoses)

* Particular concern should be exercised over the appearance of acanthosis nigricans in non-obese adults.

Necrolytic migratory erythema (associated with glucagonomata of the pancreas; gradually enlarging erythematous patches with central superficial blister formation, progressing to central crusting and healing; annular and figurate lesions result, with exudative, erosive and crusting areas especially in the perineum, groin and perioral areas; similar lesions are seen in severe zinc deficiency)

Bazex syndrome or *acrokeratosis paraneoplasia* (red to violaceous scaling, psoriatic-like patches confined to the bridge of the nose, fingers, toes and margins of the ear helices; nail folds may be red, scaling and tender with nail-grooving and onycholysis; associated with asymptomatic squamous cell carcinomata of the oral, pharyngeal, laryngeal and bronchial areas primarily in men; as the tumour progresses the rash may spread and develop, and can become very widespread)

Clubbing of the fingers (p. 201)

Hypertrophic pulmonary osteoarthropathy (clubbing in association with subperiosteal new bone formation, shafts of long bones of extremities and digits; ankles, knees, wrists and hands may be painful and swollen†)

Carcinoid erythema (eventually the flush becomes permanent and telangiectasis and tortuous veins evolve in the flushed areas—p. 403)

Urticaria pigmentosa (multiple reddish-brown or yellowish-brown macules showing Darier's sign —p. 379; may rarely be associated with myeloproliferative disorders — mast cell leukaemia, myelofibrosis, myeloid metaplasia, polycythaemia, granulocytic leukaemia)

Bowen's disease of the skin (multiple, discrete, red, scaling, flat to slightly raised patches that mimic eczematous or psoriatic patches, occurring in non-sun-exposed areas; each represents a squamous cell cancer; may progress to invasive squamous carcinoma if not excised; relationship to internal malignancy controversial; particularly associated with long-term exposure to arsenicals — well water, insecticides, industrial chemicals).

Genetic

Gardener's syndrome (multiple epidermoid and sebaceous cysts of face and scalp, fibrous tissue tumours of the skin, osteomata of the membranous bones of the face and head, and polyps of the colon and rectum; all patients develop adenocarcinoma of the bowel before the seventh decade)

Cowden's disease (numerous hamartomata of the skin, mucous membranes and internal organs; present as keratotic, warty papules and nodules on the hands, arms and central face; may be papular, cobblestone lesions on the gingiva, palate, tongue and larynx; associated with malignant neoplasms of the breast and thyroid in a high percentage of cases)

Torre's syndrome (dominant; multiple sebaceous gland tumours, sebaceous adenomata, sebaceous hyperplasia, and basal cell cancers with sebaceous differentiation; present as yellowish or red papules and nodules; associated with cancers of the colon, duodenum, ampulla of Vater, uterus and genitourinary tract)

MEN type IIb (multiple whitish to pink papular mucosal neuromata studding the lips, tip of tongue and, less often, the buccal mucosa, gingivae, palate and pharynx; neuromata on the conjunctivae and corneas; associated with medullary carcinoma of the thyroid and phaeochromocytoma—see footnote, p. 128)

Ataxia telangiectasia (recessive; telangiectasias over ears, eyelids, nose, butterfly facial area, and conjunctivae in association with progressive cerebellar ataxia, profound immunological deficiency and sinopulmonary infections; lymphoma develops in 10%; other malignancies may occur less frequently)

Wiscot–Aldrich syndrome (skin changes similar to atopic dermatitis; there may be petechiae due to thrombocytopaenia; widespread humoral and cell-mediated immunological abnormalities; 80% have lymphoma and 15% leukaemia by the age of 10 years)

Neurofibromatosis (dominant; *café-au-lait* spots,

---

† Occasionally in hypertrophic pulmonary osteoarthropathy, cutaneous thickening of the forearms and legs leads to cylindrical enlargement of the limbs. Facial features may become coarse with deep facial furrows reminiscent of acromegaly. Deep confluent skin wrinkles may evolve over the forehead and scalp, these latter features with the acromegalic features being termed, *pachydermoperiostosis*.

axillary freckles, multiple neurofibromata; 10% develop phaeochromocytoma by age of 60; acoustic neuromata and neurofibrosarcomata also associated—p. 176)

Peutz–Jeghers syndrome (dominant; numerous brown–black macules on the lips, perioral regions and hands and feet; associated with hamartomatous polyps of the small bowel, stomach and less commonly, colon—p. 236).

For colour photograph see p. 543.

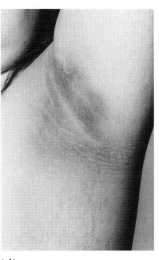
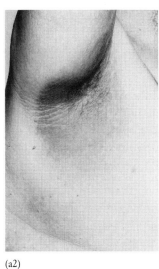
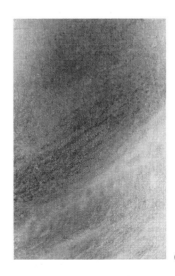

(a1) (a2) (b)

Fig. 3.186 (a1) Hyperpigmented, verrucous fold in the axilla. (2) Hyperpigmented, thickened fold in the axilla. (b) Note multiple verrucous lesions.

187 / Drusen

Frequency in survey: 0.3% of attempts at MRCP short cases.

Record
Multiple, discrete, round, yellow–white dots of variable size scattered around the macula and posterior pole of the eye.

These are retinal drusen.

Retinal drusen represent abnormal accumulations in the retinal pigment epithelium basement (Bruch's) membrane in subjects over the age of 40 years. The drusen are often precursors to visual loss from *senile macular degeneration*. The latter may lead to impairment of central vision early in its course—non-congruent central scotoma.

Retinal drusen need to be distinguished from optic disc drusen (also called hyaline bodies) which are bright excrescences at the optic disc which may be calcified. These are sometimes obvious but may be difficult to see in young persons, in whom the disc elevation they produce can be mistaken for papilloedema (*pseudopapilloedema*). Occasionally, these may be associated with tuberous sclerosis.

For colour photograph see p. 529.

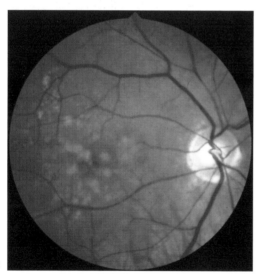

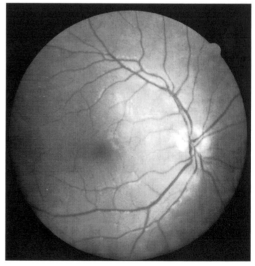

(a)

(b)

Fig. 3.187 (a) Retinal drusen. (b) Optic disc drusen in a young person leading to pseudopapilloedema (when he presented to casualty with headache, the optic disc changes were noted and an urgent CT scan was ordered; this was normal and ultrasonography of the optic disc showed up the drusen as the only abnormality).

188 / Yellow nail syndrome

Frequency in survey: 0.3% of attempts at MRCP short cases.

Record

The *nails* are thick, *excessively curved* from side to side, slow growing leaving *bulbous fingertips* uncovered and pale yellow (or greenish yellow). The *cuticles* are *lost*, the lunulae are absent and there is onycholysis (though the degree is variable).

This suggests the yellow nail syndrome (check for *lymphoedema* of the extremities which may also be present).

The yellow nail syndrome is usually associated with lymphatic hypoplasia and a number of *pulmonary conditions* may occur such as bronchiectasis, pleural effusion, chronic obstructive pulmonary disease and malignant neoplasms.

Other associations include D-penicillamine therapy, nephrotic syndrome, hypothyroidism and AIDS.

For colour photographs see p. 531.

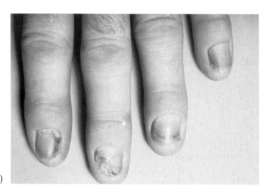
(a)

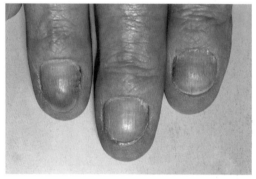
(b)

Fig. 3.188 Yellow nail syndrome. (a) Thickened nails and onycholysis. (b) No cuticles or lunula. Bulbous fingertips uncovered.

Frequency in survey: main focus in 0.3% of attempts at MRCP short cases. Hypogonadism was an additional feature in many others.

Survey note: it does not often happen, but occasionally candidates are allowed to examine the testes (see first person experience 10, p. 475, and anecdote 56, p. 499).

Record

He is *tall*, has *gynaecomastia* (may be asymmetrical), sparse body hair and has a *eunuchoid habitus*.* He has very small testes (< 2 cm length, often termed *pea-sized*; lower limit of normal for adults is 3.5 cm length).

The features suggest Klinefelter's syndrome.

See anecdote 56, p. 499.

Other features of Klinefelter's syndrome

Affects 1/400–500 men (1/20 if maternal age > 45)

Classically 47,XXY but also XXYY, more than two X (poly X) plus Y and mosaics

Azospermia and raised gonadotrophins

Though the majority have normal intelligence there is a higher than normal incidence of mental retardation (especially if greater than two X chromosomes)

Higher incidence of somatic abnormalities (especially if greater than two X chromosomes) such as hypospadias, cryptorchidism and bony abnormalities of the radius and ulna

If there is an additional Y chromosome, patients tend to be tall with very aggressive antisocial behavioural abnormalities

Less severe manifestations in mosaics (fertility has been recorded in XXY, XY)

Character and personality disorders common (may be in part related to the psychosocial consequences of androgen deficiency)

Slightly increased incidence of certain systemic diseases (diabetes, chronic obstructive airways disease, autoimmune disorders such as SLE and Hashimoto's thyroiditis, malignancy such as breast, lymphoma and germ cell neoplasms, and varicose veins).

Features of eunuchoid appearance

Average height or above (growth until mid-twenties)

Span > height†

Pubis–heel > pubis–crown

Body fat tends to be in feminine contours; broad hips, musculature poor

Sparse body hair/beard

Poorly developed genitalia

Gynaecomastia

Timid behaviour.

Causes of primary hypogonadism (with deficiency of both sperm and androgen production)

Congenital or developmental disorders

Klinefelter's syndrome and variants

Functional prepubertal castrate syndrome (congenital anorchia — no testicular tissue from birth; testes must have been active in fetal life because

---

* The degree of eunuchoidism is variable depending on the degree of androgen deficiency which is seldom complete; indeed the occasional Klinefelter's patient may have normal testosterone levels and virilization, the only abnormality being the pea-sized testes and azospermia. The patient

treated with exogenous testosterone may also be well virilized.

† In contrast to other conditions which result in prepubertal androgen deficiency, Klinefelter's patients often have disproportionate increase in lower extremity compared to upper extremity long bone growth.

the phenotype is male; hence sometimes referred to as 'vanishing testis syndrome')

Noonan's syndrome (?short stature, triangular micrognathic facial appearance and posteriorly angulated low-set ears with a thick helix, webbed neck, shield-like chest, pectus excavatum, cubitus valgus, mental retardation, right-sided cardiovascular abnormalities; often cryptorchidism as well as primary testicular dysfunction — see also p. 352).

Dystrophia myotonica — p. 159 (though most cases develop testicular atrophy with maintained androgen production but impaired spermatogenesis in middle age, 20% have manifestations of androgen deficiency as a result of primary testicular failure — testosterone in these patients may help maintain or improve muscle function)

Polyglandular autoimmune disease — see p. 279 (though much less common than autoimmune primary ovarian failure, primary testicular failure associated with antitesticular antibodies and androgen deficiency may also occur)

Complex genetic disorders (Alström, ataxia telangiectasia, Sohval–Soffer, Weinstein's and Wermer's syndromes)

NB Normal ageing (in healthy men is associated with a relative fall in testosterone with associated elevation of gonadotrophins).

Acquired disorders

Orchitis (viral, especially mumps; also gonorrhoea, leprosy, tuberculosis, brucellosis, glanders, syphilis, filariasis, bilharziasis)

Surgical and traumatic castration

Drugs (which may produce anti-androgen effects include spironolactone, ketoconazole, H_2-blockers such as cimetidine, alcohol, marijuana, digitalis, cytotoxics)

Irradiation.

Systemic disorders

Chronic liver disease — p. 84 (total testosterone low or normal, LH usually elevated, high circulating oestrogens due to impaired hepatic clearance of adrenal androgens leading to increased substrate for peripheral aromatization to oestrogens; treatment with aromatizable androgens may worsen the gynaecomastia)

Chronic renal failure (?uraemic pallor; testosterone replacement may improve the anaemia)

Malignancy (Hodgkin's disease; testicular cancer)

Sickle-cell disease

Paraplegia (transient reduction in testosterone initially)

Vasculitis (may involve the testes)

Infiltrative disease (amyloidosis, leukaemia).

Causes of secondary hypogonadism (with deficiency of both sperm and androgen production)

Congenital and developmental disorders

Isolated hypogonadotrophic hypogonadism‡ (?associated anosmia or hyposmia due to developmental failure of the olfactory lobes in which case *Kallman's syndrome*—may also exhibit other midline defects (e.g. cleft-lip or cleft-palate, colour blindness, renal agenesis, nerve deafness), cryptorchidism, and skeletal abnormalities (e.g. syndactyly, short fourth metacarpals, craniofacial asymmetry))

Isolated LH deficiency (*'fertile' eunuch syndrome*; a variant of Kallman's syndrome in which FSH secretion is preserved resulting in near normal sized testes and well-advanced, though not normal, spermatogenesis; despite the name patients are not fertile without hCG therapy)

Haemochromatosis — p. 253 (iron deposition in the pituitary selectively inhibits gonadotrophins whilst other anterior pituitary hormone secretion remains unaffected)

Complex genetic syndromes (e.g. Prader–Willi;§ Laurence–Moon–Biedl — p. 358; familial cerebellar ataxia; familial icthyosis).

---

† Differentiation from the much commoner constitutional delayed puberty is difficult. Withdrawal of androgen therapy can eventually be achieved in constitutional delayed puberty but not in hypogonadotrophic hypogonadism. Fertility can be facilitated in hypogonadotrophic hypogonadism by treatment with gonadotrophins or gonadotrophin–releasing hormone (GnRH) instead of androgens.

§ *Prader–Labhart–Willi syndrome.* Our survey has raised the possibility that this has occurred rarely as an MRCP short case. The syndrome consists of: poor fetal activity, infantile hypotonia and neonatal failure to thrive. Compulsive hyperphagia with *massive obesity* in later childhood. May be *cryptorchidism.* Thin turned down upper lips and up-slanting palpebral fissures often seen (*almond-shaped eyes*). Poor dentition is often present. Fair skin and hair darkens with age. Hands and feet characteristically small (*acromicria*). (*Cont'd*)

Acquired disorders

Hypopituitarism—p. 295

Hyperprolactinaemia (either microprolactinoma, macroprolactinoma or other large pituitary tumour causing stalk compression;‖ prolactin inhibits gonadotrophin secretion; macroadenomata may destroy pituitary gonadotrophs)

Oestrogen excess (therapy for prostatic cancer; oestrogen-producing neoplasms)

Opiate-like drugs (such as morphine, methadone and heroin) inhibit gonadotrophin production.

Systemic disorders

Cushing's — p. 231 (high levels of glucocorticoids suppress gonadotrophin secretion)

Acute stress or illness (high glucocorticoids)

Nutritional deficiency (protein–calorie malnutrition or anorexia nervosa; gonadotrophin production inhibited)

Chronic illness (malnutrition may contribute)

Massive obesity.§

Pickwickian syndrome (p. 290) may occur. Diabetes mellitus is common. Mild to severe *mental retardation* with behaviour and personality problems are usual. Hypothalamic dysfunction and *hypogonadotrophic hypogonadism* are often present. *It should be remembered that low testosterone and gonadotrophins may be found in association with any case of massive obesity.*

‖ Microprolactinomas are < 1 cm in diameter and macroprolactinomas > 1 cm. Any pituitary macroadenoma

which compresses the pituitary stalk and interferes with the prolactin-inhibiting dopaminergic neurones there may lead to hyperprolactinaemia. Serum prolactin levels > 5000 mIU l⁻¹ are not usually associated with stalk compression alone and usually reflect a true prolactinoma. Other causes of hyperprolactinaemia include central nervous system active drugs such as phenothiazines and other antipsychotic drugs, opiates, sedatives, antidepressants and stimulants.

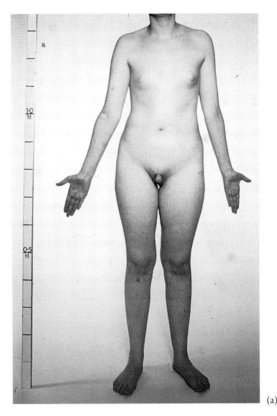

(a)

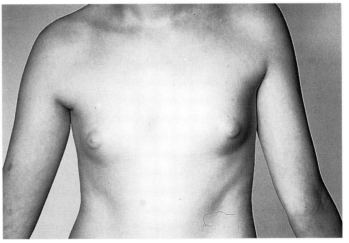

Fig. 3.189 Klinefelter's syndrome.
(a) Note the disproportionately long
lower limbs in relation to the upper
torso, the underdeveloped genitalia
and the absent axillary and pubic hair.
(b) Gynaecomastia.

(b)

190 / Keratoacanthoma

Frequency in survey: 0.3% of attempts at MRCP short cases.

Record

There is (say where—usually *sun-exposed areas*, face, backs of hands and forearms) a *round*, firm, cherry-sized, *flesh-coloured*, shell-like *tumour* with a *central crater containing horny material*. It is well demarcated and seems to be stuck on the skin.
The likely diagnosis is keratoacanthoma.

Commoner in males (3:1) also called *molluscum sebaceum*.

Microscopic appearance is so like a low grade squamous cell carcinoma that differentiation is often impossible. In keratoacanthoma (self-healing epithelioma), however, the edge is regular, the surrounding skin is undamaged and the age of onset is younger (middle-age) than in squamous cell carcinoma. The cell changes of carcinoma are absent and there is a very limited degree of invasiveness.

They begin as flesh-coloured papules that *rapidly grow* (unlike squamous cell carcinoma) to full size (may be 5 or 7.5 cm) over a period of about 6 weeks, evolving a central keratin-filled crater. The lesions remain for about 6 or 8 weeks and then undergo spontaneous involution leaving a depressed scar.

Lesions are best excised because the scars are unsightly and because of the difficulty of differentiation from squamous cell carcinoma.

For colour photographs see p. 538.

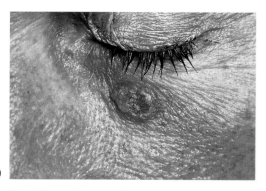

(a)

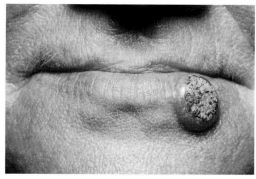

(b)

Fig 3.190 (a,b) Keratoacanthoma.

191 / Thalamic syndrome

Frequency in survey: 0.3% of attempts at MRCP short cases.

Record

The patient (who complains of *pain down one side of the body and head*) has (may have) a *hemiplegia* on the R/L side (the side of the pain), and on that side says that the *touch sensation is different* compared to the other side. Pinprick sensation was perceived as increased pain on the R/L.

These features suggest a thalamic syndrome.

Damage to the ventral posterolateral nucleus of the thalamus causes decreased sensation of all modalities on the contralateral side of the body and face. The sensory loss is often accompanied by dysaesthesias. A thalamic syndrome often appears within weeks or months of the acute thalamic damage and has been attributed to denervation hypersensitivity of sensory neurones in the midbrain reticular formation. The patient develops spontaneous pain in the distribution of the sensory loss. The quality of the pain is difficult to define. It is often exacerbated by anxiety and tends to be rather diffuse but is most marked in one limb and rarely involves the face alone. The quality of sensation on the affected side is usually distorted with diminution to all modalities and hypoalgesia. Nevertheless stimuli exceeding the sensory threshold may produce an intense exacerbation of the background spontaneous pain. Occasionally there is frank hyperalgesia. The thalamic syndrome is rare but causes a particularly unpleasant pain intractable to most therapeutic manoeuvres.

192 / Atrial septal defect

Frequency in survey: 0.1% of attempts at MRCP short cases.

Record

The pulse in this middle-aged female is irregularly irregular (onset of atrial fibrillation is usually the cause of symptoms after the third or fourth decade, otherwise asymptomatic). The JVP is not elevated (unless in right heart failure). The apex beat is just palpable and not displaced and there is a *left parasternal heave* (there may be a systolic thrill over the pulmonary area in large left to right shunts). The second heart sound is widely split (the first may also split with a loud tricuspid component), and the two-component split is not influenced by respiration (*fixed splitting*). There is an *ejection systolic murmur* (due to high flow across the pulmonary valve) over the pulmonary area. (Occasionally there may be a harsh, explosive and brief early diastolic murmur—pulmonary incompetence—and an ejection click, both due to pulmonary artery dilatation. A mid-diastolic rumble over the tricuspid area suggests a large shunt.)

The diagnosis is atrial septal defect.

Male to female ratio is 1 : 3.

Other features of atrial septal defect

Ostium secundum defect is the commonest type

Ostium primum defect is common and is in Down's syndrome (p. 337) and is associated with mitral regurgitation

rSR in the right precordial leads on ECG. Right-axis deviation is associated with an ostium secundum defect, left-axis deviation suggests an ostium primum defect

Dilated proximal pulmonary arteries and an enlarged right heart with pulmonary plethora* on chest X-ray. The aortic knuckle is small and left heart border straight. The peripheral pulmonary vascularity is replaced by clear lung fields with the advent of pulmonary hypertension. The superior vena cava is enlarged in the sinus venosus type

Paradoxical (anterior) septal movement during systole and right ventricular dilatation on echocardiography

Diagnosis confirmed by catheterization: oxygen saturation is determined serially in the superior vena cava, high, mid and low right atrium and inferior vena cava. A step-up in O_2 saturation in mid right atrium suggests a left-to-right shunt

Surgical closure for ostium secundum defect is recommended if the pulmonary to systemic flow ratio is 2 : 1 or more

Patients with pulmonary hypertension are cyanosed and may have clubbing of the fingers (Eisenmenger's syndrome—p. 205). The systolic murmur becomes faint and an early diastolic murmur with a loud P_2 appears. Operative repair is contraindicated

Usual causes of death: right heart failure, arrhythmias, pulmonary embolism, brain abscess, rupture of pulmonary artery

May be associated with acquired mitral stenosis (*Lutembacher's syndrome*).

---

* The main differential diagnosis of *pulmonary plethora* due to a left-to-right shunt is atrial septal defect, ventricular septal defect (p. 213), patent ductus arteriosus (p. 197). It may be possible to differentiate these on chest X-ray by looking at the left atrium and aorta. Small left atrium and normal aorta suggests atrial septal defect, large left atrium and normal aorta suggests ventricular septal defect, large left atrium and large or abnormal aorta suggests patent ductus arteriosus.

193 / Pyoderma gangrenosum

Frequency in survey: 0.1% of attempts at MRCP short cases.

Record

There are large *necrotic ulcers* with *ragged* bluish-red *overhanging edges* together with areas containing erythematous plaques with pustules. They are situated . . . (describe site—can occur anywhere on the body*).

The appearances are suggestive of pyoderma gangrenosum. The patient may have *ulcerative colitis* or Crohn's disease.

It may also be associated with *rheumatoid arthritis* and myeloproliferative disorders. Fifty per cent of patients with pyoderma gangrenosum have ulcerative colitis.† It is frequently an indicator of the severity of the disease. Healing often parallels that of the colitis and colectomy may allow this to be rapid. Systemic and topical corticosteroids often help. The adjunctive use of minocycline may reduce corticosteroid requirements. The histopathological findings are non-specific.

Other skin manifestations of ulcerative colitis

Aphthous ulcers
Erythema nodosum
Erythema multiforme
Perianal fistulae and abscess formation
Purpura.

Other causes of leg ulcers

Venous ulceration (only 50% have superficial varices)
Ischaemic arterial ulceration (usually anterior or lateral lower leg, pain, cold pulseless cyanotic feet, shiny hairless lower legs—p. 316)
Diabetes mellitus (see p. 168)
Vasculitis (rheumatoid arthritis or other connective tissue disorder)
Infection (acute pyogenic, tuberculous, syphilitic, cutaneous leishmaniasis)
Tumour (squamous cell, basal cell, melanoma)
Haematological (sickle-cell, thalassaemia, acholuric jaundice, paroxysmal nocturnal haemoglobinuria)
Neurological (diabetes, tabes dorsalis, leprosy, syringomyelia).

For colour photographs see p. 540.

---

* Pyoderma gangrenosum may occur as an example of *Koebner phenomenon* in which skin diseases occur in scars or sites of trauma. It may rarely complicate surgical wounds and needs to be recognized and distinguished from infection as it responds to corticosteroids.

† Pyoderma gangrenosum can precede the onset of chronic inflammatory bowel disease.

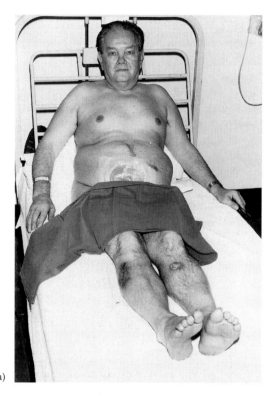

(a)

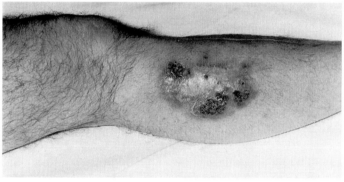

(b)

Fig. 3.193 (a) Note scarred abdomen
and ileostomy bag of this patient with
inflammatory bowel disease. (b)
Pyoderma gangrenosum on the leg of
the same patient.

194 / Multiple sclerosis

Frequency in survey: did not occur as the main focus of a short case. It was, however, considered to be the underlying cause of a short case in at least 16% of attempts at MRCP short cases.

Record 1

The patient (?a young adult) has *ataxic nystagmus* (p.171), *internuclear ophthalmoplegia* (p. 118), *temporal pallor of the discs* (p. 82), and *slurred speech* (p. 261) with *ataxia* (p. 186) and widespread *cerebellar* signs (p. 142). There are *pyramidal* signs and *dorsal column* signs.

The likely diagnosis is demyelinating disease* (a useful euphemism for multiple sclerosis).

Record 2

The legs of this (?middle-aged) patient have increased tone, they are bilaterally spastic and weak. There is bilateral *ankle clonus* and patellar clonus and the *plantars* are *extensor*. The *abdominal reflexes* are absent. The heel–shin test suggest some *ataxia* in the legs and there is slight *impairment of rapid alternate motion* in the upper limbs.

These features suggest that this *spastic paraplegia* is due to demyelinating disease. An examination of the fundi may show involvement of the discs.†

Male to female ratio is 2:3.

Features of multiple sclerosis

Rare in tropical climates

Euphoria despite severe disability (not invariable — the patient may be depressed)

Unpredictable course

May present acutely, subacutely, remittently or insidiously

Relapses and remissions (occurring in two-thirds of patients) are often a useful diagnostic pointer

May very closely imitate other neurological conditions (including neurosis)

Fatigue or a rise in temperature may exacerbate symptoms (the patient may be able to get into, but not out of, a hot bath)

Paroxysmal symptoms (e.g. trigeminal neuralgia) may occur and may respond to carbamazepine

Lhermitte's phenomenon may occur (see p. 314)

Benign course more likely if
early age of onset
relapses and remissions
onset with optic neuritis, or sensory or motor symptoms — in contrast to those of brainstem or cerebellar lesions

The visual evoked response (VER) test is useful in a patient with an isolated lesion which may be due to multiple sclerosis — e.g. spastic paraparesis,†

---

* The features in this *record* are some of those which are commonly seen in a case of multiple sclerosis. There are, of course, few neurological signs which it may not produce.

† Multiple sclerosis (MS) may present in middle-age with insidious spastic paraplegia mimicking cord compression. Signs above the level of the cord lesion may point clinically to demyelination as the cause. In this case the slight cerebellar signs are highly suggestive of MS. However, syringomyelia or a tumour at the foramen magnum could also be the cause. If the diagnosis is of a tumour there may be papilloedema. If the diagnosis is MS the discs may show global or temporal pallor (and the VERs may be delayed—even if, as is often the case, the discs are normal).

VIth nerve palsy, trigeminal neuralgia, facial palsy, postural vertigo

Cerebrospinal fluid examination may show an increase in total protein up to $1\,g\,l^{-1}$ or an increase in lymphocytes up to 50 cells mm^{-3} in 50% of patients. The IgG proportion of the total protein is increased in two-thirds of patients. Oligoclonal bands in the gamma region on agarose or polyacrylamide gel electrophoresis are seen in 90% of patients including some with normal IgG. Myelin basic protein (MBP) can be detected by radioimmunoassay and can be used as an index of disease activity

MRI scans often detect many more multiple sclerosis lesions than are suspected clinically (CT scans can also detect lesions but are much less sensitive than MRI).

195 / Felty's syndrome

Frequency in survey: did not occur as the main focus of a short case. It was, however, considered to be present in a short case in 1% of attempts at MRCP short cases.

Record

There is a *symmetrical deforming arthropathy* with *spindling* and *ulnar deviation* of the fingers, and *nodules* at the elbows. The *spleen* is enlarged at . . . cm. (Check for anaemia.)

If *neutropenia** is present (?evidence of secondary infection) this, in combination with rheumatoid arthritis and splenomegaly, would constitute Felty's syndrome.

Occurs in older patients with long-standing rheumatoid disease (5%).

Other signs and features of Felty's syndrome

Lymphadenopathy
Skin pigmentation
Vasculitic leg ulceration
Keratoconjunctivitis sicca
Thrombocytopenia
Haemolytic anaemia
Lack of relationship between the degree of haematological abnormality and the size of spleen
Tests for antinuclear factor are often positive as well as rheumatoid factor which is invariably positive.

* Splenectomy may correct the neutropenia and prevent further infections in some patients, but many do not improve.

Frequency in survey: did not occur in MRCP survey.*

Record

The pulse is regular (may be irregular if patient is in atrial fibrillation) and of normal volume (in severe cases it has a '*jerky*' character) and the JVP is not elevated (may show a prominent *a* wave). The cardiac apex is forceful in the left fifth intercostal space just outside the mid-clavicular line, there is (may be) a strong *presystolic impulse* (*double apical impulse* caused by atrial systole), and a *systolic thrill* is palpable over the left sternal border. There is a *fourth heart sound*, and an *ejection systolic murmur* (may be harsh) over the left third interspace, which radiates widely to the base and to the axilla (perhaps because it merges with the pansystolic murmur of mitral incompetence which frequently accompanies hypertrophic obstructive cardiomyopathy).

The findings suggest hypertrophic obstructive cardiomyopathy (HOCM).

Other features of hypertrophic obstructive cardiomyopathy

Patients may be asymptomatic. Severe cases are marked by symptoms such as dyspnoea, palpitations, angina, dizziness and syncope (often postural in nature or produced after cessation of exercise, cf. aortic stenosis where syncope usually occurs during exercise)

The systolic murmur may be increased by exercise, nitroglycerine and digoxin, and decreased by beta-blockers and squatting

ECG: normal in 25%. ST–T and T wave changes, tall QRS in mid-precordial leads. Q wave in inferior and lateral precordial leads (due to septal hypertrophy). Sometimes left-axis deviation

Chest X-ray may be normal, or it may show left atrial enlargement

Echocardiography characteristically shows asymmetrical septal hypertrophy, and may show systolic anterior motion of the anterior mitral valve leaflet

Angiocardiography may show marked thickening of the ventricular septum and left ventricular free wall, small left ventricular cavity, and narrow outflow tract (an hour-glass appearance). Anterior movement of the anterior mitral valve leaflet is commonly seen. In the borderline case vigorous contraction of the left ventricle may be the only suggestive feature.

---

* A case of HOCM was included in one mock Membership examination. One of the examiners commented to us that none of his prospective candidates got the correct diagnosis. It is of course possible that conditions such as HOCM did occur in the examination sittings covered by our survey, but the candidates concerned did not get, or even suspect, the diagnoses and were not enlightened by their examiners.

197 / Radial nerve palsy

Frequency in survey: did not occur in MRCP survey.

Record

There is *wrist-drop* and sensory loss over the first dorsal interosseous.*
The diagnosis is radial nerve palsy.

The hand hangs limply and the patient is unable to lift it at the wrist or to straighten out the fingers. If the wrist is passively extended he is able to straighten the fingers at the interphalangeal joints (because the interossei and lumbricals still work) but not at the metacarpophalangeal joints where the fingers remain flexed. The patient may feel that his grasp is weak in the affected hand because of lack of the wrist extension necessary for powerful grip. If the wrist is passively extended the power of grip improves. Abduction and adduction of the fingers may appear weak in radial nerve palsy unless they are tested with the hand resting flat on the table with the fingers extended.

The commonest cause (of this rare condition) is 'Saturday night paralysis' in which the patient, heavily sedated with alcohol, falls asleep with his arm hanging over the back of a chair. The nerve is compressed against the middle third of the humerus, and brachioradialis (flexion of the arm against resistance — with the arm midway between supination and pronation) and supinator are also paralysed as well as the forearm extensor muscles. Muscle wasting does not usually occur and complete recovery in a matter of weeks† is usual. If the nerve is injured by a wound in the axilla, paralysis involves triceps so that extension at the elbow is lost as is the triceps reflex.

(a)
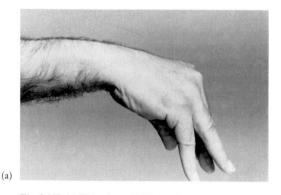
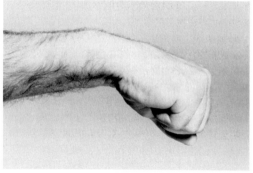
(b)

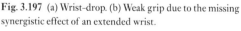

Fig. 3.197 (a) Wrist-drop. (b) Weak grip due to the missing synergistic effect of an extended wrist.

* Though the cutaneous area supplied by the radial nerve is more extensive than this (Fig. 2.1, p. 23) an overlap in supply by both median and ulnar nerves usually means that only this small area over the first dorsal interosseus has detectable impaired sensation.

† Usually damage occurs to the myelin sheath only and the Schwann cells will repair the nerve rapidly. If the pressure is prolonged and causes axonal degeneration then the peripheral nerve regeneration rate is about 1 mm day^{-1} (from the undamaged proximal nerve).

198 / Lateral medullary syndrome (Wallenberg's syndrome)

Frequency in survey: did not occur in MRCP survey.*

Record

(Assumes a lesion affecting the artery on the right.) On the right of the patient (who presented with acute vertigo†) there is (*ipsilateral*):

Horner's syndrome (descending sympathetic tract)

Cerebellar signs (cerebellum and its connections)

Palatal paralysis and diminished gag reflex (may be dysphagia and hoarseness due to a vocal cord paralysis—IXth and Xth nerves)

Decreased *trigeminal* pain and temperature sensation (descending tract and nucleus of the Vth nerve).

On the left of the patient the trunk and limbs (and sometimes the face) show (*contralateral*) decreased *pain and temperature* sensation‡ (spinothalamic tract).

The patient has a lateral medullary syndrome (produced by infarction of a small wedge of lateral medulla posterior to the inferior olivary nucleus—see Fig. 3.198) classically due to a lesion of the right *posterior inferior cerebellar artery*.§

Involvement of the nucleus and tractus solitarius may cause loss of taste. Hiccup may occur. When occlusion of the posterior inferior cerebellar artery is isolated the pyramidal pathways escape and there is no hemiplegia. In the majority of cases of lateral medullary syndrome there is also an occlusion of the vertebral artery and pyramidal signs are present. Rarely, occlusion of the lower basilar artery, vertebral artery, or one of its medial branches produces the *medial medullary syndrome* (contralateral hemiplegia which spares the face, contralateral loss of vibration and joint position sense and ipsilateral paralysis and wasting of the tongue).

Other eponymous brainstem infarction syndromes

Weber's syndrome (*midbrain*; ipsilateral IIIrd nerve palsy and contralateral hemiparesis)

Nothnagel's syndrome (*midbrain*; ipsilateral IIIrd nerve palsy and cerebellar ataxia)

Millard–Gubler syndrome (*pons*; ipsilateral VIth nerve palsy and facial weakness with contralateral hemiplegia)

Foville's syndrome (*pons*; as Millard–Gubler but with lateral conjugate gaze palsy).

These and a number of other eponymous brainstem syndromes (e.g. Claude, Benedict, Raymond–

---

* It did not occur in our surveys but it has occurred in the exam. One candidate contacted us: 'Just my luck!—one of my short cases was lateral medullary syndrome: it was your penultimate short case (in the first edition of your book) and as, according to your book, it had not occurred in the exam, it was the only short case in your book I did not study!'

† Vestibular involvement may produce nystagmus, diplopia, oscillopsia, vertigo, nausea and vomiting.

‡ Involvement of the cuneate and gracile nuclei may cause numbness of the ipsilateral (right in this case) arm.

§ Occlusion of any one of five vessels may be responsible—vertebral, posterior inferior cerebellar, superior, middle, or inferior lateral medullary arteries. The resulting clinical picture is variable and the rehabilitating patient may not show all features.

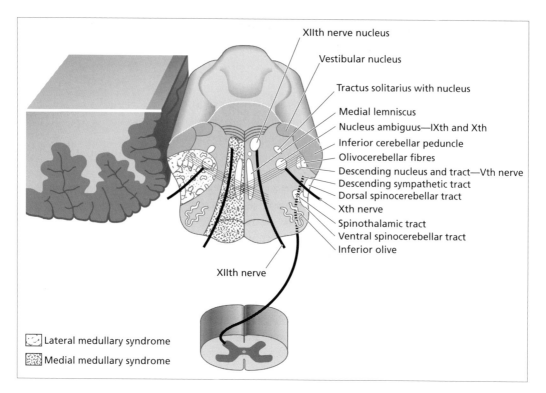

Fig. 3.198 A cross-section through the medulla at the level of the inferior olivary nucleus showing the area infarcted in the lateral and medial medullary syndromes, respectively

(adapted from Mohr, J P *et al.* in *Harrison's Principles of Internal Medicine*, 1983, 10th edn, p. 2037, by kind permission of McGraw-Hill).

Cestau) were, in their classic descriptions, mostly related to tumours and other non-vascular diseases. The diagnosis of brainstem vascular disorders is facilitated more by knowledge of the neuroanatomy of the brainstem than of these eponyms. In one analysis of 50 patients (Cornell–Bellevue series)

with brainstem infarction, only two fitted into these syndromes as originally described. The rest had an extensive mixture of signs and symptoms indicating an overlap in the areas believed to be infarcted by occlusions in specific arteries.

199 / Psychogenic/factitious

Psychogenic and factitious illnesses occur in everyday clinical practice and it would seem from the following anecdotes from our surveys that it is possible that they have also occasionally appeared in the Membership!

Anecdote 1

A candidate was asked to examine a female patient's right hand neurologically. He found normal tone but decreased power in all groups of muscles in the wrist and hand. He said there was some wasting but the examiners disputed this. The candidate thought he had better not retract, even though he felt they were probably right so he said that he thought there was some. The examiners said, 'OK'. The candidate then asked for a pin, but at that moment the bell went. The examiners told him to ask about sensory loss. The patient pointed to various places in a pattern that did not suggest organic pathology saying, 'Here, here, here . . . '. The examiner said, 'You're having difficulty, aren't you?' The candidate responded in the affirmative, trying to offer some possible explanations, but the examiners moved away chuckling to themselves. The candidate (who passed) reports 'It obviously was psychogenic!'

Anecdote 2

A candidate reports that he was taken to see a gentleman who was lying on a couch smoking and was told that he complained of being numb down one side. He felt that 'this seemed most bizarre from the start'. He was asked to examine sensation and started with light touch; this seemed to show that the patient had a sharply demarcated hemianaesthesia. Pain and joint position sensation were similar. As the bell went he was asked what he thought could cause this. He initially mumbled something about 'vascular', but then said he thought it was 'factitious'. He reports 'I'm still not sure whether my findings were correct or what the true diagnosis was' (he did not pass till his next attempt).

Anecdote 3

A candidate was shown a rash on a female patient. The rash was only in accessible areas and there were some bullae. He asked the patient a few questions and then gave a differential diagnosis of bullous lesions. The examiners asked if there were any other causes. There was a period of silence. The examiner said 'Yes, it seems to be in accessible areas'. The candidate asked the invigilating registrar later about the case and was told that 'Apparently no one yet knows the cause!' In retrospect the candidate feels it may have been a case of dermatitis artefacta.

As stated by Anderson and Trethowan,* hysterical behaviour or symptoms have a place in a spectrum at one end of which motivation, due to extreme capacity for the denial of inconvenient reality, is almost if

* Anderson EW, Trethowan WH (1973) *Psychiatry*, 3rd edn. Baillière Tindall, London.

not entirely hidden from the patient. This probably applies to no more than a tiny minority of patients. At the other end of the spectrum, and once again a minority, motivation is clear and purposive, amounting no more or less, to simulation.† The great bulk of hysterical disorders show various shades of 'awareness' in between. Thus there is no 'either/or' — it is a question of how much of each. The capacity for self-deception and denial is a common human attribute which varies greatly between individuals. In deceiving himself the hysteric supposes he can deceive others. In some this belief is justified so that even the most experienced psychiatrist or clinician may err at times. The manifestations of hysteria are legion. The symptoms can be divided into:

Physical symptoms

Pseudoneurological (including paralyses, contractures, anaesthesiae not corresponding to the sensory distribution of a nerve, hemianaesthesia of the whole side of the body,‡ hysterical gaits,§ tremors, fits, aphonia, hysterical deafness, tubular vision and many more)

Cardiovascular (pseudoanginal crises)

Respiratory (simulated asthma, hyperventilation until tetany occurs)

Gastrointestinal (globus hystericus, abdominal proptosis from downward pressure of the diaphragm and a lordotic posture, hysterical vomiting)

Gynaecological (exaggerated dysmenorrhoea; some female hysterical patients are sexually frigid and some may suffer from dyspareunia or from vaginismus).

Mental symptoms

Somnambulism (sleep walking)

Hysterical fugue

Hysterical amnesia

Pseudodementia (simulated dementia in a characteristic way — e.g. $2 + 2 = 5$, date before or after the actual one, elementary knowledge denied or given in a childishly perverted way)

Ganser syndrome (disturbances of consciousness, hallucinations, somatic conversion symptoms, and a tendency to give approximate answers — as in pseudodementia; usually occurs in those in some kind of trouble — e.g. remand prisoners; it represents an attempt to escape from an intolerable situation)

Puerilism (patient regresses to a childish level in an attempt to escape from a difficult situation, for manipulative purposes or as a form of attention seeking)

Twilight states (dream-like state of consciousness, visual pseudohallucinations, re-enactment of emotionally charged episodes; hysterical stupor, hysterical trance states; multiple personality — patient becomes at times 'a different person' claiming no knowledge of the other 'self').

Behavioural symptoms

Repeated spurious suicidal attempts (not intended to succeed; attempt to gain attention; may succeed by accident and must therefore be taken seriously)

Dermatitis artefacta‖ (self-inflicted lesions varying from redness to ulceration; absence of complete resemblance to any other disorder; lesions have an artificial and curiously bizarre appearance, pos-

---

† Frank malingering with a motive such as avoiding work which is disliked. It might be thought that compensation neurosis would fall at the frank malingering end of the spectrum. It is believed, however, that the power of human self-deception is far too strong to make this necessary. Patients suffer from complaints that they hope will bring compensation and at the same time retain their self-respect by believing in them themselves.

‡ Usually the left side; sometimes incongruously differential to different sensations, e.g. feel cold but not warm items.

§ May mimic hemiparetic (usually an atypical dragging behind of the affected leg during a series of hops or supported steps), steppage or ataxic gait disorders. The

diagnosis is obvious when the patient walks in a lurching, irregularly based, sometimes bent-forward manner, grasping anything in reach for support and reeling from side to side inconsistently. He may sink to the floor but does not usually endure a self-injuring fall.

‖ As with the other conditions mentioned, dermatitis artefacta is usually a manifestation of hysteria, with the usual minorities of cases at either end of the spectrum—at the one end the patient who not only denies knowing how the lesions developed but also may not in fact know their cause; and at the other end the frank malingerer. It should be remembered also that patients with psychotic illnesses may mutilate themselves without any obvious motive.

sessing angles and edges not associated with lesions of any other disorder; severity depends on the agent used—e.g. carbolic acid, alkalis, cigarettes, matches, sandpaper — they may be ingeniously hidden — severe burns, deep scars and ragged ulcers may be seen; hospitalization may be required to definitely discover the diagnosis and cause)

Thermometer manipulation (spurious impression of fever)

Pseudohaemoptysis or pseudohaematemesis (extraction of blood from lips, gums or pharynx)

Swallowing objects (e.g. buttons, safety pins, even cutlery).

Munchausen's syndrome

First described and named by Richard Asher (as in Appendix 5, p. 525) in 1951. Patients travel from hospital to hospital telling dramatic but untruthful stories, simulating acute illnesses and submitting to countless unnecessary operations and investigations. A few days after admission they discharge themselves and resume their travels. Common varieties include laparotomophilia migrans (acute abdominal crises), neurologica diabolica (fits, blackouts, disturbances of consciousness, etc.) and haemorrhagica histrionica (haematemesis, etc.).

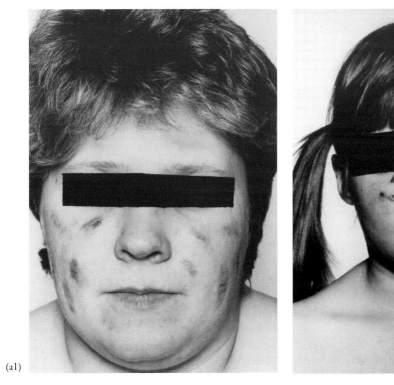
(a1)

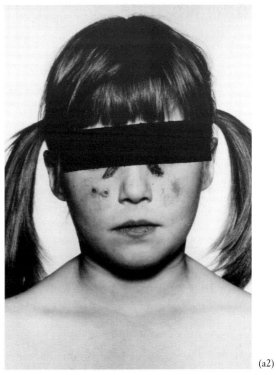
(a2)

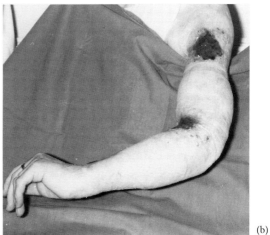
(b)

Fig. 3.199 (a1,2) Dermatitis aftefacta—self-inflicted lesions.
(b) Self-inflicted ulcers.

From the survey it is clear that the commonest reason for finding no abnormality is missing the physical signs which are present (probably anecdote 5 below and possibly anecdote 4; see also experience 51, p. 454). Nevertheless, short cases have occurred in which it seems that there was no abnormality and 'normal' was the correct diagnosis. Three or four from the original first edition survey are detailed below. The instructions to examiners show that patients without physical signs may be included in the short cases. Despite this we feel that it is likely that most cases of 'normal' will be either because the physical signs are no longer present by the time the patient comes to the examination (anecdote 1 below), or that the examiners and candidate disagree with the selectors of the cases about the presence of physical signs (may have happened in anecdote 2 below; see also experience 87, p. 459 and anecdote 50, p. 498).

Anecdote 1

A candidate was asked to examine a patient's eye movements. He found no abnormality and said so. He reports that this was confirmed by the examiners and he passed. Apparently the patient had been included in the examination because she had had internuclear ophthalmoplegia, but this was no longer present at the time of this examination.

Anecdote 2

A candidate was asked to examine the fundi. He found no abnormality and diagnosed a normal fundus. He reports that the patient had multiple sclerosis and that he knows one of the examiners who has since confirmed that her fundi were considered to be normal. He passed the examination but he felt he would have failed if he had said 'bitemporal pallor'.

Anecdote 3

A candidate was asked to examine the abdomen. She could find no abnormality and told the examiner she thought the abdomen was normal. She was asked to demonstrate the 'tests' for splenic enlargement. She passed the examination and in retrospect she still feels that it was a normal abdomen.

Anecdote 4

A candidate was asked to examine a man's abdomen. He could find no abnormality and diagnosed a normal abdomen. In retrospect he is not sure if he missed something. Though he failed the clinical he felt he had passed the short case section.

Anecdote 5

A candidate was asked to examine the heart. He could find no abnormality and said so because he thought he had to be honest. He has no idea what the diagnosis was. He failed.

Section 4
Experiences, Anecdotes, Tips, Facts and Figures, Quotations*

'I know 'cos I was there'.†

* For detailed contents of Section 4, see Appendix 7, p. 544.
† Max Boyce—referring to the victory of the Welsh rugby team in the 1970s over the All Blacks.

This section starts with a variety of MRCP short-case *experiences* and *anecdotes* (taken from the large number recounted to us by the candidates in our surveys and also including a few from those brought to us by some flies on the walls!). Because of limited space only a few full accounts are given; the remainder are extracts. Although they span the last 10–20 years (including one or two from when the exam was only 20 min long), the tragedies and triumphs do not seem to change with time.

We have placed the extracts into specific groups. If an examiner spots a weakness, such as poor observation or examination technique, he is likely to explore this further before deciding whether to pass or fail a candidate. Consequently, some of the experiences are grouped according to which aspect of the candidate's clinical competence the examiner might have been probing most. A miscellaneous group of anecdotes follows the experiences. Though the outcome was not necessarily decided by the particular short case(s) in question, for additional information we have indicated with many of the experiences and anecdotes whether the candidate passed or failed. A list of useful *tips* is given, before some further *facts and figures* which were gleaned from the original (first edition) survey. The section finishes with a selection of *quotations* from successful MRCP candidates. At the end of the questionnaire, the candidates in our survey were asked if there were any comments they would like passed on to the candidates of the future. We felt the consistencies and occasional discrepancies in the advice of such a large number of 'authorities' might be of interest to some candidates and so we present here a selection from the large number received. In order not to distort the force and intentions contained in these advisory comments, we have tended to offer them verbatim. Inevitably some of the quotations are contradictory in their opinions — as with all examinations, individuals have different experiences and offer differing advice. Our views on these discrepancies are reflected throughout the book as far as they could be dealt with.* Ultimately you will have to come to your own conclusion depending upon the circumstances of a particular case.

Experiences

'The examiners let him realize that he had missed coarctation of the aorta'.

1 In his first case (first attempt) a candidate was asked: 'Examine this man's heart'. He found a short systolic murmur in a hypertensive patient and diagnosed aortic sclerosis. He did not look for radiofemoral delay because he had been asked to examine the heart and not the cardiovascular system. The examiners let him realize that he had missed coarctation of the aorta. Filled with anger and dismay at this injustice he was taken to the next case where he was asked to listen to the *back* of a woman's chest. He had a quick look at the *front* (was not asked to) and spotted the radiation marks (he felt that the examiners were trying to hide this clue from him). He looked purposefully at the back and noted pleural aspiration marks. He therefore suspected a pleural effusion and performed the relevant clinical steps to confirm this impression. He was asked the probable cause and without hesitation gave the diagnosis of bronchial carcinoma along with the supportive evidence. He was then asked to examine a man's cranial nerves. He performed a rapid, efficient screen and reported left VIth, VIIth, XIIth nerve palsies and left lateral nystagmus but he was not asked for a diagnosis. For his fourth case he was asked to look at a man and he gave the spot diagnosis of acromegaly. When asked how to diagnose the condition he suggested imaging of the pituitary fossa, GTT with growth hormone levels, etc. Next he was asked to look at a patient's arm and he instantly recognized the 'plucked chicken skin' appearance of pseudoxanthoma elasticum in the antecubital fossa. Finally, he was asked to look at a woman's face where he saw nothing obvious until he

* For example, the discrepancies of quotations under the heading: 'Listen, obey and do not stray'—in general we support extending the examination beyond the examiner's instruction, whenever necessary, so long as this is done with intelligence and discrimination.

spotted a small left pupil and slight ptosis. He immediately diagnosed a left Horner's syndrome and was asked for, and gave, the possible causes. Though his performance in all but the first case had been impeccable he was convinced, until the result arrived, that he had failed because of that first case. In retrospect his reaction to the first case may have had a positive effect on the subsequent performance. Instead of going to pieces (e.g. experience 2, below, and quotations 52 and 55, p. 506) he felt anger at being asked to examine the heart when the key finding was at the femoral pulse. He conducted the rest of the exam with ruthless efficiency and avenged himself by looking for more than he was asked to. The parting words of the examiner were: 'You'll never miss radiofemoral delay again, will you?' (Pass)

'He looked down on two thin legs, imagined two inverted champagne bottles, and before he could stop himself, heard himself saying "Charcot–Marie–Tooth disease"'.
2 On his second attempt another candidate was asked first to: 'Examine the abdomen'. Without looking anywhere he coned down and felt the liver edge. After a long time, and some persuasion, he noticed the palmar erythema, anaemia, gynaecomastia and decreased body hair. These signs, in particular the gynaecomastia, together with the diagnosis of cirrhosis had to be dragged out of him by the examiners. The candidate had been nervous before the start and now, realizing that he had performed badly on the first case through lack of proper inspection, was already becoming engulfed in the 'downward spiral syndrome'. At the second case the examiner said: 'We haven't much time so just quickly feel the pulse and listen over the apex and base'. He was confused as he did not know where the base was so he listened at the lower left sternal edge and the apex. He did not look at the neck or at the praecordium. He felt a collapsing pulse, heard a systolic murmur and diagnosed mitral incompetence. In retrospect he thought that he must have missed mixed aortic valve disease. On the next case he was asked to examine the legs. He realized that things were going very badly and that he had to score highly from then on. He looked down on two thin legs, imagined two inverted champagne bottles and, before he could stop himself, heard himself saying 'Charcot–Marie–Tooth disease'. The examiner, who was apparently becom-

ing increasingly doubtful about the candidate's capability at performing a competent clinical examination, had to drag a hesitant, unstructured examination out of him which revealed spastic paraparesis. A discussion followed on the possible causes. In the next case the candidate looked at a fundus with whiteness around the disc and diagnosed myelinated nerve fibres. In his last case he examined a patient's hands with swollen metacarpophalangeal and proximal interphalangeal joints, tapered fingers, wasted intrinsic muscles and papery thin skin. With his morale gone, it took a long time before he saw any of the abnormalities and longer still to suggest rheumatoid arthritis (?on steroids). (Fail)

'He was side-tracked into saying that she could have hereditary haemorrhagic telangiectasia'.
3 After an indifferent start in the short cases, a candidate was asked to examine a man's pulse. He found it regular and the rate was 40 beats min^{-1}. He was then asked to listen to the precordium but he failed to comment on the variable intensity of the first heart sound which could have led him to the diagnosis of complete heart block. He was next asked to look at a woman's face. There was perioral tethering and telangiectasis, but since he had not performed a *visual survey* and his presentation was loose, he was side-tracked into saying that she could have hereditary haemorrhagic telangiectasia. It became obvious to him (he was asked to look at the hands — sclerodactyly) that the patient had scleroderma! The examiner then asked him: 'On which part of the tongue would you say the telangiectasiae would most likely be found in hereditary haemorrhagic telangiectasia, if you were teaching a class of medical students!' Having been unable to impress the examiners so far, he was asked to look at a man's neck. (The bell went almost immediately signalling the end of the exam.) The patient was lying down and his neck movements were completely restricted. The candidate diagnosed cervical spondylosis. The typical 'question mark' posture of ankylosing spondylitis only became recognizable when the patient sat up!

In his second attempt, this candidate was asked to examine a middle-aged woman with a goitre—he felt it was really quite straightforward. The goitre was asymmetrical but he annoyed one examiner by using the term 'slightly asymmetrical'. He also let out the word 'tumour' in front of the patient when asked to discuss management. (Fail)

'During the examination he was interrupted at various times'.

4 A candidate on his first attempt was asked to look at a man's legs (the examiner pulled the pyjamas to the lower end of the patella, leaving a lateral scar covered — which the candidate did not see until the end). He found a swollen, warm left leg and diagnosed a deep venous thrombosis. He was asked for other possibilities and said ruptured Baker's cyst. The examiner said he would not ask who Baker was but wanted an explanation of the term. The examiners probed for further possibilities such as cellulitis, muscle rupture and also asked about ruptured plantaris muscle. On his next case he was asked to look at some hands and describe them. He diagnosed rheumatoid arthritis and was asked to explain the reasons for ulnar deviation, subluxation and boutonnière deformity. The examiner asked: 'Why is it called boutonnière? Have you ever seen a button hook? Why is the wrist like that? What are the important functions of the hand?' He was then asked to look at the knees of the same patient. He found a swollen, painful right knee which he thought was due to synovial swelling. He said he had been about to say: 'Charcot's joint' but realized it was painful. He diagnosed rheumatoid arthritis of the knee and was then asked how he knew it was synovial swelling. At the next patient the examiners said: 'I think we would be interested in this lady's precordium'. During the examination he was interrupted at various times: 'What do you think of the pulse?'; 'What do you think of the JVP?'; and in fact they stopped him before he had finished and asked for the findings. He diagnosed mixed mitral valve disease but had missed the mitral valvotomy scar. The examiner then handed him an ophthalmoscope and said: 'We would like you to use this on the next patient'. The candidate noticed that this patient showed some incoordination and a spastic leg so he expected to find optic atrophy. When he mentioned this diagnosis the examiner asked him if he knew what sort of visual field defect he would expect and then asked him to test the visual fields. On the last case he was asked to feel the abdomen. He found an inguinal hernia, a palpable aorta and a palpable liver edge at about 2 cm below the right costal margin. He said he did not think it was hepatomegaly. The examiners asked what signs he would look for if the patient did have hepatomegaly! (Pass)

In the following examples the examiner seems to be probing the power and range of the candidate's observations

5 A candidate, in her first attempt, was somewhat uncertain about her performance in the first two short cases. She was then asked to examine the motor system of a man's legs. She found global weakness, wasting and loss of reflexes. She gave a differential diagnosis of lower motor neurone paralysis which included a disc lesion, spinal canal problems, degenerative disorders and motor neurone disease. The examiners asked her to look at the patient's tongue—it was fasciculating. She was then able to narrow the differential diagnosis to the last-mentioned possibility. (Pass)

6 A candidate was asked: 'Look at this man's chest and then examine his respiratory system'. The patient had a right mastectomy scar and the skin changes of previous radiotherapy. There was dullness to percussion and reduced breath sounds at the right base. The candidate diagnosed carcinoma of the breast and a right pleural effusion. (Pass)

7 Taken to her first short case, a candidate was asked only to listen to a patient's heart. No other cardiovascular system examination was expected. She found the features of mitral stenosis but did not notice the valvotomy scar. This was pointed out to her by the examiner. (Pass)

8 After rapid progress through the first three short cases, a candidate was asked to look at a woman's hands. He found the changes of rheumatoid arthritis. A description was not wanted, only the diagnosis. The examiner then asked him: 'Why is she wearing a cervical collar?' The candidate, who had noticed but not mentioned it, said that it could be due to atlantoaxial subluxation. (Pass)

9 After mistaking a malar flush for SLE in a patient who had mitral stenosis, a candidate was asked to examine a woman's hands. She diagnosed acromegaly. Although the patient had wasting of the thenar eminence she missed this, and the diagnosis of carpal tunnel syndrome, until the examiner told her about the patient's symptoms. The candidate

diagnosed optic atrophy, splenomegaly and hepatosplenomegaly successively in three other short cases and was then shown a patient and asked: 'On general appearance what is wrong with this man?' She thought that he had a myopathic facies and diagnosed dystrophia myotonica. The examiner asked why she thought he had a hearing aid. She looked at the head again and realized that the patient had an enlarged cranium, rather than wasted facial muscles, and diagnosed Paget's disease. (Fail)

10 At her next attempt this candidate gave a better account of herself in four short cases but missed a nodule at the elbow in a patient with rheumatoid arthritis. She was then asked to examine a man's abdomen. She found an enlarged and knobbly liver and diagnosed secondaries in the liver, but forgot to test for ascites. She was asked if there was any free peritoneal fluid. The examiners watched intently as she demonstrated the presence of ascites. (Pass)

11 A candidate was asked to examine the abdomen. He found bilateral masses in the loins and diagnosed polycystic kidneys. The patient also had a craniotomy scar for a ruptured berry aneurysm. On another case he was able to diagnose hypothyroidism by looking at a woman's face. The examiner asked why she was in a surgical ward and he suggested severe constipation as a reason. (Pass)

12 In his second attempt a candidate was asked: 'Examine this lady's cardiovascular system, commenting as you go'. He diagnosed mixed mitral valve disease but missed (cardiac) cachexia and a left mastectomy scar. The examiners wanted him to comment that she was very ill and to suggest why. They also asked for comments as to whether the mitral stenosis or mitral incompetence was dominant. (Fail)

13 A candidate was asked: 'Comment on this patient's appearance. Pretend he is sitting opposite you on the underground train and perform one clinical test'. The candidate noted frontal bossing, bilateral ptosis, deafness, missing fingers on the right hand and a saddle-shaped nose. Initially the candidate thought he had congenital syphilis and wanted to do a Romberg's test. The examiner manipulated the discussion and got him round to thinking about dystrophia myotonica. After this the candidate sug-gested a handshake as the one clinical test. He was then asked to examine the abdomen of the next patient. He found bilateral enlarged and 'lumpy' kidneys which were easily palpable and he diagnosed polycystic kidneys. The candidate was then shown the patient's left forearm and, having worked on a renal unit, he immediately recognized the presence of an arteriovenous fistula for haemodialysis. The examiners seemed quite impressed with this. (Pass)

14 Another candidate was shown the same patient with dystrophia myotonica and asked: 'What observations do you make?' He commented on bilateral ptosis, wasted sternomastoid and temporalis muscles, and after demonstrating myotonia in the hands was able to make the diagnosis. There then followed a brief viva on cardiomyopathy in dystrophia myotonica! (Pass)

15 After failing to palpate polycystic kidneys, a candidate was asked to listen to a patient's heart. He found mitral incompetence and noted that the patient's face looked acromegalic. However, he did not mention the acromegaly until he was directly asked about it. (Fail)

16 A candidate was taken to a patient with a recent laparotomy scar and asked to examine his neck. He noticed a biopsy scar and on palpation found matted glands. He diagnosed Hodgkin's disease and the examiner asked him for a differential diagnosis. (Pass)

17 In his fourth attempt a candidate was asked to make some observations on a patient with a goitre, then on his next case to feel the pulse and suggest what had happened to that patient (he had atrial fibrillation, exophthalmos and a right hemiplegia). He was then taken to the foot of the next patient's bed and asked: 'Look at this patient from here. What would you like to do now?' He noticed a man with long extremities, muscle wasting, a pustular rash, paronychia, nicotine-stained fingers and pectus excavatum. He had to be prompted to the diagnosis of Marfan's syndrome. He was then asked to look into the patient's mouth (high-arched palate) and to listen to his heart (aortic incompetence). He found both of these but did not mention the hyperextensible joints. (Pass)

18 'This lady is breathless—listen to her heart' was the opening instruction to a candidate who was appearing for the first time. He diagnosed mitral stenosis but the examiners pointed out that he had not noticed that the lady had rheumatoid arthritis as well. He was taken to his next case and told: 'This patient is breathless — examine the respiratory system'. He found crepitations and basal dullness so he diagnosed pulmonary fibrosis and pleural effusion. Having learned from the previous case, he was able to relate both to the rheumatoid arthritis which he had already observed in this patient. (Pass)

19 After having difficulty deciding whether a patient had diabetic or hypertensive retinopathy, a candidate was asked to examine another patient's neck. He diagnosed a small multinodular goitre but the examiners remained dissatisfied. They asked if the patient was thyrotoxic or not. While he examined for a tremor he noticed the gross rheumatoid arthritis in the hands. He reported that the examiners were looking for the diagnosis of autoimmune thyroid disease. (Fail)

20 A candidate was invited to look at a patient's face. The face was normal when looking straight ahead but on further examination he discovered weakness of the lower part of the right side of the face and he diagnosed a right upper motor neurone VIIth nerve palsy. He missed the surgical scar just below the jaw on the right side and, in retrospect, felt it was a partial right lower motor neurone VIIth nerve palsy. (Fail)

21 A candidate was asked to look at a patient's face. He said: 'Acromegaly'. The examiner asked if he was happy with that. The candidate realized that he should have looked for more physical signs so at once he said he would like to look for complications such as bitemporal hemianopia, hypertension, cardiomegaly, or evidence of treatment already given. The patient did, in fact, have a hemianopia. (Pass)

In the experiences that follow the spotlight seems to be on the candidate's examination technique

22 After diagnosing psoriasis and lupus pernio in fairly quick succession, a candidate was asked to examine a patient's legs neurologically. He found bi-

lateral upper motor neurone signs and was then asked the level of the lesion. The candidate proceeded to examine the arms and found upper motor neurone signs in one arm. He next tested the jaw jerk which was normal. No further questions were asked. (Pass)

23 A candidate was asked to examine a patient's abdomen. He found an enlarged organ in the left hypochondrium and thought that it was a polycystic kidney but he admits that his examination was 'cack-handed'. In retrospect he believes it was a spleen. He was later asked to look at a patient's fundi. He diagnosed choroiditis but in retrospect he feels that it was probably a diabetic retinopathy with laser burns. (Fail)

24 After an opening case of a Ramsay Hunt syndrome a candidate was asked to examine a woman's fundi, to look for pyramidal signs in her hands, and to elicit her plantar responses. He found early papilloedema on the left and an increased finger jerk and supernator jerk on the right, and an extensor planter on the right. He admitted that he had made a mess of doing the finger jerks and did not know the two ways of eliciting these; in fact the examiner had to demonstrate the tests. He was about to test the plantar response with the end of the patella hammer when he was stopped by the examiner who gave him a thin wooden orange stick! (Pass)

25 Having spoiled the first two short cases a candidate was asked to look at, and then examine, the legs of a man who complained of unsteadiness. He found ataxia, pyramidal weakness with clonus in both legs and bilateral extensor plantar responses and he diagnosed multiple sclerosis. However, the examiner was not at all happy with his neurological examination technique and, in fact, showed him how to do it! (Fail)

26 In his third attempt, a candidate missed something in two of the first four short cases (diabetic maculopathy, calcinosis in scleroderma). He was then asked to watch a patient walk and to examine his lower limbs. He could see bilateral foot-drop with wasted anterior compartments but did not make the diagnosis of Charcot–Marie–Tooth disease. The examiners criticized the way he examined the reflexes. (Fail)

27 A candidate was told: 'This man has gone off his feet. Examine the legs and say why'. He found gross wasting, fasciculation, absent ankle jerks and flexor plantar responses and he diagnosed progressive muscular atrophy (motor neurone disease). He commented to us that he had had to wait for what seemed to be 3–4 min before any fasciculation was seen, though when it did come it was very obvious. (Pass)

28 A candidate was asked to examine a patient's eyes. He was almost blind in the left eye with a left VIth nerve palsy. He commented that he might well have failed the examination had he not tested visual acuity and thus found the explanation for the absence of diplopia. (Pass)

29 A candidate was asked to examine a man's hand neurologically. The patient had gross wasting and weakness of the small muscles of the hand. Although the candidate diagnosed a T1 lesion he admitted that he looked very confused examining the hands. A little unsettled by this experience he was asked to examine another patient's abdomen and jugular venous pressure. He found a pulsatile liver and giant *v* waves. He diagnosed tricuspid incompetence but admitted that he lacked confidence and this showed in the way he carried out the examination. He was then asked to examine the chest of a patient who had a thoracotomy scar, stridor and clubbing. He did not notice the stridor and also missed the pleural effusion. (Fail)

30 On being asked to examine the abdomen of a patient a candidate found bilateral subcostal masses. He gave the findings and said the diagnosis was probably polycystic kidneys. The left-sided mass could have been a small spleen moving diagonally across the abdomen from under the rib cage on inspiration but it was bimanually ballotable. He gave the findings and persevered with the diagnosis of polycystic kidneys. The examiners persisted in discussing the possibility that the mass was a spleen but the candidate stuck to his diagnosis which he thinks was right. (Pass)

31 A candidate was asked: 'Examine this man's chest. Is there anything else you would look for?' He found ankylosing spondylitis with poor expansion

and excursion of the chest, but commented that he had to get the patient out of bed before he appreciated the ankylosing spondylitis. There was no evidence of aortic regurgitation or upper lobe fibrosis. (Pass)

32 A candidate examined the abdomen of a 35-year-old Afro–Caribbean woman and found a 6 cm spherical mass in the left upper quadrant. He commented that he was allowed to 'go through the motions'—nodes, mouth, hands, etc. He said it was not a spleen or a kidney and he explained why. He gave a brief differential diagnosis . . . 'Expressionless and without comment they led me away'. (Pass)

33 A candidate had done well in his first four short cases except that he failed to demonstrate stridor in a patient with superior vena cava obstruction. He was taken to his fifth case and asked: 'Show me how you examine the reflexes in the legs'. He found absent knee and ankle jerks and extensor plantar responses. He offered the differential diagnosis of tabes dorsalis, subacute combined degeneration of the cord and hereditary neuropathy such as Freidreich's ataxia. He was asked what else he would like to examine and he suggested the pupillary reflexes. He found small regular pupils which reacted to light and accommodation, but more to accommodation. He was asked if these were Argyll Robertson pupils and he answered: 'No'. The other examiner said: 'You said that this picture in the legs may be due to tabes dorsalis. How do you explain the extensor plantars?' He answered that this indicates pyramidal tract involvement. The examiner pointed out that this is called taboparesis, not tabes dorsalis. The candidate felt that his unfamiliarity with the different manifestations of neurosyphilis let him down, and he had failed to recognize Argyll Robertson pupils. (Fail)

34 The opening short case of a candidate in his first attempt was a patient with an obvious squint and exophthalmos. He was asked to *examine** the eyes, look at the neck and feel the pulse. He stated the obvious, but did not test the eye movements adequately and reports: 'Actually the examiner expected me to examine the eye movements prop-

* Our italics. The candidate was expected to do more than just look at the eyes.

erly and identify the muscle paralysed'. The examiner then explained that exophthalmos and goitre suggest thyrotoxicosis and that the normal sinus rhythm suggests that the latter has been treated. The candidate was also shown cases of clubbing of the fingers, cyanosis and psoriatic arthropathy, all of which he could recognize, and the examiner finally took him to a patient and asked him: 'Examine the abdomen'. He found an enlarged liver of three finger breadths and a spleen of four finger breadths and diagnosed hepatosplenomegaly. The examiner's parting comment was: 'It is no good only making a diagnosis; there is a proper method to examine the patient!' (Fail)

35 A candidate was asked to examine the back of the chest of a young man. He diagnosed bilateral pleural effusions and he felt that these were probably due to nephrotic syndrome. He believes the examiners agreed. However, he had forgotten to test for vocal resonance or tactile vocal fremitus. (Fail)

36 A candidate was asked to examine a patient's heart. He went through all the correct examination steps except that he forgot to lift up the arm and feel for a collapsing pulse. He diagnosed mixed mitral valve disease. One examiner proceeded to listen to the heart while the other examiner asked if the candidate had felt for a collapsing pulse. The candidate now wonders if he missed aortic valve disease. (Fail)

37 A candidate was asked to examine the eyes of a girl aged about 20–30 years. He went comprehensively through, checking visual acuity and visual fields before testing eye movements. He felt the examiners were impatient at the delay in finding the nystagmus which was present. The examiners asked what he wanted to examine now. The candidate, thinking that the diagnosis was likely to be multiple sclerosis, said he wanted to look at the fundi. He could not understand why the examiners seemed so irritated by this. They wanted him to demonstrate the cerebellar signs which were present. The candidate felt that this was an easy case on which he had made no great errors and yet the examiners seemed to have been unimpressed by his performance. (Fail)

38 A candidate was asked to examine a patient's legs neurologically and then to ask him some questions.

He found global aphasia and a profound right-sided spastic hemiparesis. He diagnosed a dominant hemisphere vascular lesion. He was asked: 'What might be the cause? The patient is 40'; —(pause)— 'Feel the pulse'. He was in atrial fibrillation. 'What do you think the cause is now?' (Pass)

39 A candidate was shown a woman with a spastic paraparesis which she correctly diagnosed. After she had been taken to the next case, the examiners said: 'By the way, which side of the fire does that other lady usually sit by?' Luckily, she had noticed the erythema ab igne on the legs. (Pass)

A lack of polish and fluidity may make the examiners reflect on the clinical competence of a candidate. In the following examples, the examiners seem to be endeavouring to find the real clinical depth

40 An examiner pointed to a patient with typical rheumatoid hands and said to a candidate: 'This lady had a fit 6 months ago, examine her hands'. During his examination he found no skin rash or nodules. He diagnosed SLE in view of the fit. However, in retrospect, he still wonders if the diagnosis was rheumatoid arthritis. (Pass)

41 A candidate was introduced to a man of about 40 years. The examiner said: 'This young man has started having blackouts, would you examine him and tell me why'. The candidate was in a quandary. He noticed the patient was young. He wondered whether he was diabetic or had postural hypotension, and whether they wanted a neurological examination or a cardiovascular examination. The patient interrupted his thoughts and asked which part of him he wanted to examine. He told the patient he was not sure. He started with the pulse and went on to examine the cardiovascular system and made the correct diagnosis of mixed aortic valve disease with predominant aortic regurgitation. He was asked about the pulse character and how he would assess it and he then got all this wrong. He felt that he had done a good job communicating his dilemma to the examiners! (Fail)

42 A candidate was asked to examine the cardiovascular system in a patient. He found a slow rising pulse, an ejection systolic murmur and an early diastolic murmur. He diagnosed mixed aortic valve disease with predominant aortic stenosis. The examiners asked him to guess his blood pressure. (Pass)

43 After correctly diagnosing spastic paraparesis, a candidate was asked to give the differences between upper and lower motor neurone lesions. In the next case he was asked to feel a man's pulse. He suggested slow atrial fibrillation but in retrospect he thinks it may have been complete heart block. There then followed a discussion about the differential diagnosis and the management of complete heart block with different types of pacemakers. (Fail)

44 A candidate who was taking the examination for the fourth time was taken to his first case and asked: 'Feel this patient's pulse and apex beat, and listen to the base of the heart'. He was required to give a full description of the findings and the probable diagnosis at each stage. He found pulsus bisferiens, a displaced apex, an ejection systolic and an early diastolic murmur. (Pass)

45 A candidate, who was unhappy with his examination technique and the mistakes he had made in an easy first case, was asked to examine the right arm of a 40-year-old man. He reports finding a 'flail' arm with increased reflexes. He thought his method of examination was poor and he was unsure of the diagnosis. He was then asked to examine the same man's abdomen and reports finding bilateral, large, smooth, more or less symmetrical masses in the lumbar regions which he diagnosed as bilateral hydronephrotic kidneys.* (Fail)

46 A candidate was asked to: 'Examine the eyes from a neurological point of view'. He found bilateral ptosis and a homonymous hemianopia and he said to the examiner that he could not explain the findings by one lesion. The examiner said: 'Examine the hands'. The candidate became preoccupied with the obvious rheumatoid arthritis and came up with the suggestion of rheumatoid arthritis associated with myasthenia gravis, which would explain the

ptosis but not the hemianopia. The examiner said: 'Feel the pulse'. The candidate found an irregular pulse and diagnosed atrial fibrillation causing a cerebral embolus. (Pass)

47 A candidate examined the back of the chest of a patient and found a pleural effusion. He had to go through the full examination and was asked what he was doing at every move, what each finding was caused by and how he interpreted it, e.g. breath sounds, crepitations, etc. (Pass)

Common errors
48 Having done well in his first three short cases a candidate was asked to give a running commentary as he examined the cardiovascular system. He commented on a collapsing pulse and on a mitral valvotomy scar but found no murmurs. He diagnosed mitral stenosis and got involved in a long discussion on the causes of a collapsing pulse! (Fail)

49 A candidate was asked to listen to a woman's heart. He found systolic and diastolic murmurs maximal at the base of the heart, to the left of the sternum. He diagnosed mixed aortic valve disease. In retrospect he is sure that he missed the typical machinery murmur of a patent ductus arteriosus. (Fail)

50 A candidate was asked to examine a man's chest, commenting as he went along. Though he thought the patient had chronic obstructive airways disease he was not actually asked for a diagnosis, but instead became caught up in a discussion on the distinction between a wheeze and stridor. (Pass)

51 Still flustered by two of the previous three cases which had gone badly, a candidate examined a fundus of a patient whose pupil had been dilated. He could not find much wrong and wondered if there was some vascular abnormality. He made a wild guess at diabetic retinopathy and wonders in retrospect if this was a branch retinal vein or artery occlusion. His comment was: 'I was totally lost by this time!' (Fail)

52 A candidate examined the fundi of a patient and diagnosed bilateral optic atrophy and background diabetic retinopathy. He told us he had 'blurted out my impressions before stopping and thinking'. Even

---

* We wonder if this patient had polycystic kidneys and an old cerebrovascular accident (ruptured berry aneurysm/ hypertension).

in retrospect he does not know what the diagnosis was. (Fail)

53 A candidate was asked to examine the fundi of a patient (dilated pupils, dark room). He saw haemorrhages, exudates and some whiteness around the disc. He was put off by the examiners talking in the background and by his paranoia that the examiners were thinking that he was taking too long so he stopped before he had finished. He offered the diagnosis of diabetic retinopathy and myelinated nerve fibres. One examiner looked in the fundi while the other enquired if any microaneurysms had been seen. The candidate was not sure. There was then a discussion about the treatment of diabetic retinopathy and when photocoagulation was mentioned the examiner asked if there was any evidence of this. In retrospect the candidate felt diabetic retinopathy was probably right but wonders about the possibility of having missed hypertensive retinopathy and papilloedema. He felt that if only he had continued examining longer to elicit the exact findings present he would have saved himself over £200.* (Fail)

54 A candidate was asked to feel the pulse of a patient. She was unable to feel it and guessed that atrial fibrillation must be present. (She failed) Another candidate was taken to the same patient and admitted that she could feel neither the radials, brachials nor carotids (the patient was in low output cardiac failure). Afterwards she was told by the examiners at the sherry reception (Edinburgh) that they had re-examined the patient and agreed with her. (Pass)

55 A potential candidate was asked to examine the back of the chest of a patient with bronchiectasis who had appeared in the examination. During auscultation the patient, in her enthusiasm to cooperate, breathed deeply and expired forcibly, generating upper airways wheeze.† The candidate, who already had his stethoscope in his ears, was unaware of the racket the patient was making. He

reported the finding of widespread wheeze (the basal crepitations were completely drowned) though there was no wheezing at all when the patient was asked to breath deeply in and out in a relaxed fashion.

Look first

56 A candidate was asked to listen to the back of a lady's chest. Although only asked to listen, she examined expansion, percussion, palpation and finally auscultation thinking that they would stop her if all they wanted her to do was listen. They did not interrupt. She presented her findings of bilateral mid to late inspiratory crackles up to the mid zone and her diagnosis of fibrosing alveolitis. The examiners asked: 'Look at the patient and tell us what you think is the cause in her case'. At first the candidate could see no obvious cause from the face and therefore looked at her hands and immediately *spotted the changes of systemic sclerosis*. She then looked at the face again and the telangiectasia and tight skin were evident. (Pass)

57 A candidate was taken to a plethoric man in his forties and told that he had difficulty breathing and was asked to find out why. He *did not spot the mitral valvotomy scar* and therefore started examining the respiratory system. It was only when he got to percussion of the chest that he noticed the scar. In view of the scar, he asked the examiners if he was examining the wrong system. They asked if it could be for any other operation. When the candidate said it could only be a mitral valvotomy, they asked him to examine his heart and the candidate went on to find atrial fibrillation and signs of mixed mitral valve disease. A discussion took place over the best place to hear the opening snap. (Pass)

58 A candidate was asked to examine a lady's neck. The candidate started off looking at the patient generally. No JVP was obvious. She started feeling for lymph nodes. The examiners said: 'What are you doing?' so she explained that she was looking for lymph nodes—they asked why. She explained that

---

* Correct at time of first edition.

† You can generate upper airways wheeze yourself by expiring hard at the same time as voluntarily narrowing your upper airways. If in doubt in the hysterical asthmatic, ask the patient to purse his lips as he breathes. This manoeuvre will

abolish factitious wheeze. Though the wheeze of such a patient may be heard down the corridor, the pulse is not significantly elevated in the absence of true severe asthma (unless the acute asthma is due to the inappropriate prescription of a β-blocker!).

she could not see anything else abnormal and then *spotted the glass of water* on the window sill and 'twigged'. She then started a thyroid examination and found a left thyroid nodule which was both visible and palpable on swallowing. A discussion followed about possible causes. (Pass)

59 A candidate was asked: 'Look at this lady, tell us what you notice'. The candidate thought the patient had a heliotrope rash and said so. The examiners were unimpressed. 'Have another look at her eyes' they said. The candidate then *spotted that she was jaundiced*. 'Now examine her abdomen', they said. He reported a liver edge at three fingers breadth, no spleen and ascites. He felt that he presented his findings in a rather disorganized way. They responded by feeling the liver themselves. 'That's not three fingers breadths', one of them said. 'Could you feel a spleen?' they asked, perfectly well aware that he had already said that he couldn't. The candidate reports that he stuck to his guns and said he could not feel a spleen and he presumes that he must have been right. He reports that he was 'well rattled' by this short case but went on to perform well on the other short cases. (Pass)

60 A candidate was asked to examine a patient's legs. He initially noticed gross ataxia, nystagmus and dysarthria when he went to introduce himself and shake his hand. However, he still managed to fail to make a diagnosis of Friedreich's ataxia ('youthful ignorance'!) and also ignored the examiner's prompt when he offered him a tuning fork and a patella hammer! He was then asked to look at another patient's legs. He thought he saw pes cavus and went on to do a full neurological examination being determined to show the examiners that he could do it! However, it was normal! The examiners then pointed out arachnodactyly so he changed his diagnosis to Marfan's syndrome! (Fail)

Double pathology

61 A candidate in her first attempt was asked to examine a woman's legs neurologically. She found absent ankle jerks, increased knee reflexes and equivocal plantars. She was told that the patient was a diabetic and she noticed that she was wearing a cervical collar. Her mind alerted to the possibility that there was a combination of a peripheral neuropathy and cervical spondylosis. (Pass)

62 After three successful cases a candidate was shown a patient and told: 'This patient has something wrong with his cardiovascular system. Find out in the most expeditious way'. She noticed exophthalmos and found a large abdominal scar and cardiac outflow tract obstruction. The patient later said that he had had a repair of a thoracic aortic aneurysm! (Pass)

63 After an easy first short case (splenomegaly) a candidate was asked to look at the face of a woman who presented with melaena. In retrospect he felt the patient had acromegaly and Peutz–Jeghers syndrome (!) but he had not spotted the latter condition quickly enough. He was asked to examine the visual fields and, having mentioned the presence of greasy skin, was drawn into a discussion on skin function. (Fail)

64 A candidate was asked to comment on the appearance of a patient. She had proptosis and a prosthetic eye. In addition there was also a thyroidectomy scar, evidence of thyroid acropachy and pretibial myxoedema. She had also had a recent amputation. He was asked to examine the fundi and it was obvious that she was also diabetic. (Pass)

65 A candidate who had had a genial discussion on scleroderma and its complications, was then asked to examine the legs of a man whom he was told had diabetes mellitus. He found a peripheral neuropathy and peripheral vascular disease. He also spotted that the patient had coexistent facioscapular dystrophy. (Pass)

66 In his second attempt, a candidate who had not done too well in the opening short case was then asked to examine the heart only of the next patient. He found mixed aortic valve disease. He also suspected mitral stenosis but did not mention it as he had 'not expected to find double valve pathology'. (Fail)

Tell them of the expert that told you

67 A candidate was examined on a patient with acromegaly and feels that he performed reasonably well. In the discussion as to why he had used a red pin to test visual fields, he told them that a neurologist who he had worked for had recommended it for the peripheral fields. The examiners seemed happy with that explanation. (Pass)

Apologies accepted

68 A candidate at his fourth attempt was so nervous as he went into the viva that when the examiner asked the first question, though it was easy, he found he could not speak. After a pause both examiners started writing on their pads which further increased the tension in the atmosphere. Eventually the candidate found his voice and gave a faultless performance for the rest of the viva. At the end he was still very concerned that the exam was over-shadowed by a bad start so before he left he apologized for it, saying that it was because he was so nervous. The examiners smiled and said that it was very understandable in a way which made him feel that his bad start had not had much effect on their overall judgement. He was glad he brought this up and obtained their reassurance because otherwise he feels he may still have been worrying about the viva when he went into the long and short cases. (Pass)

69 After doing well on his other short cases, a candidate was told to look in the eyes of a patient. He felt the disc margins were blurred and reported this. The examiners asked him if he could see venous pulsation. The candidate pointed out that he would not recognize it if he saw it! The candidate reports that the examiners appeared to like this response and went on to grill him on the different causes of blurred disc margins. The diagnosis was apparently hypermetropia. (Pass)

70 A candidate who had passed on her other short cases was asked to examine the fundi and reported background diabetic retinopathy. The examiners asked if she had seen laser burns. She said that she hadn't but that the eye was not dilated (which was true) and the examiners accepted this. (Pass)

71 A candidate was asked to examine the fundi of a patient who was diabetic. She explained that she could not see with her left eye and could only under-take ophthalmoscopy with her right eye. The examiners responded: 'As long as you are competent, we do not care how you do it'. (Pass)

72 A candidate who had passed on the basis of his other short cases was asked to examine the pre-

cordium of a 55-year-old female. He found atrial fib-rillation and mitral stenosis and a long discussion followed about 'How do you know it's atrial fibrilla-tion?' He reports that he forgot to mention the vari-able first heart sound. He reports that he made a big blunder when he said that the tapping apex was due to a big left atrium. Thirty seconds later, he said: 'Sir, I was wrong earlier. The tapping apex is not due to a big left atrium'. The examiner looked relieved and went on to ask where the candidate would feel for a big left atrium.* Luckily, the bell went at that moment and the candidate was not required to answer. (Pass)

73 A candidate reported to us: 'I think I probably did pass this section of the exam. Although I was a bit scrappy in my presentation I felt that I got all the diagnoses correct (eventually) and they seemed quite happy to let me retract my wrong diagnosis of diabetes mellitus in one of the patients. As in previous exams they nagged away at me and yet encouraged me when I was right. I felt that all the nagging was not just a test of my mettle but was also allowing me to show a depth of knowledge and confidence. My advice is to retract with confidence and admit areas of gaping ignorance'. (Pass)

'Even though I didn't mean to say it—I did; I opened my mouth and all this rubbish came out'

74 A candidate, nervous on his first attempt, was asked to palpate the abdomen. He found bilateral masses in the upper quadrants but states that he was interrupted before he could examine them properly. He thought they were polycystic kidneys but in the stress of the moment he found himself saying hepatosplenomegaly before he could stop himself! (Fail)

75 A candidate was asked to examine a woman's abdomen. The candidate found a deeply jaundiced woman with cachexia and a hard craggy liver. She did not detect ascites nor, convincingly, a spleen. However, when asked to give her findings, she found herself saying 'and she has a 2cm spleen'. She reports that she heard herself lying but was unable to stop herself. The examiner was not convinced

* First heart sound is palpable; left atrium is not palpable.

either and the candidate then started talking about 'a difficult to define mass in the left hypochondrium which could be hepatic'. She said the examiner seemed happier with this but did not ask how to differentiate between left hypochondrial masses. (Fail)

76 A candidate was asked on his first case to examine the cardiovascular system. He reports that he was stopped after examining the precordium before feeling the carotids and that though the signs had fitted with aortic stenosis, he was unsure whether the murmur was classically crescendo-decrescendo and he found himself giving the diagnosis of ventricular septal defect. The examiners made it obvious that they disagreed with this diagnosis. (Pass)

77 A candidate was asked to examine the fundi of a 19-year-old asymptomatic girl. On looking at the right fundus, she could not see the disc but the vessels and background were normal. She assumes now that there must have been papilloedema but it was the first case, she was in a complete panic and found herself saying that she did not know the diagnosis. She was told that she must know the diagnosis and then said: 'Hypertension'. The examiners walked out without comment leaving her feeling that she had completely messed up the case and had already failed the exam. She went on to do well enough on the other short cases to pass though was convinced after the exam that she had failed on the basis of the first short case. She stresses the importance of not giving up even if you think you have made a total mess of one short case. (Pass)

78 A candidate was told that a female patient was breathless and he was asked to examine her abdomen and to explain her breathlessness. He found massive hepatosplenomegaly plus anaemia and instead of coming out with myelosclerosis as the diagnosis, he said sarcoidosis! At this stage the examiners, who had been very pleasant until then, began to look impatient! (Fail)

79 'Examine the heart'. It would have been easy to start by saying, 'This chap, who is comfortable at rest with a midline sternotomy scar, has mitral regurgitation'. However, my mouth went into action before my brain and a load of verbal diarrhoea came out. The diagnosis was correct but the delivery was awful. (Fail)

Invigilators' diaries

80 A candidate was asked to examine the legs of a patient. He was allowed to carry out a large proportion of a full neurological examination before he became aware, with prodding from the examiner, of the large skull, hearing aid and the bowed tibiae of Paget's disease. The examiner commented that if he had *looked* at the patient first he might have saved himself the time wasted on the unnecessary neurological examination.

81 A candidate was asked to examine the eyes of a patient. He carried out most of the examination of the eye movements before he noticed the obvious blue sclerae of osteogenesis imperfecta. The examiner was irritated by this and commented that the candidate had wasted several minutes of the examiner's time by not looking at the eyes properly and noticing an obvious physical sign.

82 A candidate was asked to examine the fundi of a patient with diabetic retinopathy and laser photocoagulation scars. It was the end of the afternoon and the tropicamide drops, which had been put in that morning to dilate the pupil, had worn off. The candidate said she could see nothing and asked to take the patient into a darkened room. A side room was found but it was only semi-dark. She still said she could see nothing. The examiner was very unimpressed that she had missed what he considered to be a very easy case of diabetic retinopathy. When the invigilator tried to help save the candidate by apologizing that the drops had worn off, the examiner retorted that 'the pupils would not be dilated in the casualty department'.

83 A patient in the examination had a 'full house' of mixed mitral and aortic valve disease. The examiner commented that candidates kept failing to hear all the murmurs. He suspected that having heard one or two loud ones, they stopped listening for the others which were less obvious.

84 A candidate was asked to look at a lady's hands. He described Heberden's nodes, spindling of the fingers and proximal joint swelling, all of which the

patient had. He suggested combined osteoarthritis and rheumatoid arthritis. When the examiner asked about conditions associated with rheumatoid arthritis, the candidate looked beyond the hands and noticed the generalized pigmentation and then the palmar crease pigmentation of Addison's disease. The latter condition was the reason for the patient's inclusion in the examination—the joint changes had not been noted before.

85 A patient with a small calcified embolus in the fundus had been included amongst the patients available for one session of the examination. Before the exam, when the examiners were going around the patients by themselves, one examiner came away from this fundus and said to another examiner: 'Could you see the embolus?' 'No', said the second. 'Neither could I', replied the first: 'I'm not going to take any of my candidates on that case'. The case was used by other examiners on just one or two candidates.

86 A patient known to have Behçet's disease was included as a fundus case with optic atrophy. On fundoscopy he had optic atrophy, choroidoretinitis and also sheathing of the vessel walls. All the examiners agreed that they had not seen a fundus like it before and that it was a 'museum' case. The underlying cause was not discussed with any of the candidates who were only expected to see what was there and describe it accurately. Calling the vessel sheathing 'silver wiring', as one candidate did, was considered unacceptable.

87 Before one examination session all the examiners gathered around a patient to be shown his signs, which were said to include splenomegaly. Two or three of the examiners felt the abdomen and agreed that they could not feel the spleen. After these had moved on, another of the examiners examined the abdomen and called the invigilator over, saying: 'Put your hand here, like this—the spleen is palpable—can you feel it?'

88 A candidate was asked to examine the heart of a patient with mitral valve prolapse. Unfortunately the backrest collapsed while he was examining and could not be repaired so the patient could only be examined lying flat or sitting upright. Though the examiners accepted that this was off-putting, they

did not feel that it justified missing all the signs and getting systole and diastole the wrong way round!

89 A membership examiner was heard telling a group of students that many candidates fail to recognize atrial fibrillation. Furthermore, in his experience, about 20% of candidates cannot accurately demonstrate the second left intercostal space. He had also noticed that candidates were often poor in their technique of examining ankle jerks.

90 A candidate was asked to examine the fundi of a patient with laser-treated diabetic retinopathy. She diagnosed diabetic retinopathy but when asked if she had seen any microaneurysms or photocoagulation scars she was not sure.

91 A candidate was shown a euthyroid diabetic patient with necrobiosis lipoidica diabeticorum and was given some of the patient's historical features which were vaguely suggestive of hyperthyroidism; he was then told to assess the girl's thyroid status. Despite the normal pulse rate and lack of other supportive signs the candidate apparently managed to diagnose hyperthyroidism!

92 An examiner was watching a candidate feeling for the apex beat of a female patient. The rough handling of the patient's breast irritated the examiner who later commented: 'That sort of behaviour brings a candidate immediately to the pass/fail borderline'.

93 After observing some candidates performances on a case of rheumatoid hands, a fly on the wall advised: don't give too much prominence to the possibility of psoriatic arthropathy in an obvious rheumatoid case. Look particularly for nail changes if you are considering psoriatic arthropathy in this instance. If there are boutonnière and swan neck deformities, say so rather than spending ages describing what's happening at each metacarpophalangeal and interphalangeal joint.

94 A flustered and over-anxious candidate marked himself out by spending an inordinate amount of time fixing the patient's blanket and putting the patient's pyjamas back on rather than following the examiners to the next case—they had to come back for him twice. 'Oh heck!', he remarked at their second return for him. On another occasion he was still shaking hands with the last patient when the examiners were trying to get him to start on the next! After forgetting to listen in the neck in a patient with a systolic murmur in the aortic area, he elected to draw the examiner's attention to this without prompting: 'I'm sorry, I didn't listen in the neck!' He was generally slow and took ages describing, hesitantly, peripheral and unimportant things, digging holes when it would be better to come out immediately and say confidently: 'I think this patient has aortic incompetence'. On the rheumatoid hands he spent ages trying to describe what was happening at each metacarpophalangeal and interphalangeal joint, struggling in his panic trying to find the words when it would have been better to get straight to the diagnosis with just a few key extras such as 'boutonnière' and 'swan neck', 'ulnar deviation', etc. The examiner commented: 'He looked as though he was going to fall apart at any moment; he looked as though he was not used to examining people; I wonder if he is in public health!' It was reckoned that during the 30 min he said 'Sir' about 84 times!

95 A candidate was doing a good full chest examination when suddenly the senior examiner intervened: 'Bear in mind there are a lot of short cases to get through; don't spend too much time on general examination'. The candidate speeded up very well. The patient had bronchiectasis without clubbing but the candidate diagnosed resolving pneumonia. Afterwards the examiner commented: 'We ask the candidates what was the main system in their long case in order to try to get them to examine, between long cases and short cases, at least one each of chest, abdomen, cardiovascular system and neurology. To these four major systems we add a few small brief short cases. It is quite a task to get through the four major ones and therefore we have to keep the candidates going'.

96 A candidate was taken to see a patient with one leg which was slightly shorter and wasted compared to the other. The candidate didn't think of old polio. The examiner commented: 'A lot of young people won't have seen polio'.

97 A patient in the long cases had brought his inhaler. When the examiner was seeing the patient before the exam started, he checked the patient's inhaler technique and found it to be poor. The examiner later asked the candidate if he had checked the inhaler technique. The candidate had not.

98 A candidate was asked to examine the hands of a patient with gross generalized wasting and frontal baldness. The candidate carried out a long detailed examination of the hands before reaching the diagnosis (dystrophia myotonica) after finally being prompted to shake hands with the patient.

99 A candidate on her first case had a patient with lymphoma causing a right iliac fossa mass, splenomegaly and generalized lymphadenopathy. The candidate missed the spleen, got bogged down in standard lists of causes of a right iliac fossa mass including irrelevant ones such as appendix abscess! This all gave a very bad impression to the examiner and therefore, despite doing very well in all the other short cases, she only scored 5/12. Thus the dictum that 'you can still pass after doing very badly in one short case', may sometimes mean that you only score a bare fail on the short cases and have to make up for this by doing well elsewhere in the exam to pass overall.

100 A candidate in her long case said there were brisk reflexes in the arm when there were not. She was clumsy with the reflex testing and missed ankle clonus. The examiner commented: 'She sounded very good but got the signs wrong'. She was therefore given a borderline mark. However, at the examiners meeting, the other pairs of examiners reported that she was excellent on short cases, excellent in the viva, and she was therefore given a clear pass overall.

Fly on the wall—complete accounts

In the same way that later in this section we have some complete first-hand accounts of candidates experiences during the short cases, the following are two complete accounts from one sitting, followed by two complete accounts from the same morning of another sitting—the notes of a fly on the wall.

101 *The second examiner chipped in: 'Can you have an opening snap in the presence of atrial fibrillation?'—the candidate looked nonplussed, hesitated and did not come up with an answer.*

Short case 1. Hepatosplenomegaly and poly-cythaemia. Patient had a red face not noticed or mentioned by the candidate. Asked to look at the abdomen from the end of the bed while the patient breathed, the candidate did not notice the liver moving up and down. The fact that the liver was pal-pable was dragged out slowly. The examiner asked the candidate to mark the position of the spleen on the skin with a finger so that the size of the spleen could be verified.

Short case 2. The examiner said: 'Check pulse, JVP and precordium'; the candidate proceeded to irritate him by examining the fingernails. The patient had loud mitral stenosis. The examiner instructed: 'Diagnosis or findings—you choose'. The candidate said mitral stenosis. Examiner: 'Why mitral steno-sis?' 'Was there an opening snap?' — the candidate was unsure, asked to listen again, and said there was an opening snap. The examiner asked: 'What is an opening snap—what causes it?' As they were leaving the patient the second examiner chipped in: 'Can you have an opening snap in the presence of atrial fibrillation?' The candidate looked nonplussed, hesitated and did not come up with an answer. The examiner said afterwards he thought this was a very relevant question which the candidate ought to have been able to answer.

Short cases 3 and 4. Two short cases in one — first of all hereditary haemorrhagic telangiectasia then congenital nystagmus. The candidate moved hesi-tatingly to the diagnosis. She was asked why there was a scar on the left chest. The candidate suggested arteriovenous fistula. The examiner asked if there was a better, more commonly used term. The candidate was very slow to answer 'arteriovenous shunt and arteriovenous malformations'. She was slow to get congenital nystagmus as the cause of the nystagmus and was asked how she could tell it was congenital nystagmus and not any other cause. She did not really know but had the fact that it was present in all directions dragged out of her. The examiner (a neurologist) explained that the nystag-mus was coarse, in the same plane as the eye move-ment, of variable frequency, with the fast phase sometimes in one direction and sometimes in another. She was asked if she knew of another con-dition that went with congenital nystagmus and she did not. The examiner explained that there were

little nodding movements of the head that the patient sometimes exhibited which are called 'spasmus nutans'.

Short case 5. Psoriasis of the soles of the feet which the candidate got and also gave the differential diag-nosis, when asked, of keratoderma blenorrhagica in association with Reiter's.

Short case 6. Rheumatoid hands with swan neck and boutonnière deformities. The candidate was being asked about the cause of the swan neck deformity and started talking about the small muscles of the hand. The examiner said: 'I wouldn't have said that but since you mention it, what small muscles of the hand'! The candidate was very hesitant and eventu-ally said: 'flexor digito . . .' 'You are talking rubbish', said the examiner, 'it is the interossei and lumbri-cals'. As the examiner moved on to the next case, the candidate said that there were also boutonnière deformities.

Short case 7. The examiner was about to ask the can-didate to look into the eyes of the next patient when he stopped, reached in his pocket and pulled out an instrument and asked the candidate what the instru-ment was. She did not know. It was a two-point sen-sation discriminator. 'Can be very useful in testing sensation', said the examiner.

Short case 8. The candidate's next case was diabetic retinopathy which she got accurately including the fact that there were hard exudates near the macula.

Short case 9. In view of the previous, fairly disas-trous, abdomen, the candidate was taken to another abdomen which had hepatosplenomegaly; she got it this time and when asked the cause suggested 'a myeloproliferative disease' which was correct. She was asked to draw the edge of the spleen again.

The examiners felt that she was between a 5/12 (bare fail) and 6/12 (bare pass), but nearer the bare fail and so gave her a 5/12 over all. It was during this discussion that the examiner made his comment about the opening snap and atrial fibrillation.

She scored a 2 for her long case by one examiner, 4 by the other and scored 3/8 (bare fail) overall. The case had been one of widespread vascular disease including stroke. When asked her findings at the bedside of the long case she said two finger breadth hepatomegaly and when she was asked whether a patient may have emphysema with the liver pushed down she was struggling. She was asked to examine the visual fields of the patient in front of the examiners; it was clear from watching her that she had found visual field defect, but when she came to report her findings she said, with slight encouragement from the examiners, that the visual fields were normal! She scored 4/10 (bare fail) in the viva. With bare fail in both short and long cases she would be failed overall.

102 *Though he did extremely well scoring 7/8 in the long case and 6/10 in the viva this was not enough to save him from the disaster of the short cases . . . the short case examiners had no choice—other candidates in the same sitting had diagnosed the old choroiditis and not called it papilloedema; had diagnosed the retinopathy and not called it optic atrophy; had identified the palpable kidney and marked the correct size of the spleen, etc.*

The candidate scored brilliantly in the long case, the patient had ankylosing spondylitis and the candidate did very well. One examiner gave 6–7, the other examiner 7 and they agreed a mark of 7/8. After seeing his long case performance one expected that, continuing in the same vein, his performance in the short cases would be spectacular:

Short case 1. The first case was hepatosplenomegaly, right kidney easily palpable and left kidney scarred. The candidate started off with: 'I would like to examine the patient from nipples to knees'. He was asked to concentrate on the abdomen. He said that he had found hepatosplenomegaly. He was asked to show the edge of the spleen and said it was 6 cm and marked it as such when in fact it was just a spleen tip. It was interesting to note that when he had actually been examining the spleen one could see where he was feeling it and that he had felt the spleen tip with the patient turned on the right side; yet he went on to describe it as 6 cm. He did not mention the bimanually ballottable right kidney which presumably he thought was a liver.

Short case 2. After this bad start he did reasonably well on a patient with mitral stenosis. He was asked to examine the pulse, the JVP and the precordium. After feeling the pulse, looking at the JVP and pal-

pating the precordium the examiner stopped him and asked his findings. He gave them as those of mitral stenosis and said he expected to hear the auscultatory findings which he did. However, he got into a mess when asked to describe the venous pressure and said that it was a single wave and when asked about the relevance of this started talking about atrial fibrillation and mitral stenosis. He said: 'CV waves'. The examiner raised his eyebrows at this. The candidate did not mention tricuspid incompetence which was the cause of the neck pulsations. The examiner then asked if there was anything else he had noticed about the patient (this was not on the official documentation about the patient but the examiner was an endocrinologist) and after a struggle the candidate said chest deformity and after a further struggle kyphosis. There was more delay and struggling and then the examiner showed him the patient's axillae which had no hair. The candidate suggested maybe the patient shaved and she said that she had not had hair for many years. The examiner asked if the candidate could tie up the absent axillary hair with the chest and spinal deformities and the candidate was unable to do so. It turned out that the patient had had an early menopause and had been oestrogen deficient for many years and this is what the examiner was looking for.

Short case 3. The next case was a fundus with a patch of old choroiditis superior and just temporal to the macula. The candidate diagnosed papilloedema.

Short case 4. The patient had polyarteritis and bilateral carpal tunnel syndrome. The candidate diagnosed rheumatoid arthritis and bilateral carpal tunnel syndrome. The examiner said: 'If she had a patch of numbness on her right leg here [pointing below the knee], what would you say?' The candidate answered: 'Mononeuritis multiplex'. This was accepted by the examiner.

Short case 5. The next case was visual fields in a patient with widespread cerebrovascular disease who presumably had a right homonymous hemianopia. The candidate found a defective temporal field in the right eye but also a defective nasal field and said that both nasal and temporal fields were diminished. The candidate was asked without comment to go on and examine the legs and he said that he had found 'pyramidal weakness of the right leg'. He was asked what this meant and responded 'weakness of flexion at the hip, the knee and dorsiflexion at the foot'. This was accepted. He also said that he felt the reflexes were brisk bilaterally. The examiner (?a neurologist) asked what other reflexes could be done — in cases of doubt about the briskness of reflexes ('How can you tell if reflexes are brisk if they are bilaterally brisk?'). The candidate said, and did, the adductor reflexes. The examiner asked what it is that causes the brisk reflex. The candidate struggled and was unable to describe the reflex arc. He was then asked what causes increased tone and started talking about muscles being perpetually in contraction; and was then asked, if he meant that the muscles are contracting all the time, to which he replied: 'No'. He was asked why there could be discordance between tone and jerks.

Short case 6. The last patient had grade III hypertensive retinopathy. The candidate said there was no retinopathy but that the discs were pale.

He was scored 4/12 by both examiners independently and therefore 4/12 (definite fail) over all. He went on to do well in the viva scoring 6/10.

Though he did extremely well scoring 7/8 in the long case and 6/10 in the viva this was not enough to save him from the disaster of the short cases. At the examiners meeting the other examiners spoke highly of the candidate from what they had seen in the long case and viva, and were surprised by the account given by the short case examiners. However, the short case examiners had no choice—other candidates in the same sitting had diagnosed the old choroiditis and not called it papilloedema; had diagnosed the retinopathy and not called it optic atrophy; had identified the palpable kidney and marked the correct size of the spleen, etc.*

103 *The candidate was asked to demonstrate with his finger where the spleen edge was exactly and where the liver edge was exactly.*

The candidate had received 7/8 from both examiners on his long case (which was a patient with jaundice and positive hepatitis B serology) and not knowing this, of course, entered the short case exam.

*This case and number 100 on p. 460 show the discriminating power of the short cases.

Short case 1. His first case was a youngish woman with mixed aortic valve disease and mixed mitral valve disease though the mitral incompetence was debatable. He diagnosed mixed aortic valve disease but did not notice the mid-diastolic murmur though the examiner did not seem perturbed by this. The candidate, when asked about whether the pulse was collapsing or not, said that it was not and the examiner then asked him for the peripheral signs of aortic incompetence and the discussion moved to the nail-fold sign. The candidate was asked what this was called and he said: 'Quinke's sign' and he was asked to see if the patient had this. The candidate thought he had and the examiner answered: 'I thought so too'.

Short case 2. The next case was a patient with bronchiectasis and the candidate was asked to examine the chest. He examined the chest from the front and when he was about to move to the back the examiner said: 'Time is at a premium, could you discuss your findings so far?' During the examination the patient had given a rattly cough on several occasions. The candidate thought that the diagnosis was bronchiectasis but then went on to say that he thought the patient looked cushingoid and wondered if the patient was on steroids for obstructive airways disease. (The patient was not on steroids.) The causes of bronchiectasis were asked.

Short case 3. The candidate was asked to look at a patient with Parkinson's disease and he spotted the diagnosis correctly and said he would like to examine the gait; he was allowed to do this. The only parkinsonian feature in the gait was that one arm swung less than the other and exhibited a slight tremor. When the candidate said this, the examiner asked what features he might have had. In the ensuing discussion the candidate was asked what 'festinant' meant. He said he did not know. The examiner told him that it meant 'dancing' and asked him why he thought this word should be used to describe the parkinsonian gait.

Short case 4. The next case was a patient with diabetic fundi, multiple laser burns and debatable new vessels on the disc. The candidate during the discussions said that the discs were normal and when pressed on this stuck to his decision that they were normal.

Short case 5. The next case was a patient with CREST syndrome and he was asked: 'What is your spot diagnosis?' The candidate immediately answered: 'Tophaceous gout'. When the examiner was unhappy about this he explained that he was sorry that he had rushed to that diagnosis. The examiner told him that he should never rush to a diagnosis. The candidate then discussed systemic sclerosis and CREST syndrome and a discussion took place about difficulties with swallowing.

Short case 6. The next patient had neurofibromatosis and the candidate was asked to: 'Look at the hands and tell me what you see—spot diagnosis'. The candidate got the diagnosis at once.

Short case 7. The next patient had hereditary haemorrhagic telangiectasia and the candidate got this diagnosis at once. He was then asked if the patient had anything else and the candidate answered to the effect that the patient had gross nystagmus. On being pressed on this, he said that there was also a squint and when being pressed further for a diagnosis, he suggested that the patient had congenital nystagmus (which is what the patient had).

Short case 8. The next patient had a cerebrovascular accident, cerebellar signs and a carotid bruit. The examiner told the candidate that the patient had difficulty with walking and asked him to perform a neurological examination of the legs. The candidate started off by looking and after a brief pause the examiner asked him to: 'move on if you want to finish on time'. He examined power, and reflexes, found the reflexes diminished at the right knee compared to the left, and started discussing an L3/4 root lesion as the cause. The examiner told him to leave sensation and what else would he like to examine. The candidate did not come up with a suggestion. Eventually, the examiner suggested he checked coordination in the legs and the candidate was then led to examine for cerebellar signs in the arms. Cerebellar signs were found on the right. When asked about the possible diagnosis, the candidate suggested cerebellar signs and a lower motor neurone lesion at L3/4. The examiner suggested that this was a bizzare collection of physical signs and asked the candidate to listen to his neck. A right carotid bruit was found. The candidate then offered 'cerebellar infarction' as the cause, to which the examiner said: 'What about a middle cerebral artery stroke?' In the ensuing discussion the examiner said: 'Do you disagree with me, you can if you want to you know'.

Short case 9. The next patient had hepatosplenomegaly and the candidate started his presentation by saying that the patient was pigmented. The examiner said: 'Do you think he is pigmented? Actually he's tanned; he's just been to Cyprus for his holiday'. The candidate was asked to demonstrate with his finger where the spleen edge was exactly and where the liver edge was exactly. In the discussion on the cause myeloproliferative disease was suggested first, to which the examiner responded by saying that the patient had had the spleen for 30 years. The candidate then suggested an 'ethnic anaemia' and a discussion took place about why it was not thalassaemia minor and was not thalassaemia major and when the candidate suggested sickle-cell disease the examiner told him: 'You didn't mean that did you?' After the bell went he told the candidate that it was haemoglobin H disease but that the candidate need not worry because he was on the right lines. One examiner thought the marks should be 8 or 9 the other thought it should be 7 or 8 and the candidate was finally given 8 out of 12.

In his viva he had to discuss talking to the relatives of a patient requiring a postmortem, a homosexual with fever who turned out to be HIV positive, an 85-year-old patient with no physical signs who had just been admitted to hospital and was causing a lot of trouble in the night, and viral causes of diarrhoea. He received 5 out of 10 and passed the whole examination.

104 *She got the patient to open his mouth and put his tongue out (the inside and outside of his mouth was covered with telangiectasiae—how did she not see it?).*
Things went badly wrong in her long case. The patient had mixed mitral valve disease, cerebellar signs and polyneuropathy. There was also diabetes and the examiner had found hypertensive retinopathy. The candidate had not examined coordination, did not find any of the neurological signs and felt that the reason why the patient was confined to a wheelchair was because of low back pain. She felt that the fundi were normal and stuck to this and, more or less, to the absence of neurological signs

even when she took the examiners to the bedside. She had started the exam very confident, but as time progressed it was clear she was sensing that things had gone badly wrong. She was given 2 out of 8 by both examiners without hesitation and when she left the long case room she was clearly in a 'downward spiral' state.

Short case 1. The first short case had systemic sclerosis which she called at first (on examining the hands) psoriasis, and then dermatomyositis, before coming to the right diagnosis.

Short case 2. The next patient had hepatosplenomegaly and she got it right without problems.

Short case 3. The next one was hereditary haemorrhagic telangiectasia and she was asked to examine the back. She found a thoracotomy scar and evidence of a lobectomy (presumably removal of an AV shunt). Then in a discussion which led to the fact that 'some lung had been removed' she was asked to discuss possible reasons. (She was told the operation had been many years previously.) She suggested tuberculosis and this possible cause was accepted. 'Anything else?' She suggested there might be rheumatoid changes in the hands and this was accepted. 'Why would this lead to a thoracotomy?' The candidate started discussing pulmonary fibrosis before she realized that this would not lead to a thoracotomy. The examiner asked if she thought the patient was cyanosed. She got the patient to open his mouth and put his tongue out (the inside and outside of his mouth was covered with telangiectasiae—how did she not see it?) and she said she did not think there was cyanosis. Did she know why the patient might have had a thoracotomy? — 'No'.

Short case 4. The next patient, she was told, was unsteady on the feet and she was asked to examine the arms. The patient had cerebellar signs following a cerebrovascular accident. She initially started discussing Parkinson's disease and cog-wheeling and then retracted this. She was asked to examine the eyes for nystagmus and soon after she started doing this she was asked: 'Has she got it?', to which the candidate immediately answered: 'Yes'. 'Tell us about the nystagmus'. She was asked to examine speech and eventually got the patient to have difficulty saying, 'West Register Street'.

Short case 5. She was asked for a spot diagnosis on a patient with neurofibromatosis and she got this.

Short case 6. She was asked for a spot diagnosis on a patient with exophthalmos and got this. When asked where else to look, she eventually discussed looking at the shins for pretibial myxoedema which the patient had (debatably).

Short case 7. The next patient had a small to moderate multinodular goitre which the candidate said was a big goitre; and initially that it was diffuse, though she later said it was nodular.

Short case 8. The next patient had mixed aortic valve disease and mixed mitral valve disease. The candidate confidently diagnosed aortic stenosis but nothing else.

Short case 9. The next patient had diabetic retinopathy with laser burns and the candidate got this.

Short case 10. The next patient had Parkinson's disease which she got. A discussion then took place on the causes of Parkinson's disease and when she ground to a halt after giving a number of these, she was asked for any others — 'Have you heard of the expression "mad as a hatter"?' When she did not know what the examiner was talking about, they moved to the next case which was coarctation of the aorta. The examiner said that he wanted to put her in the area of the circulatory system but not to do a full examination of the heart because she had already done this. He led her to listen to the precordium and she heard something of a systolic murmur but the bell went before discussion could take place. She mentioned 'patent ductus' as she left the room.

One examiner gave her 4 out of 12, the other 5 out of 12 and it was left at 4 out of 12.

In the viva salicylate overdose was discussed, what is meant by meta-analysis, what the word 'Cochrane' conjures up, modes and medians, and *H. pylori*. Her overall mark for the viva was 5 out of 10, but unfortunately she had received a clear fail in both the long and short cases.

That morning the examiners only passed one out of the six candidates and that was the candidate described in experience 103 above. In the general discussion about the performance of the candidates at the examiner's meeting, one of the examiners mentioned that he did not like the attitude of one of the candidates to the patients — for instance, having asked the patient to hold his arms out in front of him for the purpose of an examination, he then proceeded to discuss things at great length whilst the patient sat there for a long period with the arms held out in front, without the candidate noticing or being concerned about the discomfort caused to the patient. The same candidate had asked a patient, when examining the aortic area, to take a deep breath in, and then breathe out; but then the candidate did not allow the patient to breathe again for an uncomfortably prolonged period and this was noted by the examiners.*

Ungentlemanly clinical methods

105 A candidate was asked to examine a patient's respiratory system. He found clubbing and basal crackles and diagnosed bronchiectasis. He confessed that he was helped along in this diagnosis because he could see it on the examiner's clipboard!

106 A candidate was asked to examine the fundi. The examiners were several yards away and as he was examining he quietly asked the patient if he was a diabetic, to which the patient answered: 'Yes'. The candidate diagnosed proliferative diabetic retinopathy with photocoagulation scars in one eye and a vitreous haemorrhage in the other. He was asked why it was difficult to see one of the fundi well and replied that it was because of the vitreous haemorrhage. (Pass)

107 A candidate reports: 'I was asked to "look at this lady's right eye". I saw laser scars, cataract and retinopathy. I said "diabetic retinopathy" — which was what I saw printed on the examiner's sheet!'. (Pass)

108 A candidate reported that while he was waiting to be examined on his long case, he got chatting to another candidate who was an Irish lad who told him the details of the diabetic patient with bilateral amputations that he had seen. The candidate then

reports that during his subsequent short case exam, he was taken to this diabetic and asked to examine his eyes. He did so and reported: 'Proliferative diabetic retinopathy with evidence of laser treatment'. This seemed to satisfy the examiners. (Pass)

109 A candidate reports: 'My last short case really made my day. Having arrived at the examination ward with little time to spare, I happened on an elderly woman going in the same direction who obviously was not a candidate and too polite to be an examiner! She asked if we were going to the same place and volunteered that she always came up for the examinations. She told me that they always looked at her eyes and shins, and then at her neck, volunteering that she had no scar but had "drunk iodine"! Sure enough, I was led to this same woman who smiled when I was told to examine her legs which had pretibial myxoedema. I went on to demonstrate the exophthalmus with lidlag, a multinodular goitre and no scar!' (Pass)

110 For one of his short cases a candidate was taken to see the patient whom he had had as a long case. He owned up to having already seen him and the examiner said, jokingly, that he would be awarded an extra mark for honesty — but only one! (Pass)

111 During her short cases a candidate was asked to examine the hands of the lady who she had already seen as a long case. She said: 'I am sorry but I have already seen this lady for my long case'. They liked that and she thinks they gave her a mark for honesty. She reported, however, that a friend of hers passed even though he did not own up when taken to see his long case as a short case. He diagnosed primary biliary cirrhosis with confidence and passed. She reports: 'He didn't even show a smirk on his face and the patient did not give the game away — risky business!'

Some experiences written in the first person

For the surveys which we undertook following publication of the first edition of this book, many of the contributors were aware of what our enterprise was about and wrote detailed accounts of their experi-

---

* The most extreme example we have heard of this type of 'fail' generating, unconcerned, behaviour towards patients, is a candidate who presented and discussed the findings in the abdomen whilst still holding on to the patient's genitalia!

ences in the first person. Some examples of these accounts are given below.

Miscellaneous 'pass' experiences

'The examiner said: "First class". This was the nicest remark made to me in the last 2 years!'

1 *Short case 1:* 'Would you examine these hands. This chap has a weakness in his hands'. The patient had an obvious bilateral *ulnar nerve palsy* and I was asked the causes.

Short case 2: 'Examine this patient's abdomen. He came in with anaemia'. There was obvious hepatosplenomegaly and I was asked for a differential including *myelofibrosis* and why it could be this condition. I said because of the size of the spleen.

Short case 3: 'Examine this patient's fundus'. There were haemorrhages and exudates with nipping. I suggested diabetic eye disease but the examiner then said: 'What if I tell you that the other eye is normal?' I then suggested a *retinal branch vein occlusion* to which the examiner said: 'First Class'. This was the nicest remark made to me in the last 2 years!

Short case 4: 'This man has a sore arm, would you examine it'. He certainly had a swollen and painful right arm and hand but with no dilated veins. However, it was slightly warm. Apparently the diagnosis was of *acute shoulder hand syndrome*. I didn't know this but the examiner told me!

Short case 5: 'Listen to this lady's heart'. There was no history given. Before I went any further I checked to see if I was allowed to palpate, etc. 'No', said the examiner, 'auscultate only'. I found a *mitral diastolic murmur* with an opening snap and ?presystolic accentuation. The examiner asked if the patient was in sinus rhythm. I said I couldn't tell just by auscultating, but the examiner said: 'What do you think?'

Short case 6: 'This lady has a rash on her thighs'. It looked like purpura but then they showed me her shins. There was no lesion visible here. 'Does this put you off a diagnosis of purpura?' 'Yes', I said. 'Quite right', said the examiner. 'What if I told you she had pains in her joints and trouble with her kidneys?' I suggested polyarteritis nodosa. 'No', said the examiner, 'but don't worry. I have only seen it once before!' (Apparently it was *Fabry's disease*.)

Short case 7: This patient was in a side room which gave me a clue. The examiner said, 'This young man has lost weight and noticed these lesions on his chest. What are they?' They were definitely *Kaposi's sarcomata*. I was then asked the mechanism of diarrhoea in *AIDS*.

Short case 8: 'Examine this patient's abdomen'. There were polycystic kidneys. The examiner asked me if I would like to ask the patient some questions.

Short case 9: 'Examine this patient's visual fields'. There was a homonymous hemianopia (Pass—sixth go!)

'As we left the room, we heard a round of applause from the man behind us and at this point, I was really beginning to enjoy myself!'

2 I was first taken into a room where there were three ladies. I was asked to examine two of these patients. The first was an elderly lady with widely dilated pupils. I was asked to look at her fundi. I tested her pupil reactions to light but not to accommodation and elicited a light reflex. I then examined the right fundus. It was obviously *background diabetic retinopathy* and after approximately 20 seconds I looked up and asked if they wanted me to specifically look into the left fundus. He said: 'Not if you are ready to present your findings'. I did present the findings, gave the diagnosis and emphasized that there were no proliferative or hypertensive changes or laser burns. I was then taken to a young woman with a mitral valvotomy scar, atrial fibrillation and the murmurs of *mixed mitral valve disease*. She was not short of breath or cyanosed. I presented the findings and continued to give my reasons why I believed the stenotic component was predominant. I was asked if the murmurs were haemodynamically significant. I replied that they were not and again gave my reasons. The examiners and the patients all appeared pleased. In fact, on leaving the room the first lady commented loudly upon 'what a nice young man' I was and how I had 'said it all so nicely!'

I was then led into a day room with five seated men. The first had obvious *severe rheumatoid arthritis* and evidence of previous joint replacements. I was asked to describe what I saw and then to look for additional evidence of rheumatoid arthritis, i.e. nodules. There were none present so they asked me where else they might be found. I replied: 'I would look on a chest X-ray'. We then moved on and I got the impression that the examiners were now on my side.

The next patient had pronounced *exophthalmos* and the examiner began by asking me to describe what I could see, saying: 'You can be as rude as you like to Mr L.' to which the patient laughed. I demonstrated the examination of exophthalmos and lid lag and said that I could feel a goitre (which I think was present though not large). The examiner did not appear completely convinced but conceded to my observation. I was asked to assess the thyroid state clinically. He was *euthyroid* and I gave my reasons for this. We then proceeded to walk out of the day room, but, in passing, I was asked to give a 'spot' diagnosis on a gentleman by the door. He had subtle, but definite, *acromegaly*. I gave a one-word answer and was told 'very good'. As we left the room we heard a round of applause from the man behind us and at this point I was really beginning to enjoy myself!

There was then a change-over and the previously silent examiner took me to the next patient who was laid in bed with a cervical collar on. I was asked to examine his legs neurologically because 'he has difficulty walking'. He had a smaller, wasted, areflexic left leg suggestive of *old polio* and a very brisk set of reflexes in the right leg. I suggested that he had old polio of the left leg with superimposed *cervical myelopathy* affecting the right leg. I was then asked to examine the back of another man's chest. There was dullness to percussion and reduced chest wall movement on the right side, but the air entry was not diminished greatly in comparison to the left side. I gave a tentative diagnosis of a right *pleural effusion* but added why I was not certain. I was then asked to examine his abdomen 'because my intern informs me that he has *hepatomegaly*'. The liver margin was in fact easily palpable. However, on percussion it appeared low lying and I therefore suggested this and the examiner appeared to agree. I was then taken to my last case and asked to palpate the precordium only. There was a systolic apical thrill. I was asked to give a differential diagnosis but at this point my concentration was somewhat flagging and I could only mention mitral regurgitation and forgot the *ventricular septal defect*. He asked again if there was anything else of note on palpation—eek! I had nearly missed his bilateral *gynaecomastia*. I was asked what drugs might be the cause in this particular case. I gave a reasonable list but could not think of spironolactone. He repeated the question but somehow mixed up his words and actually said: 'What are the spiros . . .' I began to laugh as did both the patient and the other examiner who had been observing at this point. As the bell had now sounded they said that they would let me go. I thanked them and shook hands—phew! (Pass)

'I was asked if I would have worried about mouth-to-mouth resuscitation in case the patient had AIDS'.
3 This lady came in to have her varicose veins done and something else was noted incidentally. 'Please examine her abdomen and tell us what you find that is abnormal'. On examination there was gross visible splenomegaly with mild anaemia. I was asked the causes of massive splenomegaly and the definition of splenomegaly. She in fact had *myelofibrosis*.

I was then taken to a *resuscitation dummy* and the examiner said: 'You walk on to a ward and a nurse calls you to a patient who has arrested, what would you do? Show us'. I said that I would check that the patient had truly arrested and would call the crash team. I would give a sternal blow and start bag and mask ventilation and cardiac massage whilst 'taking a history' and obtaining a trace, or I might defibrillate the patient anyway. The examiner gave me various 'what ifs' like 'the nurse faints' and 'suppose it happened in the street'. I was asked if I would have worried about mouth-to-mouth resuscitation in case the patient had AIDS. 'No', I said. Also they were constantly checking to see that I was getting the right light coming up on the machine (green for correct ventilation, orange for correct cardiac massage, and red for incorrect ventilation and massage). I was asked about the possible damage from an incorrect technique. I was also asked if I had had much experience with cardiac arrests and I said I had spent a year on the acute crash team. They wanted to know what my immediate success rate was. I said it varied with the circumstances, i.e. coronary care unit versus surgical ward and what the patient's pathology was and they spent quite a long time on this aspect. I said my success rate was probably 30% for the initial resuscitation back to a spontaneous rhythm.

I was then taken on to the next short case. The examiner said: 'This man has a cough and fever. Examine the respiratory system'. He was an Asian chap who was clubbed and dyspnoeic at rest. He had superb signs. There was dullness to percussion with increased breath sounds (bronchial breathing) and there was increased vocal resonance at the left upper zone/apex. I was asked for a differential diagnosis and because he was Asian I said tuberculosis and, because he was a smoker as detected by the discoloration of his nails, I also suggested carcinoma of the lung. The examiner told me that he did not like my technique for testing for tracheal deviation (thumb to each side separately) and he showed me his way of doing it and asked me to try it. I had to admit that the trachea probably was deviated to the left. There was then a long dissertation from the examiner regarding the physical findings in the left upper lobe, i.e. collapse versus consolidation, and I was not really asked to contribute at all to this conversation!

I was then taken to see a gentleman who had a white stick and the examiner said: 'This man is almost blind, please examine his eyes'. I found no cataracts or corneal problems but there was gross choroidoretinitis. I desperately tried to find evidence of diabetic retinopathy to make this into laser therapy but I couldn't. Therefore, I thought it could be retinitis pigmentosa though I had never seen it before. I told this honestly to the examiners who agreed that the treatment of diabetic eye disease would be the commonest cause of this type of thing but that (a) it was a bit different and (b) this is Membership! It was in fact *retinitis pigmentosa*. I wondered if it could have been a *Refsum's syndrome* as the Whittington Hospital does have a willing case of this.

My last patient was a lady and the examiner said: 'Tell me about her hands'. I had to be very quick as the bell had gone but she had gross *nodular rheumatoid*. I described the features as I was examining and I was also expected to perform a functional assessment. The examiners at the end said: 'Very good', and let me go. (Pass)

'I know this patient well, Sir, this is Mrs L. and I biopsied her liver last year!'
4 *Short case 1*: I was asked to examine the precordium. She had *mitral stenosis* and atrial fibrillation. I was criticized for not actually counting the apical rate and only giving a guestimate of 130/min. I was then asked the complications of mitral stenosis.

Short case 2: 'This girl was admitted with an acute asthmatic attack. Can you find a cause for it?' After some prompting I noticed a slight excoriation on the flexor creases and this was the only physical sign. I thought it was probably *atopic eczema*. The examin-

ers then asked me what I would tell this girl's mother about her prognosis.

Short case 3: 'Look at this patient's skin'. There were *café-au-lait* spots on the forearms and *neurofibromata* on the abdomen.

Short case 4: 'Examine this patient's legs'. I recognized this patient—so I said: 'This is Mrs G. and she has *Charcot–Marie–Tooth disease!*'

Short case 5: 'Examine this patient's abdomen'. 'I know this lady as well, Sir. This is Mrs L. and *I biopsied her liver* last year!' The examiner said: 'Have you worked in this hospital before?' and I replied: 'Well, er, yes!'

Short case 6: 'Palpate this patient's chest. No, feel again, there!' There was *aortic stenosis* with a systolic thrill which I missed initially. I was asked for further investigations so I mentioned echo and Doppler together with cardiac catheterization.

Short case 7: 'Look at this man's face'. He had definite facial flushing and we then discussed the features of the *carcinoid syndrome* and its treatment. The patient had had hepatic artery embolization.

I had been allocated to a hospital in which I had worked the previous year. My consultants advised me not to change as the examiners would not be prejudiced and I would not be at any disadvantage. However, I recognized two of the patients and I admitted to this. Although I was given credit for honesty it meant I missed out on the examination of two very good cases. The examiners told me afterwards at the sherry reception that they had sat on the fence for the clinical but that I had passed comfortably on the other sections. I would advise any candidates finding themselves in a similar position to inform the college and to ask for a re-allocation. Events such as this might easily upset one's whole performance. (Pass)

'Just because you are cool, it doesn't mean that you know the answers. But perhaps it helps convince the examiners that you do!'
5 *Short case 1*: *Gross acromegaly*. 'Examine this lady's hand. What do you notice?' The diagnosis was easy. He asked me to enumerate the features found in the hand in an acromegalic. 'And what else do you notice?' I listed all the facial features. 'What would you find in the other systems?' Again I gave a nice list. 'What are the treatments for this condition?' This was the perfect start to the short cases. I felt the

examiners warmed to me and it was all quite easy from here on.

Short case 2: *Ventricular septal defect*. 'Listen to this boy's heart'. He looked like a healthy teenager. Inspection of the apex was normal and his pulses were normal; however, palpation revealed a systolic thrill and on auscultation he had a systolic murmur only. I listened to his back. 'Why did you do that?' 'Because if he has a patent ductus the murmur would be loudest at the back'. (The real reason was that I am terrible at interpreting murmurs and it gave me an extra few seconds to think.) Afterwards the examiner went back to listen.

Short case 3: *Choroiditis*. 'Look in this woman's eye. What do you see?' As I started to inspect her eye he said. 'No, just look at the fundus'. To begin with I could see nothing wrong but just as I turned to look away she changed her direction of gaze and I saw the gross lesion. The moral must be to look everywhere in the retina.

Short case 4: *Maculopathy*. This was difficult. I learned subsequently from one of the examiners that the ophthalmologist had sent the patient along as an interesting example of some obscure eye pathology. There were some abnormalities at the macula so they had decided that maculopathy was acceptable!

Short case 5: *Clubbing* of the fingers. This was easy. I was allowed to ask some questions so I inquired how long the lady had had fingers like this. She was healthy and the answer was familial clubbing. I was then asked to recite the causes of clubbing.

Short case 6: Classical *dermatomyositis*. I had never seen this except in photographs and I almost missed it. She looked 'autoimmune' with white hair, pale skin and purplish eyelids and knuckles. I pointed this out but couldn't give a diagnosis. I was then asked to examine her arms where she had a healing, small surgical scar over one triceps. Once I had clicked that this was a muscle biopsy the diagnosis was easy. By now I was thoroughly enjoying myself and I turned to one of the examiners and said. 'I almost missed that'. 'Yes', he said, 'but you didn't!'

Short case 7: *Paget's disease*. This was bizarre. It was a lady of about 70 years whose radius and ulna of the right forearm were bent at 90°. I asked her if she had broken the arm and had a poor result from healing but the answer was no. I knew that there

is a congenital cause of forearm deformity (Madelung's?*) but this wasn't it so that left Paget's which I was told was the correct diagnosis.

Short case 8: *IIIrd nerve palsy*. It was a complete IIIrd nerve palsy. The examiner asked me to give the likely cause and the visible craniotomy scar gave me the answer.

Short case 9: *Malignant melanoma* with metastases. I was asked to examine this man's abdomen. He was deeply jaundiced and had a big knobbly liver. I was then asked to describe the surface anatomy of the normal liver since his extended across to the left subcostal area and at first I thought he also had splenomegaly. However, the examiner demonstrated to our mutual satisfaction that he had hepatomegaly only. 'Now look in his eyes'. One was in the light and one was in shade so I looked at the one in the light. 'He is deeply jaundiced', I said. I was then asked why and instructed to look in both eyes. One had a white sclera! On asking the patient how long he had had his glass eye he said about 10 years and that he had had a tumour at the back of the eye! At this point the examiners didn't ask me the diagnosis but simply thanked me and wished me good luck in the rest of the test. (Pass)

Afterwards the attending registrar said to me that I looked remarkably relaxed and cool under fire. I replied: 'Just because you're cool it doesn't mean that you know the answers'. But perhaps it helps convince the examiners that you do!

'The first thing I noticed was a puncture mark over the right lower chest suggesting a recent pleural aspiration'.
6 My first patient was introduced to me as a lady who was short of breath and would I do a cardiovascular examination to find out why she was breathless. Just as I was about to listen to the lung fields at the end of my routine I was stopped. My examiner asked if I had finished. I said: 'Yes'. And then I realized that I hadn't listened for an aortic diastolic murmur but the examiner kindly allowed me to go back to do this. I was then asked for the diagnosis and I offered *mixed mitral valve disease* with a previous valvotomy. I was then asked which valve lesion was dominant. I plumped for stenosis by virtue of the loud first heart sound and was then pushed as to

---

* *Madelung's deformity*—the arm is bent over the radial side due to the developmental overgrowth of the ulna.

whether I wanted to change my mind. I didn't so we passed on to the next case.

This was a lady whose neck I was asked to examine. It was obvious that she had a *goitre* but I tried to stop myself immediately going for this before checking for other abnormalities. I showed them that I was examining for retrosternal extension and bruits and then I was about to look for signs of hypo- or hyperthyroidism when I was asked to describe my findings. As with the other cases they let me start to show that I would extend my examination further and this seemed to impress but they always then stopped me in mid-flow. I told them I had found a smoothly enlarged thyroid goitre and they then questioned as to whether I was sure it was smooth. I was about to go back and re-examine but then realized that this would not look impressive. I did think it was smooth and so stuck to my original findings. I later discovered another candidate had been pushed on the same point and had also stuck firm.

I was then taken to a gentleman with frontal balding, mild ptosis and some facial muscle wasting and I was asked to hazard a diagnosis. I suggested *dystrophia myotonica* and I was asked why. I explained my findings and made the mistake of saying 'myopathic facies'. My examiner looked puzzled and asked me what I meant. I explained about the muscle wasting that I could see though retracted my description of 'myopathic facies' as an unhelpful statement so he didn't push me further.

I was then taken to a young lady with a large intravenous cannula in her right antecubital fossa and was asked to examine the back of her chest. The first thing I noticed was a puncture mark over the right lower chest suggesting a recent pleural aspiration. I quickly found a right *pleural effusion* and was asked to explain what brought me to that diagnosis and what was the most likely cause. In view of her age and the intravenous cannula I suggested pneumonia and was then asked the most likely microbiological cause for this lady and the most suitable antibiotic treatment.

I was then taken to another lady and was asked to examine her fundi and to describe my findings. I found early cataract formation, indistinct disc margins, arterial narrowing and patchy black *pigmentation* particularly in the *macular* region. I was asked where in the left eye there was a particularly dense black deposit. Unlike my first attempt I didn't try to pull the wool over their eyes with bluffing my way out. I was honest in saying I didn't know where the densest deposit was and they allowed me a second look. I was then asked to hazard an attempt at putting all these features together and I was utterly stumped. However, my examiner just asked the cause of black pigmentation and passed on to the next case.

I was asked to look at, and examine, a lady's hands. There was obvious *osteoarthrosis* but I didn't want to be put off by this so I quickly checked for muscle wasting, clubbing and for a sensory loss. I was about to examine the elbows for gouty tophi and rheumatoid nodules, when I was stopped and directed to discuss my findings. I was asked what were the eponymous names for the swellings of the proximal and terminal interphalangeal joints.

I was finally taken to a middle-aged lady with a complete left *ptosis*. I was asked what I saw from the end of the bed and for the possible causes. I was then asked to examine further. I made a bit of a mess of this case. I examined the pupils and then proceeded to examine for diplopia which I was very ham-fisted about. I was desperately trying to keep the left eye lid open and examine visual movements by asking her to follow my finger and I got my arms all in a muddle! The examiner quickly intervened and asked me what I had found. I mentioned the pupillary reactions and the down and out position of the left eye and so he asked me for a diagnosis. I told him it was a *complete IIIrd nerve palsy* and he then requested me to ask the lady some questions to elucidate the cause. I asked about headache thinking of a posterior communicating artery aneurysm and that seemed to cause some surprise in the examiner. I then asked about diabetes. The lady was in fact diabetic but I was told in her case this was irrelevant and asked to hazard one more question. Fortunately, I was inspired to ask how long she had had the ptosis and discovered it was congenital. I was pushed on the difference between a complete and partial IIIrd nerve palsy and after describing the probable findings was asked the anatomical difference in the lesions. I thought I was being asked something esoteric and was somewhat annoyed when it transpired that all he wanted me to say was that in a partial nerve palsy only some of the IIIrd nerve fibres are affected!

My advice is to keep your head even when you have made a mistake. If you know you've made a mistake be quick to say so before your examiner has a chance to capitalize on it. If your examiner challenges, don't assume it means you have said something wrong. He may just be testing to see if you'll stick firm to your diagnosis because you are absolutely certain of it. Practise, practise and practise particularly in front of people who make you nervous. Also I found it helpful to regard some of my out-patients as potential short cases. I think some of them had never been so thoroughly examined! Make every effort to show the examiner you can put the patient at ease. Introduce yourself and ask their permission to examine them and tell them exactly what you are going to do. Don't forget to thank them afterwards. It gives you time to calm down and think—and also it impresses the examiners. (Pass)

'*The patient sounded most alarmed and said she hoped her daughter wouldn't get it*'.

7 *Short case 1*: The first patient was an elderly, rather slow lady—'Examine this lady's heart and chest'. (It'll take hours I thought!) I was almost panicked into combining my examination but then started doing the cardiovascular system alone. She was deaf and I felt I wasn't being very slick. I distinctly remember a wave of panic/fear that this was it! Anyhow I found *mixed mitral valve disease* (MR > MS) and *aortic regurgitation*. I stood back and said this. The examiner nodded and said we'd not bother with the chest. (My hands were cold when I started and the patient jumped which didn't help my composure!)

Short case 2: A young man with widespread *psoriasis* and a moon face. 'What do you think of this man?' I asked him if he'd had any treatment, then stood back and said he had widespread psoriasis and could have been on systemic steroids. The examiner nodded, pointed out his palms and soles and asked what I would call the type of psoriasis. I answered: 'Pustular'. They agreed and moved on.

Short case 3: An ill-looking, jaundiced, old lady in a rather dim bay. 'Examine this abdomen'. The examiners listened intently with me to my percussion but otherwise didn't hastle me. I said I should like to go on to test for shifting dullness and to do a rectal exam, but didn't attempt to move her for the former because she looked so grotty. They accepted this and moved away from the bedside. I said I'd found *hepatosplenomegaly* in a jaundiced patient and

that I had noticed inguinal and supraclavicular nodes and a node biopsy scar in her groin. I suggested chronic myelocytic or lymphocytic leukaemia/non-Hodgkin's, or metastatic carcinoma as the differential diagnosis. They asked how I would tell a student to examine the spleen and what its characteristic features were. (I wondered had I done it all wrong or felt a kidney instead!)

Short case 4: A lady with dilated pupils. 'Examine this fundus', they said and then wandered away a little. I looked in one eye and then asked if I could look in the other and got a rather non-commital 'if you must' expression. But I did anyway. I said I'd found *grade II hypertensive retinopathy* with silver wiring and AV nipping but no sign of haemorrhages, exudates or papilloedema. The examiner just said: 'Yes' and moved on.

Short case 5: A lady with florid *hereditary haemorrhagic telangiectasia* (HHT). 'What's the diagnosis?' When I got my tongue round it, I said the diagnosis in full! They said: 'What question would you like to ask?' and I asked if anyone in the family had it. She said: 'No', and the examiners asked if I was surprised. I said it was an autosomal dominant trait and tended to run through the generations, to which the patient sounded most alarmed and said she hoped her daughter wouldn't get it. The examiners placated her saying there was a 50% chance. I felt annoyed that it reflected badly on me upsetting her but surely the patient must have heard of it running in families before!

Short case 6: A lady with *neurofibromatosis*. They asked for a diagnosis and then for any neurological complications. I replied: 'Epilepsy, cord compression, carpal tunnel syndrome, tumours'.

Short case 7: A grossly *acromegalic* man. 'What's the diagnosis? And what features would you like to demonstrate?' I described his facies, jaw and hands. They led me on to *carpal tunnel syndrome* and got me to demonstrate wasting and to try to show any sensory loss (intact!) and to talk about testing for median nerve motor function.

Short case 8: An old lady with denuded blisters and mouth lesions. The diagnosis was *pemphigus*. He asked me: 'Where's the split in the skin?' I said it was at the intraepidermal level.

Overall my short cases went quite fluently. My worse moments were when I surprised a patient with my ice cold, stress-induced hands, and when I apparently upset the lady with HHT for mentioning it ran in families. One examiner questioned my use of 'He/she probably has . . .' when the diagnosis was obvious from just looking. By the end I was being more dogmatic which seemed to go down better. Even with no disasters it was hard to treat each case afresh but I'm sure that's the knack of scoring highly. (Pass)

'Yes', said the examiner, 'tell me about the precursors of bilirubin?'
8 I was first asked what I had seen for my long case. When I told the examiners that it had been a patient with mitral valve disease they said: 'OK we won't see anything like that!'

Short case 1: 'Examine this man and shake hands with him'. The diagnosis was obviously *dystrophia myotonica*. The examiner asked me what else I would like to ask the patient. I suggested asking about family history and the examiner said: 'Good'.

Short case 2: 'Look at this man, what is the diagnosis?' He had *pseudoxanthoma elasticum* and the examiner again said: 'Good'. He asked me what the description of the skin was and I replied: 'Plucked chicken skin' and again he said: 'Good! 'What would you expect to hear listening to his heart? That is what he is really here for'. I replied mitral valve prolapse. 'That's right', said the examiner.

Short case 3: 'Look at this girl, what do you think? She is 25 years old'. I said: 'If she will forgive me she is rather short'. 'That's right', said the examiner, 'what would you like to ask her?' I asked her how tall her parents were. 'Anything else?' said the examiner. I asked her when her periods started, if at all. The examiner said: 'That's a good question, what do you think of her face? She has *Crohn's disease*'. I replied that she had a cushingoid moon face, and that steroids had probably been the cause of her short stature. 'Yes', said the examiner, 'in association with the malabsorption'.

Short case 4: 'Look at this man'. He had obvious *acromegaly*. I was asked to examine his fundi and I found a pale left disc. 'Yes', said the examiner, 'I thought he had. Would you like to examine for a scotoma?' I produced a red hat pin and the patient volunteered that it changed colour. The examiners seemed satisfied.

Short case 5: 'What is the diagnosis?' The patient had obvious *hereditary haemorrhagic telangiectasia* so I looked in the patient's mouth, which pleased the examiner. The examiner asked me what the other

name of the condition was and I replied: 'Osler–Weber–Rendu syndrome'.

Short case 6: 'What do you think about this man's feet?' He had definite *pustular psoriasis*. 'That's right', said the examiner, 'look at his hands'. He had the worst onycholysis that I have ever seen. 'Yes', said the examiner, 'that's the third time this has happened to this poor chap'.

Short case 7: 'Look at this woman. What strikes you about her?' I replied that she appeared green in colour. 'That's right', said the examiner, 'why do you think that she is this colour?' I replied that I didn't know but that perhaps it was very severe *jaundice*. 'Yes', said the examiner, 'tell me about the precursors of bilirubin?' I replied that it was biliverdin.

Short case 8: 'Look at this woman's rash—this part in particular'. Some parts of the rash looked bullous and others appeared to have target lesions. I looked in her mouth. My first thought was that it was pemphigoid but eventually I came out with the right diagnosis of *erythema multiforme*.

Short case 9: 'Look at this patient's hands'. I rolled up her sleeves that had been left down to her elbows and this revealed many *neurofibromata*. There was also partial amputation of several of her fingers.

I felt that I had passed the short cases. However, I only had one examiner as the other had just been admitted to hospital. Also is nine short cases any sort of a record?* (Pass)

'The other examiner, who seemed annoyed at his colleague, took over and took the bull by the horns!'
9 *Short case 1*: The first examiner dithered and was an irritatingly slow 'Dove'. He asked me to examine the respiratory system. I introduced myself, stood at the end of the bed and thought of the Newport course! He allowed me to examine fully both the anterior and posterior chest. I found an area of posterior consolidation on the right, with what I felt to be an area of anterior effusion. He mumbled something about 'over diagnosing' but agreed with the *consolidation*.

Short case 2: The next case was a nightmare. I was asked to examine a man's legs neurologically. Again, I introduced myself and observed. I examined extensively and found a loss of proprioception only. The examiner agreed and told me that that was correct and that sensation was otherwise normal. He

* No; many candidates see nine short cases.

asked me to look at the man's face. He had a left-sided eye patch. Underneath he had a partial ptosis. No further examination was allowed and I was asked for my thoughts on a possible diagnosis. This really stumped me and there was an embarrassing pause of several seconds. My only thought was of luetic disease but he was not satisfied. Again a number of long pauses. In the end he just wanted a polyneuropathy! I was told subsequently by the registrar running the exam that this was the *Guillain–Barré Miller–Fisher variant*. Most neurologists I've talked to disagree!

Short case 3: At this point the half-way bell went and the other examiner, who seemed annoyed at his colleague, took over and took the bull by the horns. At the next cubicle he asked me to look at a man and tell him immediately if I had a diagnosis. It was clear from the patient's expression (or lack of it) that he had *Parkinson's*. We quickly left the room.

Short case 4: The fourth case was again a spot diagnosis. The lady had glasses, a *marfanoid appearance* and a high-arched palate. I gave the diagnosis and he agreed, whisking me out.

Short case 5: I was then asked to: 'Listen only', to a man's heart. I palpated the carotid but that wasn't much help. There was a very, very soft ejection systolic murmur at the left sternal edge with no radiation to the neck. I got up and he asked specifically for a diagnosis. I told him (quickly) my findings and plumped for early *aortic stenosis*. He said nothing but hurried me to the next case.

Short case 6: I was asked to look at the fundus of a lady doing some knitting close to her face. She had no cataracts, and on inspection of the fundus she had what I'm sure was *retinitis pigmentosa* albeit not as typical as I had seen before.

Short case 7: With glee he then gave the same instruction for the lady sitting next to her, also knitting but showing no family resemblance. She too had a very pigmented retina but this time it was *panretinal photocoagulation* scars.

Short case 8: For the eighth case I was asked to examine a lady's conjugate eye movements. She had a *bilateral VIth nerve palsy*. He agreed and asked me for the possible causes. I said the causes of mononeuritis multiplex and he seemed happy.

Short case 9: My last case was an elderly man with striking jaundice and firm irregular *hepatomegaly* with no spleen. He asked the most likely cause and I said malignancy. He agreed.

I can't believe anybody comes out of the short cases thinking they have passed. My second case was, in my own mind, a disaster, but I don't think the other examiner was happy with the case chosen, and did everything in his power to show me many more. I think it all comes down to how you look and the air of confidence you give. I heard them commenting on my good technique (learnt in Gwent) and I'm sure this was the overriding factor that passed me. Being given cases of retinitis pigmentosa and diabetes photocoagulation scars side by side was a cheeky little number, a neat trick! Finally, if disasters occur early, it is *not* all over. I survived and now have 'MRCP' to tell the tale! (Pass)

'He had small, irregular pupils which did not react to light'.

10 The first patient was an elderly lady who was sitting upright. She was breathless at rest and quite cachectic. The examiner said to me: 'This lady is not very well so could you examine her chest from the back only?' I looked quickly at her hands and she had gross clubbing. The left side of her chest didn't move on inspiration and it was dull to percussion. The examiner stopped me at this point and asked for a diagnosis so I said there was a large left *pleural effusion* but it could be consolidation. He agreed and asked the most likely cause. I replied: '*NG*', as the patient was listening, and he agreed with me.

The next patient was a woman who was lying flat and I was asked to examine her abdomen. I looked at her hands, eyes, mouth, neck and axillae quite quickly and then moved on to the abdomen. She had *hepatosplenomegaly* but there was no ascites on testing for shifting dullness. The second examiner said that I shouldn't bother to do shifting dullness if she was not stony dull in the flanks to percussion. I nodded. 'What do you think the diagnosis is?' I said that it was probably a lymphoreticular problem such as chronic lymphatic leukaemia or chronic myeloid leukaemia in view of the patient's age (she was about 60–70). 'What else could it be?' I suggested lymphoma but there were no nodes or it could be cirrhosis, malaria or another infection. The examiner said: 'No', to all of these suggestions so I have no idea what they were really after.

The third patient was another elderly woman sitting upright. The examiner asked me to feel her pulse. It was about 100 beats min^{-1} in atrial fibrillation. 'Is there anything else?' said the examiner.

'No', I replied. 'OK', he said, 'then feel her apex beat'. Again it was about 100 beats min⁻¹ in atrial fibrillation and forceful. 'Forceful?' asked the examiner. 'Yes', I said. 'OK, carry on and listen to her heart'. I started to position the patient correctly at 45°, etc. but the other examiner said to me: 'Don't bother with that, it wastes time. We want to take you to see as many patients as possible'. So I just listened. My findings were that she had *isolated mitral stenosis*. I told them this and they nodded.

The next patient was a young boy about 20 years old and he was grossly overweight. I was asked to look at his abdomen and to say what I thought the scar was due to. It was a horizontal scar midway between the umbilicus and the groins. If he had been older I would have said it was for an aortic aneurysm but it was a bit too low so I eventually told them that I had never seen a scar like that before. The examiner said that it was an *apronectomy* and he asked me why I thought he had had it done. The patient did not look cushingoid so I said it was probably for obesity as I didn't think any surgeon would perform such an operation for a reversible metabolic cause. He laughed and said that was one way of looking at it! He asked if I thought he had *gynaeco-mastia*. I felt for breast tissue and said that there was. He then asked me to examine his testes which were very small. They took me outside and asked what I thought the diagnosis was. I said: 'Was it due to alcoholism?' They said: 'No'. I explained why I thought it wasn't Cushing's. They nodded: 'What else?' I suggested *Klinefelter's syndrome* because he was very tall. 'Yes', they said.

The fifth patient was sitting in a darkened room with about four other patients. 'Look at his fundi', they said. I thought he had proliferative diabetic retinopathy with extensive laser burns. However, there was no reply from the examiner. 'What else could it be?' I said it could be retinitis pigmentosa but explained how it looked different as the vessels were not usually traversed. 'Yes, but what else?' '*Choroidoretinitis* is another possibility but it isn't usually circumferential'. 'Yes', they said.

The sixth patient was another gentleman in the same room. 'Examine his visual fields'. I pulled up a chair and sat opposite to the patient at arm's length. I started to examine his visual fields but the examiners were walking about and talking and generally distracting the patient. I kept telling him to ignore them and to look at my nose! He had a *left homony-mous hemianopia*. They asked me for the site of the lesion. He had no other gross signs of facial weakness or hemiplegia so I said it was probably a right middle cerebral artery cerebrovascular accident but that the lesion could be anywhere along the optic radiation and they agreed with this.

The next patient was a man of about 50 lying in bed. 'Examine this man's legs', they said. He had a grossly deformed right ankle joint. I asked him if it was painful. He replied that it wasn't and never had been. I then said that it was a *Charcot's joint*. 'Due to what?' they asked. 'Probably due to *luetic disease*'. 'Yes, OK, what else would you like to examine?' I started to test the legs for sensation which was normal and for joint position sense which he did not allow me to do. 'What else?' The patient started to lift one of his feet and wiggle it about. 'Coordination', I suggested. 'Yes, OK'. I found that he was ataxic. 'What else would you like to examine?' The patient started winking at me. 'I'd like to examine his eyes, please'. He had small, irregular pupils which did not react to light. 'Does that confirm your suspicions?' I replied that it did and that was the end of the exam.

The examiners were very nice and helpful to me and seemed to want to pass me. I was really very fortunate to have had such a pleasant experience. (Pass)

'I would advise candidates that, whenever they are on call, to practise examining patients. I had the clinical on a Monday and was on call all weekend. As it turned out, this was very good practise'.

11 My first patient was a cyanosed elderly man with clubbing and basal crackles. I said that *fibrosing alveolitis* was the most likely diagnosis. The examiner said: 'What else could it be?', so I suggested *occupational lung disease* and this seemed to suffice. The examiner then showed me the chest X-ray and expected me to describe the reticular pattern. He asked me for the Latin name for lacy! I didn't know the word so the examiner moved on quickly.

The next patient was a young Asian man with an old ulcer on his shin. I was asked to say what had caused this so I suggested *sickle-cell disease* and this was correct.

The next patient was an old, pale man with *hepatosplenomegaly*. The examiner asked how I knew that it was not polycystic kidney disease. I initially bluntly replied that I had not formally examined for the kidneys (which I had in fact forgotten to do) and the examiner looked a bit taken aback. However, I went on to say that he had no evidence for dialysis (shunts or peritoneal) and I could not get above the masses, etc. I feel that although I had forgotten to formally examine the kidneys he had obviously not noticed and my straightforward admission got me off the hook.

The next patient was a young lady and I was asked to examine her right hand. I noticed that both forearms seemed wasted distally. The right hand had both hypothenar and thenar wasting with clawing. I was asked first to describe this and then what I thought it could be due to (having briefly gone through a neurological motor and sensory examination and had demonstrated the most likely nerve lesions). I felt that it could be *hereditary motor* and *sensory neuropathy* extending to the arms and said I would want to see the legs. In retrospect I think that this must have been correct. The examiner did not seem displeased but then asked for other possibilities. We got on to peripheral nerve lesions, brachial plexus lesions and syringomyelia, each of which I had to justify.

The next patient had *proliferative diabetic retinopathy*. The examiner asked me where the microaneurysms were so I said between the vessels. He then asked me why they were not right by the vessels. Seeing me struggle he asked about Harvey's theories at which I realized that they must be aneurysms of the capillaries.

The next patient had complicated heart murmurs including *aortic regurgitation* and *mitral stenosis/ Austin Flint murmur* plus *mitral regurgitation*. She had had previous surgery and we got into a discussion about the indications for warfarinization and artificial pig valves.

The last patient was a straightforward *psoriatic arthropathy*.

The first examiner took me rapidly through the cases. Immediately I got the diagnosis or answered the question he would move on which suited me fine. I would advise candidates that, whenever they are on call, to practise examining patients. I had the clinical on a Monday and was on call all weekend. As it turned out this was very good practice as when seeing patients I would just concentrate on one particular system. (Pass)

'There was a loud stenotic murmur so I didn't mention that I had heard the regurgitant jet'.

12 'Examine this man's abdomen'. I started with the hands and was told (not unkindly) to move on. As soon as I had demonstrated the *spleen* they stopped me. 'What is your finding?' I said a large spleen. 'What is the cause in this man?' He was about 70–80 and I had to modify my list accordingly which I did rather poorly.

The second patient had a *diabetic retinopathy* with laser scars. The examiner asked me about his visual fields and whether the scars involved the macula. 'Yes', I said. 'So I expect a scotoma and a constrictive field defect'. 'Examine them then'. Of course I found the patient to have a completely normal blind spot and full fields!

The next patient had *optic atrophy*. It was an old man with hydrocephalus. I was asked what had caused his underlying optic atrophy and I replied that it was probably due to chronic raised intracranial pressure. I had the impression that this was a case that they weren't sure about including as they seemed pleased that I had made something of it.

I was then taken to the next patient and asked to feel the pulse. It was a collapsing pulse and I was then asked to examine the precordium. I heard the regurgitant murmur in the aortic area only. There was a loud stenotic murmur so I didn't mention that I had heard the regurgitant jet. (I do not know why!) I said he had *aortic stenosis* but why the pulse? 'I would like to see the blood pressure', I said. This was 190/40. 'He must have *aortic regurgitation*'. The examiner said: 'Uuuh. Listen again'. Which I did and heard it again. (This time it was very loud!) However, I had been allowed to re-listen to this patient. I felt that I could have done much better here in summing up the signs more sensibly.

The next patient was an elderly lady with a resting tremor, an intention tremor, titubation, a mini tracheostomy and clasp-knife tone. The examiner said: 'What do you notice?' I said: 'She has a mini tracheostomy'. 'Yes', said the examiner, 'the last candidate missed that'. My brief examination demonstrated all the above findings. The examiner said: 'What nerve supplies the larynx?' There was then a brief discussion on brainstem syndromes and I discovered afterwards that the eventual diagnosis here had been the *olivocerebellopontine degeneration syndrome*! (Pass)

'I said "infectious mononucleosis" before I could stop myself'.

13 I was asked to examine the language function of a patient. This went well as she had an *expressive dysphasia*. I was then asked to examine her visual fields and she had an *homonymous hemianopia*. I was asked about the general management of stroke patients and the factors involved in their prognosis. They seemed happy with my answers. I was then asked to examine the next patient's heart. I therefore listened and felt the carotid pulse at the same time. There was a plateau pulse plus aortic stenosis. I gave my findings and asked for the blood pressure. I was told it was 120/80. I made a diagnosis of *aortic stenosis* and had to explain why it was not aortic sclerosis. I was told that the patient had presented as a collapse so we then talked about syncope secondary to aortic stenosis. I then got on to arrhythmias and Stokes–Adams attacks. I know that they were trying to change my mind about the diagnosis but I said clinically my diagnosis was of aortic stenosis and that an ECG and an echo and possibly catheter studies would help confirm this. I am sure I would have failed if I had changed my mind.

We went on to the next patient and I was asked to examine the abdomen and to explain what I was doing and to give my findings as I went along. They stopped me after I had found *hepatosplenomegaly* and then asked me for a differential diagnosis. I gave alcoholic liver disease with portal hypertension and infection. 'What sort of infection?', they asked. I said 'infectious mononucleosis' before I could stop myself and the examiner laughed and said: 'Is it likely?' I said: 'No, because the patient is in the wrong age group', and they seemed satisfied. I mentioned chronic myeloid leukaemia and they asked me about enzyme markers and that went OK.

For the next patient I had to examine the neck. There were large pulsating masses on both sides which were possibly *carotid aneurysms*. I examined the neck and then the examiner handed me my stethoscope! I presented my findings but was not asked for a diagnosis.

We moved on to the next patient: 'Examine these fundi'. The right fundus was normal but the left fundus had optic atrophy plus a small area of choroidoretinitis. They seemed surprised when they asked me to describe what I had seen. Then they asked for the diagnosis. I thought they meant of the *optic atrophy* and the *choroidoretinitis*. So I said:

'Toxoplasmosis!' They laughed and said: 'No, the patient went suddenly blind'. I then offered a diagnosis of temporal arteritis. The examiner obviously did not know about the choroidoretinitis. I saw the patient afterwards and he told me that they'd had another look. I hope they saw it!

Both the examiners were very pleasant. I know my examination technique was fine but sometimes I was a bit hesitant when answering their questions. (Pass)

'I thought the examiners were probably a little the worse for lunch. Don't be fooled by their jovial attitude (if they are like that) into becoming frivolous yourself'.

14 The first patient had bilateral *polycystic kidney disease* and I was asked to examine the abdomen. I went straight to the hands and the examiners asked what I was looking for. They wanted to know if I had found any of these features and before I could say that they were in fact normal I was jovially accused of not having really looked but I firmly stated that I had. When I asked the patient if he had any pain in the tummy they said: 'He soon will have'. I was then told: 'We have to get our entertainment this afternoon somehow'. There was eventually a discussion on how polycystic kidneys present.

The second patient had *mitral stenosis* and *aortic regurgitation*. Again the examination was interspersed with quips from the examiners. They expected me to have felt the trachea to check the position of the mediastinum. I hadn't and was told: 'Naughty, naughty'. A look of horror must have crossed my face as they said: 'Don't worry, you're doing very well'. The instruction for this patient had been: 'Examine this woman's chest from the cardiovascular point of view'.

The third patient had *diabetic retinopathy*. It was fairly uncomplicated except that the examiners fell around laughing when, having asked the patient if I could look in the first eye, I then asked if I could look in the left eye. The instruction had been: 'Examine this patient's eyes' (whilst they were handing me an ophthalmoscope) so I had asked if they only wanted fundoscopy and they had said: 'Yes'.

The next patient had *titubation* and *nystagmus* in all planes. The instruction was: 'Examine this patient's eyes'. I got the Snellen chart from your book and they were delighted, clapping their hands and saying: 'Bonus points for that!' The rest of the examination of this patient was unremarkable and there was a brief discussion on possible causes.

The fifth patient had a *spastic paraparesis* and I was asked to examine the legs. It was uneventful until just before the plantars. I was asked which way they were going to go and I said: 'Up'. He said: 'OK, make them go up like a real neurologist'. They went up and at that point I couldn't resist a broad grin. There was a brief discussion on possible causes.

The last patient had *clubbing, pigmentation* and *kyphosis* and we talked about a possible aetiology.

I thought the examiners were probably a little the worse for lunch. Don't be fooled by their jovial attitude (if they are like that) into becoming frivolous yourself. When I started the exam they said: 'What are you good at? Don't tell me, everything I suppose'. I said: 'Well, I have been practising', and they roared with laughter. (Pass)

'The delayed fundal question ploy I thought—I was ready for that!'

15 Examiner 1 (male): 'What do you think the skin lesion is on this leg?' (discoloured, purple/pink with marked scaling) 'Psoriasis', I said, 'but there are no other plaques'. 'No — think again', 'Drug reaction?' 'No', said the examiner who appeared exasperated. 'How about infection?' 'Well it could be *cellulitis*,' I said. 'Yes, at last. Well perhaps you'll do better on the others'. (I'd never imagined they would put a cellulitis in, especially an atypical one.)

'Examine this man's leg and talk as you go through it. You may ask him questions'. I grappled with demonstrating a *paraplegia* whilst speaking (which was difficult). 'What do you think of his speech?' (Heck! I realized it wasn't the content but the speech character they wanted me to note.) I asked a question and noted his *dysarthria*. 'Would you like to demonstrate the plantars!' I said I would normally do them and showed they were upgoing. (By this time I was despondent but determined.)

'Examine this girl's cardiovascular system quickly.' It went smoothly. I presented it clearly and discussed the *ventricular septal defect* or mitral regurgitant murmur. 'Do you think the VSD is significant?' 'Well, no because there . . .' I said. 'Don't say why just say yes or no' (exasperated examiner). 'No'. 'Fine', he said.

Examiner 2 (male, but more friendly): 'Look at this man. Perhaps it is easier if he stands up. Tell me what you think'. 'He has a *marfanoid appearance*,

Sir'. 'Yes, what would you look for?' 'Aortic and mitral regurgitation', I replied. 'Which valve is most likely to be affected?' '*Aortic regurgitation*'. The examiner pulled back the shirt trumphantly to demonstrate the aortic valve replacement scar (Bingo!).

'Examine this fundus'. There was a background *diabetic retinopathy*. I confidently presented my prepared speech. 'Yes', and we walked away. *Then* he said: 'And were there any laser scars?' 'No', I said. 'And were there cotton-wool spots?' 'No'. 'Correct'. (The delayed fundal question ploy I thought—I was ready for that!)

'Examine the abdomen of this girl'. There was a *liver and spleen* palpable so I gave these signs succinctly. We moved away and the examiner noticeably relaxed filling time. 'What do you think is the cause?' 'Hodgkin's is most likely', I said. 'Yes, anything else — how about biliary cirrhosis? 'There are no signs of chronic liver disease and the spleen goes against this', I said. 'Yes, but it is *biliary cirrhosis*', and he shrugged his shoulders! (Pass)

'I have already made a diagnosis. Do you want me to continue?'

16 I was asked to examine the arms of a man who was complaining of weakness. He had the facial appearance of *dystrophia myotonica*. I shook hands with the patient and said: 'I have already made a diagnosis. Do you want me to continue?' I then had to demonstrate how to examine power in the arms. I was asked if I wanted to ask the patient any questions. I asked him about family history and the effects of cold.

I was then asked to examine another patient's fundi. He had grade II *hypertensive retinopathy* with marked AV nipping.

The third patient was an 'Examine the respiratory system'. He had dyspnoea, cyanosis, clubbing and the fine inspiratory basal crackles suggestive of *fibrosing alveolitis*. I was asked to give the causes and differential diagnoses of fibrosis of the lungs. I was then shown the patient's chest X-ray and asked to comment. It showed bilateral lower zone fibrotic changes.

Next, I was asked to examine a patient's abdomen. There were bilateral *polycystic kidneys* and an AV fistula in the arm. I was asked to demonstrate one of the kidneys. The examiner seemed satisfied, and asked me the single most useful investigation. I answered: 'Ultrasound', and he nodded.

I was taken to the next short case and asked to examine the heart and to tell the examiner what the diagnosis was. The pulse was of normal character and there was a long *systolic murmur* all over the praecordium maximal at the left sternal edge. I said I was unsure of the diagnosis and gave a differential of mitral regurgitation and aortic sclerosis. He asked me what the heart sounds were like. I could not remember them clearly and said 'normal'. He then said he thought the second sound was quiet. I wondered whether I had missed aortic stenosis. We then got into a discussion between aortic sclerosis and stenosis. I admitted that I thought aortic sclerosis was a bad term and wished I had never mentioned it! He asked me what I would do in the clinic if presented with such a murmur, and I said an ECG, chest X-ray and an echocardiogram. He nodded.

My advice is to stay as calm as possible and hope that the first case goes well. Always look at the patient's surroundings and general appearance before starting your specific examination. It is impressive if you can make the diagnosis, for example, of dystrophia myotonica from the end of the bed and it saves time too. (Pass)

'What they really wanted me to notice were the old-fashioned controls'.
17 For my next case I was asked to examine a patient's abdomen. I thought I could get over the mass in the left hypochondrium and so I said the diagnosis was of polycystic kidneys. I then looked for dialysis marks on the arms. In retrospect, it was so clearly *hepatosplenomegaly*. In fact I can still feel my fingers jumping over the sharp edge of the liver. I really don't know why I said polycystic kidneys. If I had been the examiner I would certainly have failed me!

We then moved on to the next patient. The examiner said: 'What do you notice about this woman?' There was half a minute's pause. 'She's in a wheel-chair', I said. 'What does that tell you about the chronicity of her disease?' 'If it's an NHS wheel-chair then she will have been waiting some time!' (They liked this.) What they had really wanted me to notice were the old-fashioned controls. They went on: 'Examine her fundi'. She had the whitest discs that I have ever seen. 'What would you like to

test next?' They obviously thought I wasn't extending my examination quickly enough. What they really meant was: 'Examine her gait', which I eventually did and she was grossly ataxic. 'What is your diagnosis?' '*Multiple sclerosis*'. It had taken a long time to drag me through this case! (Pass)

'She must have had cystic fibrosis presenting with a cerebral abscess'.
18 For my next case I was asked to examine a lady's abdomen. She was about 40 years old. I performed a standard abdominal routine and found that she had a large mass on the right side which I could get above. It moved with respiration and was hollow to percussion. I thought it was most likely to be a polycystic kidney but since I could not feel one on the other side I suggested that I would investigate it further. The examiner said: 'Well it is a *polycystic kidney*, and I wouldn't worry too much about being able to feel one on the other side'.

The last short case was a 30-year-old lady. I was told that she had come to casualty last week having had several fits. She had papilloedema and the examiners had done a CT scan. They then asked me to examine her chest. She had clubbing with a Hickman line *in situ* and she also had a left thoracotomy scar. There was a left pleural effusion with thickening and a right pleural rub. The examiner said: 'Can you piece it all together?' I went: 'Um, um, um', and then the bell went. The examiner said: 'Come on'. I went: 'Uhh . . . uhh . . .' He said: 'OK, forget it!' I think she must have had *cystic fibrosis* presenting with a cerebral abscess.

One must look interested in the cases themselves and take time to be nice to the patients. I said: 'Excuse me' to one of the examiners while pointing to an open curtain behind him before examining a young lady's chest. He said: 'Sorry' and closed the curtains! (Pass)

You never know you've failed until the list is published

The following examples illustrate the extent to which the candidate's assessment of what is happening can be very different from the examiners. Though the examiners may appear rude and hawkish, and you may feel that you are doing badly, you may be performing well—at least well enough to get the bare fail which can be compensated for from other sections of the exam!

19 For my first case I was asked to examine the abdomen of a 60-year-old female. I found a large *mass on the left side of the abdomen*, there was no anterior notch, I could not get above it or below it. I thought it was probably a kidney or a spleen but to this day I don't know what it was. I told the examiners I thought it was probably a renal mass and gave reasons why but I feel I was probably wrong. They said nothing and looked displeased.

For the next case, they took me to a 70-year-old male and asked me to 'listen to the back of the chest only'. There were bilateral basal fine expiratory crackles and clubbing. I told the examiners that there was *pulmonary fibrosis* and it was probably idiopathic. This was followed by: 'For goodness sake woman, calm down!' 'What is the diagnosis?' I told them the same diagnosis again. 'What does he have?' I told them again! 'What is the cause?' I told them again and got upset and said 'I'm sorry but . . .' The examiner said: 'Look at him again'. I looked and could see nothing so I said that. He eventually hinted at connective tissue diseases so I asked the patient to open his mouth — he had *scleroderma*! In retrospect, I feel that this was not obvious and that the examiner was unduly harsh in his attitude.

The next patient was a 35-year-old female and I was asked to examine the cardiovascular system. I heard *some sort of murmur*. I noticed a sternotomy scar and a funny pulse. I was still shaking from my experience in the second case and was by now even more nervous. It was either mitral valve disease or combined aortic valve disease — I obviously got it wrong as the examiner listened and looked cross. The examiners muttered between themselves and I felt completely useless by this stage. The only saving grace was that I had examined the cardiovascular system of the patient efficiently.

The next patient was a 50-year-old male and I was asked to look at his fundi. The room was light and the pupils were not fully dilated. I used my own ophthalmoscope which was a great help. I reported early background *diabetic retinopathy* in the left eye only and they moved on. In the meantime, in a loud voice, the first examiner said: 'Well, I would never employ this woman — would you?' If I had been nervous before, I was even worse now and felt certain that I had failed.

The next patient was a 60-year-old male with a harsh *pansystolic murmur* at the left sternal edge and a displaced apex. I again examined thoroughly and described what I had heard in response to the instruction 'Feel the pulse, listen at the apex'. I was asked the diagnosis and said ventricular septal defect because of the apex and the harsh quality. He wanted to know the differential diagnosis and how I would differentiate them clinically. The examiner was still unhappy. I think it must have been mitral regurgitation.

The next patient was a 60-year-old female. I was told to: 'Look at this face — what do you see?' '*Cushingoid*', I responded. 'Name three causes in a woman of this age'. I gave three. 'Anything else you notice?' '*Basal cell carcinoma*'. 'What else?' I could see nothing else so I pointed out a second basal cell carcinoma which I had already seen. They then both walked off muttering.

The examiners were rude and unpleasant. My only advice to future candidates is to pretend you are in the accident and emergency department and ignore the examiners. (Pass!)

'The examiners looked surprised when I said the tone was increased. I was asked to demonstrate and therefore withdrew my rash and foolish remark and finally concluded with possibilities for combined upper and lower motor neurone lesions'.

20 'Examine this lady's *legs and gait*': a disaster! Gait: partly obscured by long nightgown — ?steppage or ?right foot-drop. Examination on the bed: tone (patient nervous) seemed increased but reflexes and plantars could not be illicited, the power was reduced, and the testing of sensation was laborious and inconclusive. I was uncertain when to say I had finished. There were pitying looks from the examiners. I blurted out some findings. The examiners looked surprised when I said the tone was increased. I was asked to demonstrate and therefore withdrew my rash and foolish remark and finally concluded with possibilities for combined upper and *lower motor neurone lesions*.

We passed on (with much relief) but scarcely more success. 'Examine this patient's knees': on inspection the knees were clearly swollen, left more than right, and the quadriceps were wasted. On palpation, the knees were warm but I failed to elicit fluid even though effusions were obviously present. The examiners raised their eyebrows as I recounted my findings. 'Please show me how you look for fluid'. On this second attempt, I clearly elicited the patella tap sign. Causes for the *swollen knees* were not discussed. We passed on (with increasing confusion on my part). 'Listen to this man's heart!' I heard and reported *aortic incompetence*, having noted the cannula in the patient's arm. I was asked for the aetiology and suggested subacute *bacterial endocarditis* which seemed to be what they wanted—at last (!) but surely I was beyond redemption.

'Look at this lady's neck': I inspected the plucked chicken skin and gave the diagnosis of *pseudoxanthoma elasticum*. I was not asked any more and we passed on and I noted Resuscitation Annie on an adjacent bed but we passed her by.

'Examine this man's chest': on inspection he was blue, bloated and very breathless and I proceeded with palpation, percussion and auscultation though the examination was punctuated by bouts of severe coughing which I thought would lead to his death at any moment! The examiners seemed understanding as I asked if he wished me to continue. My diagnosis of exacerbation of *chronic obstructive airway disease* was accepted.

I was grateful to get to the next patient. 'Examine this man's abdomen': I was going through my normal procedure when the bell sounded which is always offputting and I sought to reach a hasty conclusion. I suggested that there was a non-tender 2 cm *liver edge* and then hazarded that there was a mass in the right iliac fossa. The examiners eyebrows were raised again in response to this. I am not sure whether there was a mass. A colleague who saw the patient, told me later that he had only felt a liver edge. The short cases ended with ears ringing and I was convinced of failure.

Of my six short cases. two went smoothly. two were barely mediocre (not least because the bronchitic threatened to expire at the end of every breath) and two were terrible and I had to repeat the part of the examination which I got wrong. So I strongly emphasize that the odd calamity need not mean failure. The candidate is probably very poorly placed to decide how he or she is doing (even if this is the best evidence we have about the exam). (Pass)

'The examiners were continually unnerving me and making me feel that my answers were wrong'.
21 I was asked to examine the hands of the first patient. They looked rheumatoid but the patient also seemed to have tophi. There were no nodules at the elbow and I eventually said it was inactive

rheumatoid arthritis. One examiner asked what I would think if his uric acid was 0.6 mmol l⁻¹. I said that was because he had *gout* as well! On walking to the next case, they asked me about treatment and I managed to discuss this satisfactorily.

I was asked to talk to an elderly man with nasogastric feeding in process. He had dysarthria. They stopped me before I got any further and asked what I thought. I said that with dysarthria and nasogastric feeding, which was probably as a result of dysphagia, he had bulbar palsy. They asked me how I would differentiate pseudobulbar from bulbar palsy — I said I would look at his tongue—it was small and fasciculating. I therefore diagnosed *bulbar palsy*. As they moved away, they asked me the cause—I could only think of multiple cerebrovascular accidents. I forgot this would not do for the bulbar palsy I had just diagnosed!

For the next case, I was asked to look at the fundi. I could see lots of *laser burns* but no signs of diabetic retinopathy and so I said so. They asked me what I thought of the vessels. When I was looking, I did think there was AV nipping but thought that I would be better not mentioning this. However, as they were actually asking me, I said that there was AV nipping which I had not mentioned because I thought it was a 'soft sign'. They didn't seem to like this. I then said that there may be hypertension as well. They didn't respond. I was beginning to get unnerved!

I was next asked to look at a lady's eyes. She had *gross unilateral exophthalmos* and ophthalmoplegia. They soon stopped me and asked me what I thought. The only thing I could think of was thyrotoxicosis. They said she was euthyroid and pointed to a scar just above the nose and eye. I didn't have a clue what it was. They asked me what was directly behind the centre of the forehead. I told them the pituitary and that the exophthalmos might be due to a space-occupying lesion. They asked me what type. I noticed the patient was quite hirsute but by this stage the examiners had walked away and I couldn't think so I didn't say anything.

They showed me a man with a *large mole* on his left arm. I didn't know what it was. Although it didn't look like a melanoma, this was the only thing I could think of so I said that the lesion should be excised and biopsied. They told me that the patient had had the lesion for years and that he had another one on his leg and they asked me what I thought about this. I said that I didn't know and that I would still biopsy the lesion! It seemed that I was arguing with the examiner and as I realized this, it made me feel even worse!

I was next asked to examine the cardiovascular system of a middle-aged female. She had a midline and lateral thoracotomy scar and *prosthetic heart sounds* with no murmur at the apex — he stopped me before I could listen further. I said that she had a prosthetic valve without any murmurs and with the two scars she had probably had a mitral valvotomy and later a valve replacement. One examiner asked me if this was likely in view of the fact that she was in sinus rhythm. I said that one expects atrial fibrillation but the sinus rhythm was possible. The examiner laughed! They asked me about the aortic area — I said I hadn't listened there as I hadn't had time. The bell went and I was allowed to go. I felt like walking out and giving up.

I thought I did very badly. The examiners were continually unnerving me and making me feel that my answers were wrong. I was made to feel very unsure and I felt that it was very difficult to keep going. By the third and fourth case, I had semi given up. As I was told time and time again prior to the exam, I am sure the main thing is to keep going despite what happens — you never know you've passed or failed until the letter comes through the door! (Pass)

'Still to this day I think I got it wrong and really should have failed the exam'.

22 I was next taken to a jaundiced lady who had *large masses in her abdomen*. I said that they were bilateral palpable kidneys and that the diagnosis was of polycystic kidney disease. The examiner said that they thought the masses were dull to percussion. I replied that my initial impression, noting her to be jaundiced, was that the masses ought to be hepato-splenomegaly but that when I found that they were not dull and were, I thought, ballottable masses then I had had to say that they were kidneys. Still to this day I think I got it wrong and really should have failed the exam, especially as the next case was a *hepatosplenomegaly*! I was not sure whether this was done to see if I could actually diagnose hepato-splenomegaly but I tried not to be flustered by my previous case and so carried on. I really thought I had done well until this case and that now I had probably failed. I couldn't really imagine how anyone could pass a candidate who mistook hepato-splenomegaly for polycystic kidneys. I may have got the diagnosis wrong but my general impression after the first three or four cases was that they quite liked me and thought that I was a reasonable candidate. They weren't so particular over details once they were satisfied with my overall standard. I think the examiners make their minds up quite quickly and also I think they like to see you being nice and chatty with the patients. (Pass)

'I felt like going home there and then but I am glad I didn't'.

23 'Listen to this man's heart — no, go straight to the precordium'. I was not given any history. I was so completely confused by the murmurs which were systolic and diastolic that I could not make head nor tail of them. Some findings were eventually coaxed out of me and a conclusion forced upon me. I felt like going home there and then but I am glad I didn't. I was forced into saying that this was *aortic valve disease* with dominant regurgitation. I haven't a clue if I was right or wrong. I was then asked to look at a man's hands. There was gross *clubbing* with no apparent cause, i.e. he was not cyanosed and there wasn't a Horner's, etc. I was asked for more possibilities — they eventually told me that this was pachydermoperiostitis — I admitted that I had never seen it before!

'Look at this man's fundi'. I thought I saw a *pigmented lesion in the choroid* which was well demarcated and single. I was asked for more possibilities and to say what it actually was. I plumped for a melanoma.

I was then asked to look at another man's hands. He had *gouty tophi* but there was nothing on the ears or the elbows. They seemed satisfied with this. The next patient was an 'Examine this man's abdomen'. I felt a *4 cm liver* and they asked me if I could feel a spleen. I said: 'No'.

I was then taken to a lady and asked to look at her — 'What do you see?' She was pigmented and mildly jaundiced with leuconychia and xanthelasma. She also had hepatomegaly and ascites. I was then shown her hands again and I had missed her liver palms but that was after I had already given the diagnosis of *primary biliary cirrhosis*!

My last short case was another 'Look at this man's hands' and he was *another case of gouty tophi*. The examiners told me that I was correct. I was absolutely convinced that I had made an irretrievable mess of the short cases. I still can't understand how they passed me! (Pass)

Survivors of the storm

'I found hepatosplenomegaly and told the examiner this. He then turned to the patient and said: "What operation have you just had?" and the patient answered: "A splenectomy!"'

24 'What's the diagnosis in this patient?' I noticed he had both *neurofibromatosis* and finger *clubbing*. The examiner asked me if I could relate the two conditions. I said: 'No' and the examiner said: 'Neither can I!' I was then asked to examine a fundus. I found *optic atrophy* and *resolving papilloedema*. The examiner suggested that I should look at the patient's neck and I found a ventriculoperitoneal shunt present. The next patient had an abdomen to be examined. There was a recent mid-line scar. I found *hepatosplenomegaly* and told the examiner this. He then turned to the patient and said: 'What operation have you just had?' and the patient answered: 'Splenectomy!' I was then asked to examine a patient's cardiovascular system. I found atrial fibrillation, *mixed mitral valve disease* (it was a restenosis as there was an old valvotomy scar), *pulmonary hypertension* and *tricuspid regurgitation*. There were pronounced CV waves in the neck and a pulsatile liver. I am sure I scored extra marks by feeling the abdomen. I was then asked to discuss the waveforms of the JVP and I even had to draw a diagram! (Pass)

'The examiners appeared irritated by all my answers and when we had finished the female examiner shook her head scornfully!'

25 The first two patients were in a dark room. Both had dilated pupils and I was asked to look at their fundi. I did not get the diagnosis with the first patient. I said the vessels looked thin and the retina was dark and wondered whether it was *optic atrophy*.

The second patient definitely had a *diabetic retinopathy* and the examiner asked whether there were any hypertensive changes as well.

The third short case was a female patient with a small, smooth *goitre* and eye signs. I was asked to examine the patient and say why I was performing each action. I was then asked if the patient was *euthyroid* or not.

Next I was taken to a 30-year-old patient and asked to feel her abdomen. There was a *mass in the*

right loin. I was asked what a horseshoe kidney would feel like, and I was then asked to give my findings before I had finished palpating the kidneys. So I just carried on feeling until I had finished.

I was then asked to examine another patient's heart and again I was asked for the findings when I had only listened at the apex and the left sternal edge. The patient was a lady in her eighties. She had peripheral cyanosis, atrial fibrillation and *right ventricular hypertrophy* but I could hear no murmurs. I said that the diagnosis was probably tight pulmonary stenosis but I should really have said tight mitral stenosis or an atrial septal defect. I was really taken to task on the following points: Was the patient cyanosed? What other signs of cyanosis do you know? How common is pulmonary stenosis in this age group? What is the commonest cause of pulmonary stenosis? The examiners appeared irritated by all my answers and when we had finished the female examiner shook her head scornfully!

The last patient was a lady aged about 30. I was asked to examine her pulses and to comment on them. She appeared to have *peripheral vascular disease* and *aortic stenosis*. (Pass)

'I found that if my first answer was incorrect, the examiners continued questioning until I got the right answer; and if my first answer was correct, then they took the questioning a little further'.

26 'Look at this patient. What do you notice?' There was pallor, mild jaundice and bruising. I thought the diagnosis could possibly be *pernicious anaemia* and the examiners asked why. 'Because it looks like it', I replied. (Stupid answer!) I tried again and said: 'The patient is the right sex and age'. The examiner went on to ask me to examine the fundi. There were haemorrhages present which were obviously secondary to the pernicious anaemia but I said it was probably diabetic retinopathy!

My second short case was a *ventricular septal defect* in a 25-year-old but I said I thought he had hypertrophic obstructive cardiomyopathy and we discussed the symptoms and findings, and finally the examiner said: 'What else could it be?' I said a ventricular septal defect and then he seemed happy!

The third patient had *rheumatoid arthritis* with *subluxation of the cervical spine* causing a *spastic paraparesis*. I was asked to examine the legs neurologically. I found this difficult as all the patient's joints were incredibly painful. Therefore, tone and power were hard to test. I had noted the rheumatoid arthritis and the upper motor neurone signs in both legs but failed to put two and two together to come up with subluxation of the spine.

The fourth patient had a complete left *IIIrd nerve palsy*. I demonstrated the findings and suggested all the causes of a IIIrd nerve palsy but unfortunately failed to see a scar which indicated that she had had an aneurysm clipped!

The fifth patient had finger clubbing and a marked tremor. I noted these findings and suggested *thyroid acropachy*. I was then asked to find whether she was in fact hyperthyroid. I concluded she was euthyroid and found out later that that was correct.

My last patient had *psoriasis* of the hands with an *arthropathy*. I described the nail changes and the skin changes but in my panic forgot to demonstrate the terminal interphalangeal arthritis. I found that if my first answer was slightly incorrect the examiners continued questioning until I found the right answer; and if my first answer was correct then they took the questioning a little further. (Pass)

'I was harassed continually by the examiners saying: "Why are you doing x, y, z?" despite the fact that I was trying to tell them!'

27 'Examine this man's cardiovascular system and talk us through it. You've no need to do the BP'. I was harassed continually by the examiners saying: 'Why are you doing XYZ?', despite the fact that I was trying to tell them! For example: 'Why did you roll him on to the left side?' My final diagnosis was of *tricuspid incompetence* in a patient with right heart failure. I told the examiners that I would like to look for a pulsatile liver and they said: 'Show us'.

I was then taken round the corner to the next case and the examiner said: 'This lady has just collapsed, resuscitate her'. It was the *Resuscitation Annie*. It went very well and at the end I was asked for the survival figures in our hospital from cardiac arrest and I knew this, thank goodness!

'This gentleman is from Mauritius, examine his chest'. My findings were of clubbing with bronchial breath sounds at the left upper zone. I said that the most likely diagnosis was a mitotic lesion in the left upper zone. Examiner: 'Tell me where the trachea is'. Whoops, I had fogotten to feel, so I said I had forgotten to look for it. Examiner: 'Would you like to?' I said: 'OK, yes, it's displaced to the left'. Examiner: 'This gentleman has had these signs for 20 years'. I

suggested that the most likely diagnosis was of *post tuberculous bronchiectasis with collapse of the left upper lobe*. Examiner: 'Correct. Why, if the upper lobe collapses, do you get bronchial breath sounds but if the lower lobe collapses you only get reduced breath sounds?' I said: 'It depends in either case on whether there is patency of a major airway'. Examiner: 'No, it is because the upper airways are less dependent'. All I could say was: 'Oh!'

I was then taken to a side room with the lights put out. Examiner: 'Examine this lady's eyes with the ophthalmoscope'. I did so and found *background diabetic retinopathy*. Examiner: 'Tell me about the pupils'. (We were in a pitch black room!) I had to tell him that I hadn't examined the pupils properly as he had asked me to look at the fundi. Examiner: 'Put on the lights and have a look'. I did so. 'The right eye is dilated and the left eye is constricted', I said. Examiner: 'Look at the eyelids'. I was staring in desperation. Examiner: 'Do you think she has a left sided ptosis?' I said: 'No'. Examiner: 'Well, she has. She has a left *Horner's* and midriatics in the right eye'. What a case to end on!

The Resuscitation Annie was the turning point as they were impressed by my performance and said so but then I had practised at work on a similar dummy. (Pass)

'Two stone-faced, non-committal, silent, disapproving examiners! Despite expecting this, it still threw me a bit'.

28 Two stone-faced, non-commital, silent, disapproving examiners! Despite expecting this, it still threw me a bit. The first case — *hepatosplenomegaly* in a patient with *polycythaemia rubra vera*. I got the signs, then was asked for a differential — was told he had polycythaemia rubra vera and was asked the symptoms. This unnerved me.

The second case was a fundus — just the right one. At first, all I could see were a couple of haemorrhages. They said: 'Would you like another look?' I was convinced I had failed. I then asked if I could use my own ophthalmoscope (with a beam just down from a laser!) and found a *retinal artery branch occlusion* which I described, although I had never seen one before. This satisfied them and they asked me to do his visual fields which was easy and I demonstrated the *unilateral left lower quadrantopia*. Still convinced I had failed I was taken to a patient and told to examine the legs as expeditiously as possible.

I checked the foot pulses, then did a neurological exam. I demonstrated a mixed motor and sensory distal neuropathy, but the plantars kept going up! I said this was probably *subacute combined degeneration of the cord* in an elderly lady, and said why it wasn't motor neurone disease or Friedrich's but that syphilis was possible. They asked how else I could demonstrate a plantar response. I did Oppenheimer's test but they still looked vexed as the toes went up. They asked how else I could demonstrate plantars but I couldn't think of another answer. We went on!

Convinced I had failed, we went to a lady with a malar flush. I was asked to examine the pulse and I found slow atrial fibrillation. I then described the face. They then asked me to auscultate only. I picked up *mixed aortic* and *mixed mitral valve disease*. They asked me the cause, and I said rheumatic heart disease. They gave no impression if I was right but asked if she was in heart failure. I replied that they hadn't allowed me to listen to the lung bases or to look for ankle oedema, but that her pulse was not fast and there was no third heart sound. I then looked at the JVP and pointed out the systolic waves of *tricuspid incompetence*. Then the bell went.

I felt that having only seen four cases (although all were 'long' short cases) I might not have done enough. Presumably, I passed because I had my routines completely 'off pat', so I didn't hesitate while examining; I got the signs because I'd been to so many practice sessions and had seen everything except retinal artery branch occlusion before. Also I had always practised presenting the cases in a loud, clear voice on the grounds that if I was wrong, I might as well sound good and that if I was right I would come across as being confident in my diagnostic ability. (Pass)

'Nothing else was said and they didn't introduce themselves'.
29 The examiner's opening remarks for the short cases were: 'Your initials are SM, Oh no its N, N for nothing'. He then said: 'We'll start you off with "9" as "9" is a lady's mark'. Nothing else was said and they didn't introduce themselves. The first patient was a young woman with a long laparotomy scar which was pointed out to me and a distended abdomen. I was asked to examine the abdomen and to suggest an explanation. She had a *palpable liver*. I suggested it was a staging laparotomy but in fact it

was a splenectomy scar. They wanted to know the reason so I suggested haemolytic anaemia.

I was then asked to examine the cerebellum in a man who was unable to sit up. He had nystagmus, pass pointing, dysdiadokokinesis and internuclear ophthalmoplegia. They wanted a cause so I gave *multiple sclerosis*. They wanted to know what one would look for in the lower limbs so I suggested a pendular knee jerk after they had discarded my original suggestion of looking at the gait.

The next patient was a young woman with a *palpable thyroid* and a nodule at the isthmus (however, it was also diffusely enlarged according to the examiner). She was clinically euthyroid with exophthalmos. However, when I examined her I thought she had a staring appearance without exophthalmos. The examiner wanted to know the histology of Graves' disease.

I was then asked to examine a man who was short of breath and to look particularly at the cardiovascular system. He had a collapsing pulse, was in sinus rhythm, had a carotid pulsation, a displaced heaving apex beat with an early diastolic murmur and an ejection systolic murmur at the aortic area radiating to the carotids. So I suggested *mixed aortic valve disease* with mainly incompetence. They didn't say anything and moved straight to the next case.

The last patient was a man and I was asked to examine the abdomen. He had *hepatosplenomegaly* and they asked me how big the spleen was. I said it was eight finger breadths so they made me go back and measure it. I made it 15 cm but they made it 8 cm! (Pass)

'For some perverse reason, my mouth said pseudobulbar palsy'.
30 The first case was a young lady with *multiple sclerosis*. I had to examine her legs, gait and fundi. They interrupted me continuously and wanted firm, quick decisions and some common sense. The case was easy and went well.

They then gave me a little case history. 'This gentleman was admitted as an emergency with newly diagnosed diabetes mellitus. Would you feel his abdomen'. I was given all of 30 seconds to feel his abdomen and they wanted to know what I would put my money on as the cause of the firm *mass in the epigastrium*. I don't think they really cared if it was correct but just that I had logically reached a reasonable differential.

We then went on to the next patient. The examiner said: 'This is a quick one. Just look at this fundus'. In retrospect, he had *senile macular degeneration* but I did not get it at the time. The chap was very restless indeed thus making examination tricky so I just described what I had seen but said that I couldn't make a diagnosis.

I was then shown a gentleman with an *axillary vein thrombosis*. This was easy as he had a heparin pump. The examiners laughed about this when I came straight out with the diagnosis. They then wanted a few investigations that I'd do and this was really quite straightforward.

The next case was a disaster! They gave me a short history of the man's symptoms. He had classical *bulbar palsy* because of the nasal regurgitation and dysphagia, etc. However, for some perverse reason, my mouth said pseudobulbar palsy though I did immediately correct myself. I then got mixed up over which way the uvula deviates with a unilateral palsy. The examiner then corrected me and I just kept smiling!

The last case was my redemption. We only had a few minutes left so I was asked to 'quickly auscultate'. She had *mixed aortic and mitral valve disease* which I diagnosed almost immediately. They slowed me down and asked me to explain which murmurs I had heard. I am sure that I had got them right looking back on it. I actually overheard the examiners discuss me as I walked away (I've got very acute hearing!). They were agreeing that my general performance was OK and excusing the pseudobulbar disaster as nerves! (Pass)

Some 'fail' experiences

Examiners rarely let the candidate know whether their diagnosis is right or wrong or whether their clinical examination technique is professional. In the same way that candidates may perceive they have performed poorly and yet pass as illustrated above, candidates may also think that they have performed well and yet fail. Such candidates may feel that the exam is unfair without being aware of the imperfections in the performance they gave, or that some of their diagnoses were wrong. In the following accounts, some of the candidates recognized that they were failing but some did not.

'If she had Huntington's at that age, would she be doing the crossword puzzle in the newspaper?'

31 The first patient that I was taken to see was an elderly woman. The examiner said: 'This woman came to the thyroid clinic, what would you write in the notes after examining her eyes?' I tried to test visual acuity but was told to examine the eye movements. I thought she had a left VIth cranial nerve palsy but the examiner seemed unhappy with this. I then said that she had a thyroid ophthalmoplegia. He asked whether it bothered me that the *proptosis* was in the other eye? I wasn't sure!

The next patient was a sitting case. It was a middle-aged woman with *eruptive xanthomata* over the elbows and knees.

We then moved on to the next case. This was an elderly woman who was constantly fidgeting with either choreiform or athetoid type movements. I was asked to have a few words with her. She sounded a bit dysarthric. I was asked for the diagnosis and I wanted to say Huntington's chorea but did not wish to say so in front of the patient. So I tried to say a hereditary chorea. The examiner said: 'Like what?' So I said: 'Huntington's'. He said if she had Huntington's at that age, would she be doing the crossword puzzle in the newspaper? I said: 'No'. I hadn't actually noticed that she was doing this beforehand. He asked me for another diagnosis. I hesitated but got *drug-induced dyskinesia* out eventually.

The female examiner then took over. She showed me a man with very *deformed arthritic hands*. I pushed up his sleeves and showed the *psoriatic plaques* on the forearms and elbows. The disease looked burnt out so when she asked me what I would treat this man with, I said non-steroidals. She looked irritated and said: 'What else?' I suggested coal tar or dithranol for the skin. She was still not satisfied and walked off to the next case.

'Examine the cardiovascular system'. I examined the patient in silence and she then asked for my findings. Initially I just said *mitral incompetence*. So she then said: 'as manifest by . . .?' I then gave her my findings. The other examiner asked me if the pulse was in atrial fibrillation and I said it wasn't.

The next patient was a respiratory system. I thought the percussion was a bit dull at the left base and said that there was a small left pleural effusion. They made me examine the *trachea* again. I still did not think it was *displaced*. She then told me to percuss out the chest again. By this time the bell had gone. They did not seem at all pleased about this last case. The Senior Registrar who led me away said: 'Don't worry about the chest — it's a tricky one'. He also said there was nothing to worry about before the long cases as they were all straightforward. However, my long case was a diagnostic nightmare! Throughout the short cases both examiners were rather distant and cold. (Fail)

'If I were examining the examiner, he would have failed!'

32 The examiner asked me to look at a woman's neck. She was sitting in a chair and she had obvious *proptosis and a goitre*. I went straight to the neck and told the examiner that she had a visible goitre. He seemed irritated by this, but I thought he was just trying to put me off my stride, so I continued with what I thought was a faultless presentation. The same rotten examiner, who was young and abrasive, then asked me to examine a woman's cerebellum. I asked for her address and he shouted: 'What are you doing?' 'Examining her speech, Sir', I replied. 'But we have quotes for that', he retorted. Again I thought he was just seeing if I would crack up. So I replied: 'Yes Sir, but I can hardly walk up to the lady and say, "Hello Mrs J., I am Dr S. and can you say hippopotamus?"'! I moved on to finger–nose testing which demonstrated *gross ataxia*. I looked for nystagmus which I couldn't find but was asked about vertical nystagmus. I also demonstrated dysdiadochokinesis. He asked me to examine her legs so I began with: 'May I see the lady walk?' He gave me a curt reply: 'She can't walk'. I then tested power, tone, heel–shin test, and he stopped me again abruptly. 'This lady has had some injections years ago, what other system do you want to examine?' I confessed that I had no idea as I thought that I was looking at a cerebellar problem. He then said: 'Posterior columns'. I still don't know what the connection was but it went as so: firstly, I examined joint position sense — I thought I would get some extra marks here as I had demonstrated the technique to the patient and she complied well. Then I did vibration sense — I examined sternal sensation first and then the sensation peripherally. 'What else?', he said. I retorted: 'Two-point discrimination, Sir'. 'Yes, yes, what else?' He was obviously irritated and I said I didn't know what he meant. So he said: 'Deep pain', and then he grabbed the woman's heels. If I were examining the examiner, he would have

failed! However, I still felt he was trying to rile me so I continued still believing I was doing well.

The next two cases were a *mixed mitral valve disease* and *psoriatic arthropathy* and I had no problems with either of these.

The final case was then a patient with *hepatosplenomegaly* and nodes, which was possibly chronic lymphatic leukaemia and again I had no problems here.

Overall I felt that I had coped with the examination and I went home feeling fairly confident that I had passed. However, I failed. I wrote to the college and they told me that I had failed on my neurology case. I talked to a local examiner and when I told him what had happened he said that the examiner must be new and that it all sounded very unfair. I still feel that he was unfair and now having passed the exam on the fifth attempt without doing anywhere near as good as on this attempt I will still say that the whole exam is very unfair.* (Fail)

'I was asked about the severity of the lesion (aortic incompetence), how long it had been present and whether an operation was indicated. I was totally unprepared for this'.

33 I was initially taken to a young, well-looking patient and I was asked to listen to the heart. He had a systolic murmur at the apex, normal heart sounds and no click. I volunteered a *mitral valve prolapse*. The examiner asked about the heart sounds which I said were normal. I think I was right on this case.

I was then asked to look at a patient's fundus having been told that he was completely blind. I found a *cataract* and *retinitis pigmentosa*. I stood up and the examiner asked if I had a diagnosis. I told him my findings and he asked about *optic atrophy*—I hadn't even looked! I said the discs were normal but they can't have been.

The next case was: 'Please examine this man's chest from the front'. There was a slightly red patch on the right side of his chest. I watched him take a deep breath and was stopped and asked for my findings. All I had found was the red area which I suggested might be due to radiotherapy for a bronchial neoplasm. I then found that the trachea was deviated to the left. Also the left hemithorax expanded poorly and the percussion note was impaired. I was then stopped and asked for the diagnosis. For some reason I said neoplasia. I am sure he had *old*

*For our comments on this, see Introduction, p. xiv.

tuberculosis at the left apex, and the mark on the right was incidental.

I was then taken to the next patient and told that this patient's GP had referred him to my clinic because he had a heart murmur and wondered about mitral incompetence. I found signs of lone *aortic incompetence* and thought that the diagnosis alone would satisfy the examiners. The signs were so straightforward that 99% of candidates would get them right. I was asked about the severity of the lesion and how long it had been present and whether an operation was indicated. I was totally unprepared for this and answered badly.

I was told that my next patient had been referred to me with anaemia and that I should examine her abdomen to find out why. The examiners 'tutted' as I looked at her hands, mouth, neck glands, etc., and impatiently hurried me on. She had *hepatosplenomegaly* and although I was exceedingly gentle and explained what I was doing she winced repeatedly. I appealed to the examiners — should I carry on?—but they remained impassive! I gave a list of different lymphoproliferative disorders to the examiners as I had found numerous *lymph nodes in her axillae*.

I was taken to my last patient and was instructed to ask her some questions. I asked her for her name and she replied with a *cerebellar dysarthria*. I was asked for one other sign that I would like to look for and I proceeded to demonstrate that she had finger–nose ataxia. I volunteered cerebellar disease and suggested demyelination as the cause. One examiner grunted and the other wandered off! (Fail)

'The last patient had polycystic kidneys which I called hepatosplenomegaly. This was probably the final nail in the coffin'.
34 For my first patient I was asked to look in the eyes. I found *optic atrophy*. It was the first time I had ever seen it and I nearly said so! However, I had failed to notice the white stick and the aphakic spectacles. I was then asked to look at a lady's face. I found *Horner's syndrome* and again it was the first I had ever seen. I just managed to give a few causes.

For my third patient I was asked to examine a chest. I had no idea what the matter was with it so I re-examined the front. There was dullness to percussion with reduced expansion and *coarse crepitations at the right upper zone*. I suggested fibrosis, tuberculosis or asbestosis. However, the patient also

had an *ataxia*. I was hampered by the examiners asking for my findings at 10-second intervals!

I was then taken to a patient and asked to: 'Listen here' (they pointed to the left sternal edge, fifth intercostal space). There was *mixed aortic valve disease* and I had been asked to auscultate only. There were no problems here and I was not asked for any causes or investigations or treatment.

The last patient had *polycystic kidneys* which I called hepatosplenomegaly. This was probably the final nail in the coffin. (Fail)

'I felt it was tapping and said so. This was a big error as it wasn't'.
35 'This man has been referred by his GP because of a heart murmur. Examine his cardiovascular system and say what you think'. I was allowed to make a full examination and diagnosed *aortic stenosis*. They didn't seem happy and asked: 'Did you hear any other murmurs?' I hadn't and said so.

For the second patient I was given the same history. I was only allowed to feel the pulse briefly before being told that it was normal and being asked to feel the *apex beat*. This was abnormal and slightly *displaced*. I felt it was tapping and said so. This was a big error as it wasn't. On auscultation I had to amend my diagnosis. There followed a discussion about the different types of apex beat and I was able to answer all their questions well but I knew I had done badly on the first two cases.

I was then asked to look at a man's hands. He had classical *dermatomyositis* and I described it as such. However, I had to be prompted to test for muscle power which was much reduced.

For the next patient I was asked to examine the abdomen. It was a young man with *massive splenomegaly* and no other abnormalities. I was asked for a possible diagnosis so I said that it was possibly a myeloproliferative or lymphoproliferative disorder. They told me that it wasn't and asked for other diagnoses. I started to say: 'In a tropical country . . .' but was stopped. The examiner suggested that hepatic disease might cause such splenomegaly. I answered that it would be unusual to cause such massive splenomegaly and they agreed. I subsequently found out that the diagnosis was *sarcoid*.

I was then asked to examine a patient's fundi. The first retina showed scarring that did not look typically like laser burns. I gave a differential diagnosis of diabetes with laser treatment or choroidoretinitis.

They asked me to look in the other eye but not to take so long about it this time. The second retina showed similar scarring but also small haemorrhages giving the diagnosis of a *diabetic retinopathy*. I was asked what I thought of my differential diagnosis of choroidoretinitis and answered that I thought it had been a mistake!

The last patient was a complicated one with heart failure, a high JVP and a pleural effusion. I now know the diagnosis was of *constrictive pericarditis* (from my college tutor). I cocked this short case up badly and knew that I had failed the short cases outright. (Fail)

'They asked for a diagnosis. I tentatively said SBE (I later found out it was hereditary haemorrhagic telangiectasia)'.

36 *Short case 1*: Probable *diabetic fundus*. The patient had very thick glasses on and the examiners asked me to take them off. The ophthalmoscope was one I had not come across before and I could not focus it. I was too nervous to remember I had brought one with me in my handbag! (Incidentally, I would advise all females not to take a handbag—they are just a nuisance.) I saw a few exudates and haemorrhages but was very unsure. This was a very bad start.

Short case 2: I was asked to examine a young man's chest. In retrospect I found that it was *ankylosing spondylitis*. However, I managed to convince myself that he had unilateral signs consistent with an effusion and so I presented them. The examiners just said: 'Ummmm . . .', and moved me on!

Short case 3: I was asked to examine a man's cardiovascular system. He had atrial fibrillation, *prosthetic heart valve noises* and also I thought a systolic murmur. However, I was very unsure what it all was. They said: 'So you don't think there is a diastolic murmur?' I said: 'No', and we moved on (in retrospect I found out that he had *aortic valve disease!*).

Short case 4: I was asked to examine a man's abdomen. They did not let me look at hands, etc. He had *hepatomegaly*. However, I could not palpate a spleen although I did not turn him over or bimanually palpate. In retrospect he was deathly pale and presumably had a myelo- or lymphoproliferative disorder. They then showed me what I thought was senile purpura — they dragged out of me that he might be on steroids and asked the mechanism for the discoloration. I talked about capillary fragility but he said: 'No, no, it's all to do with macrophages', in a tone of voice that made me feel really stupid for not knowing.

Short case 5: I was asked to examine a poorly lady with *ascites* and *deep jaundice*. I was asked just to assess what I thought was the most important thing from a practical point of view. So I looked for a *liver flap*. They asked about other causes for a flap.

Short case 6: I was shown a lady with cyanosis, clubbing and multiple petechiae and splinter haemorrhages (I thought!). They asked for a diagnosis. I tentatively said SBE and they then gave me another chance but I could not come up with anything so we moved on. I later found out it was *hereditary haemorrhagic telangiectasia*.

Short case 7: I was shown a young woman with a burn on her hand and an amputated finger. I suggested a sensory problem but they then gave me a clue by telling me that she was unable to move her hand away from trauma in time. I then asked her to grip my hand and she had obvious *myotonia*.

Short case 8: Young boy with a *Horner's syndrome*. I was asked what question I would like to ask him and I asked if he had had any neck surgery.

Short case 9: Elderly lady with *osteoarthritis*.

Short case 10: Elderly lady with *CREST syndrome*. (Fail)

'My first patient looked as if she was of Mediterranean origin. I thought she had polycystic kidneys'.

37 My first patient looked as if she was of Mediterranean origin. I thought she had *polycystic kidneys*. The examiners asked me why it wasn't a large spleen and had I thought of thalassaemia as she looked Greek. I was a little uncertain after this but said to the examiners I felt I could get above the masses. Most of the other candidates that I spoke to afterwards thought this was polycystic disease but the registrar on duty would not comment.

The second patient had a corrected *Fallot's tetralogy* and was a young fit man. There was a mid-systolic murmur loudest all along the left sternal edge. Initially I said it was aortic stenosis despite the fact that there was an easily visible sternotomy scar. I was asked if it was usual to have a stenotic murmur after a cardiac operation and the penny eventually dropped!

The third patient had *diabetic retinopathy*. It was a simple background retinopathy and the pupils had been dilated for me.

The fourth patient had *rheumatoid hands*. I was just asked to describe the findings and not to examine. I began saying that she had a symmetrical deforming polyarthropathy and was then dragged off to the next patient who had pulmonary fibrosis. I was asked to list the possible causes and what was the most likely cause in this patient. I said idiopathic *fibrosing alveolitis*. It was a well, middle-aged female with no other problems. 'What one question would you ask?' I suggested asking what her occupation was and they said that would be more appropriate if the patient was male. 'Anything else?', they said. I asked her if she kept any animals and they led me away.

The next patient had a *spastic paraparesis*. I was asked to examine the legs and the examiners were very pleased when I asked to see the patient walk first but I then got myself into a discussion about the various types of gait. 'Would you like to do anything else?', they asked. 'I would like to examine the fundi and the spine', I replied. 'Good', they said. They asked me what the most likely cause was, so I said: 'Demyelinating disease'. The examiner asked me what I meant by that so I said: 'Multiple sclerosis'. The other examiner who was just approaching us at that moment said: 'Never say that, say demyelinating disease!'

Once again the short cases were late. The examiners seemed very fed-up and cross right from the start. I was questioned *en route* between patients whilst I was trying to keep up with them. At one point the examiner in the front turned abruptly to look at the examiner coming up behind me and said: 'What did she say?' The examiner behind me (who was really fed-up) said: 'How should I know'. I said: 'Shall I start again?' and they both roared: 'No time!' (Fail)

'During auscultation one examiner pulled me from the patient by the back of my suit!'
38 'This patient is breathless, find out why as quickly as possible'. I did not spot the *flattening of the apex on the right* and was asked to look again. I thought that the trachea was central, even on re-examination, but then said that I would not argue with the chest X-ray! The examiner seemed displeased.

The next case was: 'Examine the patient cardiovascularly'. There was fast atrial fibrillation at a rate of approximately 120 beats min^{-1} together with *mitral facies and a thoracotomy scar*. There was also a median sternotomy scar. The JVP was difficult to see and I was told to move on. During auscultation one examiner pulled me from the patient by the back of my suit! I described the findings and said that I didn't know what the underlying diagnosis was. I was told to give a diagnosis: 'Come on—three, two, one, going, going, gone!'

The next patient had a large spleen with no lymphadenopathy or hepatomegaly. The diagnosis, I thought, was *myelofibrosis*. The examiner wanted a list of the other possible diagnoses which I gave them. When we got to the fourth patient the examiner said: 'Examine this patient's eyes'. We were in a darkened room so I asked whether just to look at the fundi. They said: 'Look at everything'. I asked for the lights to be turned up in order to check acuity, fields, pupils and movements. There was no abnormality found. However, the patient had classic *optic atrophy* in the left eye on fundoscopy. I was asked for a differential diagnosis and the possible significance of the field defect. (Apparently he had a *bitemporal hemianopia* and a *pituitary tumour*.)

For the last patient I was again asked to examine the cardiovascular system. There was a collapsing pulse. I was stopped and asked what the diagnosis was. I said this could be *aortic regurgitation* and listed the findings that I would expect. I finished examining the patient and confirmed the findings of aortic incompetence. We then discussed the Austin Flint murmur.

The examiners were quite rude. Their initial response to my attempts to introduce myself to the patient was: 'Now you've made us miss the best cases!' Even if my examination technique was not good enough to pass the exam I do not expect to be grabbed by the back of the suit. The examiners should not use their unfair advantage to behave in a way which would be completely unacceptable in public! (Fail)

Four months later I re-sat the exam. My first short case was: 'Examine this man's abdomen'. I said I would like to move the bed in order to examine him from the correct side. Their response was: 'Extra marks for moving the bed in a Part II!' When the bed came apart in their hands and I had re-assembled it and then moved it, the examiner said: 'Extra marks for knowing how the bed works!' The findings were eventually of *hepatosplenomegaly* and a small amount of *ascites*. There were no stigmata of chronic liver disease or lymphadenopathy. I said that the possible diagnoses were . . .

When we arrived at the second patient the examiner said: 'Examine this patient's hair'. She had a full head of hair and eyebrows but little on her forearms and none in her axillae. I was then allowed to ask if she had ever had hair here, and she said: 'Yes'. She looked mildly cushingoid and the skin was fine and thin. I thought the diagnosis was of *panhypopituitarism* in a patient who had been given steroid replacement. I said: 'The possible causes are . . . and would you like me to check the visual fields?'

The third patient had *proliferative retinopathy* and *maculopathy*.

For the next patient the examiners said: 'This man is breathless. Would you examine him?' He looked as though he had *ankylosing spondylitis* so I asked him to look up and he couldn't! I said this was likely to be the diagnosis and described the possible associated features of upper lobe fibrosis and kyphosis with a restrictive deficit. The examiner then asked me to examine his eyes. I found *proptosis* with no lid lag or exophthalmos. He was clinically euthyroid with no goitre and I said the most likely diagnosis was of dysthyroid eye disease. The examiner asked if there was any connection and I said: 'No'.

I was then asked to listen to a patient's heart. I felt the apex and the carotid pulse which I then used to time the murmur at the same time as assessing its character. I found *mitral stenosis* and also the patient was in sinus rhythm. I said that the patient had mitral stenosis because of the loud first heart sound and the middiastolic murmur with a presystolic accentuation. There was no evidence of pulmonary hypertension.

I was then taken to a patient with a *skin rash*. I described it and said it didn't have the characteristics of psoriasis, eczema or lichen planus, etc. I said I really didn't know what it was. The examiners said they didn't either and were going to biopsy it!

The last patient had an asymmetrical oligoarthropathy in the small joints of the hands. The examiners seemed to like the quick routine I had been shown which assessed function of all joints, grip and power, pincer and opposition, and fine finger movements. She was a West Indian girl with patchy pigmentation on the face. I said the dif-ferential diagnosis of oligoarthropathy included *SLE* which turned out to be the actual diagnosis.

On this occasion the examiners were very pleasant and no one grabbed me by the back of my suit! (Pass)

Downward spirals

'I completely collapsed when one of my short case examiners introduced herself as Dr X'.

39 I had heard the previous day from a colleague who had also been examined at Newham General that he had encountered a woman examiner who had given him a really difficult time. My anxiety about this was increased when someone else reported: 'I hope it isn't Dr X, she fails everyone!' followed by a few other stories. I completely collapsed when one of my short case examiners introduced herself as Dr X.

Short case 1: cardiology — a young West Indian woman and the examiner said: 'Examine the CVS'. I thought she had mixed *mitral and aortic valve disease*. There was absolutely no feedback from the examiners as to whether this was right or wrong.

Short case 2: neurology — a young Asian man. 'Examine these legs'. There was a *spastic paraparesis* and a *peripheral neuropathy*. I got heavily criticized for attempting to demonstrate cerebellar signs in someone who was obviously very weak but I attempted to defend this. I then became very flustered when asked to list the causes of this combination of signs. I handled this all very badly and even when pushed on the issue of the man's ethnicity and what I should be considering (presumably tuberculosis causing a cord compression) I remained pretty inarticulate. From here on there was a complete loss of confidence and everything was badly handled.

Short case 3: abdomen — an old, wasted, ill-looking lady. 'Examine the abdomen'. I found a *hepatic mass* and *1 cm splenomegaly*. There was no ascites. I described the findings as above. The examiner started pushing me on the causes of the mass (which was attached to, but discrete from, the liver). I felt uncomfortable as he had not moved away from the patient's bed and to my horror I ended up saying what I had kept avoiding saying, i.e. the word 'tumour' in front of the patient. I knew this was a disaster.

Short case 4: chest — a middle-aged, obese man. 'Examine the respiratory system'. I found *clubbing* as well as very traumatized nails (multiple peripheral splinters). There was poor chest wall movement bilaterally with inspiratory and expiratory crepitations. I suggested *fibrotic lung disease* with an intercurrent infective exacerbation. There was no feedback at all from the examiners. (Fail)

'The examiner was aware I was bluffing and asked for more and more detail'.

40 I was first taken to a gentleman and asked to examine his abdomen. I grabbed for his hand after introducing myself but was told firmly, though politely, to stick to the abdomen. I found a *small spleen* and at this point the examiner stopped me and asked for my findings. He then asked me to ask the patient three questions to elucidate a cause. I asked about alcohol abuse and travel abroad (in particular malaria) and then I was stumped so I asked a daft question about rheumatoid arthritis (thinking of Felty's syndrome). This was daft because I had already had a look at the gentleman's hands! It annoyed the examiner because it was at the bottom of his differential diagnosis!

I was then led on to a fully dressed lady and asked to listen to her aortic area and to decide whether she had aortic incompetence. They didn't like it when I tried to take her sweat shirt off to examine her properly. They expected me to examine her around her clothing. I wasn't sure whether I could hear an aortic incompetent murmur since I had never been convinced by one in the past! So I did a daft thing again and said I thought there was one. He then asked me what other features I would look for on general examination. We went through all of these and of course she didn't have any of them. At this point he asked me to look at her generally and it was then that I noticed her malar flush and peripheral oedema. He suggested these were more in keeping with mitral valve disease and asked me to listen for this. I heard a *mitral incompetent murmur*. I was very uptight over my errors from the last case and annoyed because I felt I had been deliberately misled.

I was then taken to the one case I particularly dread, *diplopia*, and was asked to examine the visual movements. I totally went to pieces and did this very badly. I was unable to establish what the lesion was even after the examiner tried to help. He seemed particularly interested in the *nystagmus* and the direction in which it was maximal. I wondered if I had missed ataxic nystagmus and the diplopia of multiple sclerosis.

I was then taken to a lady and asked to examine her fundi. She had definite *diabetic retinopathy* and after stepping back ready to say this, the examiner said to me that there were no prizes for the diagnosis. It was obviously diabetic retinopathy but could I describe in detail what I saw and where each feature was! I should probably have admitted defeat but instead I strung together what I had seen and made up the position of these relative to the disc. The examiner was aware I was bluffing and asked for more and more detail.

He then took me to a lady and announced that she had had atrial fibrillation and asked me to suggest a cause. I noticed a *thyroidectomy scar* and so offered thyrotoxicosis. I was asked to examine for this and found her clinically euthyroid but with *exophthalmos*. Presumably she had had thyrotoxicosis treated in the past. He then asked for another cause so I suggested mitral valve disease and then noticed a midsternal scar. He asked me to listen to her mitral valve which I did literally. At this point I got a sarcastic comment: 'Can you pretend this is the Membership and examine the heart properly?' Exasperated by now I retorted that he had asked me to *listen* to the mitral valve and he did concede this. I proceeded to listen to the precordium and heard a *prosthetic valve* but was unable to remember how to distinguish between mitral and aortic prostheses. Again I bluffed and probably got it wrong. With very little comment I was dismissed.

I was thrown in this attempt by the fact that although the cases were relatively straightforward, either the questions or the approach to each case was not. There seemed to be the deliberate attempt to confuse and lead me astray. I found it useful the second time round to think about the different ways a short case could be presented other than the straightforward, 'Examine this cardiovascular system'. I also learnt by experience that it is helpful to have some 'questions' ready relating to lists of common causes of, for example, splenomegaly. This paid off in my second attempt (see first person experience 6, p. 470) when I was shown a IIIrd nerve palsy and asked to ask some questions. (Fail)

'I forgot to assess her speech and only knew one way to demonstrate dysdiadochokinesis'.

41 I was taken to the first patient and the examiner said: 'Examine this lady's cardiovascular system'. After I presented my findings of lone *mitral* *incompetence* he said: 'Did you hear mitral stenosis?' My reply was: 'No'. He said: 'Did you hear aortic valve disease?' Again my reply was: 'No'.

We went on to the next patient. The examiner said: 'Examine this lady's *cerebellar signs* from the waist up'. This was the start of the downward spiral syndrome. I forgot to assess her speech and only knew one way to demonstrate dysdiadochokinesis. The examiner was *not* impressed.

For the third case he said: 'Look at this lady's hands'. She had *rheumatoid arthritis* and I even remembered to look for, and noticed, the cushingoid facies. However, the follow-up question was a 'killer'. 'Outline your surgical options here'. I was stuffed!

The fourth case was: 'Look at this *fundus*'. I couldn't see a bloody thing. She was middle-aged and therefore I went for diabetic retinopathy. I still don't know whether I was right or not.

The examiner led me on. 'Look at this lady's hands'. She had *hereditary haemorrhagic telangiectasia*. We talked about inheritance, presentation and management. At last I'd had a decent case!

The final patient was: 'Examine this man's abdomen'. He had massive *splenomegaly and lymphadenopathy*. All my examiner wanted to know was what I knew about *Waldenström's macroglobulinaemia*! (Fail)

'The examiners were very upset and so was I'.
42 I was asked to examine a lady's chest and I hurt her during the examination. The examiners were very upset and so was I. The whole exam went downhill from there onwards. This particular patient, however, had a *right lower lobe fibrosis* from tuberculosis.

The examiners then said to me: 'What does that man have?' They were pointing to a gentleman who was disappearing through a door at the time. I correctly replied *ankylosing spondylitis*.

I was then taken to another gentleman and asked if he needed treatment. He had a definite *parkinsonian tremor* with rigidity and a little bradykinesia but was walking very well. I said 'not at the moment' and explained why.

I was then asked to comment on another patient's rash. It was a fading *erythema nodosum* on the legs of a girl of 20 years. They asked the commonest cause in this age group. I said Crohn's and ulcerative colitis and the examiners replied: 'Good'.

I was then taken on to the next patient and asked to examine his eyes. I really cocked this up! I asked to test his visual acuity and he had not brought his reading glasses with him. I then missed a *central scotoma* and *optic atrophy*!

The next patient was an 'examine this lady's abdomen'. She had a 2 cm liver and a 4 cm spleen. They uncovered her chest and asked the diagnosis. She had multiple spider naevi so I suggested *chronic liver disease*. At last the examiners seemed happy!

I was taken on to the next patient. 'Your house officer thinks this man has had a CVA, do you agree?' I thought he had had a *cerebrovascular accident* affecting the left side but they weren't happy that the right side was normal. I did not look for fasciculation and I wondered if he actually had motor neurone disease.

The last patient was a spot diagnosis and I was asked to just look. It was a girl who was covered from her shoulders downwards. She had a positive Corrigan's sign and I said that she probably had *aortic regurgitation*. They asked if she needed surgery so I said: 'Yes', after feeling a collapsing pulse. (Fail)

Anecdotes

1 A candidate was told: 'This gentleman presented with headaches seven years ago. Examine his abdomen'. The candidate tried to start with the hands but the examiners stopped him and made him concentrate on the abdomen. He found polycystic kidneys, reported this and was then asked to ask the patient a further relevant question. The candidate asked the patient about his urinary symptoms (he had become anuric seven years previously) and questions relating to possible subarachnoid haemorrhage in the past. The examiner then showed him the AV fistula on his arm and explained that this was why he stopped him looking at the patient's hands before examining the patient's abdomen! (Pass)

2 A candidate was asked: 'Examine the back of this man's chest'. He found a left thoracotomy scar in a man in his thirties. Even though the examiners were standing in front of it, trying to stop him seeing it, he managed to spot the sputum pot and diagnosed bronchiectasis. (Pass)

3 While examining the fundi, the candidate pressed the wrong button on the new type of ophthalmoscope that he had been given and the batteries fell out! The examiners handed him an older ophthalmoscope with which he was more familiar and he went on to diagnose proliferative diabetic retinopathy with a lot of fibrosis. (Fail)

4 A candidate was taken to a patient with gross acromegaly. The examiners were laughing as they approached and said 'pre second MB stuff, eh?' The candidate said: 'Yes, "examine this man's hands"?' The examiners replied: 'No, what do you observe about him?' They had to drag out of the candidate the fact that the patient was 6ft 7inches tall. The candidate described that this may mean that the growth hormone had been high since pre-puberty and the candidate then turned to the patient and asked: 'How tall are your brothers and sisters?' The examiners were apparently delighted with this. The candidate then reports: 'They then asked me "What is the meaning of acromegaly?" and I replied "akros, an extremity like acropolis — the extremity of the town". The examiners then said "Very good, how did you know that?" I replied, "classical Greek at school Sir!" (Pass the sick bag.) The examiners were beaming'. (Pass)

5 A candidate was asked to examine the abdomen. She started with the hands but was told: 'No, just the abdomen'. There was a 15 cm spleen palpable with an obvious notch and liver just palpable on deep inspiration. After presenting her findings, she was asked why she had auscultated. She said that listening to bowel sounds was part of her normal examination of the abdomen. They asked if it was relevant to the patient in question and she answered: 'No'. They then asked that if she had auscultated over the spleen what she might have heard. She was then asked about the significance of a splenic rub! The likely diagnosis was discussed though it is not clear whether or not the patient actually had a splenic rub. (Pass)

6 After being asked to examine the heart, a candidate found a mid-diastolic murmur and diagnosed mitral stenosis. The examiners asked for the cause and he said rheumatic heart disease. They asked for another cause and he said atrial myxoma. The examiners said: 'Good', and then let him go. (Pass)

7 A candidate was asked to feel a patient's abdomen. He found a mass in the left hypochondrium which felt like a polycystic kidney but was dull to percussion, moved medially with respiration and was not ballottable. The examiners asked him what he thought it was. The candidate said that he was unsure and expressed his dilemma based on the signs he had found. The examiners said: 'If you could ask one question, what would it be? The candidate said: 'Does anyone in your family have kidney disease?' The patient answered: 'Yes'. The candidate asked the patient: 'Is it polycystic kidneys?' The patient answered: 'Yes'. The candidate turned to the examiners and said: 'I am sorry, I asked two questions'. The examiners laughed and at that moment the bell went. (Pass)

8 A candidate was told: 'Examine this young lady's abdomen'. She found a 20–30-year-old female with obvious abdominal distension who otherwise looked well. There was slight hirsutes, no lymphadenopathy, no mouth signs and a mass arising from the pelvis. There was no spleen on palpation or percussion and no palpable liver or kidneys. The examiners asked: 'What do you think this is?' The candidate summarized the findings and said she thought that the patient might be pregnant. 'Do you think we would include a pregnant woman in the MRCP exam?', asked the examiners. 'You might', the candidate replied. One of the examiners said: 'Yes we might, its an unfair exam!' 'Would you like to re-examine her to see if there is a spleen?' The candidate demonstrated again that there was not. The candidate reports that she was led away feeling unsure of what she had missed. She later rang the organizing registrar who said that the diagnosis was not known but that she had a pelvic mass and an enlarged spleen on ultrasound. (Pass)

9 A candidate was unsettled by his rather mediocre performance in the first two short cases. The examiner then asked him to examine a patient's hands and knees. He found hypoplastic nails and absent patellae but admitted that he had no idea what the diagnosis was (nail–patella syndrome). (Fail)

10 After having seen a West Indian lady who had a wig and a Bell's palsy, a candidate got the Bell's palsy and was then asked to look at her head. She had severe scarring alopecia and he was asked to give some possible causes. He suggested trauma and autoimmune disease but was not really sure what the correct diagnosis was. When he got home his mother told him that she believes she would have got that one right—it follows attempts to straighten the hair! (Pass)

11 A candidate was asked to examine the chest of a patient 'from the front only'. She found all the findings compatible with a left upper zone fibrosis/collapse and suggested that this could be due to previous tuberculosis. She was then allowed to inspect the patient's back which revealed a thoracoplasty scar. The candidate was told that she was correct. (Pass)

12 A candidate was asked to examine a chest from the back only. He noticed a left lower thoracotomy scar but failed to mention it or to piece the whole situation together. He told us the examiners took the opportunity to hang him, draw him and then quarter him. (Fail)

13 A candidate was asked to examine a woman's legs and found erythema ab igne. The examiners then asked for the differential diagnosis of reticular rashes on the legs and for the different skin biopsy appearances! (Pass)

14 A candidate was shown a patient and asked to look at the skin over her knees. It was a young girl who said: 'I am double-jointed, doctor'. The candidate found 'cigarette paper' scars over both knees and diagnosed Ehlers–Danlos syndrome. There then followed a discussion about heredity and complications. He was then shown his next short case and was told that this patient had had a car accident 3 weeks ago. He found a healing, abnormal scar over the left shin and he again diagnosed Ehlers–Danlos syndrome. The examiners asked if he would be surprised to learn that the patients were related — the candidate answered: 'No'. (Pass)

15 A candidate was asked to examine a patient's cardiovascular system. He found several murmurs and suggested patent ductus arteriosus but he is still not sure whether that was correct. He commented that the examiners were irritated because he felt the pulse first. They seemed to want him to go straight to the precordium, though they had asked for a 'cardiovascular system' examination. (Pass)

16 While giving her findings of a case of aortic regurgitation a candidate mentioned Corrigan's pulse. The examiner asked: 'Who was Corrigan?' She felt the examiners did not seem to be too serious when asking this! They then went on to ask her the causes of aortic regurgitation and they thought that she should have mentioned degenerative valve disease higher up on her list. (Pass)

17 A candidate was asked to examine a patient's eyes and then the neck. He found unilateral proptosis and a goitre and diagnosed thyrotoxicosis. He reported that he did not notice the proptosis until he looked from above. (Pass)

18 A candidate was asked to examine a lady's left fundus as she had deteriorating vision in the left eye. He started to examine the right eye and the examiner said: 'Actually, I have told you that the problem is in her left eye!' The diagnosis was a branch retinal artery occlusion. (Fail)

19 After seeing a patient with motor neurone disease a candidate was asked to examine an abdomen. He found a palpable left kidney which he suspected to be either polycystic or hydronephrotic. There was also a mass in the right iliac fossa which he thought was probably a transplanted kidney. (Pass)

20 After an opening case of rheumatoid hands, a candidate was asked to look at the hands of another patient. He found purple, swollen fingers with no arthritis, nail involvement or evidence of scleroderma but he noted some telangiectasis on his face and lips. He was told that he could ask the patient some questions to determine the cause. He said he thought the patient had Raynaud's disease but wondered retrospectively if this may have been a case of CRST syndrome. He reported: 'The examiners wanted the causes of Raynaud's phenomenon and for me to look for evidence of diseases such as scleroderma, SLE, etc. They wanted me to ask the patient if he worked with vibrating tools and what happened to his hands if he put them into cold water'. (Pass)

21 'Look at this man's abdomen and describe what you see'. The candidate found a distended abdomen in a middle-aged man with tattoos, an everted

umbilicus, reduced body hair and purpura. 'What else would you look for?' He said: 'Jaundice, spider naevi, Dupuytren's contractures and leuconychia'. He was then told to look for these signs which were all present. Then he was asked to examine his abdomen. This revealed marked ascites and a tender, two finger breadth liver but no splenomegaly. As they were walking away they asked him the likely cause of his signs and he answered, 'alcohol-related liver disease'. The examiners asked him why he thought this and he replied that he was wearing a T-shirt advertising Foster's beer! They smiled. (Pass)

22 A candidate was asked to look at a patient's legs and found erythema nodosum. He was asked to discuss the histology of this condition which he did not know. He was then shown an ECG of another patient which showed a supraventricular tachycardia with a 2:1 block. (Pass)

23 A candidate who had made reasonable progress through his first five short cases, was briefly shown a patient with parkinsonian facies who had a parenteral nutrition infusion in progress. He was asked to comment on the type of line used for feeding and to describe the procedure.* (Pass)

24 A candidate was asked to examine a patient's abdomen. He found hepatosplenomegaly. The examiners then showed him the arteriovenous shunt and asked him to re-examine the abdomen. His diagnosis then became polycystic kidneys! He was sure he had failed outright but tried to keep his head, remembering that it was possible to get by with one disaster! (Pass)

25 A candidate was asked to examine the abdomen of a woman with jaundice and hepatosplenomegaly. The examiners got annoyed when he started with examining her hands. (Pass)

26 A candidate reported that his examiners started 5 min late and he was not given any extra time. He had to undress three of the patients and get them positioned correctly. He also found explaining his findings as he went along difficult especially as one of the examiners appeared very deaf. (Pass)

*We presume the patient had Steele–Richardson syndrome.

27 A candidate was asked to examine the respiratory system of a patient with chronic bronchitis and emphysema. He was asked if there was loss of cardiac dullness. He examined for this and found that there was. (Pass)

28 A candidate was asked: 'Look at this rash in a 16-year-old girl'. There was a maculopapular rash on the limbs but not on the trunk. There was no involvement of the eyes, nails, joints or mouth. He was asked what the diagnosis was and if he would like to ask the patient some questions. The condition had been present for 5 years and the joints were painful. He offered the differential diagnosis of juvenile chronic arthritis or SLE. In retrospect he feels it was the former (Still's disease). (Pass)

29 Until a candidate reached his fifth short case his only blemish was that he took a minute in counting the respiratory rate of a patient with dyspnoea and clubbing. He was asked to examine the abdomen of a woman who weighed 'about 20 stone'. He found two subcostal masses and diagnosed hepatosplenomegaly. In retrospect he was sure that they were polycystic kidneys and that arguing the case for hepatosplenomegaly made matters worse and wasted a lot of time. (Fail)

30 A candidate reported that he lost 5 min because the examiners had been deliberating on the previous candidate's long case for longer than usual. He entered the short cases while the others were starting on their third patient! The examiner said: 'This gentleman is icteric, please examine his abdomen'. He found hepatomegaly and a mid-line laparotomy scar. He presented these findings. 'Does he have ascites?' He told the examiner that his findings were equivocal and that an ultra-sound was needed to define this. 'Does he have splenomegaly?' He replied that he couldn't feel a spleen but there was a dullness to percussion over the splenic area. He was counselled after he had failed the exam. Apparently the liver that he had felt was a palpable gallbladder. The examiner's comments were: 'He refused to commit himself as to the presence of ascites and hedged on the presence of splenomegaly'. (Fail)

31 A candidate was asked to examine a patient's left eye with the ophthalmoscope provided. He reported

that he found optic atrophy, a detached retina, laser photocoagulation scars and aphakia. He suggested that the patient had had a diabetic cataract previously. The examiner asked about primary and secondary optic atrophy and then asked about the refractive error of the patient—covering the head of the ophthalmoscope with his hand as he did so! (Pass)

32 A candidate was asked to look in a patient's eye. He could find no abnormality and said so. He was then informed that he had looked into the left eye, whereas he had actually been asked to look into the right eye! The examiners were both laughing although he was embarrassed and very apologetic. The right eye showed obvious optic atrophy and he was then asked for a differential diagnosis of this. (Pass)

33 A candidate was asked to examine a patient who had a right pleural effusion — the patient was very deaf and every time he asked him to say '99' he took a deep breath instead! (Pass)

34 A candidate was told: 'Examine this rash but don't rub it'. He found a brownish macular rash on a young, healthy-looking woman. He had no idea what the diagnosis was. In retrospect he thinks it must have been mastocytosis. (Fail)

35 A candidate was told that a patient had a chronic cough. On examination he found right upper lobe consolidation and offered a differential diagnosis of tumour or tuberculosis. He was then shown the patient's chest X-ray which showed a cavity with a crescentic upper border and he diagnosed a mycetoma. (Pass)

36 A candidate was asked to examine a heart and found isolated aortic incompetence. Two cases later he was asked to examine the heart in a different patient and was surprised to again find isolated aortic incompetence. (Pass)

37 In his second attempt a candidate was asked to listen to a heart. He heard a mid-diastolic murmur and came up with the diagnosis of mitral stenosis. The examiner asked him to auscultate again; on doing this he could also hear an early diastolic murmur. (Fail)

38 'Ask this lady some questions and find out what the problem is' was the instruction addressed to a candidate. He found a rather garrulous lady with senile dementia. He did not ask her questions very well and the examiner stepped in to help. The diagnosis was discussed and the examiner apparently agreed that it was difficult. Afterwards the candidate was told by the organizing registrar that they had had difficulty finding good cases — otherwise this dementia case would probably not have been included in the examination. (Pass)

39 A candidate was asked to examine the pulse of a patient and found a right brachial artery aneurysm. He reports that the examiner expected him to find the right radial pulse reduced in volume compared to the left but that he could not confirm this. The possible causes he offered were traumatic, iatrogenic or mycotic and in retrospect feels that it was most likely to have been a mycotic aneurysm due to subacute bacterial endocarditis many years before. (Pass)

40 A candidate was asked to look at a man's face. He found herpes zoster in the left ear and in the distribution of the mandibular division of the trigeminal nerve. He also reported a left facial nerve paralysis and wasting of the left side of the tongue with deviation of the protruded tongue to the left. He diagnosed Ramsay Hunt syndrome plus herpes affecting the Vth and XIIth cranial nerves. He was asked if such extensive involvement was possible and answered: 'It appears so'. (Pass)

41 A candidate was asked to examine the fundus of a patient. He found that the lens had been removed because of a cataract. It was very difficult to see the fundus so he guessed the diagnosis of diabetic retinopathy which he still believes was correct. (Pass)

42 After being asked to examine the heart on his first short case, a candidate reported mitral stenosis with an opening snap. The examiners asked him to point out the second left intercostal space. 'That's too high' said one examiner—'It's here!' 'No it's not, it's here' said the second. 'Well it's a silly landmark anyway' said the first. 'I agree' said the second, 'Let's move on!' (Pass)

43 A candidate was asked to examine a man's abdomen. The patient had several signs of chronic liver disease and ascites. After much deliberation, the candidate said he could not feel the liver though he expected it to be there. He was criticized for his technique of examining the spleen (which the candidate says had been taught to him by an experienced examiner) and he was told the cyanosis was not a sign of liver disease. This all proves that examiners are only human. (Pass)

44 A candidate was brought to an old lady with an obvious left hemiparesis and catheter *in situ*. He offered the diagnosis and said why and was then asked to examine the legs neurologically. He found this very difficult as she was demented and would not cooperate. However, he managed to demonstrate some findings in keeping with the left hemiparesis. They were about to lead him to the next case when he commented on the marked tibial bowing (sabre tibia) and volunteered a differential diagnosis. The examiners looked pleased and said: '10 marks off the organizing registrar and 10 marks to candidate'. He felt that by making his comments on the tibia he may have made the difference with regard to passing and failing. (Pass)

45 A candidate was asked to examine the abdomen of a woman. He had to help her get undressed and the examiners appeared to be getting annoyed. She started examining peripherally looking at the hands and checking for nodes but was told just to go to the abdomen. However, by this time she had already noticed the generalized lymphadenopathy. In the abdomen there was easily palpable splenomegaly. Unfortunately, she performed less well on other short cases on this attempt. (Fail)

Some anecdotes in the first person

46 I was asked to: 'Look at this man's hands'. He had clubbing and the examiner asked me the causes. I looked at his feet but could not see any clubbing there. However, I noted abnormalities in the left tibia and diagnosed osteomyelitis. The patient nodded encouragingly but the examiner looked really cross! (Pass)

47 'This man is diabetic and he has a peripheral neuropathy. Do you see anything in his fundi which would make you want to refer him to an eye specialist?' The patient had no background retinopathy. There was one very small vessel near the right disc which could have been a new vessel but was unlikely. He said: 'Do you think that's likely with no background retinopathy?' I said: 'No'. He looked pleased and said: 'Good. So what is the cause of his peripheral neuropathy . . .' (Silence) '. . . in Scotland?' 'Oh', I said: 'alcohol', to which the examiner again said: 'Good'. I was then taken to the next patient and asked if I would like to examine his peripheral pulses. Both femorals were present but there was nothing palpable below that, i.e. there were no popliteal dorsalis pedis or posterior tibial pulses. The examiner then said: 'What other pulses in the leg would you like to look for?' I still don't know the answer! (Pass)

48 'This man has some strange feelings in his feet and legs, would you examine them?' The patient was totally bald and was wearing some sort of corset around his waist. He had a peripheral neuropathy but I had expected to find a dermatome pattern because of the corset. I really got into a mess! The examiner told me that the corset was for an incisional hernia following a splenectomy. I suggested he had pernicious anaemia as a cause for the splenomegaly and neuropathy, then possibly that he had diabetes in association with the alopecia. I eventually worked out that he had had vincristine for leukaemia! The examiners were very good-natured throughout all of this. (Fail)

49 'Please examine this abdomen'. I did so and found definite splenomegaly. 'What is the diagnosis?' the examiner said. I replied that he most likely had CML but the examiner blew a fuse and said that he had just wanted me to say that he had a 'large spleen'! (Fail)

50 The short cases went very well. The examiners were extremely pleasant and they even carried my ophthalmoscope box for me! I felt confident and very much in command. However, for my fifth short case I was asked to examine a chest. I could find no physical signs at all and I said so. The examiner said: 'That's very honest'. I was devastated. Whilst walking away the other examiner whispered to me: 'Never mind, we couldn't hear anything either when we listened this morning!' In fact it was an upper

lobe collapse that had resolved. (I passed the short cases but failed the exam.)

51 The next patient was a 60-year-old male and I was asked to examine his abdomen. I found polycystic kidneys and liver and I demonstrated the scars of the dialysis fistula. The examiners laughed when I went on to test for a spleen as they said that to find a patient with polycystic kidneys, liver and spleen, was an examiner's dream! (Pass)

52 I was asked to examine the legs, neurologically, of a 50-year-old man. The examiners just said that he had a burning sensation in his feet but does not drink. The patient then said that he did drink until he had got diabetes! We all laughed and they then said: 'Show us how you would have proceeded anyway!' (Pass)

53 The neurological case that I was asked to examine would not initially come out from under the bed clothes! I think that most people would have panicked but given appropriate coaxing the patient was eased into a suitable position! (Pass)

54 On entering the hall for the exam I encountered an old chap who I thought was the exam hall caretaker from the hospital. I said to him: 'I'm fairly nervous. Is there a toilet nearby?' So he laughed and pointed through the examination hall and said: 'Do not listen!' He later took me for the short cases! But the greatest piece of luck was that I felt he liked me. He asked me to examine a woman's legs neurologically. He said that she had become very weak but was now getting better. The unfortunate lady was totally deaf and I was almost shouting to make her hear my examination requests. At each point during the examination I was stopped and asked what I had thought, and what I would do next. The sensory testing was an absolute nightmare. She seemed to have a fairly global weakness with absent reflexes and a patchy sensory loss. I thought the diagnosis was probably Guillain–Barré syndrome. The examiner agreed and then held my arm and said that he appreciated that it was very difficult! (Pass)

55 I definitely did *not* think that I had passed the short cases. I thought I had got it all wrong. I stuttered and stammered throughout and all the correct answers were dragged out of me painfully. They asked me to explain everything I did throughout the exam. This was something no one had ever asked me to do before in teaching sessions. (Pass)

56 I was asked to look at a man's chest. 'What do you see?' said the examiner. There was bilateral gynaecomastia. He said: 'If you were in the clinic what would you want to examine next?' 'The liver', I said. 'Go on then'. I struggled to demonstrate a normal-sized liver. 'What would you examine next?' he said. 'His testes', I answered. 'Go on then'. He had bilateral flaccid testes the size of peas. 'What's the diagnosis?' said the examiner. There then followed a nasty discussion about testosterone replacement and its relation to hair, skin texture and gonadal size. I suspect that I was making a pig's ear somewhere along the line! (Pass)

57 I was asked to examine a patient's abdomen. I started at the hands but was told to go straight to the abdomen. There was a renal transplant in the left groin and a left radial fistula with tenderness in the left loin, and I thought there was a palpable kidney. I did not palpate too firmly because it was painful and they did not mind this. The patient was also cushingoid. I felt the diagnosis was a left renal transplant with a ?polycystic kidney and that he was cushingoid due to the steroids. At this stage the patient put his thumbs up! We then went on to the next patient and I was asked to examine her cranial nerves. It was an old lady with a complete right ptosis and her eye was looking down and out. Before I had completed the examination of the IIIrd, IVth and VIth cranial nerves she started to vomit. Therefore we left her! However, we continued to discuss the causes of a IIIrd nerve palsy. I said that diabetes was the commonest cause and they said multiple sclerosis was. We then went through the entire list! They asked for investigations and I offered a blood glucose and a CT scan. (Pass)

58 'This man has been short of breath recently, could you examine his chest to find out why?' The expansion seemed reduced on the right side but the breath sounds were reduced at the left base. I could not recover from this conflicting information and completed my examination not having a clue what I was going to say. I couldn't go back over the findings as they were rushing me. I stood up and confidently gave the signs for a left pleural effusion. They said: 'Some people, when they say "left" really mean "right", are you sure this is left'? I realized I had got the wrong side but I couldn't retract what I had said so I repeated that I had carefully examined the patient and felt the signs were on the left. Then the bell went. I obviously got my last short case completely wrong but it would appear that you can get away with a gross error if you appear confident throughout the rest of the exam. Whenever they tell you to speed up—slow down. (Pass)

59 Examiner: 'Feel this woman's pulse and tell me what you find'.
Answer: 'There is atrial fibrillation'.
Examiner: 'and . . . this is the Membership, not finals'.
Answer: 'The pulse is of good volume and possibly collapsing in character'.
Examiner: 'and?'
Answer: [Long silence — you could hear a penny drop!] 'I did not count the rate'.
Examiner: 'No you didn't but what is it approximately?'
Answer: '80 beats per minute'.
Examiner: 'Now continue to examine the precordium and tell us what you find'.
Answer: 'There are no thrills, nor a palpable heart sound. The apex beat is displaced to the anterior axillary line and there is a loud pansystolic murmur of mitral regurgitation. There are no clinical signs to suggest mitral stenosis but this could be silent so I would arrange for an echocardiogram'. (Pass)

60 The short case exam was held in an ordinary ward which was receiving at the time! It was chaos! For my final short case the examiner said: 'Quickly listen to this heart'. I was not given any history. However, at this stage the tea lady appeared with empty cups for the entire ward and announced the choice of beverages beside my patient's bed. All I could hear was the deafening rattle of cups. My advice is to shoot the tea lady! (Pass)

61 The examiner handed me an ophthalmoscope. 'This patient is having trouble with her vision. Would you examine her eyes?' I commented on the cataract and then described hard exudates, both blot and flame haemorrhages, AV nipping and microaneurysms. I said that the features were consistent

with both diabetes mellitus and hypertension. This did not please one of the examiners who said that hypertensive retinopathy should have more superficial flame haemorrhages. I stood my ground and said that she did in fact have quite numerous flame haemorrhages, but otherwise the appearances suggested diabetes. He finally asked me what her refractive index was. When my answer was rather quick at +4 dioptres, he tried to trip me up by saying that I had not included my own refractive error. However, I was able to point out that I had contact lenses and so I was perfectly corrected! (Pass)

62 I was asked to examine a man having been told that he had weak hands. On inspection he had wasted small muscles bilaterally in a distal rather than a proximal distribution. There was no Horner's or fasciculation of the tongue and there was no sensory loss. The feet were also involved. There was a discussion then about findings that looked like a pure motor neuropathy. It could have been Charcot–Marie–Tooth but I opted for porphyria as this was Professor Goldberg's unit in Glasgow! The examiners smiled for the one and only time—either in absolute amusement at the ridiculous answer, or because I was correct! (Pass)

63 My last case would have been an easy cardiovascular system case except for the patient's stomach which must have been the loudest rumbling stomach in history — audible at 100 paces! I think she had atrial fibrillation, mixed mitral valve disease and aortic regurgitation. It would have been OK if I could have heard the blessed murmurs without the orchestrations from her gut! (Pass)

64 My very first patient was a lady with Graves' eye disease with a VIth cranial nerve palsy. I found trying to examine her pupils and eye movements rather difficult because she was silhouetted against the back drop of a bay window — perhaps I should have turned her round. (Pass)

65 I lost the membrane off my stethoscope during case 2. It was a patient with a pleural effusion. I was very puzzled finding a completely quiet chest — something which I had never seen beforehand. I suspected a pleural effusion from the percussion and vocal resonance. However, I discovered the faulty stethoscope at the very end of the examination. The

examiners wanted to hear first what I thought, but did eventually agree to a second listening! (Pass)

66 'What's the diagnosis?' I was given no history. However, the diagnosis was obvious as there was evidence of psoriatic plaques together with arthropathy and nail changes. I was asked what was atypical about the patient and so I mentioned that the plaques did not have any scales. The examiner asked why and I suggested that it had been treated. The examiner then said something to me in Latin and asked what it meant. I didn't have a clue. The examiners both laughed but said nothing except that the exam was now over! (Pass)

67 I was asked to examine a patient's fundi. They were very abnormal but goodness knows what the diagnosis was! I said hypertensive retinopathy because no laser burns were present, and I couldn't imagine someone having such terrible diabetic retinopathy without having had photocoagulation! (Pass)

68 After my first three cases the dove took over. I was taken to a man and told that he recently had a problem with his eyesight but that things were now improving. 'Would you like to examine his fundi?' I hadn't a clue what was going on. He seemed to have a mixture of disc swelling and atrophy but I said that I was very unsure about the degree of swelling. The examiner said that if he told me that the disc definitely swollen what would be my differential diagnosis. At this point the head of my ophthalmoscope fell off! I said that partially treated benign intracranial hypertension or a tumour treated with radiotherapy would both give this appearance. As we walked to the next patient the head of my ophthalmoscope fell off again. I said how awful it must be for them to take candidates like me around! (Pass)

Useful tips*

1 Practise, again and again, on short case material and when you think you've done enough—do more!

2 Practise being harassed. Get some 'mock' examiners to put you under stress. Nervousness gets no credit: the examiner is more likely to think that in a real emergency you would not rise to the challenge (though see experience 68, p. 457).

*From candidates in our surveys.

3 In every spare moment practise talking short case *records* (not just reading them) and talking lists (not just writing them). Get the order of lists right—give the common and uncontroversial ones first. Avoid controversial causes.

4 Practise presenting cases as much as examining them. If you can present clearly and quickly it is as impressive as examining well.

5 You have got to really practise doing short cases with senior registrars, consultants, friends — even the dog! You've got to be able to examine without thinking and to then come up with sensible diagnoses from your clinical findings.

6 Dress smartly and conservatively.

7 Take to the examination a stethoscope, a pen torch, red-headed hat pin (dip a white-headed one in red paint if necessary), a tape measure, some cotton wool and some orange sticks.

8 Be polite to the patient and the examiners; say 'Please' and 'Thank you'. The occasional use of 'Sir' will not do any harm (but do not overdo it—see experience 94, p. 459!).

9 Do not repeat the examiner's questions.

10 Do not hurt the patient, especially during the abdominal examination. Look at the patient's face during deep palpation.

11 Make sure that during the examination of the patient you let the examiner see that you are doing the correct things—as one does in a driving test.

12 Do not be put off by any of the examiner's mannerisms.

13 Think *whilst* you are examining. Extend the end of the examination by a few seconds, if necessary, to give you time to put the findings together, and to prepare what you are going to say to the examiner.

14 Don't panic if you find very little in a patient. It is better to miss something subtle than to make up something that isn't there.

15 Practise having to comment on your findings as you examine a patient.

16 Do not let your tie or hair dangle in the patient's face. When you have finished be sure to leave the patient adequately covered up (but do not overdo it—see experience 94, p. 459, again!).

17 Present cases to the examiner as if you are speaking to an equal about an easy case.

18 Be confident—but not over-confident. A supercilious attitude is fatal.

19 Look at the examiner rather than at the patient or the floor when answering, and speak clearly and fluently (do not mumble).

20 Take time to think before opening your mouth.

21 Keep cool even when interrupted and have a systematic examination technique to fall back on if you cannot make a spot diagnosis from the start.

22 Be aware that the stress of the examination can cause you to 'blurt out' things you do not really mean (see experiences 2, 52 and 74–79, pp. 448, 454 and 457–8). Keep calm and think before you speak.

23 Remember common things are common. Beware of thinking that because it's MRCP it's likely to be rare. Study the frequencies we have provided and start at the top of the list not the bottom.

24 Do not talk while the examiner is talking and be wary of arguing with him. If you make a mistake be prepared to say: 'I withdraw that', rather than try to defend it. Remind yourself that the examiner is the judge and the jury!

25 Do not try to pull the wool over the examiner's eyes. He is eminent and intelligent or he would not be an examiner, and he will resent it if you treat him as a fool.

26 Do not guess or waffle. Cut your losses and admit if you do not know.

27 Avoid strange mannerisms of speech and action including using your hands excessively when speaking. Avoid 'ers' in your speech as much as possible.

28 Do not be casual. Say 'myocardial infarction' rather than 'heart attack' or 'MI'; stand properly without leaning on the bed or putting your hands in your pockets.

29 Avoid using drug trade names—always use the proper pharmacological name.

30 Do not mention dubious or 'slight' physical signs (e.g. starting your presentation on a case of mitral stenosis with: 'The pulse is slightly collapsing').

31 At the end say: 'Thank you', in a sincere manner.

32 Be careful in your choice of hotel for the night before the exam. A candidate recalls: 'For my first attempt at the written, I booked a random hotel and ended up with a room in a cheap hotel overlooking a road which was busy all night, with burglar alarms going off. The walls were thin and the television and other loud noises of the neighbour could be heard going on throughout most of the night. For subsequent exam visits, I was very careful with my choice of hotel and always rang up to plead for a room in a corner, well away from any roads or other sources of noise, explaining to the hotelier that I had an exam to do. I believe this important strategy is essential'.

33 I had an appalling night's sleep before the exam. Book a hotel where your friends have been before and which they can recommend.

Facts and figures

These facts and figures are from the *original first edition survey*. However, we have not seen anything in our surveys since the first edition to suggest that there has been any significant change since then.

1 It is often said that the more short cases you see the better. For what it is worth, the average number of 'main focus' short cases seen in our survey on a *Pass* attempt was 6.1 (range 4–10) *Fail* attempt was 5.5 (range 3–8).

It is possible that part of this difference was due to some candidates in the survey forgetting some of their fail attempt short cases because of the time lapse between the exam sitting and filling in the questionnaire.

2 It is often said that if you are going to pass MRCP Part II, you are much more likely to do so on your first attempt. In our survey the percentage of successful candidates by number of attempts was:

65% passed on their first attempt

16% passed on their second attempt

12% passed on their third attempt

5% passed on their fourth attempt

0.5% passed on their fifth attempt

0.5% passed on their sixth attempt.

These figures have to be interpreted with caution because (i) the participants in the survey were self-selected (e.g. candidates who endured the exam several times may have been less inclined to recall unpleasant experiences and fill in a larger number of questionnaires), and (ii) we have no information on the numbers who fail and never sit again at each attempt (e.g. we do not know whether the 5% who passed on their fourth attempt were the vast majority or the tiny minority of those sitting the examination for the fourth time).

3 According to our survey, as you enter the examination room on any one attempt at the short case, you have an:

86% chance of meeting *mitral* and/or *aortic* valve disease

86% chance of meeting either palpable *kidney*(s) or *liver* and/or *spleen*

80% chance of meeting one of the following six conditions which you may be able to spot at once:

exophthalmos

chronic liver disease

Paget's disease

systemic sclerosis

hemiparesis

acromegaly

74% chance of meeting one of:

diabetic retinopathy

optic atrophy

hypertensive retinopathy

retinitis pigmentosa

papilloedema

choroidoretinitis

68% chance of meeting one of:

rheumatoid hands

wasting of the small muscles of the hand

systemic sclerosis

psoriasis/psoriatic arthropathy

ulnar nerve palsy

57% chance of meeting one of:

pleural effusion

fibrosing alveolitis

old tuberculosis

carcinoma of the lung

chronic bronchitis and emphysema

bronchiectasis

33% chance of meeting thyroid disease.

4 Candidates are not often asked to look at investigations such as X-rays during the short cases, as such skills are tested in the written section of the examination. Nevertheless 6% of candidates in our survey were shown an X-ray or ECG. This broke down approximately into:

Chest X-ray 4.5% (pleural effusion, bilateral hilar lymphadenopathy, hilar shadow, pulmonary hypertension, mycetoma)

X-ray of legs 0.5% (Paget's)

CT scan 0.5% (occipital infarct)

ECG 0.5% (SVT with 2:1 block).

Quotations*
Adopt good bedside manners

1 The examination is the same as the final MB but with no help or encouragement from the examiners. Your approach to the patient is *very* important.

2 Don't panic; don't let them hassle you; be kind to the patient.

3 Always introduce yourself by name to the patient and explain what you are going to do (in lay terms!). Position the patient correctly and check whether the part is painful. Do not be afraid to ask the examiner if you can examine a 'remote' part if you consider this necessary (he can always say no).

4 For women I would like to suggest that you wear something comfortable which will accommodate your stethoscope, and leave your handbag in a cloak-room. There is enough stress without worrying if your buttons are undone!

5 Remember to suggest moving away from the

* From candidates in our survey.

patient when having to use words like 'tumour' or 'multiple sclerosis'.

6 Play the game. Introduce yourself to the patients and explain what you are going to do. Always expose the patient fully and stand back and look at them before starting. They also say that you fail the exam if you hurt the patient. However, I grabbed somebody by the hand — it was obviously sore and the patient shouted out. I apologized profusely and got away with it.

7 The short cases went well. However, the lack of feedback was very difficult to cope with. The examiners, though, seemed happy with my simple but confident answers. I think I appeared caring and was polite to the patients. I smiled a lot at the examiners and tried to be relaxed yet professional. It all seemed to work!

Practise clinical examination and presentation

8 Don't try the MRCP too soon. See as much as possible—'cushy' jobs are not helpful in the end.

9 My theoretical knowledge was good enough but I lacked short-case practice (failed attempt).

10 Senior colleagues and consultants had prepared me for the psychological torture I was about to endure!

11 Go to as many clinical courses for Membership as possible. Work out the best method for the examination of each system and practise it until it is second nature to you. Be as direct and positive in your answers as possible (even if they are wrong!)

12 I know I passed the written and the viva but I failed badly on the short cases. Don't take the examination unless you can properly prepare for it. I was very anxious and was not thinking while I was examining. I kept imagining that the cases were supposed to be difficult, rare or complex.

13 Talk through as many short cases as possible before the examination with someone who has been through it recently, or with someone who is used to teaching, and preferably do this on a one-to-one basis.

14 Practising the technique of examination is essential so that it becomes second nature under stress. Persuade colleagues to grill you mercilessly on cases and differential diagnoses. Certain 'favourite' topics seem to recur so make sure you know these. Also don't make any statements unless you can back them up.

15 The most important point is to look professional — as if you have done it quickly and thoroughly a hundred times before. You do not need to know much. Take your own equipment as you know how it works and you don't have to ask for it and wait.

16 Before the examination I spent 6 weeks getting registrars to take me on short cases and then questioning me under examination conditions. Be meticulous about examination technique and don't be fooled by the apparent relaxed nature of the examiners — examine everything properly. Don't listen to tutors about one mistake making a failed exam.

17 Get together with someone else doing the exam and practise until you are bored with reciting the appropriate litany. I only just practised enough and wished I had started 2 months earlier. It is the only way, especially if you can get someone senior (and preferably nasty!) to put you through it!

18 The more practice at presenting short cases the better.

19 I had a lot of practice presenting short cases to a 'hawk' of a senior registrar. This experience was invaluable.

20 Adopt a systematic approach to the examination of all the major systems and have the features of the common clinical states at your finger tips, e.g. upper and lower motor neurone lesions, the auscultatory findings of various valvular lesions, etc. A well integrated, comprehensive system is needed for presenting the findings to examiners. Do not rush the presentation thereby omitting important points.

21 It's important to have a method for examining each system. I don't think the examiners necessarily want you to make a diagnosis but just to describe the signs.

22 Be very professional in your presentation. I agree it's an easy exam—it's easy to fail!

23 The Resuscitation Annie came completely out of the blue—be prepared.

24 The short cases are so variable that it is impossible to prepare! Don't believe any of this rubbish about: 'It's just like being in clinic'. It is oppressive and unpleasant.

Get it right
25 Do not rush a case—they were very keen to stop me once they considered that I had enough information to make a diagnosis.

26 If you are unsure of the diagnosis then describe the findings and give a differential diagnosis.

27 Do not be afraid to allow a few seconds of silence to pass before answering a question whilst you collect and organize your thoughts.

28 Know the diagnosis before you leave the patient and state it confidently. Be prepared for further questions on the physical signs and the management of the disease.

29 When examining fundi don't stop until you have finished and have thought of what to say.

30 Don't pass comments that cannot be substantiated. Everything will be challenged if you are on the borderline.

31 The examiners already had in their mind what answers they would accept and they kept on until they got the actual wording they wanted.

32 Try not to be obtuse in the short cases or to pick on unimportant details, as the examiners may then draw you into a frustrating and often irrelevant discussion as to what you mean or sidetrack you from the main issue.

33 If you know the diagnosis (i.e. scleroderma), there seems to be a ritual series of questions and answers (swallowing, etc.).

34 At the sherry reception, a friend was told that more than 50% of candidates had reported non-existent laser scars and non-existent proliferative retinopathy on the diabetic fundus patient and had failed at once on this patient alone.

35 I missed optic atrophy on my last short case. Moral: ask yourself a direct question—'Is there optic atrophy?'

36 In general, I found that getting the diagnosis right was not as important as I had been led to believe. Examining the patient with a systematic plan in mind and having a good differential diagnosis at each stage was much more important.

37 The examiners were very pleasant all the time and as I got more cases right I became more confident—and then I even started to enjoy myself. The examiners did not harass me but seemed concerned to let me get as much right as possible in 30 min—a stark contrast to my first attempt!

38 The short cases went really well. After the first short case they didn't ask any more aggressive questions. I think I had already satisfied them on the first case. Start well and look confident even if you don't know anything!

Listen, obey and do not stray
39 Just stick to what they ask, don't mess around. For example, don't start checking the temperature just because you hear a murmur. It seems to irritate them.

40 Do only what is asked of you. Give positive and concise answers to questions, unless a differential diagnosis is requested.

41 Always do a full examination of the system asked — show off your technique. Do not be put off by 'dead-pan' examiners. The result comes as a particular shock when you have been sitting exams for many years *without* failing them.

42 I think I passed (third attempt) because I could carry the examiner's instructions one step further, i.e. feeling the pulse of someone who has a dysphasia. Perhaps that is the secret!

43 Look at the patient as a whole and not just the system you are examining.

44 They may ask you just to listen to the heart so that you cannot get clues from the pulse and palpation.

45 I suspect that they liked the way I examined the first patient (a neurological case in which I extended the examination beyond the legs) and then decided that I was probably competent. From then on they seemed to be on my side. Most of the time I didn't get asked for a diagnosis, just for the signs, and they didn't then continue to corner me. All was surprisingly amiable!

46 Perform the examination and answer questions as requested. Try asking patients as much as possible; my examiners made *no* attempt to stop me. For example, I asked the patient in whom I had to look at the fundus, if he was a diabetic. I was left with the impression that the examination, although difficult, was fundamentally *fair*.

One wrong does not make one fail

47 Treat each short case individually and put your apparent disasters behind you.

48 Don't be put off by messing up one short case; keep trying! Be sure you understand whether a full system examination, or only part of an examination, is required. The examiners may appear irritable and unsympathetic—don't worry!

49 Don't be put off if you get a few things wrong. I made a lot of mistakes (that I know of!) and still passed.

50 Do not be distracted by mistakes made (or imagined) in preceding cases or by the examiners' mannerisms or approach.

51 The old adage is: 'Be generally observant'. Being very nervous does not necessarily fail you; one bad case should not put you off.

52 I was put off right from the beginning after they stopped me during the examination of the first case —a vague, non-specific instruction was given and I had not found enough to be sure of. I was on the downward slope from then on. I might have passed had I pulled myself together and put the experience of case 1 behind me.

53 At the time and until I received my result, I was convinced I had failed. I think the experience of my previous attempt helped considerably, because I consciously reminded myself to put each bit behind me after I had done it, and not to dwell on my mistakes.

54 Never, never, never give up. I made many mistakes and thought I'd had it but I still passed. You don't have to get it all (or even mostly) right if you can appear logical, caring and reasonably sensible. The examiners were *totally* non-commital and obviously trying to see how confident I was. I nearly failed myself!

If you say less they want more

55 After the first case there was a long silence as if they were waiting for me to say more — I went to pieces after this.

56 Be prepared for supplementary questions and for examiners who disagree or argue with your comments.

57 Be complete in your examination — examine everything even if it doesn't seem relevant. For example, all hearts need to be listened to for early diastolic and mid-diastolic murmurs even if you think you already have the diagnosis. Every possible aspect of eyes needs to be looked at if asked to examine the eyes, unless something in the instruction suggests otherwise.

58 I was shown a patient with a IIIrd cranial nerve palsy (and possibly a IVth) following transfrontal surgery. I was asked why the eye was down and out. I was a bit shaky on this—one takes it for granted that the pupil is dilated without asking why! I was getting really hot under the collar at this stage.

If you know it — say it

59 When you know the diagnosis—say it.

60 Offer a diagnosis if you are reasonably confident of it — this way you can save time from having to discuss a differential diagnosis and you will get through more cases. Try not to let the examiners rush you from case to case, thus forcing you to take short cuts in your examination technique.

61 Have a system for examining. Think, don't rush and don't say more than you have to.

62 Mention all the things you notice especially if they are obvious — even if asked about something else.

Humility is more persuasive than self-righteousness
63 Be kind and confident but humble in the short cases.

64 Don't argue your case too strongly. Beware of polycystic kidneys in obese ladies! (anecdote 29, p. 496)

65 By far the major problem was keeping my head and holding my ground *politely* when we disagreed.

66 Learn good examination techniques for all systems. Do not argue with the examiners and be polite to the patients.

67 If you know you have made a glaring error retract the remark and start again — if you're right (or at least think you are) stick to your answer.

68 The MRCP short cases are not a test of your medical knowledge. Mine is not profound. It is simply a test of whether you are competent at your job. If you think that you are and can convince the examiners of that then you will pass.

Keep cool: agitation generates aggression
69 'Panic not'. This is greatly helped if you have practised a lot of short cases under stress and seen most things before.

70 A good start is a great help. It's like skating on thin ice — if you keep going and don't fall through, you make it.

71 The most off-putting aspect of each case is the lack of feedback from the examiners as to whether you are right or wrong. This is much more disconcerting than criticism.

72 Stay calm and talk sensibly even when the diagnosis appears unclear (easy to say — difficult to do!).

73 I only saw four cases and at the end of it I was sure I had failed as I did not have a clue what was wrong with patient 2 and did not do very well on patient 4 either. However, I was wrong in my pass/fail self-assessment. A factor in my pass mark must have been that I did not lose my nerve and remained calm, even after the mistakes. After all, it is as much an exam of your nerve as your knowledge.

74 I didn't feel confident enough to think I had passed, but I thought I had a reasonable chance. It is so important to start well, keep calm, score points when you can and treat each case independently. I didn't do that in my first attempt and failed as a result; I maintained my concentration (with a supreme effort of will!) in the second attempt and it paid off.

75 Relax — and enjoy what are predominantly easy but beautifully classical signs.

Simple explanations raise simple questions
76 Very simple, straightforward answers seem to prompt straightforward questions.

77 They appear to want simple basic signs and physical examination but I am sure they penalize heavily if obvious signs are missed. They seemed quite happy for me to ask the patient questions. It is also a great relief when the answers are what you want (also gives one time to think when the patient is answering).

78 The examiners seem to be impressed by short definitive answers and not with long lists of differential diagnoses. I think it is best to answer questions as directly as possible and get on to the next case.

79 Don't be clever — give simple answers to simple questions. The examination is unfortunately an extremely unfair lottery — there is no substitute for luck.

80 Always be honest—it pays in the end (experience 54, p. 455).

Think straight, look smart and speak convincingly

81 If the diagnosis is obvious focus down and elicit all relevant signs regardless of the generality of the instruction. If the diagnosis is not immediately obvious, examine the relevant parts systematically and hope for the best. Do not be put off by mistakes or be paranoid about your performance (I was, and suffered for it).

82 Beware of dual pathology. Don't wait for the examiners to tell you what to do, just go ahead and do it. Shake hands with the patient and introduce yourself; this gives you a chance to exclude finger clubbing, etc. and to see whether the patient is deaf or disorientated.

83 Be definite about the positive findings, i.e. do not hedge your answer with 'possibly', 'almost', 'perhaps'. If there is no obvious first-choice answer then give a sensible and relevant differential diagnosis.

84 I think I failed because of hesitancy; I gave no impression of confidence and blurted out statements without thinking.

85 You must be quick and comprehensive in your examination; it looks bad if you need to go back to do something which you forgot.

86 Don't change your mind half way through—as long as you are sure you are right.

87 The initial impression is important. If the first few cases go well then you get them on your side.

You have seen it all before

88 My cases were more straightforward than I had been led to expect. In fact nothing was particularly rare.

89 It is easy to be daunted by the feeling that there will be conditions you have never heard of and that the cases will be difficult and rare. In fact after my experience in these four attempts it seems that in most cases the same old conditions keep recurring

and they are mostly straightforward if you can only keep calm.

90 The cases are simple (the ones I saw were!). It is the candidate who makes them difficult and he may fail himself.

91 This was a much more enjoyable and interesting exam than Part I. With a single-minded approach to passing an exam rather than learning everything about medicine it is much more staightforward than people think. Remember that the majority of the consultant's knowledge outside their own field is unlikely to be much greater than your own (after revising!) particularly about details. As long as you can justify your answers it will be difficult to fault you. After all, what more is the exam for than to re-assure consultants that they can stay at home while you are looking after their patients!

92 When you come out of the exam you realize that after months and months of hard work and swatting the amount of knowledge you actually used could be written on a postage stamp!!

Use your eyes first and most

93 One of the short cases—pretibial myxoedema—was given away by the eyes. I think from talking to other people that there is often an obvious 'clue' in the short cases.

94 Spend at least 10–15 seconds just looking at the patient before even attempting an examination. Speak slowly and clearly and look the examiners in the eye.

95 Always look at the patient as well as the part in question. In one case (skin lesions in a black person) my first impulse was to suspect a tropical disease (?cutaneous leishmaniasis!) but the presence of exophthalmos gave me the diagnosis (pretibial myx-oedema). Don't be put off by examiners who are (as mine were) totally non-commital.

96 Do exactly what is asked but give yourself a second or two to look at the whole patient from the end of the bed.

97 Remember to look at the bedside for clues—in my case I missed the tablet containers which would

have suggested hypertensive retinopathy. When examining fundi, keep looking until you've covered all areas and try not to panic if you think you're taking too long.

Doing and forgetting

98 They then asked me to listen to her heart. I lost concentration and did not register the findings.

99 I examined the patient in an orderly sequence looking for the right things but for some reason, when I came to presenting the case, I couldn't recall my findings with regard to the stigmata of chronic liver disease. I couldn't even remember whether she was jaundiced!

100 The examiners were fair and did not try to unsettle me. I felt I fell down on presenting my findings and should have practised this more. In the heat of the moment, I went through the routine and then discovered I could not remember what I had found! I had also had a car crash driving up to the exam (it was a right–off) so that did not help to steady the nerves! Advice—don't drive!

Examiners are different

101 The examiners were very pleasant and wanted to see how confident I was when faced with a problem. They could have failed me on many things but appeared to be wanting to see how my mind worked. They like you to be slick, thorough, and to present your findings precisely without dithering. I am sure they assess you very quickly on the first two cases and decide whether they would like you to be in charge of their patients. Stay relaxed and be honest.

102 I felt that the examiners unnecessarily rushed me. Some patients were not undressed and not on their bed. This seemed to frustrate them as well as myself though I didn't let it show and I tried to take it all in my stride. I had very little indication from their expression as to whether I was saying or doing the right thing. I found the lack of feedback to be very disconcerting but I knew it was to be expected and therefore I didn't let it upset me.

103 Both of my examiners were very aggressive and sarcastic in their approach. Also the way they interrupted and corrected me made me feel completely incompetent and stupid after only a few minutes.

104 It was very unnerving not getting any feedback and on one or two occasions they said: 'I see', which always sounds very ominous!

105 Don't get flustered. If you say something silly retract it quickly and continue to talk. They are aggressive and try to hurry you. Don't let them! Look smart and be nice to the patients.

106 Try to be calm and imagine that you are seeing the cases in a clinic and carrying out a routine examination. The examiners made me very nervous especially with their comments which, in retrospect, I should have tried to ignore as they were only trying to test my knowledge and physiological comprehension of the physical signs I had elicited.

107 There was nothing difficult. The examiners were polite, unobtrusive, to the point and clear with their instructions. They were also amazingly expressionless throughout.

108 I wish the examiners were a little more friendly and did not interrupt every 10–15 seconds!

109 Don't be bullied by the examiners. There is no substitute for experience. You can pass even if you make a mess of one short case.

110 Don't let them rattle you. Never think you have failed until you get the letter.

111 Don't let the examiners rush you as you are then likely to make mistakes and this just surrenders all control to them. They can't fail you for a methodical examination.

112 The patients were all most helpful. However, I did not examine them thoroughly enough — I felt that the examiners wanted me to be quick and so I think I missed things that they had expected me to find and I failed the exam. The examiners were most polite throughout and did not hassle me at all.

113 I was shown a patient with von Recklinghausen's syndrome. It was obvious. I tried to enter into a discussion on the types and associations as per the recent *BMJ* leader. There were blank faces — they obviously had not read it!

114 In general, in the examination as a whole and especially in the short cases, it is hard to avoid an odd sense of dissociation (almost *jamais vu*). Everything has a somewhat dream-like quality and one feels unable to control one's actions. I am sure this is an important cause of underperforming but I don't quite know how to tackle it. My examiners seemed to encourage me and having got through seven and got them right, even while hardly demonstrating any signs at all, I felt very confident about that and the whole exam. I failed the exam on the viva but I may have been too confident in the short cases.

115 There were no interesting incidents in my particular exam except that I overheard another candidate say to his examiner that a patient with mitral stenosis had a gap between the second sound and the opening snap of 80 milliseconds exactly. The examiners went mad!

116 The examiners kept asking me if I was sure of my findings as though they were trying to put me off. I wish I was this good always!

Appendices

1 / Checklists

1 / Heart

1 *Visual survey*
  (a) breathlessness
  (b) *cyanosis*
  (c) pallor
  (d) *malar flush*
  (e) carotids
  (f) jugulars
  (g) *valvotomy scar*, mid-line scar
  (h) ankle oedema
  (i) clubbing; splinter haemorrhages.
2 Pulse (rate and rhythm).
3 Lift up the arm (?collapsing).
4 Radiofemoral delay.
5 Brachials and carotids (?slow rising).
6 Venous pressure.
7 Apex beat.
8 Tapping impulse.
9 Right ventricular lift.
10 Other pulsations, thrills, palpable sounds.
11 Auscultation (time heart sounds, etc.; turn patient onto left side; lean patient forwards).
12 Sacral oedema (?ankle oedema).
13 Lung bases.
14 Liver.
15 Blood pressure.

2 / Abdomen

1 *Visual survey* (pallor, jaundice, spider naevi, etc.).
2 Pigmentation.
3 Hands (Dupuytren's contracture, clubbing, leuconychia, palmar erythema, flapping tremor).
4 Eyes (anaemia, icterus, xanthelasma).
5 Mouth (cyanosis, etc.).
6 Cervical lymph nodes.
7 Gynaecomastia.
8 Spider naevi.
9 Scratch marks.
10 Body hair.
11 Look at the abdomen (pulsation, distention, swelling, distended abdominal veins).
12 Palpation (light palpation, internal organs, inguinal lymph nodes).
13 Percussion.
14 Shifting dullness.
15 Auscultation.
16 Genitalia.
17 Rectal.

3 / Fundi
Observe
1 *Visual survey* (medic-alert bracelet, etc.).
Ophthalmoscopy
2 Lens.
3 Vitreous.
4 Disc (optic atrophy, papillitis, papilloedema, myelinated nerve fibres, new vessels).
5 Arterioles and venules (AV nipping, silver wiring).
6 Each quadrant and macula (haemorrhages, microaneurysms, exudates, new vessels, photocoagulation scars, choroidoretinitis, retinitis pigmentosa, drusen).
7 Do not stop until you have finished and are ready.

4 / Hands
Observe
1 Face (*systemic sclerosis*, Cushing's, acromegaly, arcus senilis, icterus and spider naevi, exophthalmos).
2 Inspect the hands (rheumatoid, sclerodactyly, wasting, psoriasis, claw hand, clubbing).
3 The joints (swelling, deformity, Heberden's nodes).
4 The nails (pitting, onycholysis, clubbing, nailfold infarcts).
5 The skin (colour, consistency, lesions).
6 The muscles (wasting, fasciculation).
Palpate and test
7 Hands (Dupuytren's contracture, nodules, calcinosis, xanthomata, Heberden's nodes, tophi).
8 Sensation (light touch, pinprick, vibration, joint position).
9 Tone.
10 Power.
11 Pulses.
12 Elbows.

5 / Legs
Observe
1 *Visual survey* (*Paget's disease*, hemiparesis, exophthalmos, nystagmus, thyroid acropachy, rheumatoid hands, nicotine-stained fingers, wasted hands, muscle fasciculation).
2 Obvious lesion (see group 1 diagnoses).
3 Bowing of the tibia.
4 Pes cavus.
5 One leg smaller than the other.
6 Muscle bulk.
7 Fasciculation.
Test
8 Tone.
9 Power
  (a) lift your leg up (L1, 2)
  (b) bend your knee (L5, S1, 2)
  (c) straighten your leg (L3, 4)
  (d) bend your foot down (S1)
  (e) cock up your foot (L4, 5).
10 Coordination (heel–shin).
11 Tendon reflexes (clonus).
12 Plantar response.
13 Sensation (light touch, pinprick, vibration, joint position).
14 Gait (ordinary walk, heel-to-toe, on toes, on heels).
15 Rombergism.

6 / Chest
1 *Visual survey* — general appearance (cachexia, superior vena cava obstruction, systemic sclerosis, lupus pernio, kyphoscoliosis, *ankylosing spondylitis*).
2 Dyspnoea.
3 Lip pursing.
4 Cyanosis.
5 Accessory muscles.
6 Indrawing (intercostal muscles, supraclavicular fossae, lower ribs).
7 Chest wall (upward movement, asymmetry, scars, radiotherapy stigmata).
8 Clubbing (tobacco staining, coal dust tattoos, rheumatoid deformity, systemic sclerosis).
9 Pulse (flapping tremor).
10 Venous pressure.
11 Trachea (deviation, tug, notch–cricoid distance).
12 Lymphadenopathy.
13 Apex beat.

14 Asymmetry.
15 Expansion.
16 Percussion (don't forget clavicles, axillae).
17 Tactile vocal fremitus.
18 Breath sounds.
19 Vocal resonance.
20 Repeat 14–19 on back of chest (feel for lymph nodes in the neck).

7 / 'Spot' diagnosis
1 *Visual survey*.
2 Retrace the same ground more thoroughly
  (a) head (*Paget's*, *dystrophia myotonica*)
  (b) face (*acromegaly*, *Parkinson's*, *hemiplegia*, dystrophia myotonica, tardive dyskinesia, hypopituitarism, Cushing's, hypothyroidism, systemic sclerosis)
  (c) eyes (*jaundice*, *exophthalmos*, ptosis, Horner's, xanthelasma)
  (d) neck (*goitre*, Turner's, spondylitis, torticollis)
  (e) trunk (pigmentation, ascites, purpuric spots, spider naevi, wasting, pemphigus)
  (f) arms (choreoathetosis, psoriasis, Addison's, spider naevi, *syringomyelia*)
  (g) hands (acromegaly, *tremor*, clubbing, sclerodactyly, arachnodactyly, claw hand, etc.)
  (h) legs (bowing, purpura, pretibial myxoedema, necrobiosis)
  (i) feet (pes cavus).
3 Abnormal colouring (*pigmentation*, *icterus*, pallor).
4 Break down and scrutinize (especially face).
5 Additional features.

8 / Eyes
Observe
1 Face (e.g. myasthenic, tabetic, hemiparesis).
2 Eyes (exophthalmos, strabismus, ptosis, xanthelasma, arcus senilis).
3 Pupils (Argyll Robertson, Horner's, Holmes–Adie, IIIrd nerve).
Test
4 Visual acuity.
5 Visual fields.
6 Eye movements (ocular palsy, diplopia, nystagmus, lid lag).
7 Light reflex (direct, consensual).
8 Accommodation reflex.
9 Fundi.

9 / Face

1 *Visual survey* of patient.
2 Scan the head and face.
3 Break down and scrutinize the parts of the face:
   (a) eyelids (ptosis, rash)
      eyelashes (scanty)
      cornea (arcus, interstitial keratitis)
      sclerae (icteric, congested)
      pupils (small, large, irregular, dislocated lens, cataracts)
      iris (iritis)
   (b) face (erythema, infiltrates)
      mouth (tight, shiny, adherent skin; pigmented patches, telangiectasia, cyanosis).
4 Additional features.

10 / Arms

Observe

1 Face (hemiplegia, nystagmus, wasting, Parkinson's, Horner's).
2 Neck (pseudoxanthoma elasticum, lymph nodes).
3 Elbows (psoriasis, rheumatoid nodules, scars, deformity).
4 Tremor.
5 Hands (joints, nails, skin).
6 Muscle bulk.
7 Fasciculation.

Test

8 Tone.
9 Arms out in front (winging, myelopathy hand sign, sensory wandering).
10 Power
   (a) arms out to the side (C5)
   (b) bend your elbows (C5,6)
   (c) push out straight (C7)
   (d) squeeze fingers (C8,T1)
   (e) hold the fingers out straight (radial nerve, C7)
   (f) spread fingers apart (ulnar nerve)
   (g) piece of paper between fingers (ulnar nerve)
   (h) thumb at ceiling (median nerve)
   (i) opposition (median nerve).
11 Coordination (rapid alternate motion, finger–nose).
12 Reflexes.
13 Sensation (light touch, pinprick, vibration, joint position).

11 / Neck

1 *Survey* the patient (eyes, face, legs).
2 Look at the neck (swallow).
3 Palpate the thyroid (swallow; size, consistency, etc., pyramidal lobes).
4 Lymph nodes (supraclavicular, submandibular, postauricular, suboccipital, axillae, groins, spleen).
5 Auscultate the thyroid (distinguish from venous hum and conducted murmurs).
6 Assess thyroid status.

12 / Ask questions

1 *Visual survey* (from top to toe, ?obvious diagnosis).
2 Specific questions (Raynaud's, systemic sclerosis/CRST, hypo- or hyperthyroidism, Crohn's, nephrotic syndrome).
3 General questions (name, address).
4 Questions with long answers (last meal).
5 Articulation ('British Constitution', 'West Register Street', 'biblical criticism').
6 Repetition.
7 Additional signs.
8 Comprehension ('put out your tongue', 'shut your eyes', 'touch your nose', 'smile').
9 Nominal dysphasia (keys).
10 Orofacial dyspraxia.
11 Higher mental function.

13 / Pulse

Observe

1 Face (malar flush, thyroid facies).
2 Neck (Corrigan's pulse, raised JVP, thyroidectomy scar, goitre) and chest (thoracotomy scar).

Palpate and assess

3 Pulse.
4 Rate.
5 Rhythm (?slow atrial fibrillation).
6 Character (normal, collapsing, slow rising, jerky).
7 Carotid.
8 Opposite radial.
9 Radiofemoral delay.
10 All the other pulses.
11 Additional diagnostic features.

14 / Visual fields

Observe

1 *Visual survey* (acromegaly, hemiparesis, cerebellar signs).

Test

2 Peripheral visual fields by confrontation.
3 Central scotoma with a red-headed hat pin.
4 Additional features.

15 / Skin

1 *Visual survey* (regional associations; scalp, face, mouth, neck, trunk, axillae, elbows, hands, nails, legs, feet).
2 Distribution (psoriasis on extensor areas, lichen planus on flexural areas, etc.).
3 Lesions: look for characteristic features (scaling, Wickham's striae, etc.).
4 Associated lesions (arthropathy, etc.).

16 / Gait

1 *Visual survey* (cerebellar signs, Parkinson's, Charcot–Marie–Tooth, ankylosing spondylitis).
2 Check patient can walk.
3 Observe ordinary walk (ataxia, spastic, steppage, parkinsonian).
4 Arm swing (Parkinson's).
5 Turning (ataxia, Parkinson's).
6 Heel to toe (ataxia).
7 On toes (S1).
8 On heels (L5).
9 Romberg's test (sensory ataxia).
10 Gait with eyes closed.
11 Additional features.

17 / Rash

1 *Visual survey* (scalp to sole).
2 Distribution.
3 Surrounding skin (?scratch marks).

4 Examine the lesion (colour, size, shape, surface, character).
5 Additional features.

18 / Legs and arms

As appropriate from *checklists* 5 and 10.

19 / Cranial nerves

1 Look.
2 Smell and taste (I, VII, IX).
3 Visual acuity (II).
4 Visual fields (II).
5 Eye movements (III, IV, VI).
6 Nystagmus (VIII, cerebellum and its connections).
7 Ptosis (III, sympathetic).
8 Pupils (light, accommodation—III).
9 Discs (II).
10 Facial movements (VII, V).
11 Palatal movement (IX, X).
12 Gag reflex (IX, X).
13 Tongue (XII).
14 Accessory nerve (XI).
15 Hearing (Weber, Rinné—VIII).
16 Facial sensation (including corneal reflex—V).

20 / Thyroid status

1 *Visual survey* (exophthalmos, myxoedematous facies, goitre, thyroid acropachy, pretibial myxoedema).
2 Composure (fidgety, normal, immobile).
3 Pulse.
4 Ankle jerks.
5 Palms.
6 Tremor.
7 Eyes (lid retraction, lid lag).
8 Thyroid (look, palpate, auscultate).
9 Questions.

2 / Examination frequency of MRCP short cases

Short case	Frequency Main focus (%)	Additional feature (%)	Page no.
1 Diabetic retinopathy	34	—	65
2 Hepatosplenomegaly	24	8	69
3 Mitral stenosis (lone)	20	—	71
4 Rheumatoid hands	17	7	73
5 Mixed mitral valve disease	16	—	76
6 Dullness at the lung base	14	4	78
7 Splenomegaly (without hepatomegaly)	14	2	80
8 Optic atrophy	14	4	82
9 Chronic liver disease	13	3	84
10 Polycystic kidneys	12	2	86
11 Paget's disease	12	1	87
12 Psoriatic arthropathy/psoriasis	11	1	90
13 Other combinations of mitral and aortic valve disease	11	—	93
14 Mixed aortic valve disease	11	—	94
15 Systemic sclerosis/CRST syndrome	11	1	96
16 Exophthalmos	11	8	98
17 Hepatomegaly (without splenomegaly)	10	9	101
18 Spastic paraparesis	10	2	102
19 Fibrosing alveolitis	10	1	103
20 Aortic incompetence (lone)	9	1	104
21 Hemiplegia	9	3	106
22 Old tuberculosis	8	—	108
23 Acromegaly	8	1	109
24 Aortic stenosis (lone)	8	—	112
25 Graves' disease	8	8	114
26 Ocular palsy	8	3	117
27 Mitral incompetence (lone)	7	—	121
28 Motor neurone disease	7	1	123
29 Goitre	7	6	126
30 Ulnar nerve palsy	7	—	129
31 Visual field defect	6	3	131
32 Peripheral neuropathy	6	5	134
33 Hypertensive retinopathy	6	1	136
34 Resuscitation Annie	6	—	138
35 Cerebellar syndrome	6	6	142
36 Retinitis pigmentosa	6	—	144
37 Carcinoma of the bronchus	5	4	145
38 Parkinson's disease	5	—	148
39 Chronic bronchitis and emphysema	5	1	150
40 Hypothyroidism	5	1	152
41 Osler–Weber–Rendu syndrome	5	—	155
42 Abdominal mass	4	3	157

continued

Short case	Frequency Main focus (%)	Additional feature (%)	Page no.
43 Dystrophia myotonica	4	—	159
44 Bronchiectasis	4	1	161
45 Wasting of the small muscles of the hand	4	11	162
46 Generalized lymphadenopathy	4	6	165
47 Papilloedema	3	2	166
48 Diabetic foot	3	2	168
49 Nystagmus	3	2	171
50 Old choroiditis	3	—	174
51 Neurofibromatosis (von Recklinghausen's disease)	3	1	176
52 Erythema nodosum	3	—	178
53 Horner's syndrome	3	1	180
54 Old polio	3	1	182
55 Ankylosing spondylitis	3	—	184
56 Abnormal gait	3	3	186
57 Irregular pulse	3	22	189
58 Single palpable kidney	3	3	190
59 Ascites	3	5	191
60 Sturge–Weber syndrome	3	—	193
61 Necrobiosis lipoidica diabeticorum	3	—	195
62 Ventricular septal defect	3	1	197
63 Lower motor neurone VIIth nerve palsy	3	—	198
64 Clubbing	2	13	201
65 Retinal vein thrombosis	2	—	203
66 Eisenmenger's syndrome	2	1	205
67 Crohn's disease	2	—	207
68 Mitral valve prolapse	2	—	209
69 Cervical myelopathy	2	2	211
70 Patent ductus arteriosus	2	—	213
71 Tricuspid incompetence	2	2	214
72 Purpura	2	3	215
73 Xanthomata	2	2	218
74 Drug-induced extrapyramidal syndrome	2	—	220
75 Bilateral parotid enlargement/Mikulicz's syndrome	2	—	221
76 Primary biliary cirrhosis	2	—	222
77 Lupus pernio	2	—	224
78 Muscular dystrophy	2	—	226
79 Prosthetic valves	2	1	228
80 Addison's disease	2	—	229
81 Cushing's syndrome	2	3	231
82 Friedreich's ataxia	2	—	234
83 Peutz–Jeghers syndrome	2	—	236
84 Systemic lupus erythematosus	2	—	237
85 Superior vena cava obstruction	2	—	239
86 Vasculitis	2	2	241
87 Deep venous thrombosis/Baker's cyst/cellulitis	2	—	244
88 Cor pulmonale	1	—	247

continued

Short case	Frequency		Page no.
	Main focus (%)	Additional feature (%)	
89 Myelinated nerve fibres	1	—	248
90 Charcot–Marie–Tooth disease	1	—	249
91 Cataracts	1	4	251
92 Idiopathic haemochromatosis	1	—	253
93 Chest infection/consolidation/pneumonia	1	?	255
94 Coarctation of the aorta	1	1	256
95 Bulbar palsy	1	—	257
96 Choreoathetosis	1	2	258
97 Dysarthria	1	1	260
98 Dysphasia	1	1	261
99 Ehlers–Danlos syndrome	1	—	263
100 Erythema ab igne	1	—	265
101 Marfan's syndrome	1	—	267
102 Myasthenia gravis	1	1	269
103 Osteoarthrosis	1	—	272
104 Raised jugular venous pressure	1	?	274
105 Pretibial myxoedema	1	3	275
106 Retinal artery occlusion	1	—	277
107 Vitiligo	1	—	279
108 Tophaceous gout	1	—	282
109 Fallot's tetralogy with a Blalock shunt	1	—	284
110 Slow pulse	1	1	285
111 Guillain–Barré syndrome	1	—	286
112 Pneumonectomy/lobectomy	1	—	288
113 Obesity/pickwickian syndrome	1	?	290
114 Dermatomyositis	0.9	—	293
115 Hypopituitarism	0.9	0.6	295
116 Swollen knee	0.9	1.5	297
117 Pseudobulbar palsy	0.9	—	299
118 Pemphigus/pemphigoid	0.9	—	300
119 Syringomyelia	0.9	—	303
120 Tuberculosis/apical consolidation	0.9	—	305
121 Rheumatoid lung	0.9	?	307
122 Tuberous sclerosis/adenoma sebaceum	0.9	—	308
123 Proximal myopathy	0.9	—	310
124 Pseudoxanthoma elasticum	0.8	—	311
125 Radiation burn on the chest	0.8	4	313
126 Subacute combined degeneration of the cord	0.8	0.4	314
127 Holmes–Adie–Moore syndrome	0.8	—	315
128 Peripheral vascular disease	0.8	?	316
129 Transplanted kidney	0.8	—	318
130 Glaucoma/peripheral field loss	0.8	—	320
131 Nephrotic syndrome	0.7	—	322
132 Jugular foramen syndrome	0.7	—	323
133 Herpes zoster	0.7	2	325
134 Henoch–Schönlein purpura	0.7	?	327

continued

Short case	Frequency Main focus (%)	Additional feature (%)	Page no.
135 Polymyositis	0.6	—	329
136 Argyll Robertson pupils	0.5	0.4	330
137 Congenital syphilis	0.5	—	331
138 Carpal tunnel syndrome	0.5	0.8	333
139 Cerebellopontine angle lesion	0.5	—	335
140 Dextrocardia	0.5	—	336
141 Down's syndrome	0.5	0.6	337
142 Gynaecomastia	0.5	1.6	338
143 Absent ankle jerks and extensor plantars	0.5	1	340
144 Lichen planus	0.5	—	341
145 Lateral popliteal (common peroneal) nerve palsy	0.5	—	343
146 Ptosis	0.5	5	345
147 Osteogenesis imperfecta	0.5	—	348
148 Pulmonary stenosis	0.5	—	349
149 Raynaud's phenomenon	0.5	2	350
150 Turner's syndrome	0.5	—	352
151 Mycosis fungoides	0.5	—	354
152 Morphoea	0.5	—	356
153 Laurence–Moon–Bardet–Biedl syndrome	0.5	?	358
154 Short stature	0.5	—	360
155 Pseudohypoparathyroidism	0.5	—	362
156 AIDS related	0.5	—	365
157 Porphyria	0.5	—	368
158 Lupus vulgaris	0.5	—	370
159 Cannon waves	0.5	—	372
160 Polycythaemia rubra vera	0.5	—	373
161 Asteroid hyalosis	0.4	—	374
162 Pernicious anaemia	0.4	—	375
163 Dermatitis herpetiformis	0.3	—	377
164 Urticaria pigmentosa (mastocytosis)	0.3	—	379
165 Pneumothorax	0.3	—	380
166 Tabes	0.3	0.8	381
167 Tylosis	0.3	—	383
168 Klippel–Feil syndrome	0.3	—	385
169 Pendred's syndrome	0.3	—	387
170 Secondary syphilis	0.3	—	389
171 Ectodermal dysplasia	0.3	—	391
172 Old rickets	0.3	—	393
173 Partial lipodystrophy	0.3	—	395
174 Fabry's disease	0.3	—	397
175 Subclavian-steal syndrome	0.3	—	399
176 Reiter's syndrome/keratoderma blenorrhagica	0.3	—	401
177 Carcinoid syndrome	0.3	—	403
178 Infantile hemiplegia	0.3	—	404
179 Pulmonary incompetence	0.3	—	406
180 Hereditary spherocytosis	0.3	—	408

continued

Short case	Frequency Main focus (%)	Additional feature (%)	Page no.
181 Juvenile chronic arthritis	0.3	—	409
182 Cystic fibrosis	0.3	—	411
183 Infective endocarditis	0.3	—	413
184 Malignant melanoma	0.3	—	415
185 Leg oedema	0.3	?	417
186 Acanthosis nigricans	0.3	—	419
187 Drusen	0.3	—	422
188 Yellow nail syndrome	0.3	—	423
189 Klinefelter's syndrome/hypogonadism	0.3	—	424
190 Keratoacanthoma	0.3	—	428
191 Thalamic syndrome	0.3	—	429
192 Atrial septal defect	0.1	—	430
193 Pyoderma gangrenosum	0.1	—	431
194 Multiple sclerosis	—	16	433
195 Felty's syndrome	—	1	435
196 Hypertrophic obstructive cardiomyopathy	—	—	436
197 Radial nerve palsy	—	—	437
198 Lateral medullary syndrome (Wallenberg's syndrome)	—	—	438
199 Psychogenic/factitious	see p. 440	see p. 440	440
200 Normal	see p. 444	see p. 444	444

Some short cases which occurred as 'main focus' only once in the survey for the first edition

Hemiballismus

Diabetic with pallor

Nail–patella syndrome (anecdote 9, p. 494)

Repaired thoracic aortic aneurysm (experience 62, p. 456)

Hyperlipidaemia (xanthelasma, arcus, ischaemic heart disease)

Cyanosis

Primary pulmonary hypertension

Rash on hands and lower arm ?cause

Unilateral lower motor neurone XIIth nerve lesion

Absent knee jerk

Takayasu's disease

Multiple abcesses on the thigh

Elbow flexion contraction due to haemophilia

Brisk reflexes and normal plantar responses

Pigeon chest, scoliosis and torticollis in a patient with ?pulmonary stenosis

ECG with 2:1 block (anecdote 22, p. 496)

?Steele–Richardson syndrome (total parenteral nutrition was the subject of short case rather than the condition) (anecdote 23, p. 496)

Aortic sclerosis

Epidermolysis bullosa congenita

Acne rosacea

Patient with proliferative diabetic retinopathy who also had a partial iridectomy

Thalidomide victim with psoriasis

Chest infection due to decreased immunity in a patient with hepatosplenomegaly (this may have occurred more than once)

Multiple surgical scars and hepatomegaly

A diabetic with cervical myelopathy and peripheral neuropathy (experience 61, p. 456)

Axillary vein thrombosis

Brachial artery aneurysm (anecdote 39, p. 497)

Left ventricular aneurysm

Sickle-cell stigmata

'Heart failure'

Aphakia

Senile dementia (anecdote 38, p. 497)

Torticollis

Left VIth, VIIth, XIIth cranial nerve lesions and nystagmus (experience 1, p. 447)

Absent radial pulse due to heart failure (experience 54, p. 455)

3 / Examination frequency of examiners' instructions

Instruction	Frequency (%)	Page no.
'Examine this patient's heart'	97	10
'Examine this patient's abdomen'	79	14
'Examine this patient's fundi'	67	18
'Examine this patient's hands'	58	20
'Examine this patient's legs'	54	24
'Examine this patient's chest'	49	28
'What is the diagnosis?'	41	31
'Examine this patient's eyes'	32	35
'Examine this patient's face'	20	37
'Examine this patient's arms'	15	38
'Examine this patient's neck'	12	42
'Ask this patient some questions'	8	43
'Examine this patient's pulse'	7	46
'Examine this patient's visual fields'	6	48
'Examine this patient's skin'	5	49
'Examine this patient's gait'	4	51
'Examine this patient's rash'	4	53
'Examine this patient's legs and arms'	3	54
'Examine this patient's cranial nerves'	3	55
'Assess this patient's thyroid status'	2	58

Some other instructions which occurred more than once in the survey for the first edition

Instruction	Possible diagnoses (in order of frequency)
'Examine this patient's tongue' (2%)	1 Bilateral lower motor neurone XIIth nerve lesion
	2 Motor neurone disease
	3 Unilateral lower motor neurone XIIth nerve lesion
	4 Pseudobulbar palsy
'Examine this patient's JVP' (2%)	1 Tricuspid incompetence
	2 Raised JVP—cause not asked
	3 Cor pulmonale
'Examine this patient's hands and chest' (2%)	1 Cryptogenic fibrosing alveolitis
	2 Carcinoma of the bronchus
	3 Pulmonary fibrosis and Raynaud's
'Examine this patient's mouth' (2%)	1 Osler–Weber–Rendu
	2 Peutz–Jeghers syndrome
'Examine this patient's hands and face' (2%)	1 Systemic sclerosis/CRST
	2 Cyanosis
	3 Dermatomyositis
	4 Systemic lupus erythematosus
'Examine this patient's abdomen and chest' (1%)	1 Myeloproliferative disease leading to immune deficiency and chest infection
'Examine this patient's arms and abdomen' (1%)	1 Polycystic kidneys with dialysis scars or fistulae
	2 Chronic liver disease with spider naevi
'Examine this patient's hands, legs and eyes' (1%)	1 Thyroid acropachy, pretibial myxoedema, exophthalmos
	2 Peripheral neuropathy, Charcot's joints, necrobiosis lipoidica diabeticorum, diabetic retinopathy, cataracts
'Look at the patient, now examine the abdomen' (1%)	1 Jaundice, hepatomegaly and related signs
'Look at the hands; now ask the patient some questions' (1%)	1 Raynaud's
	2 Systemic sclerosis/CRST
'Examine this patient's pupils' (1%)	1 Optic atrophy (consensual reflex but not direct)
'Examine this patient's visual fields and fundi' (1%)	1 Retinal artery occlusion
	2 Retinitis pigmentosa
'Examine this patient's knee/knees' (1%)	1 Swollen knee
'Examine this patient's feet' (1%)	1 Diabetic foot
'Examine this patient's gait and legs' (1%)	1 Spastic paraparesis
	2 Charcot–Marie–Tooth disease
'Look at the patient; now examine the heart' (1%)	1 Fallot's tetralogy with a Blalock shunt
'Examine this patient's cerebellar system' (1%)*	1 Cerebellar syndrome

* Our surveys for the second edition suggest this instruction may have a higher frequency than 1%.

4 / Pocket Snellen's chart

This pocket Snellen's chart held 2 m from the patient's eyes (i.e. just beyond the end of the bed) can be used to gain some bedside information about the visual acuity. It gives only an approximation because 6 m is the least distance at which the effects of accommodation can be ignored (hence visual acuity is normally tested at 6 m with a Snellen's chart three times as big as this). Remember that the commonest cause of diminished visual acuity is a refractive error so that to gain information about other pathology in the eye (e.g. diabetic maculopathy), the corrected visual acuity needs to be assessed (with glasses on or through a pinhole).

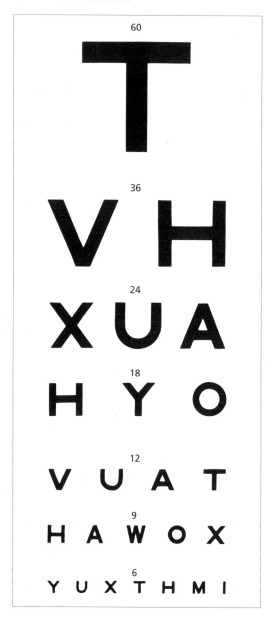

5 / Texidor's twinge and related matters

The following excerpt from the Richard Asher's book* is surely compulsory reading for all prospective members of the Royal College of Physicians. No physician's training is complete until the messages contained therein have been assimilated:

'It is pleasant to believe that the facts of medical science are there whether or not we name them; that the truth about clinical medicine exists quite independently of the names we bestow upon it. If that were so, our only responsibility would be to agree upon symbols or words for facts that already existed. That theoretical ideal is hardly ever fulfilled. A little patient thinking will soon convince the enquirer that it is not just a simple matter of finding words to fit the facts, but just as often of finding facts to fit the words. When christening a baby we wait for the child to be born and then we find a name for it. When christening a disease we sometimes wait for the name to be born and then we try to find a disease to suit it. With children we announce their names in the birth columns of The Times *and with diseases we announce their names in the original articles of the medical journals. The only difference is that children's names have to be registered. There is no such procedure with medical terms. There is no Medical Registrar-General of Terminological Births and Deaths. Only medical dictionaries and the international list of classified diseases. These do not include every living medical term, and they list many that have died or that ought to be painlessly put away. There is something about a name, particularly an eponymous term, which brings into being things which never seemed to be there before. In creation the word may come first: the opening sentence of the Gospel of Saint John is—"In the beginning was the Word".*

Take, for instance, Pel Ebstein fever. Every student and every doctor knows that cases of Hodgkin's disease may show a fever that is high for one week and low for the next week, and so on. Does this phenomenon really exist at all? If you collect the charts of 50 cases of Hodgkin's disease and compare them with the charts of 50 cases of disseminated malignant fever, do you really believe you could pick out even one or two cases because

of the characteristic fever? I think it is very unlikely indeed. Yet if, by the vagaries of chance, one case of Hodgkin's did run such a temperature, the news would soon travel round: "There's a good case of Hodgkin's disease in Galen Ward. You ought to have a look. It shows the typical Pel Ebstein fever very well".

The chart might be copied for teaching purposes, or even put in a book. The mere description and the naming of a mythical fever leads inevitably to its occurrence in textbooks. One popular textbook for nurses depicts particularly classical temperature charts, attributed to various fevers. I asked the author how many hospital notes she had combed before she found such beautiful examples: "Oh, there was no trouble about that", she replied, "I made them up out of my head".

I wonder whether any examples of Pel Ebstein and other fevers in textbooks have similar origins. It does not matter whether or not Pel Ebstein fever exists, my contention remains the same: the bestowal of a name upon a concept, whether real or imaginary, brings it into clinical existence.

Out of curiosity I looked up the original papers, and Dr Burrows kindly translated them for me. Both describe patients with chronic relapsing fever and splenomegaly but there is nothing in either paper to suggest any of them had Hodgkin's disease. Both describe cases of undulant fever and Ebstein suggested the name chronic relapsing fever, but it was very probably one of abortus fever.

An important example of the creation of a thing beginning with the word is gallstone colic. There is no such thing. Colic is a pain continuously waxing and waning, like the colonic cramps of food poisoning. Gallstone pain after its onset steadily climbs to an agonizing peak without any fluctuation, and then passes off. But the label colic has been so firmly stuck on to this pain that the pain is expected to be colic, assumed to be colic, believed to be colic and finally bullied into being colic, so that a man with gallstone pain will be described as having colicky pain, however steady it may be.

Contrariwise, if something has no individual descriptive term it has far less chance of clinical acceptance or clinical recognition. A rose without a name may smell as sweet, but it has far less chance of being smelt. Suppos-

* From the book *Talking Sense*, edited by Sir Francis Avery Jones (Pitman Medical, 1972).

ing we take an unnamed fever and an unnamed pain to contrast with the examples I have given. In untreated pernicious anaemia there is often quite a high fever. Sixty per cent of cases with red cell counts under 1.5 million show a fever over 101°F. This invariably settles to normal levels within a week of one adequate injection of B_{12}. I make no assertion that this fever is of great importance. What I do assert is that had it been called the Addison–Castle fever or hypo-cyanocobalminic fever there is not a medical student in the land who would not have heard of it, many doctors would be afraid to diagnose pernicious anaemia without its presence, and the proportion of patients showing the fever would rise sharply once the name got into nurses' textbooks (because if they did not show the fever they would have their thermometers put back in their mouths until they behaved themselves).

Now for a pain without a name. Have any of you ever had a very brief, sharp needle-like pain near the apex of the heart: acutely localized to one point seemingly inside the chest wall, but feeling as if something was adherent to it? Breathing sharpens it, so there is often a disinclination to take a deep breath while it lasts. It comes out of the blue, it passes off in a few minutes, and although acute it is not at all distressing.

Enquiries among my friends showed that quite a lot of them occasionally had this pain, but, till they knew other people had it too, they did not mention it; espe-

cially because it has no official name, and also because it did not bother them.

I circulated various doctors I knew, and also circularized 50 recently elected Fellows of the College of Physicians—to see if it was reasonably common. It was ... So if any of you happen to have it, you are not branding yourselves as either grievously neurotic or grossly hypochondriacal if you admit to having it.

[In the second of the Lettsomian lectures, on which this essay is based, with the permission of the President of the Medical Society of London, Dr Asher asked his audience of medical men whether any of them had encountered anything closely resembling this pain in either themselves or their friends, and if they had, to raise their hands. Over a third of the audience held up their hands.]

There seems no doubt that this condition exists, yet, because it has no name, it has no official clinical existence. We cannot discuss it or investigate it or write about it. Whether or not the condition should be named I am unable to say.* Though the naming of disease is not in any way restricted or supervised it ought not to be undertaken lightly. A fertile medical author can easily beget a large number of clinical progeny by describing and naming them, but some of his youngsters may turn out to be illegitimate, and with others there may be much doubt about their paternity if others claim to have begotten them years ago.'

* In a foreword to *Sense and Sensibility* the author explained that the pain had been described and named four years previously by A.J. Miller and T.A. Texidor (1955) in the *Journal of the American Medical Association*, and that it might in future be known as *Texidor's twinge*.

6 / Colour photographs of some MRCP short cases

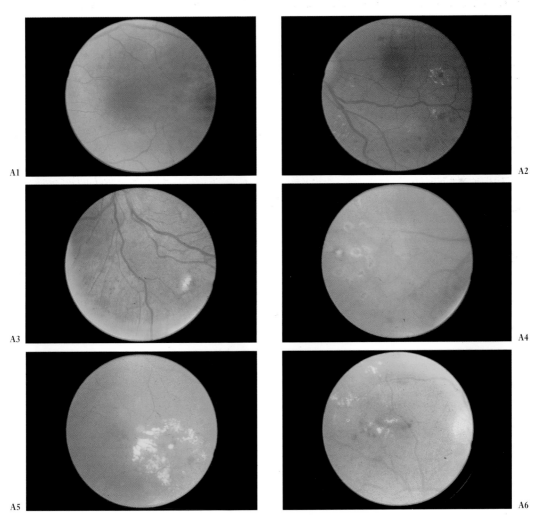

A1

A2

A3

A4

A5

A6

A1 Diabetic retinopathy—early background changes of microaneurysms and blot haemorrhages.

A2 Diabetic retinopathy—extensive background changes (note small circinate temporal to the macula).

A3 Diabetic retinopathy—the soft exudate in the lower right of the picture indicates ischaemia which is the stimulus to new vessel formation.

A4 Diabetic retinopathy (note photocoagulation scars).

A5 Diabetic retinopathy—the large circinate temporal to the macula indicates oedema in that area.

A6 Diabetic retinopathy—haemorrhages and exudates at the macula (maculopathy).

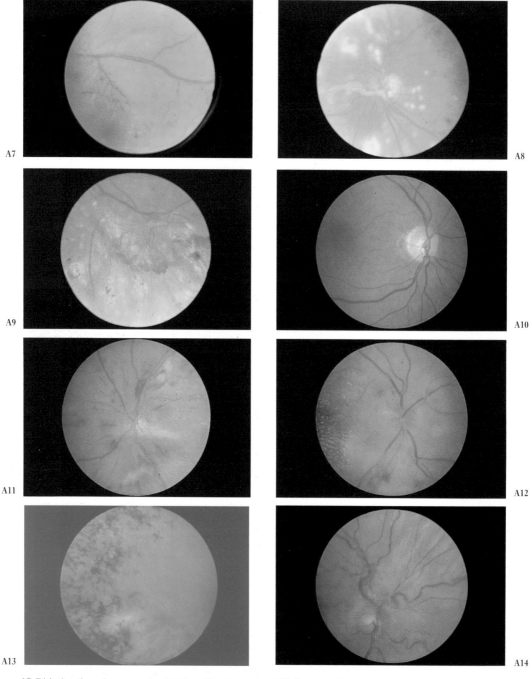

A7 Diabetic retinopathy—venous irregularity and beading (preproliferative sign).

A8 Diabetic retinopathy. The leash of new vessels protruding into the vitreous is in focus, whereas the retina with its photocoagulation scars is further away and therefore slightly out of focus. Note the leash of fibrous tissue accompanying the new vessels (previous haemorrhage).

A9 Diabetic retinopathy—peripheral new vessels which are haemorrhaging (note photocoagulation scars—same patient as A8).

A10 Optic atrophy.

A11 Hypertensive retinopathy—grade 4 (note papilloedema, flame-shaped haemorrhages and cotton wool spots).

A12 Hypertensive retinopathy—grade 4; part of a macular star can be seen.

A13 Retinitis pigmentosa.

A14 Papilloedema (benign intracranial hypertension).

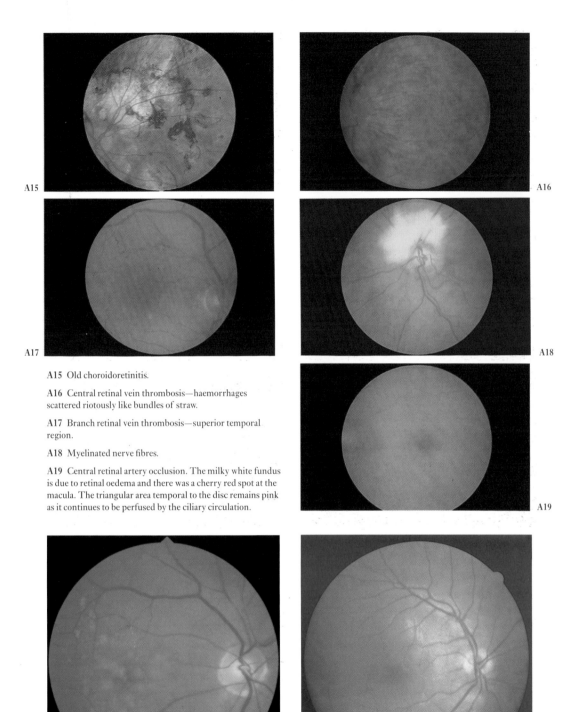

A15 Old choroidoretinitis.

A16 Central retinal vein thrombosis—haemorrhages scattered riotously like bundles of straw.

A17 Branch retinal vein thrombosis—superior temporal region.

A18 Myelinated nerve fibres.

A19 Central retinal artery occlusion. The milky white fundus is due to retinal oedema and there was a cherry red spot at the macula. The triangular area temporal to the disc remains pink as it continues to be perfused by the ciliary circulation.

A20 (a) Retinal drusen; (b) optic disc drusen in a young person leading to pseudopapilloedema. When he presented to casualty with headache, the optic disc changes were noted and an urgent CT scan was ordered. This was normal and ultrasonography of the optic disc showed up the drusen as the only abnormality.

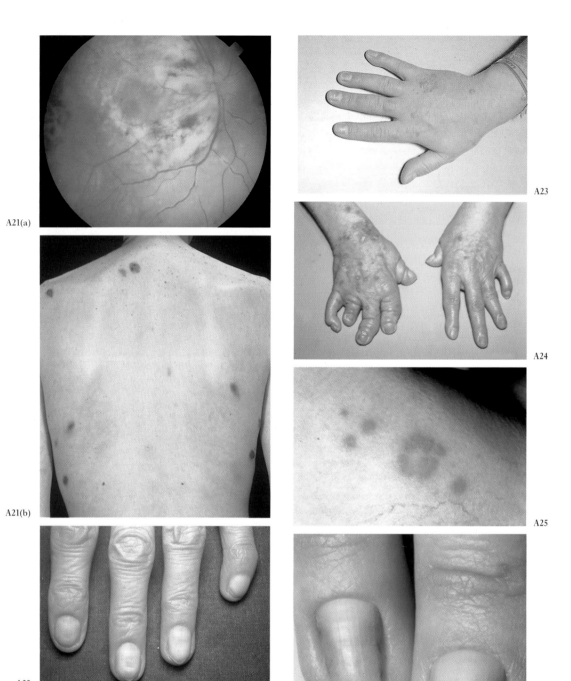

A21 (a) Cytomegalovirus retinitis—'scrambled egg and tomato sauce'. (b) Kaposi's sarcoma.

A22 Leuconychia.

A23 Psoriasis with nail pitting on the index fingers.

A24 Psoriasis in arthritis multilans. Note the telescoping of the fingers on the left.

A25 Granuloma annulare.

A26 Ectodermal dysplasia—thin, ridged, discoloured nails.

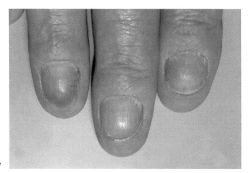

A27

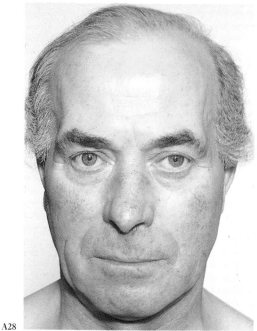

A28

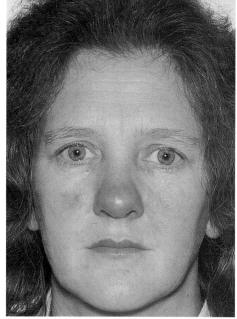

A29

A30

A27 Yellow nail syndrome—there are no cuticles or lunula. The bulbous fingertips are uncovered.

A28 Malar flush (mitral stenosis).

A29 Malar flush (myxoedema).

A30 Lupus pernio.

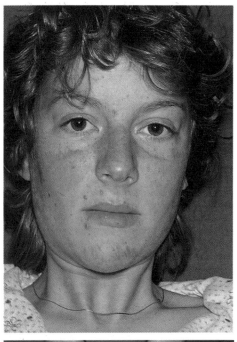

A31

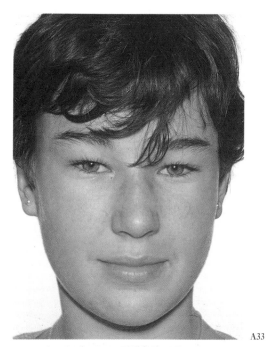

A33

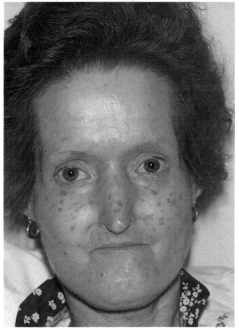

A34

A31 Systemic lupus erythematosus.

A32 Dermatomyositis—Gottron's papules.

A33 Dermatomyositis—note oedema and heliotrope discoloration around the eyes.

A34 Systemic sclerosis (note the tight, shiny skin, pinched nose and telangiectasia).

A32

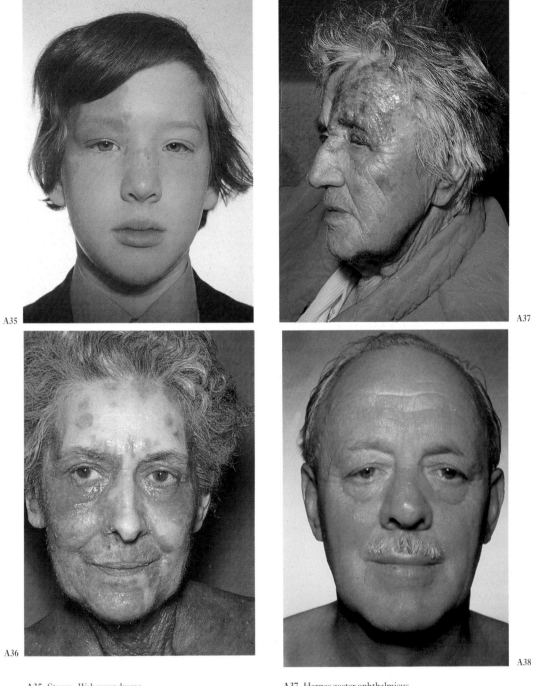

A35 Sturge–Weber syndrome.

A36 Pemphigus.

A37 Herpes zoster ophthalmicus.

A38 Polycythaemia rubra vera.

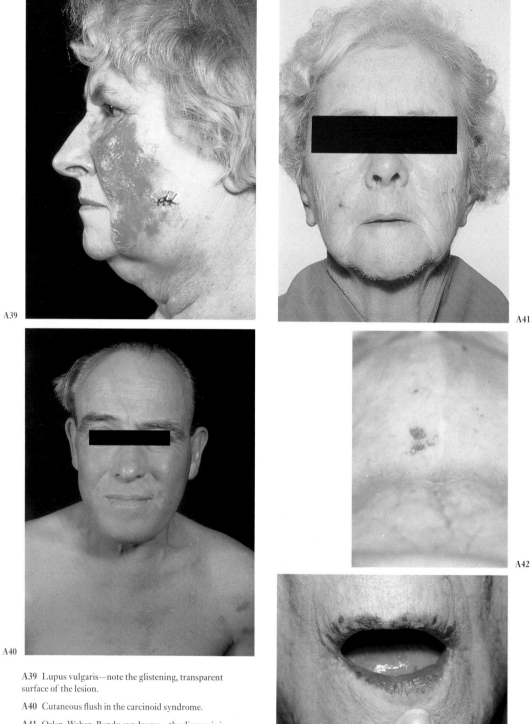

A39 Lupus vulgaris—note the glistening, transparent surface of the lesion.

A40 Cutaneous flush in the carcinoid syndrome.

A41 Osler–Weber–Rendu syndrome—the diagnosis is confirmed on looking inside the mouth.

A42 Osler–Weber–Rendu syndrome—the soft palate of the same patient as A41.

A43 Peutz–Jeghers syndrome.

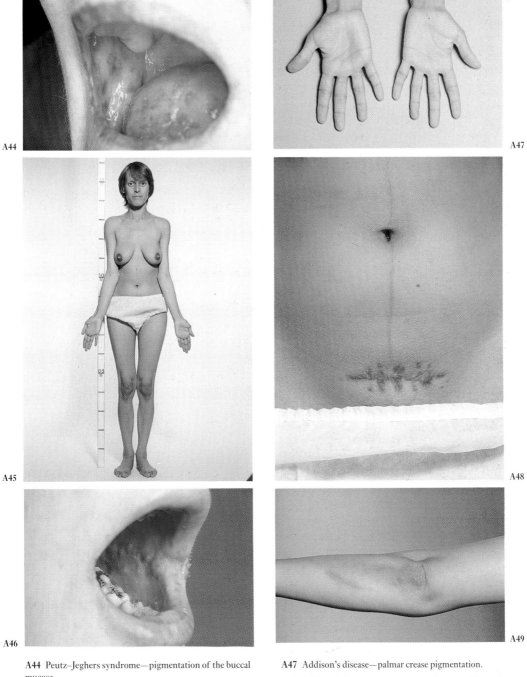

A44 Peutz–Jeghers syndrome—pigmentation of the buccal mucosa.

A45 Addison's disease (note pigmentation of the nipples).

A46 Addison's disease—pigmentation of the buccal mucosa.

A47 Addison's disease—palmar crease pigmentation.

A48 Addison's disease—pigmentation of scar and linea alba.

A49 Addison's disease—pigmentation at the elbow (a pressure point).

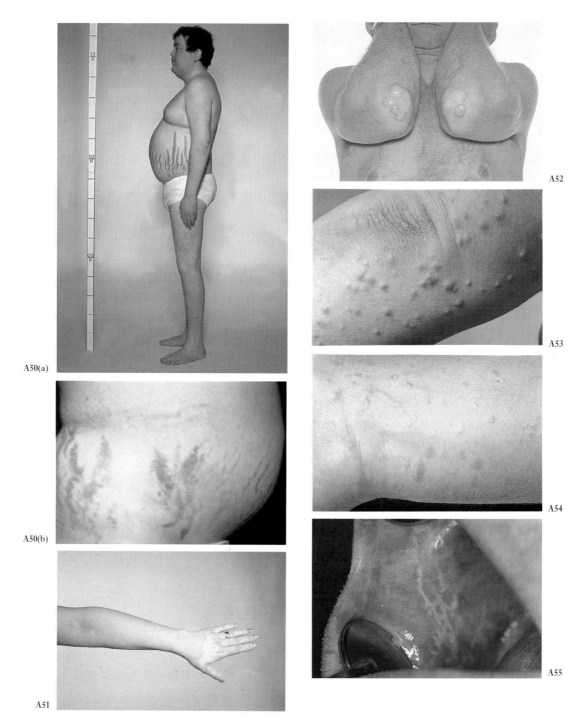

A50(a)

A50(b)

A51

A52

A53

A54

A55

A50 (a) Cushing's syndrome; (b) abdominal striae.

A51 Vitiligo.

A52 Tuberous xanthomata.

A53 Eruptive xanthomata.

A54 Lichen planus—flat-topped, violaceous, polygonal papules on the wrist. Note Wickham's striae.

A55 Lichen planus—white, lacy pattern on the buccal mucosa.

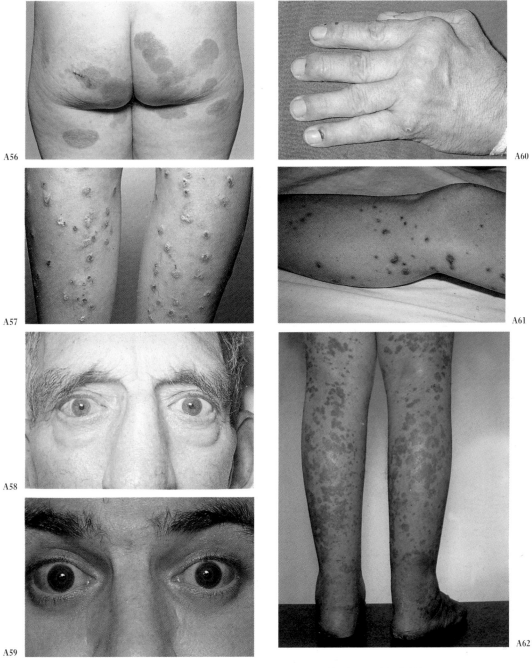

A56 Mycosis fungoides.

A57 Dermatitis herpetiformis.

A58 Episcleritis (rheumatoid disease).

A59 Blue sclerae of osteogenesis imperfecta.

A60 Vasculitis (rheumatoid arthritis).

A61 Vasculitis.

A62 Henoch–Schölein purpura.

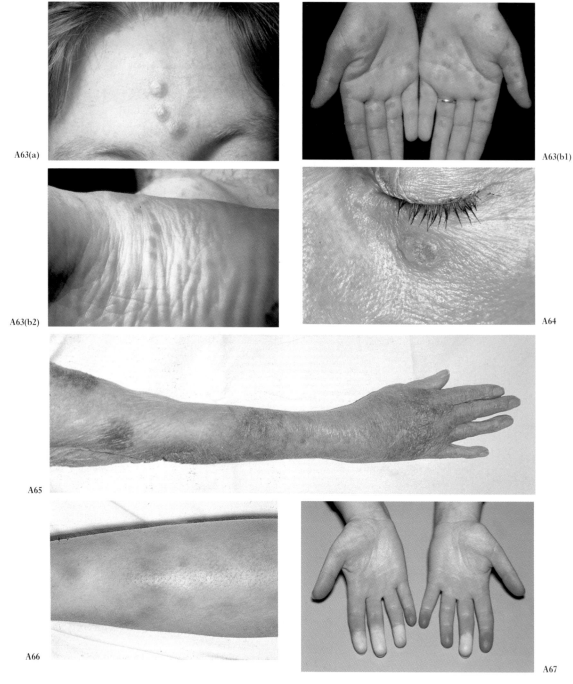

A63(a)

A63(b1)

A63(b2)

A64

A65

A66

A67

A63 (a) Round papules of secondary syphilis—note the fine scaling on the surface; (b) well-demarcated round and oval papules: (1) palms and (2) soles.

A64 Keratoacanthoma.

A65 Purpura (steroid therapy for rheumatoid arthritis).

A66 Erythema nodosum.

A67 Raynaud's phenomenon.

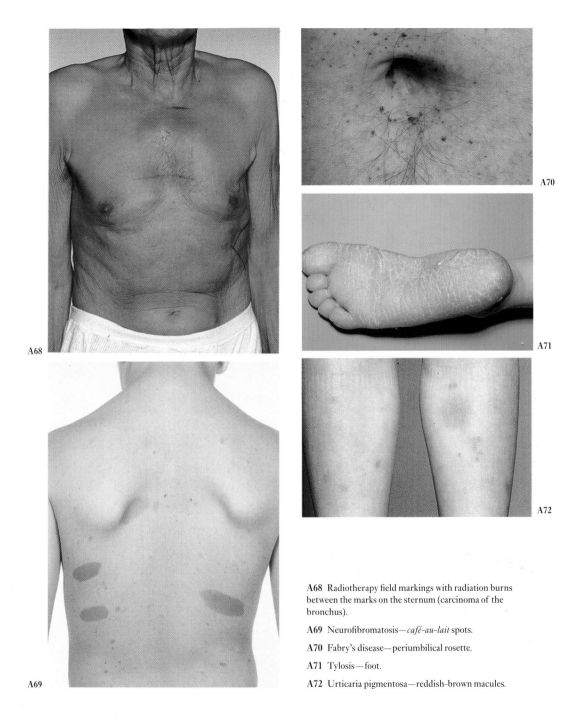

A68 Radiotherapy field markings with radiation burns between the marks on the sternum (carcinoma of the bronchus).

A69 Neurofibromatosis—*café-au-lait* spots.

A70 Fabry's disease—periumbilical rosette.

A71 Tylosis—foot.

A72 Urticaria pigmentosa—reddish-brown macules.

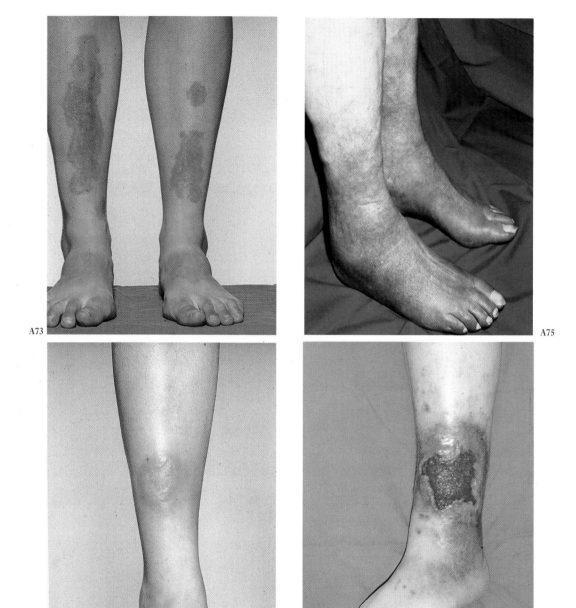

A73 Necrobiosis lipoidica diabeticorum.

A74 Pretibial myxoedema.

A75 Peripheral vascular insufficiency.

A76 Pyoderma gangrenosum (note ragged, bluish-red edge to the ulcer).

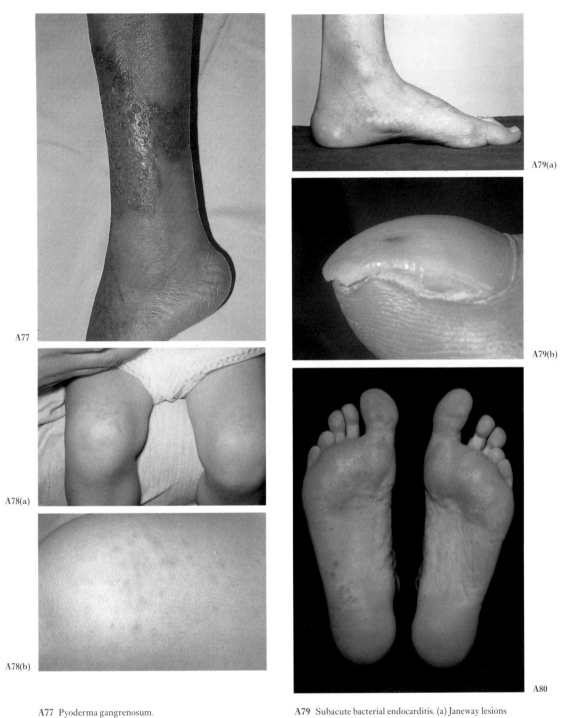

A77 Pyoderma gangrenosum.

A78 Chronic juvenile arthritis. (a) Arthropathy affecting the knees. Note a crop of characteristic macular lesions. (b) Close up view of the rash.

A79 Subacute bacterial endocarditis. (a) Janeway lesions above the ankle; (b) splinter haemorrhage.

A80 Keratoderma blenorrhagica.

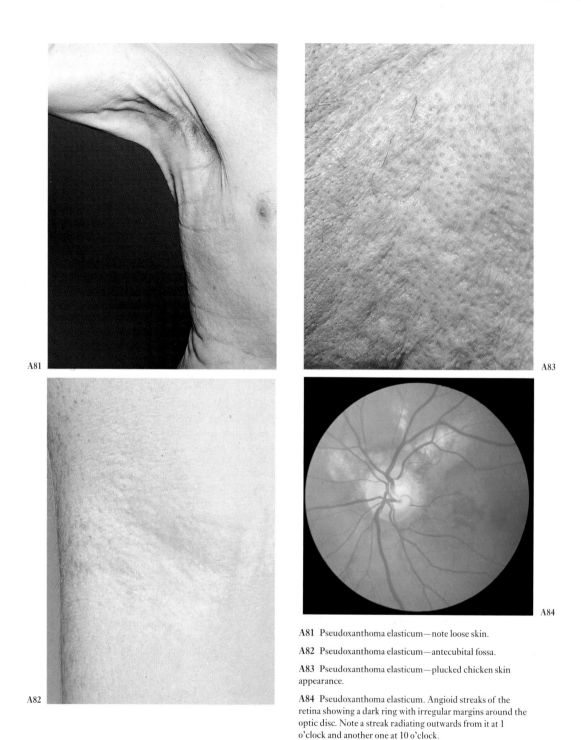

A81   Pseudoxanthoma elasticum—note loose skin.

A82   Pseudoxanthoma elasticum—antecubital fossa.

A83   Pseudoxanthoma elasticum—plucked chicken skin appearance.

A84   Pseudoxanthoma elasticum. Angioid streaks of the retina showing a dark ring with irregular margins around the optic disc. Note a streak radiating outwards from it at 1 o'clock and another one at 10 o'clock.

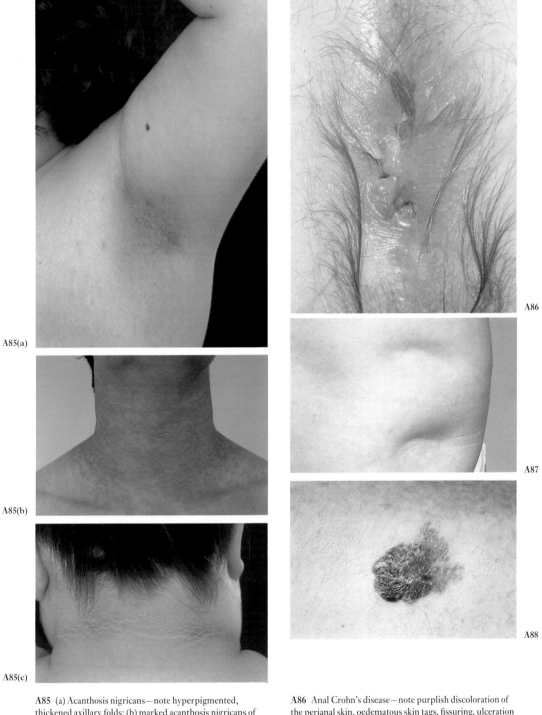

A85(a)

A85(b)

A85(c)

A86

A87

A88

A85 (a) Acanthosis nigricans—note hyperpigmented, thickened axillary folds; (b) marked acanthosis nigricans of the neck; (c) less marked acanthosis nigricans at the back of the neck in an overweight female.

A86 Anal Crohn's disease—note purplish discoloration of the perianal skin, oedematous skin tags, fissuring, ulceration and fistula formation.

A87 Morphoea—depression caused by the atrophy of the underlying tissues.

A88 Malignant melanoma.

7 / Detailed contents of Section 4

Index

Page numbers in **bold** refer to examination routines and short cases; those followed by an 'n' refer to footnotes

carcinoid 420
necrolytic migratory 420
Erythema ab igne **265–6**
Erythema gyratum repens 146
Erythema multiforme, hands 51
Erythema nodosum **178–9**, 538
Erythropoietin production 373
Essential tremor, benign 149
Eunuchoidism 424, 424n
Euthyroid Graves' disease 98
Examinations 4–6
  examination 'nerves' 5
  examination *routines* 4, 7–59
  reactions of examiners 5–6
  simulated practice 3–4
Examiners' instructions, examination frequencies 522–3
Exophthalmic ophthalmoplegia 118
Exophthalmometry 98
Exophthalmos **98–100**, 114n
  malignant 98
  pulsating 98
  see also Graves' disease; Thyrotoxicosis
Experiences 447–93, 544–5
Extrapyramidal syndrome, drug-induced **220**
Eyes, examination **35–6**
  accommodation–convergence reflex 36, 36n
  checklist 514
  congenital abnormalities 193
  diagnosis frequencies 35
  during thyroid status assessment 58
  facial inspection 35
  movement assessment 36
    cranial nerve examination 56
  routine **35–6**
  variations of instructions 35
  see also Fundi, examination; Pupils; Visual fields, examination

Fabry's disease **397–8**, 539
Face, examination **37–8**
  checklist 515
  diagnosis frequencies 37
  during arm examination 39
  during pulse examination 47
  eyes examination 38
  routine 38
  skin 50
  variations of instruction 37
Facial movements, during cranial nerve examination 56
Facial sensation, testing 57
Facio-scapulo-humeral muscular dystrophy 226, 227
Factitious illnesses **440–3**
Facts and figures 502–3
Fallot's tetralogy
  with Blalock shunt **284**
  differences from Eisenmenger's syndrome 206
Familial polyposis coli 236n
Fasciculation 22, 123, 182n, 249
Feet
  diabetic
  skin examination 51
Felty's syndrome 73, **435**
Femoral pulse, right 48
'Fertile' eunuch syndrome 425
FET (forced expiratory time) 31, 31n
Fibrosing alveolitis 31n, **103**, 161, 161n, 307, 307n
Finger(s)
  shortening 362, 364
  triggering 73
  see also Clubbing
Fistulae, anal 207

Fixed splitting, atrial septal defect 430
Flaccid dysarthria 260
Flushing, cutaneous, carcinoid syndrome 403, 403n, 534
Folate deficiency 375n, 376
Foot drop 187, 343
Forced expiratory time (FET) 31, 31n
Foster–Kennedy syndrome 132n, 166n
Fourth nerve palsy 118
Foville's syndrome 438–9
Frank's sign 12n
Friedrich's ataxia 102, 142, **234–5**, 340
Froment's 'thumb sign' 129n
Functional prepubertal castrate syndrome 424–5
Fundi, diabetic 174
Fundi, examination **18–20**
  checklist 513
  diagnosis frequencies 18
  routine **18–20**
  variations of instruction 18
  see also Eyes, examination
Fundoscopy 56

Gag reflex, during cranial nerve examination 57, 57n
Gait
  abnormal **186–8**
  ataxic 52, 186–7
  hysteric 441n
Gait apraxia, elderly 188
Gait examination **51–2**
  checklist 516
  diagnosis frequencies 52
  during leg examination 27
  routine **52**
  variations of instructions 52
Gallstone pain 525
Ganser syndrome 441
Gardener's syndrome 420
Gastrocnemius rupture 417
Gaucher's disease 69
General paralysis/paresis of the insane (GPI) 102, 260, 381n
Generalized lymphadenopathy **165**
Genitalia
  external, examination 17
  skin examination 51
  testicular atrophy 159
Giant cell arteritis 241, 277
Glaucoma 82, **320–1**
Global dysphasia 261, 261n
Glomerulonephritis, post-streptococcal 322n
Glutamate toxicity 123n
Gluten-sensitive enteropathy, dermatitis herpetiformis
    association 377
Goitre 42, 100, **126–8**
  associated autoimmune disorders 126n
  congenital 387
  with deafness 387
  multinodular 114n, 126, 127
Goitrogens 126
Gonadotrophin deficiency 338
Gordon's reflex 26n
Gottron's papules 51, 293, 294, 532
Gout, tophaceous **282–3**
GPI (general paralysis/paresis of the insane) 102, 260, 381n
Graham–Steell murmur 71, 71n, 406, 406n
Granuloma annulare 195, 530
Graves' disease **114–16**, 126n, 127
  euthyroid 98, 114
  and exophthalmos 98
  hyperthyroid 98, 126
  hypothyroid 98, 152

Proliferative diabetic retinopathy 68
Prosthetic heart valves **228**
   complications 228
Proximal myopathy **310**
Pruritus 53, 53n
   primary biliary cirrhosis 222
Pseudoathetosis 212
Pseudobulbar palsy 260, **299**
Pseudodementia 441
Pseudogout 297
Pseudohaematemesis 442
Pseudohaemoptysis 442
Pseudohypertrophic muscular dystrophy 226
Pseudohypoparathyroidism 361, **362–4**
Pseudopapilloedema 422
Pseudoporphyria 368, 368n
Pseudoptosis 347
Pseudotumour cerebri (benign intracranial hypertension) 166, 166n
Pseudoxanthoma elasticum **311–12**, 542
Psoriasis **90–2**
   on the hands 22, 530
   like Reiter's syndrome 401n
Psoriatic arthropathy **90–2**
Psychogenic illnesses **440–3**
Ptosis 56, **345–7**
Puberty, constitutional delayed 425n
Puerilism 441
Pulmonary embolus and infarction 78
Pulmonary fibrosis, with alveolitis, associated disorders 103
Pulmonary heart disease, causes 247
Pulmonary hypertension 13, 247, **274**, 406, 407
Pulmonary incompetence **406–7**
Pulmonary plethora 430, 430n
Pulmonary stenosis **349**
Pulse
   bisferiens 48
   carotid artery 141
   collapsing 12, 47, 48
   Corrigan's sign/pulse 12, 104
   irregular **189**
      differential diagnosis 189
   jerky 436
   peripheral 48
   radial 23, 48
   right femoral 48
   slow **285**
   slow rising 12, 47–8
   water-hammer 47
Pulse, examination **46–8**
   character (waveform) 47–8
   checklist 515
   diagnosis frequencies 47
   during cardiac examination 12
   irregular **189**
   radial pulse 48
   rate and rhythm 47
   right femoral pulse 48
   routine **47–8**
   slow **285**
   slow rising 12, 47–8
   variations of instruction 46
Pulseless (Takayasu's) disease **316–17**
Pupils
   examination 36
   light reflexes 36
      during cranial nerve examination 56
   nerve supply 181
Purpura **215–17**, 538

Pustules, definition 54
Pyoderma gangrenosum **431–2**, 540, 541

Questions, to the patient *see* Patient questioning
Quincke's sign 104n
Quotations 503–10, 545

Radial nerve palsy **437**
Radiation, and cataracts 251
Radiation burn, chest **313**, 539
Radiofemoral delay 12, 48
Ragged red fibres 345n
Raised jugular venous pressure **274**
Ramsay Hunt syndrome 198, 200, 325, 325n, 326
Rash, examination **53–4**
   checklist 516
   diagnosis frequencies 53
   lesion distribution 53
   routine **53–4**
   surrounding skin 53
   see also Skin, examination
Raynaud's disease
   idiopathic 350, 350n
   patient questioning 44
Raynaud's phenomenon **350–1**, 538
Reaven's syndrome 291n
Records 4–5, 61–444
Rectum, examination 17
Refsum's disease 135, 144, 235
Reiter's syndrome **401–2**
Renal cell carcinoma 86
Renal disease
   hypertensive 318
   and partial lipodystrophy 395
Resuscitation Annie **138–41**
Retinal artery occlusion **277–8**, 529
Retinal vein thrombosis **203–4**, 529
Retinal venous pulsation 167
Retinitis pigmentosa **144**, 251, 528
Retinopathy
   diabetic 19, **65–8**
   hypertensive 19, **136–7**
   non-proliferative 68
   proliferative and preproliferative 68
Retro-orbital tumours 98
Rhabdomyomata 308
Rhagades, congenital syphilis 331
Rheumatic heart disease 112, 121, 214
Rheumatoid arthritis
   corticosteroid therapy 233
   hands 21, **73–5**, 162, 162n, 164
   peripheral neuropathy 134
   psoriatic arthropathy like 90, 92
   swollen knees 297
   vasculitis 73n, 75, 242, 243, 537
Rheumatoid hands **73–5**
Rheumatoid lung **307**
Rib cage, hyperinflated 150, 151, 412
Rib notching 256, 256n
Rickets
   bowed tibia 88
   old **393–4**
Right ventricular lift 13
Riluzole 123n
Rinné test 57n
Rodent ulcer 50
Romberg's sign/test 27, 52
   SACD 314
   tabes dorsalis 330

MRCP— 'it teaches more than it tests'